# STATISTICAL HANDBOOK ON INFECTIOUS DISEASES

# STATISTICAL HANDBOOK ON INFECTIOUS DISEASES

**Sarah B. Watstein**
**and John Jovanovic**

An Oryx Book

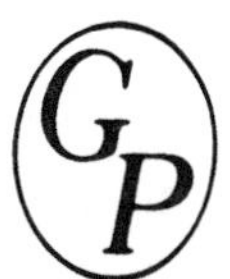

Greenwood Press
Westport, Connecticut London

**Library of Congress Cataloging-in-Publication Data**

Watstein, Sarah.
Statistical handbook on infectious diseases / Sarah B. Watstein and John Jovanovic.
p. ;cm.
Includes bibliographical references and index.
ISBN 1–57356–375–7 (alk. paper)
1. Communicable diseases—Statistics—Handbooks, manuals, etc. 2. Epidemiology—Handbooks, manuals, etc. I. Jovanovic, John. II. Title.
[DNLM: 1. Communicable Diseases—epidemiology—Handbooks. 2. Vaccination—statistics & numerical data—Handbooks. WC 39 W343s 2002]
RA643.W33 2003
614′.07′27—dc21 2002022055

British Library Cataloguing in Publication Data is available.



Library of Congress Catalog Card Number: 2002022055
ISBN: 1–57356–375–7

First published in 2003

Greenwood Press, 88 Post Road West, Westport, CT 06881
An imprint of Greenwood Publishing Group, Inc.
www. greenwood.com

Printed in the United States of America

The paper used in this book complies with the Permanent Paper Standard issued by the National Information Standards Organization (Z39.48–1984).

10 9 8 7 6 5 4 3 2 1

**Acknowledgements:**
From John S. Jovanovic and Sarah Barbara Watstein:
We would like to thank Eleanora Von Dehsen, our acquiring editor,
with thanks for your guidance, support, and most of all, your patience;
We would also like to thank the following for helping us ferret out and format information—
Louveller Luster, formerly Head, Government Documents, Virginia Commonwealth University, VCU Libraries
&
Mary Horman, Government Information Specialist, Virginia Commonwealth University, VCU Libraries
&
Pascal Calarco, Head, Library Information Systems, Virginia Commonwealth University, VCU Libraries

**Dedication:**
From John S. Jovanovic
To Emily and Ethan, who fill each of my days with joy

From Sarah Barbara Watstein
To my family and friends, and especially to Dr. R.,
who believed that there was light at the end of the tunnel

# Contents

# List of Tables

## A. NATIONALLY NOTIFIABLE DISEASES

## B. HUMAN IMMUNODEFICIENCY VIRUS (HIV) AND ACQUIRED IMMUNODEFICIENCY SYNDROME (AIDS)

## C. MALARIA

### 1. General Surveillance Data



### 2. Data by *Plasmodium* Species



### 3. Area of Acquisition



### 4. Imported Malaria Cases by Interval between Arrival in the United States and Onset of Illness



### 5. Purpose of Travel



## D. SEXUALLY TRANSMITTED DISEASE

### 1. *Healthy People 2000*



### 2. Summary Data



### 3. Chlamydia



### 4. Gonorrhea

## E. TUBERCULOSIS

### 1. Trends



### 2. Case Rates by Selected Characteristics



### 3. Cases by Form of the Disease



### 4. Cases by Subpopulation



### 5. TB and HIV

## F. FOODBORNE DISEASES

### 1. Foodborne Diseases by Etiology



### 2. Foodborne Diseases by Etiology and Month of Occurrence



### 3. Foodborne Diseases by Place Where Food Was Eaten



### 4. Vehicle of Transmission



### 5. Etiology and Contributing Factors



### 6. Significant Foodborne Diseases

## G. WATERBORNE DISEASES

### 1. Classification of Investigations of Waterborne-Disease Outbreaks



### 2. Waterborne Disease and Drinking Water



### 3. Waterborne Disease and Recreational Water



## H. INFECTIOUS DISEASE WORLDWIDE: PRESENT ISSUES, EMERGING CONCERNS

### 1. Global Estimates and Surveillance



### 2. Targeted Diseases

## I. VACCINE-PREVENTABLE DISEASES

### 1. Vaccines and Vaccine Development



### 2. Incidence of Disease



### 3. Immunization Coverage



### 4. U.S. Childhood Immunization



### 5. Vaccination in Developing Countries



### 6. Spending



## J. INFECTIOUS DISEASE ELIMINATION AND ERADICATION

### 1. Target Dates and Cost of Eradication

# Preface

## SEPTEMBER 11, 2001.
## THE UNTHINKABLE HAPPENED.

Since the terrorist attacks in the United States on September 11, 2001, the potential of biological terrorism has loomed large in the minds of government officials and a frightened public. Rising public concern, even hysteria, over the dangers of biological terrorism is increasingly evident. This concern is fueled by an increased awareness of the myriad challenges posed by severe outbreaks of infectious disease, whether natural or manmade. Attention has focused on two threats above all others: the germs that cause anthrax and smallpox. Both are hardy and highly lethal, making them good weapons for inflicting mass casualties. The consequences of such an attack include deaths conceivably reaching into the tens of hundreds of thousands.

Fears of anthrax are in many ways understandable. Among some 30 biological agents that have been studied as potential weapons, anthrax may be the most likely choice for terrorists because it is easier to acquire than most and is so lethal, killing 80% to 90% of all unvaccinated people who are not treated promptly. The anthrax spore is also very durable, able to survive for decades in the soil or other areas protected from direct sunlight. However, anthrax does not spread from one victim to another, which limits its impact to those who inhale the aerosols. One authoritative group, using worst-case assumptions, estimated that a plane spreading anthrax over a big city might kill 100,000 people. Another suggested the figure might even be three million. But the only real-world precedent—a leak of anthrax spores from a biological weapons plant in Russia in 1979—killed just 68 people, perhaps because the amount released was so small. Individuals can be protected by a vaccine given in a series of six doses followed by annual boosters, a cumbersome regimen. But the only vaccine currently available is for military use—and even that is controversial, with some service members refusing to take it for fear of side effects and because of doubts about its effectiveness. Nevertheless, alarmed citizens have been besieging the sole manufacturer to make the vaccine available, which is an impossibility, since the company is unable to meet military needs.

Antibiotics, including Cipro, penicillin, and doxycycline, can also treat anthrax if they are administered within days of exposure. Panicky citizens have been trying to obtain and hoard Cipro or other drugs to use if the unthinkable happens.

Fears of smallpox are, in many ways, like fears of anthrax, understandable. Indeed smallpox is an even bigger worry for some experts because of the global pandemic it could trigger. Unlike anthrax, smallpox is contagious, spreading from person to person through the air, and it kills about 30% of unvaccinated victims. The disease was eradicated from the globe in 1977, and routine vaccinations stopped in the United States in 1972. By one estimate, more than 40% of the American public has not been vaccinated, and those who were vaccinated only once in earlier years are almost certainly now vulnerable. Should smallpox be reintroduced in the United States, it could move progressively through the population and, in today's highly mobile world, flash back to hit the rest of the planet as well.

However, the smallpox virus should be extremely difficult to obtain. Once the disease was eradicated, the World Health Organization made a concerted effort to concentrate all remaining samples of the virus in two laboratories, one in the United States and one in Russia. Questions remain: Were all samples really destroyed elsewhere? Have disaffected scientists in Russia made the virus available to other countries? Do rogue nations have clandestine supplies?

There is no treatment for smallpox, but there is an effective vaccine. As of October 2001, the United States currently has 15 million doses and has ordered an additional 40 million to be delivered in 2002. That might be enough to contain an outbreak in a single city by vaccinating those at risk of infection, but many experts believe the nation needs more than 100 million doses to truly be ready. The U.S. government plans to keep amassing the vaccine until it has enough for everyone in the country. Virtually all experts agree that it would make no sense for most citizens to take the vaccine in advance of any smallpox outbreak. The threat is simply too remote, and the vaccine's side effects could kill or cause brain damage in some of those vaccinated.

Threats that were once remote—such as the possibility of severe outbreaks of disease, whether natural or manmade, or the possibility of a global infectious disease pandemic—are no longer so remote. Today it is not difficult to envision how a germ such as the causal agents of anthrax or smallpox, once reintroduced in a given locale, could move progressively through a population and possibly over the planet.

The events of September 11, 2001, underscore how important it is for individuals to be able to access reliable and dependable information about infectious disease. The editors therefore dedicate this *Handbook* to all citizens, with a shared belief that information alone has the power to strengthen our ability—as individuals and as nations—to cope with severe outbreaks of disease.

# Introduction

## RATIONALE

This statistical handbook is designed to offer students, researchers, practitioners, and the general adult population a comprehensive statistical overview of the status of infectious disease worldwide. In recent years there has been a dramatic increase in the availability of statistical information on both infectious diseases as a whole and individual epidemic-prone infectious diseases on the Internet. On one hand, the dramatic increase in the availability of this information has made it more convenient for students, researchers, practitioners, and the general adult population to access information on these subjects. On the other hand, however, the vast array of statistical information available on the Internet is often difficult to find, access, and use. Both individuals needing quick descriptive information and those demanding quantitative and authoritative data that put into context the thinking and analysis of their fields of interest and study are often frustrated by the challenge of "surfing the Web." This book, with its large yet accessible array of statistical information, will, we hope, inspire readers to further study and investigation.

## DEFINITION AND SCOPE

Infectious diseases are defined as any of the many diseases or illnesses (caused by bacteria or viruses) that can be transmitted from person to person, from animal to animal, or from organism to organism by direct or indirect contact. The common cold and AIDS are infectious diseases, whereas illnesses such as diabetes and gout are not. Infectious diseases thus include any communicable diseases. Epidemic-prone infectious diseases are individual contagious diseases that have high epidemic potential. Note that an epidemic is an occurrence of cases of a disease in excess of usual expectations for a particular population. An outbreak of influenza that affects thousands of people in a month in a nation and a half dozen cases of a rare form of liver cancer affecting industrial workers in a chemical plant over a period of years are both examples of epidemics. A single case of a rare and dangerous contagious disease that has never occurred before or has long been absent from a community represents a potential epidemic, as does a small cluster of cases of a disease such as typhoid in an urban community with good sanitation. Infectious pathogens (bacterial and viruses) cause most epidemics, while some are caused by a toxic industrial process or toxic substance in food or water.

Because infectious diseases do not discriminate, this *Handbook* covers the incidence of infectious diseases in the United States and worldwide.

## HEALTHY PEOPLE

In the United States, national objectives for public health provide both a road map for the country and a vision of public health for its citizens. Quantified ten-year objectives for disease prevention and health promotion have proved to be a useful guidepost for many federal agencies, state governments, and even local organizations since 1980. The publication in that year of *Promoting Health/Preventing Disease: Objectives for the Nation in 1980* represented a turning point in the articulation of health challenges and goals in the United States.[1] These 226 measurable objectives were established to help achieve the broad goals of a health strategy articulated in 1979 with the publication of *Healthy People: The Surgeon General's Report on Health Promotion and Disease Prevention*.[2] This set of five challenging goals, intended to reduce mortality among four age groups—infants, children, adolescents, and young adults, and adults—and increase independence among older adults, was supported by objectives with 1990 targets that drove action. Those objectives for 1990 and the ten-year plan that they set in motion for disease prevention and health promotion contributed enormously to a new sense of purpose and focus for public health and preventive medicine.

*Healthy People 2000* was released in 1990. It is a comprehensive agenda organized into 22 priority areas, with 319 supporting objectives. The Objectives for the Year 2000[3] build on the foundation of the objectives for 1990 and offer a vision for the new century, characterized by significant reductions in preventable death and disability, enhanced quality of life, and greatly reduced disparities in the health status of populations within society. Three overarching goals are to increase years of healthy life, reduce disparities in health among different population groups, and achieve access to prevention health services. Objectives relative to infectious disease are found throughout the document, in which separate chapters are allotted to food and drug safety, HIV infection, sexually transmitted diseases, and immunization and infectious diseases. Progress on *Healthy People 2000* objectives is monitored in a series of tracking profiles.[4]

Selected tables, figures, and charts in this book include reference points that monitor progress toward some of the *Healthy People 2000* national health status objectives for a particular disease.

Readers interested in exploring new baselines and targets for objectives as well as changes in population data tables and text will want to keep up with this series. Note that *Healthy People 2010* was published in January 2000.[5]

## ORGANIZATION AND CONTENT

Data and information on infectious diseases designated as notifiable at the national level during 1999 are presented first. Note that the official statistics for the reported occurrence of a given infectious disease are often published one to two years after surveillance data are collected and compiled. This is due to the manner in which statistics are collected, recorded, reported, finalized, and published. Concerning nationally notifiable diseases, it is noted that the *MMWR Summary of Notifiable Diseases, United States, 1999* was published April 6, 2001. Here, readers will find historical trends, summary data, and data on selected diseases. The following chapters highlight selected nationally notifiable diseases: HIV/AIDS, malaria, sexually transmitted diseases, and tuberculosis. Because of the increased awareness of foodborne and waterborne diseases, we have included separate chapters on these topics as well.

The focus then shifts to the status of infectious diseases worldwide. Chapter H opens with summary data on the problem and highlights several diseases that the world health community considers new or significant health threats. Vaccine-preventable diseases are the focus of the next chapter. Here, readers will find data and information on vaccines and vaccine development, immunization coverage, childhood immunization, vaccination in developing countries, and spending. A chapter then follows on disease elimination and eradication, providing information on those diseases that the World Health Organization (WHO) has formally targeted for elimination. Bioterrorism is the subject of the final chapter in the *Handbook.*

Many diseases could have appeared in multiple chapters. For example, polio is a vaccine-preventable disease that the world community has targeted for elimination. Cholera, which WHO considers a reemerging health threat, is also vaccine preventable. In order to prevent confusion and duplication, statistics on the incidence of diseases that are new, reemerging, or targeted for elimination are discussed in these chapters even if they are also vaccine preventable. We have included information on vaccine coverage for these diseases in the vaccine chapter.

Each chapter on a specific disease contains background on the disease, including a short description of the transmission process, clinical features, and other characteristics of the disease that are important for surveillance. The available data are described, as well as the strengths and weaknesses of the surveillance system. Explanatory commentary from the original document is included, as is the source of the data. The statistical tables follow. Detailed source information on each table, figure, or chart allows the user to begin digging both for further information and for the stories behind the numbers.

The *Handbook* concludes with a glossary of key terms, a topical bibliography that is also a guide to information sources available on the Internet, and a detailed keyword index.

## SOURCES AND DATA

The editors have provided data on a variety of infectious diseases recognized as nationally notifiable by the Centers for Disease Control and Prevention (CDC), as well as those recognized by the most recent edition of the *International Statistical Classification of Diseases and Related Health Problems* (ICD) developed by the World Health Organization (WHO). The ICD defines infectious diseases to include those diseases generally recognized as communicable or transmissible as well as a few diseases of unknown but possibly infectious origin.

The statistical tables, charts, and figures in the *Handbook* are reproduced from a variety of print and Web-based sources, including federal government sources, international government sources, and non-government publications. In each case, data quality and data availability influenced the selection of sources.

The surveillance of an infectious disease is fundamental for disease prevention and control. To the extent possible, the editors have drawn on the most recent surveillance data. As noted earlier, the most recent surveillance data may in fact be one or two years old, due to the manner in which the official statistics for the reported occurrence of a given infectious disease are collected, recorded, reported, finalized, and published. Readers are advised, however, that there is considerable variety in national, regional, and global epidemiological surveillance of both infectious diseases and individual infectious epidemic-prone diseases. Causative factors include differences in epidemic intelligence and differences in national, regional, and global health regulations, as well as differences in surveillance itself, such as differences in surveillance assessments and action plans, surveillance standards, surveillance tools, and differences in field epidemiology. Differences in surveillance support functions such as training and supervision, disease-specific laboratory networks, communications, and resource management may also affect global and regional epidemiological surveillance of individual infectious epidemic-prone diseases. Note too that certain infectious diseases may have specialized surveillance needs. The variety in the surveillance of infectious diseases and individual infectious epidemic-prone diseases poses a special challenge for the reader seeking consistency in data reporting, data analysis, and response.

The editors have attempted to point out the strengths and weaknesses of the data; however, in all cases, more detailed information (both data and analyses) is available from the original source.

## NOTES

1. U.S. Department of Health and Human Services. *Promoting Health/Preventing Disease: Objectives for the Nation* (Washington, DC: U.S. Department of Health and Human Services, 1980).
2. U.S. Department of Health and Human Services. *Healthy People: Surgeon General's Report on Health Promotion and Disease Prevention* (Washington, DC: U.S. Department of Health, Education and Welfare, 1979).
3. U.S. Department of Health and Human Services. *Healthy People 2000: National Health Promotion and Disease Prevention Objectives* (Washington, DC: U.S. Department of Health and Human Services, 1990).
4. Visit the Healthy People 2000 Web site at http://odphp.osophs.dhhs.gov/pubs/hp2000. Every product since the *Healthy People 2000 Midcourse Review and 1995 Revisions* is available on the Web site.
5. U.S. Department of Health and Human Services, *Healthy People 2010, 2nd ed. With Understanding and Improving Health and Objectives for Improving Health*, 2 vols. (Washington, DC: U.S. Government Printing Office, 2000).

# A. Nationally Notifiable Diseases

## BACKGROUND

The collection of morbidity reports on infectious diseases in the United States has its roots in 1878, when Congress authorized the U.S. Marine Hospital Service (the forerunner of the Public Health Service) to collect morbidity reports regarding cholera, smallpox, plague, and yellow fever from U.S. consuls overseas. The intention was to use this information to institute quarantine measures to prevent the introduction and spread of these diseases into the United States. In 1879, a specific congressional appropriation was made for the collection and publication of reports of these notifiable diseases. Congress expanded the authority for weekly reporting and publication of these reports in 1893 to include data from states and municipal authorities. To increase the uniformity of the data, Congress enacted a law in 1902 directing the Surgeon General to provide forms for the collection and compilation of data and for the publication of reports at the national level. In 1912, state and territorial health authorities, in conjunction with the Public Health Service, recommended immediate telegraphic reporting of five infectious diseases and the monthly reporting, by letter, of 10 additional diseases.

The first annual summary of *The Notifiable Diseases* in 1912 included reports of 10 diseases from 19 states, the District of Columbia, and Hawaii. By 1928, all states, the District of Columbia, Hawaii, and Puerto Rico were participating in national reporting of 29 specified diseases. At their annual meeting in 1950, state and territorial health officers authorized the Council of State and Territorial Epidemiologists (CSTE) to determine which diseases should be reported to the Public Health Service. In 1961, the Centers for Disease Control and Prevention (CDC) assumed responsibility for the collection and publication of data concerning nationally notifiable disease.

## SURVEILLANCE

As of January 1, 1999, a total of 58 infectious diseases were notifiable at the national level.[1] A notifiable disease is one for which regular, frequent, and timely information regarding individual cases is considered necessary for the prevention and control of the disease.

Public health officials at state health departments and CDC collaborate in both compiling and revising the list periodically. The Council of State and Territorial Epidemiologists (CSTE), with input from CDC, makes recommendations annually for additions and deletions. However, state reporting of nationally notifiable diseases to CDC is voluntary. Legislation or regulation only at the state and local level currently mandates reporting. Thus, the list of diseases considered notifiable varies slightly from state to state. All states generally report the internationally quarantinable diseases (i.e., cholera, plague, and yellow fever) in compliance with the World Health Organization's International Health Regulations.

The list of 58 infectious diseases designated as notifiable at the national level during 1999 is as shown in this table.

**Infectious Diseases Designated as Notifiable at the National Level during 1999**

| | | |
|---|---|---|
| Acquired immunodeficiency syndrome (AIDS) | *Haemophilus influenzae*, invasive disease | Rabies, human |
| Anthrax | Hansen disease (leprosy) | Rocky Mountain spotted fever |
| Botulism | Hantavirus pulmonary syndrome | Rubella |
| Brucellosis | Hemolytic uremic syndrome, postdiarrheal | Rubella, congenital syndrome |
| Chancroid | Hepatitis A | Salmonellosis |
| *Chlamydia trachomatis*, genital infection | Hepatitis B | Shigellosis |
| Cholera | Hepatitis C; non-A, non-B | Streptococcal disease, invasive, group A |
| Coccidioidomycosis | Human immunodeficiency virus (HIV) infection, adult | *Streptococcus pneumoniae*, drug-resistant, invasive disease |
| Cryptosporidiosis | HIV infection, pediatric | Streptococcal toxic-shock syndrome |
| Cyclosporiasis | Legionellosis | Syphilis |
| Diphtheria | Lyme disease | Syphilis, congenital |
| Ehrlichiosis, human granulocytic | Malaria | Tetanus |
| Ehrlichiosis, human monocytic | Measles | Toxic-shock syndrome |
| Encephalitis, California serogroup viral | Meningococcal disease | Trichinosis |
| Encephalitis, eastern equine | Mumps | Tuberculosis |
| Encephalitis, St. Louis | Pertussis | Typhoid fever |
| Encephalitis, western equine | Plague | Varicella (chickenpox) |
| *Escherichia coli* O157:H7 | Poliomyelitis, paralytic | Varicella deaths |
| Gonorrhea | Psittacosis | Yellow fever |
| Rabies, animal | | |

*Note*: Although varicella (chickenpox) is not a nationally notifiable disease, the Council of State and Territorial Epidemiologists recommends reporting cases of this disease to CDC.
*Source:* Centers for Disease Control and Prevention. *Summary of Notifiable Diseases*, United States, 1999. MMWR 1999, 48, no. 53. http://www.cdc.gov/mmwr/PDF/wk/mm4853.pdf.

Data regarding all nationally notifiable diseases are reported to CDC through the National Notifiable Diseases Surveillance System (NNDSS).[2] Note that the numbers of reported cases of individual diseases presented in other chapters in this *Handbook* might differ from data presented in this chapter because of differences in the collection and transmission of data. Additionally, and in general, NNDSS receives less detailed clinical and epidemiological data regarding specific diseases than do other disease-specific surveillance systems.

## DATA SOURCES

The CDC publishes the statistical summary of notifiable diseases in the United States to accompany each volume of the *Morbidity and Mortality Weekly Report (MMWR)*. Provisional data concerning the reported occurrence of notifiable diseases are published weekly in *MMWR*. After each reporting year, staffs in state health departments finalize reports of cases for that year with local or county health departments and reconcile the data with reports previously sent to CDC throughout the year. These data are compiled in final form in the *MMWR Summary of Notifiable Diseases, United States*. The data are published for use by state and local health departments; schools of medicine and public health; communications media; local, state, and federal agencies; and other agencies or persons interested in following the trends of reportable diseases in the United States. This publication also documents which diseases are considered national priorities for notification and the annual number of cases of such diseases.

Data in the *MMWR Summary of Notifiable Diseases, United States* were derived primarily from reports transmitted to the Division of Public Health Surveillance and Informatics, Epidemiology Program Office, CDC, from health departments in the 50 states, five territories, New York City, and the District of Columbia through the National Electronic Telecommunications System for Surveillance (NETSS).

Final data for selected diseases are from the surveillance records of selected CDC programs. These include the National Center for Health Statistics, Office of Vital and Health Statistics Systems (deaths from selected notifiable diseases); the National Center for Infectious Diseases, Division of Bacterial and Mycotic Diseases (toxic-shock syndrome; Streptococcal diseases, invasive, group A; Streptococcal toxic-shock syndrome; and laboratory data regarding botulism, *Escherichia coli* O157:H7, salmonellosis, and shigellosis); the National Center for Infectious Diseases, Division of Viral and Rickettsial Diseases (animal rabies; Hantavirus pulmonary syndrome); the National Center for HIV, STD, and TB Prevention, Division of

HIV/AIDS Prevention—Surveillance and Epidemiology (acquired immunodeficiency syndrome [AIDS]); the National Center for HIV, STD, and TB Prevention, Division of Sexually Transmitted Diseases Prevention (chancroid, chlamydia, gonorrhea, and syphilis); the National Center for HIV, STD, and TB Prevention, Division of Tuberculosis Elimination (tuberculosis); and the National Immunization Program, Epidemiology and Surveillance Division (poliomyelitis, *Haemophilus influenzae*, invasive disease, type B, and varicella).

Notifiable disease reports are the authoritative and archival counts of cases. The appropriate epidemiologist from each submitting state or territory must approve them before they are published in the *MMWR Summary of Notifiable Diseases, United States*.

## INTERPRETING DATA

The data are useful for analyzing disease trends and determining relative disease burden. As with all data presented in this volume, these data must be interpreted in light of reporting practices. For example, the degree of completeness of data reporting varies from disease to disease. In a similar vein, the uniformity of data collection also varies from disease to disease.

Disease totals for the United States, unless otherwise stated, do not include data for American Samoa, Guam, Puerto Rico, the Virgin Islands, or the Commonwealth of the Northern Mariana Islands. Population estimates for the states are from July 1, 1999, estimates by the U.S. Department of Commerce, Economics, and Statistics Administration, Bureau of the Census, Population Division, Population Distribution Branch, Internet press release ST-99-1, December 29, 1999. Population numbers for territories are 1998 estimates from Bureau of the Census press release PR-99-1 and CB98-219. More information regarding census estimates is available at http://www.census.gov/.

Rates are presented as incidence rates per 100,000 population, based on data for the U.S. total-resident population. Population data from states in which diseases were not notifiable or disease data were not available were excluded from rate calculations.

## TABLE OVERVIEW

**A1.1–A1.6. Historical Trends** The first cluster of tables offers data on notifiable diseases from 1968 through 1999. The last table (A1.6) presents figures on deaths from selected notifiable disease for 1980–1998. The diseases included in each table vary, reflecting the periodic revision of the list.

**A2.1–A2.6. Summary Data** This suite offers the most recent data available on notifiable diseases. Tables report cases by month, by geographic division and area, by age group, by sex, by race, and by ethnicity. The data are final totals as of August 15, 2000, unless otherwise noted. Nationally notifiable diseases that are reported in fewer than 40 states do not appear in these tables. In all tables, leprosy is listed as Hansen disease, and tickborne typhus fever is listed as Rocky Mountain spotted fever. Additionally, because no cases of anthrax, human rabies, or paralytic poliomyelitis were reported in the United States during 1999, these diseases do not appear in the tables in this series.

**A3.1–A3.19. Selected Diseases** The graphs and maps in this suite focus on selected nationally notifiable diseases of high interest or for which we present worldwide information in later chapters.

**A3.1. Cholera** Although cholera has been primarily a disease of travelers to Latin America, Asia, and Africa in recent years, cases are occasionally acquired in the united States from contaminated seafood.

**A3.2. Diphtheria** Diphtheria is a potentially fatal disease that was a major killer in the United States until the development of a vaccine. Since 1988, all confirmed cases in the United States have involved visitors or immigrants. There were no probable or confirmed cases reported in 1999.

**A3.3. Haemophilus influenzae** In 1999, a total of 261 cases of *Haemophilus influenzae* (Hi) invasive disease among children under 5 years were reported. Before a vaccine was introduced in 1987, approximately 20,000 cases of *H. influenzae* type b (Hib) invasive disease occurred among children annually.[3] The sharp decline in the number of Hib cases is attributed to the widespread use of the Hib vaccine among preschool-aged children. Among the 71 cases of Hib invasive disease reported in children aged under 5 years, 30 (42%) were among children aged under 6 months, which is too young to have completed a three-dose primary Hib vaccination. Twenty-three (56%) of the 41 children who were old enough to have completed a three-dose primary series were incompletely vaccinated (20 children) or their vaccination status was unknown (3 children). These cases might have been prevented with age-appropriate vaccination.[4]

**A3.4. Hansen Disease (leprosy)** In 1999, a total of 108 cases of Hansen disease was reported in the United States. The number of cases peaked at 361 in 1985, during an increased influx of Indo-Chinese refugees as a result of conflicts in the area. Since 1988 the number of cases has remained relatively stable.

**A3.5–3.6. Hepatitis A, B, and C** Hepatitis A, B, and C are all considered nationally notifiable. The overall rate of hepatitis A reported during 1999 (17,047 cases) was the lowest recorded. Routine immunization or the natural variability in infection rates may be the cause of this low rate. However, because hepatitis A rates tend to vary from year to year and from region to region, determining whether this low rate is caused by either is impossible.

A total of 7,694 cases of hepatitis B were reported in 1999. Note that because most infections among infants and young children are asymptomatic, reported cases underestimate the incidence of disease in these groups. Regardless of this, the number of reported acute hepatitis B cases has decreased by more than 60% during the past decade, from 21,102 cases in 1990 to 7,694 cases in 1999. This downward trend is expected to continue as a national strategy for eliminating hepatitis B virus (HBV) transmission is implemented. Components of this strategy include screening pregnant women for hepatitis B surface antigen and providing postexposure immunoprophylaxis to infants of infected women; routinely vaccinating infants; providing catch-up vaccinations for children aged under 19 years; and targeting vaccinations to children, adolescents, and adults at increased risk for infection.

Hepatitis C virus (HCV) is the most common chronic bloodborne infection in the United States. During 1999, 3,111 cases of HCV were reported. Note however that cases of hepatitis C reported to the National Notifiable Disease Surveillance System (NNDSS) are considered unreliable because (1) there is no serologic marker for acute infection and (2) most health departments do not have resources to determine if a positive laboratory report for hepatitis C virus (HCV) infection represents acute infection, chronic infection, repeated testing of a person previously reported, or a false-positive result.

**A3.7. Lyme Disease** In 1999, a total of 16,273 cases of Lyme disease were reported. Lyme disease occurs primarily in the northeastern and north-central United States. In December 1998, the U.S. Food and Drug Administration approved a new Lyme disease vaccination.

**A3.8. Measles** In 1999, a total of 100 confirmed cases of measles was reported. Of these cases, 33 were imported from outside the United States, and exposure to these case-patients caused 33 additional cases. The remaining 34 cases were of unknown source. An attack of measles almost invariably confers permanent immunity. In 1999, CDC convened a panel of expert consultants who concluded that measles is not currently endemic in the United States. However, because of the continued threat of imported measles, high population immunity must be maintained to continue low levels of transmission.

**A3.9. Meningococcal Disease** Meningoccal disease rates have remained stable since the 1960s, with 2,501 cases reported in 1999. However, case fatality rates remain high; of the 1,091 patients with outcome reported in 1999, a total of 12.5% died.

**A3.10. Mumps** In 1999, a record low of 387 mumps cases was reported, meeting the *Healthy People 2000* objective of 500 cases per year.

**A3.11–3.12. Pertussis** In 1999, a total of 27% or 7,288 reported cases of pertussis occurred among children aged under 7 months, who were too young to have received the recommended three doses of pertussis vaccine. Eleven percent of cases were among preschool-aged children (i.e., those aged 1–4 years), and 28% were among children aged 10–19 years. Since 1995, the coverage rate with at least three doses of pertussis vaccine has been 95% among U.S. children aged 19–35 months (*MMWR 2000* 49:585–89). Because vaccine-induced immunity wanes approximately 5–10 years after pertussis vaccination, adolescents can become susceptible to disease. Since 1990, the incidence among preschool-aged children has not changed, but the incidence among adolescents has increased in some states.[5]

**A3.13. Plague** In the roster of nationally notifiable diseases, one disease—plague—is particularly notable in that its agent, *Yersinia pestis*, was recently designated as a potential agent of biological terrorism. In 1999, nine cases of plague among humans were reported in the United States. In recognition of the fact that *Yersinia pestis* was recently designated as a potential agent of biological terrorism, CDC is collaborating with other public health and federal agencies to develop guidelines for responding to bioterrorism events involving *Y. pestis*.

**A3.14. Poliomyelitis, Paralytic** A sequential schedule of inactivated poliovirus vaccine (IPV) and live, attenuated oral poliovirus vaccine (OPV) was introduced in 1997 for routine childhood polio vaccination in the United States. Since implementation of this schedule, five cases of vaccine-associated paralytic poliomyelitis (VAPP) with onset in 1997 and two cases with onset in 1998 have been confirmed. Before the sequential schedule, the average annual number of VAPP cases was eight, suggesting that VAPP has declined since introduction of the sequential schedule. Note that preliminary findings may be skewed by potential delays in reporting. Further reductions are expected because the Advisory Committee on Immunization Practices (ACIP) has approved an all-inactivated polio vaccine (IPV) intended to eliminate the risk for VAPP.

**A3.15. Rabies** Rabies is not, in the natural sense, a disease of humans. Human infection is incidental to the reservoir of disease in wild and domestic animals. Consequently, data for the number and distribution of cases of rabies in domestic animals provides the best estimates of the impact of rabies on a country. Over the last 100 years, rabies in the United States has changed dramatically. More than 90% of all animal cases reported annually to CDC now occur in wildlife; before 1960 the majority were in domestic animals. The principal rabies hosts today are wild carnivores and bats. The number of rabies-related human deaths in the United States has declined from more than 100 annually at the turn of the century to one or two per year in the 1990s.

**A3.16. Rubella** During the 1990s, rubella cases declined substantially in the United States, from 1,124 reported cases in 1990 to 267 reported cases in 1999. Since 1997, approximately 19 rubella outbreaks have occurred in the United States, mostly among persons born in countries that do not have routine rubella vaccination programs or that have only recently implemented such programs. During the decade, fewer than 10 cases of congenital rubella syndrome have been reported annually; most cases were among infants born to mothers outside the United States.

**A3.17. Tetanus** The CDC reported 40 cases of tetanus in 1999. Five cases (12.5%) were among persons under 25 years, 22 (55.0%) were among persons aged 25–59 years, and 13 (32.5%) were among persons over 59 years. Seven of the cases among persons aged 25–59 years were reported in intravenous drug uses; two of these cases were fatal. Two cases were in children (aged 4 and 5 years) who had never been vaccinated against tetanus because of their parents' philosophic objection to vaccination. The percentage of cases among persons aged 25–59 has increased during the last decade; previously most cases were among persons over 59 years.

**A3.18. Typhoid Fever** In 1999, typhoid fever was diagnosed in 346 persons in the United States. Despite the availability of effective vaccines, NNDSS reports 300–400 cases each year. Approximately 80% of these cases occur among persons who report international travel during the preceding six weeks. Persons traveling to and from their country of origin appear to be at high risk (*Journal of the American Medical Association* 283 (2000): 2668–73). In many areas of the world, *Salmonella Typhi* strains have acquired resistance to multiple antimicrobial agents, including ampicillin, chloramphenicol, and trimethoprim-sulfamethoxazole (*Journal of the American Medical Association* 283 (2000): 2668–73).

**A3.19. Varicella (chickenpox)** In 1995, varicella vaccine was licensed in the United States. During 1999, vaccine coverage among children aged 19–35 months was 59%. Varicella is not a nationally notifiable disease, but the Council of State and Territorial Epidemiologists recommends reporting cases of this disease to the CDC. Seven states maintained adequate levels of reporting by reporting varicella cases constituting greater than or equal to 5% of their birth cohort during 1990–1995. Although the number of cases varied annually, the number declined steadily in these states during 1997–1999. The marked decline in reported cases in 1999 is consistent with data from active varicella surveillance and is suggestive of vaccine impact.

## NOTES

1. As of November 2001, the 1999 annual figures were the most recent available from the *MMWR Summary of Notifiable Diseases*, Published by the *Morbidity and Mortality Weekly Report* from the Centers for Disease Control.
2. For a description of NNDSS, see S.M. Teutsch, "Considerations in Planning a Surveillance System, Appendix 2A, Description of National Notifiable Disease Surveillance System in the United States," in S.M. Teutsch, and R.E. Churchill, eds., *Principles and Practice of Public Health Surveillance* (New York: Oxford University Press, 1994).
3. *Journal of the American Medical Association (JAMA)* 269 (1993): 221–26.
4. *Morbidity and Mortality Weekly Report (MMWR)* 47 (1999): vii.
5. Güris, D., P. Strebel, and B. Bardenheier et al. "Changing Epidemiology of Pertussis in the United States: Increasing Reported Incidence Among Adolescents and Adults, 1990–1996." *Clinical Infectious Diseases* 28 (1999):1230–37.

## Table A1.1. Reported Incidence Rates of Notifiable Diseases per 100,000 Population, United States, 1989–1999

| Disease | 1989 | 1990 | 1991 | 1992 | 1993 | 1994 | 1995 | 1996 | 1997 | 1998 | 1999 |
|---|---|---|---|---|---|---|---|---|---|---|---|
| AIDS* | 13.58 | 16.72 | 17.32 | 17.83 | 40.20 | 30.07 | 27.20 | 25.21 | 21.85 | 17.21 | 16.66 |
| Amebiasis | 1.34 | 1.38 | 1.23 | 1.21 | 1.21 | 1.20 | | | † | | |
| Anthrax | — | — | — | 0.00 | — | — | — | — | — | — | — |
| Aseptic meningitis | 4.14 | 4.77 | 6.26 | 5.18 | 5.39 | 3.71 | | | † | | |
| Botulism, total (includes wound and unspecified) | 0.04 | 0.04 | 0.05 | 0.04 | 0.04 | 0.06 | 0.04 | 0.05 | 0.05 | 0.04 | 0.06 |
| Foodborne | 0.01 | 0.01 | 0.01 | 0.00 | 0.01 | 0.02 | 0.01 | 0.01 | 0.02 | 0.01 | 0.01 |
| Brucellosis | 0.04 | 0.03 | 0.04 | 0.04 | 0.05 | 0.05 | 0.04 | 0.05 | 0.04 | 0.03 | 0.03 |
| Chancroid | 1.90 | 1.70 | 1.40 | 0.80 | 0.54 | 0.30 | 0.20 | 0.15 | 0.09 | 0.07 | 0.06 |
| Chlamydia§ | | | | ¶ | | | 182.60 | 188.10 | 196.80 | 236.57 | 254.10 |
| Cholera | — | 0.00 | 0.01 | 0.04 | 0.00 | 0.02 | 0.01 | 0.01 | 0.01 | 0.01 | 0.00 |
| Cryptosporidiosis | | | ¶ | | | | | | 1.12 | 1.61 | 0.92 |
| Diphtheria | 0.00 | 0.00 | 0.00 | 0.00 | — | 0.00 | — | 0.01 | 0.01 | 0.00 | 0.00 |
| Encephalitis, primary | 0.40 | 0.54 | 0.40 | 0.30 | 0.36 | 0.28 | | | † | | |
| Postinfectious | 0.04 | 0.04 | 0.03 | 0.05 | 0.07 | 0.06 | | | † | | |
| Encephalitis, California serogroup viral | | | | | ¶ | | | | | 0.04 | 0.03 |
| Eastern equine | | | | | ¶ | | | | | 0.00 | 0.00 |
| St. Louis | | | | | ¶ | | | | | 0.01 | 0.00 |
| Western equine | | | | | ¶ | | | | | 0.00 | 0.00 |
| *Escherichia coli* O157:H7 | | | ¶ | | | 0.82 | 1.01 | 1.18 | 1.04 | 1.28 | 1.77 |
| Gonorrhea | 297.36 | 276.60 | 249.48 | 201.60 | 172.40 | 168.40 | 149.50 | 122.80 | 121.40 | 132.88 | 133.20 |
| Granuloma inguinale | 0.00 | 0.00 | 0.01 | 0.00 | 0.00 | 0.00 | | | † | | |
| *Haemophilus influenzae*, invasive disease | ¶ | | 1.10 | 0.55 | 0.55 | 0.45 | 0.45 | 0.45 | 0.44 | 0.44 | 0.48 |
| Hansen disease (leprosy) | 0.07 | 0.08 | 0.06 | 0.07 | 0.07 | 0.05 | 0.06 | 0.05 | 0.05 | 0.05 | 0.04 |
| Hepatitis A | 14.43 | 12.64 | 9.67 | 9.06 | 9.40 | 10.29 | 12.13 | 11.70 | 11.22 | 8.59 | 6.25 |
| Hepatitis B | 9.43 | 8.48 | 7.14 | 6.32 | 5.18 | 4.81 | 4.19 | 4.01 | 3.90 | 3.80 | 2.82 |
| Hepatitis C; non-A, non-B** | 1.02 | 1.03 | 1.42 | 2.36 | 1.86 | 1.78 | 1.78 | 1.41 | 1.43 | 1.30 | 1.14 |
| Hepatitis, unspecified | 0.93 | 0.67 | 0.50 | 0.35 | 0.24 | 0.17 | | | † | | |
| Legionellosis | 0.48 | 0.55 | 0.53 | 0.53 | 0.50 | 0.63 | 0.48 | 0.47 | 0.44 | 0.51 | 0.41 |
| Leptospirosis | 0.04 | 0.03 | 0.02 | 0.02 | 0.02 | 0.02 | | | † | | |
| Lyme disease | ¶ | | 3.80 | 3.93 | 3.20 | 5.01 | 4.49 | 6.21 | 4.79 | 6.39 | 5.99 |
| Lymphogranuloma venereum | 0.08 | 0.10 | 0.19 | 0.10 | 0.10 | 0.10 | | | † | | |
| Malaria | 0.51 | 0.52 | 0.51 | 0.43 | 0.55 | 0.47 | 0.55 | 0.68 | 0.75 | 0.60 | 0.61 |
| Measles | 7.33 | 11.17 | 3.82 | 0.88 | 0.12 | 0.37 | 0.12 | 0.20 | 0.06 | 0.04 | 0.04 |
| Meningococcal disease | 1.10 | 0.99 | 0.84 | 0.84 | 1.02 | 1.11 | 1.25 | 1.30 | 1.24 | 1.01 | 0.92 |
| Mumps | 2.34 | 2.17 | 1.72 | 1.03 | 0.66 | 0.60 | 0.35 | 0.29 | 0.27 | 0.25 | 0.14 |
| Murine typhus fever | 0.02 | 0.02 | 0.02 | 0.02 | 0.01 | 0.01 | | | † | | |

## Table A1.1. *(Continued)*

| Disease | 1989 | 1990 | 1991 | 1992 | 1993 | 1994 | 1995 | 1996 | 1997 | 1998 | 1999 |
|---|---|---|---|---|---|---|---|---|---|---|---|
| Pertussis (whooping cough) | 1.67 | 1.84 | 1.08 | 1.60 | 2.55 | 1.77 | 1.97 | 2.94 | 2.46 | 2.74 | 2.67 |
| Plague | 0.00 | 0.00 | 0.00 | 0.01 | 0.00 | 0.01 | 0.00 | 0.01 | 0.01 | 0.00 | 0.00 |
| Poliomyelitis, paralytic | 0.00 | 0.00 | 0.00 | 0.00 | 0.00 | 0.00 | 0.00 | 0.01 | 0.01 | 0.00 | — |
| Psittacosis | 0.05 | 0.05 | 0.04 | 0.04 | 0.02 | 0.02 | 0.03 | 0.02 | 0.02 | 0.02 | 0.01 |
| Rabies, human | 0.00 | 0.00 | 0.00 | 0.00 | 0.00 | 0.00 | 0.00 | 0.01 | 0.01 | 0.00 | — |
| Rheumatic fever, acute | 0.13 | 0.09 | 0.12 | 0.06 | 0.08 | 0.09 | | | † | | |
| Rocky Mountain spotted fever | 0.25 | 0.26 | 0.25 | 0.20 | 0.18 | 0.18 | 0.23 | 0.32 | 0.16 | 0.14 | 0.21 |
| Rubella | 0.16 | 0.45 | 0.56 | 0.06 | 0.07 | 0.09 | 0.05 | 0.10 | 0.07 | 0.13 | 0.10 |
| Salmonellosis, excluding typhoid fever | 19.26 | 19.54 | 19.10 | 16.04 | 16.15 | 16.64 | 17.66 | 17.15 | 15.66 | 16.17 | 14.89 |
| Shigellosis | 10.07 | 10.89 | 9.34 | 9.38 | 12.48 | 11.44 | 12.32 | 9.80 | 8.64 | 8.74 | 6.43 |
| Syphilis, primary and secondary | 18.07 | 20.10 | 17.26 | 13.70 | 10.40 | 8.10 | 6.30 | 4.29 | 3.19 | 2.61 | 2.50 |
| Total, all stages | 44.94 | 53.80 | 51.69 | 45.30 | 39.70 | 32.00 | 26.20 | 19.97 | 17.39 | 14.19 | 13.07 |
| Tetanus | 0.02 | 0.03 | 0.02 | 0.02 | 0.02 | 0.02 | 0.02 | 0.02 | 0.02 | 0.02 | 0.01 |
| Toxic-shock syndrome | 0.16 | 0.13 | 0.11 | 0.10 | 0.08 | 0.10 | 0.07 | 0.06 | 0.06 | 0.06 | 0.05 |
| Trichinosis | 0.01 | 0.05 | 0.02 | 0.02 | 0.01 | 0.01 | 0.01 | 0.01 | 0.01 | 0.01 | 0.00 |
| Tuberculosis | 9.46 | 10.33 | 10.42 | 10.46 | 9.82 | 9.36 | 8.70 | 8.04 | 7.42 | 6.79 | 6.43 |
| Tularemia | 0.06 | 0.06 | 0.08 | 0.06 | 0.05 | 0.04 | | | † | | |
| Typhoid fever | 0.19 | 0.22 | 0.20 | 0.16 | 0.17 | 0.17 | 0.14 | 0.15 | 0.14 | 0.14 | 0.13 |
| Varicella (chickenpox)†† | 121.77 | 120.06 | 135.82 | 176.54 | 118.54 | 135.76 | 118.11 | 44.13 | 93.55 | 70.28 | 44.56 |
| Yellow fever | — | — | — | — | — | — | — | 0.00 | — | — | 0.00 |

* Acquired immunodeficiency syndrome (AIDS).

† No longer nationally notifiable.

§ Chlamydia refers to genital infections caused by *C. trachomatis.*

¶ Not previously nationally notifiable.

**Anti-HCV (hepatitis C virus) antibody test became available May 1990.

†† Not nationally notifiable.

Note: Rates <0.01 after rounding are listed as 0.00. Data in the *MMWR Summary of Notifiable Diseases, United States* might not match data in other CDC surveillance reports because of differences in the timing of reports, the source of the data, and the use of different case definitions.

*Source*: Centers for Disease Control and Prevention. *Summary of Notifiable Diseases, United States, 1999. MMWR* 1999, 48, no. 53. http://www.cdc.gov/mmwr/PDF/wk/mm4853.pdf.

## Table A1.2. Reported Cases of Notifiable Diseases, United States, 1992–1999

| Disease | 1992 | 1993 | 1994 | 1995 | 1996 | 1997 | 1998 | 1999 |
|---|---|---|---|---|---|---|---|---|
| AIDS | 45,472 | 103,691 | 78,279 | 71,547 | 66,885 | 58,492 | 46,521 | 45,104* |
| Amebiasis | 2,942 | 2,970 | 2,983 | | | † | | |
| Anthrax | 1 | — | — | — | — | — | — | — |
| Aseptic meningitis | 12,223 | 12,848 | 8,932 | | † | | | |
| Botulism, total (includes wound and unspecified) | 91 | 97 | 143 | 97 | 119 | 132 | 116 | 154 |
| Foodborne | 21 | 27 | 50 | 24 | 25 | 31 | 22 | 23 |
| Infant | 66 | 65 | 85 | 54 | 80 | 79 | 65 | 92 |
| Brucellosis | 105 | 120 | 119 | 98 | 112 | 98 | 79 | 82 |
| Chancroid | 1,886 | 1,399 | 773 | 606 | 386 | 243 | 189 | 143§ |
| Chlamydia¶ | | ** | | 477,638 | 498,884 | 526,671 | 604,420 | 656,721§ |
| Cholera | 103 | 18 | 39 | 23 | 4 | 6 | 17 | 6 |
| Cryptosporidiosis | | ** | | | | 2,566 | 3,793 | 2,361 |
| Diphtheria | 4 | — | 2 | — | 2 | 4 | 1 | 1 |
| Encephalitis, primary | 774 | 919 | 717 | | | † | | |
| Postinfectious | 129 | 170 | 143 | | | † | | |
| Encephalitis, California serogroup viral | | | | ** | | | 97 | 70 |
| Eastern equine | | | | ** | | | 4 | 5 |
| St. Louis | | | | ** | | | 24 | 4 |
| Western equine | | | | ** | | | — | 1 |
| *Escherichia coli* O157:H7 | ** | | 1,420 | 2,139 | 2,741 | 2,555 | 3,161 | 4,513 |
| Gonorrhea | 501,409 | 439,673 | 418,068 | 392,848 | 325,883 | 324,907 | 355,642 | 360,076§ |
| Granuloma inguinale | 6 | 19 | 3 | | | † | | |
| *Haemophilus influenzae*, invasive disease | 1,412 | 1,419 | 1,174 | 1,180 | 1,170 | 1,162 | 1,194 | 1,309 |
| Hansen disease (leprosy) | 172 | 187 | 136 | 144 | 112 | 122 | 108 | 108 |
| Hepatitis A | 23,112 | 24,238 | 26,796 | 31,582 | 31,032 | 30,021 | 23,229 | 17,047 |
| Hepatitis B | 16,126 | 13,361 | 12,517 | 10,805 | 10,637 | 10,416 | 10,258 | 7,694 |
| Hepatitis C; non-A, non-B†† | 6,010 | 4,786 | 4,470 | 4,576 | 3,716 | 3,816 | 3,518 | 3,111 |
| Hepatitis, unspecified | 884 | 627 | 444 | | | † | | |
| Legionellosis | 1,339 | 1,280 | 1,615 | 1,241 | 1,198 | 1,163 | 1,355 | 1,108 |
| Leptospirosis | 54 | 51 | 38 | | | † | | |
| Lyme disease | 9,895 | 8,257 | 13,043 | 11,700 | 16,455 | 12,801 | 16,801 | 16,273 |
| Lymphogranuloma venereum | 302 | 285 | 235 | | | † | | |

## Table A1.2. *(Continued)*

| Disease | 1992 | 1993 | 1994 | 1995 | 1996 | 1997 | 1998 | 1999 |
|---|---|---|---|---|---|---|---|---|
| Malaria | 1,087 | 1,411 | 1,229 | 1,419 | 1,800 | 2,001 | 1,611 | 1,666 |
| Measles | 2,237 | 312 | 963 | 309 | 508 | 138 | 100 | 100 |
| Meningococcal disease | 2,134 | 2,637 | 2,886 | 3,243 | 3,437 | 3,308 | 2,725 | 2,501 |
| Mumps | 2,572 | 1,692 | 1,537 | 906 | 751 | 683 | 666 | 387 |
| Murine typhus fever | 28 | 25 | | | † | | | |
| Pertussis (whooping cough) | 4,083 | 6,586 | 4,617 | 5,137 | 7,796 | 6,564 | 7,405 | 7,288 |
| Plague | 13 | 10 | 17 | 9 | 5 | 4 | 9 | 9 |
| Poliomyelitis, paralytic§§ | 6 | 4 | 8 | 7 | 5 | 5 | 1 | — |
| Psittacosis | 92 | 60 | 38 | 64 | 42 | 33 | 47 | 16 |
| Rabies, animal | 8,589 | 9,377 | 8,147 | 7,811 | 6,982 | 8,105 | 7,259 | 6,730 |
| Rabies, human | 1 | 3 | 6 | 5 | 3 | 2 | 1 | — |
| Rheumatic fever, acute | 75 | 112 | 112 | | | † | | |
| Rocky Mountain spotted fever | 502 | 456 | 465 | 590 | 831 | 409 | 365 | 579 |
| Rubella | 160 | 192 | 227 | 128 | 238 | 181 | 364 | 267 |
| Rubella, congenital syndrome | 11 | 5 | 7 | 6 | 4 | 5 | 7 | 9 |
| Salmonellosis, excluding typhoid fever | 40,912 | 41,641 | 43,323 | 45,970 | 45,471 | 41,901 | 43,694 | 40,596 |
| Shigellosis | 23,931 | 32,198 | 29,769 | 32,080 | 25,978 | 23,117 | 23,626 | 17,521 |
| Syphilis, primary and secondary | 33,973 | 26,498 | 20,627 | 16,500 | 11,387 | 8,550 | 6,993 | 6,657§ |
| Total, all stages | 112,581 | 101,259 | 81,696 | 68,953 | 52,976 | 46,540 | 37,977 | 35,628§ |
| Tetanus | 45 | 48 | 51 | 41 | 36 | 50 | 41 | 40 |
| Toxic-shock syndrome | 244 | 212 | 192 | 191 | 145 | 157 | 138 | 113 |
| Trichinosis | 41 | 16 | 32 | 29 | 11 | 13 | 19 | 12 |
| Tuberculosis | 26,673 | 25,313 | 24,361 | 22,860 | 21,337 | 19,851 | 18,361 | 17,531¶¶ |
| Tularemia | 159 | 132 | 96 | | | † | | |
| Typhoid fever | 414 | 440 | 441 | 369 | 396 | 365 | 375 | 346 |
| Varicella (chickenpox)*** | 158,364 | 134,722 | 151,219 | 120,624 | 83,511 | 98,727 | 82,455 | 46,016 |
| Yellow fever | | ††† | | | 1 | — | — | 1 |

* Total number of acquired immunodeficiency syndrome (AIDS) cases reported to the Division of HIV/AIDS Prevention—Surveillance andEpidemiology, National Center for HIV, STD, and TB Prevention (NCHSTP) through December 31, 1999.

† No longer nationally notifiable.

§ Cases were updated through the Division of Sexually Transmitted Diseases Prevention, NCHSTP, as of August 8, 2000.

¶ Chlamydia refers to genital infections caused by *C. trachomatis.*

** Not previously nationally notifiable.

†† Anti-HCV (hepatitis C virus) antibody test was available as of May 1990.

§§ Numbers might not reflect changes based on retrospective case evaluations or late reports (see *MMWR* 1986; 35:180–2).

¶¶ Cases were updated through the Division of Tuberculosis Elimination, NCHSTP, as of May 3, 2000.

*** Varicella was taken off the nationally notifiable disease list in 1991. Many states continue to report these cases to the CDC.

††† Last indigenous case of yellow fever reported in 1911; last imported case reported in 1999.

Note: Data in the *MMWR Summary of Notifiable Diseases, United States* might not match data in other CDC surveillance reports because of differences in the timing of reports, the source of the data, and the use of different case definitions.

*Source*: Centers for Disease Control and Prevention. *Summary of Notifiable Diseases, United States, 1999. MMWR* 1999, 48, no. 53. http://www.cdc.gov/mmwr/PDF/wk/mm4853.pdf.

## Table A1.3. Reported Cases of Notifiable Diseases, United States, 1984–1991

| Disease | 1984 | 1985 | 1986 | 1987 | 1988 | 1989 | 1990 | 1991 |
|---|---|---|---|---|---|---|---|---|
| AIDS* | 4,445 | 8,249 | 12,932 | 21,070 | 31,001 | 33,722 | 41,595 | 43,672 |
| Amebiasis | 5,252 | 4,433 | 3,532 | 3,123 | 2,860 | 3,217 | 3,328 | 2,989 |
| Anthrax | 1 | — | — | 1 | 2 | — | — | — |
| Aseptic meningitis | 8,326 | 10,619 | 11,374 | 11,487 | 7,234 | 10,274 | 11,852 | 14,526 |
| Botulism, total (includes wound and unspecified) | 123 | 122 | 109 | 82 | 84 | 89 | 92 | 114 |
| Foodborne | † | 49 | 23 | 17 | 28 | 23 | 23 | 27 |
| Infant | † | 70 | 79 | 59 | 50 | 60 | 65 | 81 |
| Brucellosis | 131 | 153 | 106 | 129 | 96 | 95 | 82 | 104 |
| Chancroid | 665 | 2,067 | 3,756 | 4,998 | 5,001 | 4,692 | 4,212 | 3,476 |
| Cholera | 1 | 4 | 23 | 6 | 8 | — | 6 | 26 |
| Diphtheria | 1 | 3 | — | 3 | 2 | 3 | 4 | 5 |
| Encephalitis, primary | 1,257 | 1,376 | 1,302 | 1,418 | 882 | 981 | 1,341 | 1,021 |
| Postinfectious[§] | 108 | 161 | 124 | 121 | 121 | 88 | 105 | 82 |
| Gonorrhea | 878,556 | 911,419 | 900,868 | 780,905 | 719,536 | 733,151 | 690,169 | 620,478 |
| Granuloma inguinale | 30 | 44 | 61 | 22 | 11 | 7 | 97 | 29 |
| Hansen disease (leprosy) | 290 | 361 | 270 | 238 | 184 | 163 | 198 | 154 |
| Hepatitis A | 22,040 | 23,210 | 23,430 | 25,280 | 28,507 | 35,821 | 31,441 | 24,378 |
| Hepatitis B | 26,115 | 26,611 | 26,107 | 25,916 | 23,177 | 23,419 | 21,102 | 18,003 |
| Hepatitis C; non-A, non-B | 3,871 | 4,184 | 3,634 | 2,999 | 2,619 | 2,529 | 2,553 | 3,582 |
| Hepatitis, unspecified | 5,531 | 5,517 | 3,940 | 3,102 | 2,470 | 2,306 | 1,671 | 1,260 |
| Legionellosis | 750 | 830 | 980 | 1,038 | 1,085 | 1,190 | 1,370 | 1,317 |
| Leptospirosis | 40 | 57 | 41 | 43 | 54 | 93 | 77 | 58 |
| Lymphogranuloma venereum | 170 | 226 | 396 | 303 | 185 | 189 | 277 | 471 |
| Malaria | 1,007 | 1,049 | 1,123 | 944 | 1,099 | 1,277 | 1,292 | 1,278 |
| Measles | 2,587 | 2,822 | 6,282 | 3,655 | 3,396 | 18,193 | 27,786 | 9,643 |
| Meningococcal disease | 2,746 | 2,479 | 2,594 | 2,930 | 2,964 | 2,727 | 2,451 | 2,130 |
| Mumps | 3,021 | 2,982 | 7,790 | 12,848 | 4,866 | 5,712 | 5,292 | 4,264 |
| Murine typhus fever | 53 | 37 | 67 | 49 | 54 | 41 | 50 | 43 |
| Pertussis (whooping cough) | 2,276 | 3,589 | 4,195 | 2,823 | 3,450 | 4,157 | 4,570 | 2,719 |

## Table A1.3. *(Continued)*

| Disease | 1984 | 1985 | 1986 | 1987 | 1988 | 1989 | 1990 | 1991 |
|---|---|---|---|---|---|---|---|---|
| Plague | 31 | 17 | 10 | 12 | 15 | 4 | 2 | 11 |
| Poliomyelitis, total | 9 | | | | ¶ | | | |
| Paralytic | 9 | 8 | 10 | 9 | 9 | 11 | 6 | 10 |
| Psittacosis | 172 | 119 | 224 | 98 | 114 | 116 | 113 | 94 |
| Rabies, animal | 5,567 | 5,565 | 5,504 | 4,658 | 4,651 | 4,724 | 4,826 | 6,910 |
| Rabies, human | 3 | 1 | - | 1 | - | 1 | 1 | 3 |
| Rheumatic fever, acute | 117 | 90 | 147 | 141 | 158 | 144 | 108 | 127 |
| Rocky Mountain spotted fever | 838 | 714 | 760 | 604 | 609 | 623 | 651 | 628 |
| Rubella | 752 | 630 | 551 | 306 | 225 | 396 | 1,125 | 1,401 |
| Rubella, congenital syndrome | 5 | - | 14 | 5 | 6 | 3 | 11 | 47 |
| Salmonellosis, excluding typhoid fever | 40,861 | 65,347 | 49,984 | 50,916 | 48,948 | 47,812 | 48,603 | 48,154 |
| Shigellosis | 17,371 | 17,057 | 17,138 | 23,860 | 30,617 | 25,010 | 27,077 | 23,548 |
| Syphilis, primary and secondary | 28,607 | 27,131 | 27,883 | 35,147 | 40,117 | 44,540 | 50,223 | 42,935 |
| Total, all stages | 69,888 | 67,563 | 68,215 | 86,545 | 103,437 | 110,797 | 134,255 | 128,569 |
| Tetanus | 74 | 83 | 64 | 48 | 53 | 53 | 64 | 57 |
| Toxic-shock syndrome | 482 | 384 | 412 | 372 | 390 | 400 | 322 | 280 |
| Trichinosis | 68 | 61 | 39 | 40 | 45 | 30 | 129 | 62 |
| Tuberculosis | 22,255 | 22,201 | 22,768 | 22,517 | 22,436 | 23,495 | 25,701 | 26,283 |
| Tularemia | 291 | 177 | 170 | 214 | 201 | 152 | 152 | 193 |
| Typhoid fever | 390 | 402 | 362 | 400 | 436 | 460 | 552 | 501 |
| Varicella (chickenpox) | 221,983 | 178,162 | 183,243 | 213,196 | 192,857 | 185,441 | 173,099 | 147,076 |
| Yellow fever | | | | ** | | | | |

* Acquired immunodeficiency syndrome (AIDS).

† Not reported as distinct categories during this period.

§ Beginning in 1984, data were recorded by date of report to state health departments. Before 1984, data were recorded by onset date.

¶ Categories other than paralytic are no longer reported.

** Last indigenous case of yellow fever reported in 1911; before 1996, the last imported case was reported in 1924.

Note: Data in the *MMWR Summary of Notifiable Diseases, United States* might not match data in other CDC surveillance reports because of differences in the timing of reports, the source of the data, and the use of different case definitions.

*Source*: Centers for Disease Control and Prevention. *Summary of Notifiable Diseases, United States, 1999. MMWR* 1999, 48, no. 53. http://www.cdc.gov/ mmwr/PDF/wk/mm4853.pdf.

## Table A1.4. Reported Cases of Notifiable Diseases, United States, 1976–1983

| Disease | 1976 | 1977 | 1978 | 1979 | 1980 | 1981 | 1982 | 1983 |
|---|---|---|---|---|---|---|---|---|
| Amebiasis | 2,906 | 3,044 | 3,937 | 4,107 | 5,271 | 6,632 | 7,304 | 6,658 |
| Anthrax | 2 | — | 6 | — | 1 | — | — | — |
| Aseptic meningitis | 3,510 | 4,789 | 6,573 | 8,754 | 8,028 | 9,547 | 9,680 | 12,696 |
| Botulism, total (includes wound and unspecified) | 55 | 129 | 105 | 45 | 89 | 103 | 97 | 133 |
| Brucellosis | 296 | 232 | 179 | 215 | 183 | 185 | 173 | 200 |
| Chancroid | 628 | 455 | 521 | 840 | 788 | 850 | 1,392 | 847 |
| Cholera | - | 3 | 12 | 1 | 9 | 19 | — | 1 |
| Diphtheria* | 128 | 84 | 76 | 59 | 3 | 5 | 2 | 5 |
| Encephalitis, primary | 1,651 | 1,414 | 1,351 | 1,504 | 1,362 | 1,492 | 1,464 | 1,761 |
| Postinfectious[†] | 175 | 119 | 78 | 84 | 40 | 43 | 36 | 34 |
| Gonorrhea | 1,001,994 | 1,002,219 | 1,013,436 | 1,004,058 | 1,004,029 | 990,864 | 960,633 | 900,435 |
| Granuloma inguinale | 71 | 75 | 72 | 76 | 51 | 66 | 17 | 24 |
| Hansen disease (leprosy) | 145 | 151 | 168 | 185 | 223 | 256 | 250 | 259 |
| Hepatitis A | 33,288 | 31,153 | 29,500 | 30,407 | 29,087 | 25,802 | 23,403 | 21,532 |
| Hepatitis B | 14,973 | 16,831 | 15,016 | 15,452 | 19,015 | 21,152 | 22,177 | 24,318 |
| Hepatitis, unspecified | 7,488 | 8,639 | 8,776 | 10,534 | 11,894 | 10,975 | 8,564 | 7,149 |
| Legionellosis | 235 | 359 | 761 | 593 | 475 | 408 | 654 | 852 |
| Leptospirosis | 73 | 71 | 110 | 94 | 85 | 82 | 100 | 61 |
| Lymphogranuloma venereum | 365 | 348 | 284 | 250 | 199 | 263 | 235 | 335 |
| Malaria | 471 | 547 | 731 | 894 | 2,062 | 1,388 | 1,056 | 813 |
| Measles | 41,126 | 57,345 | 26,871 | 13,597 | 13,506 | 3,124 | 1,714 | 1,497 |
| Meningococcal disease | 1,605 | 1,828 | 2,505 | 2,724 | 2,840 | 3,525 | 3,056 | 2,736 |
| Mumps | 38,492 | 21,436 | 16,817 | 14,225 | 8,576 | 4,941 | 5,270 | 3,355 |
| Murine typhus fever | 69 | 75 | 46 | 69 | 81 | 61 | 58 | 62 |
| Pertussis (whooping cough) | 1,010 | 2,177 | 2,063 | 1,623 | 1,730 | 1,248 | 1,898 | 2,463 |
| Plague | 16 | 18 | 12 | 13 | 18 | 13 | 19 | 40 |
| Poliomyelitis, total | 10 | 19 | 8 | 22 | 9 | 10 | 12 | 13 |
| Paralytic[§] | 10 | 19 | 8 | 22 | 9 | 10 | 12 | 13 |
| Psittacosis | 78 | 94 | 140 | 137 | 124 | 136 | 152 | 142 |
| Rabies, animal | 3,073 | 3,130 | 3,254 | 5,119 | 6,421 | 7,118 | 6,212 | 5,878 |
| Rabies, human | 2 | 1 | 4 | 4 | — | 2 | — | 2 |
| Rheumatic fever, acute | 1,865 | 1,738 | 851 | 629 | 432 | 264 | 137 | 88 |
| Rocky Mountain spotted fever | 937 | 1,153 | 1,063 | 1,070 | 1,163 | 1,192 | 976 | 1,126 |
| Rubella | 12,491 | 20,395 | 18,269 | 11,795 | 3,904 | 2,077 | 2,325 | 970 |
| Rubella, congenital syndrome | 30 | 23 | 30 | 62 | 50 | 19 | 7 | 22 |
| Salmonellosis, excluding typhoid fever | 22,937 | 27,850 | 29,410 | 33,138 | 33,715 | 39,990 | 40,936 | 44,250 |
| Shigellosis | 13,140 | 16,052 | 19,511 | 20,135 | 19,041 | 19,859 | 18,129 | 19,719 |
| Syphilis, primary and secondary | 23,731 | 20,399 | 21,656 | 24,874 | 27,204 | 31,266 | 33,613 | 32,698 |
| Total, all stages | 71,761 | 64,621 | 64,875 | 67,049 | 68,832 | 72,799 | 75,579 | 74,637 |
| Tetanus | 75 | 87 | 86 | 81 | 95 | 72 | 88 | 91 |
| Trichinosis | 115 | 143 | 67 | 157 | 131 | 206 | 115 | 45 |
| Tuberculosis | 32,105 | 30,145 | 28,521 | 27,669 | 27,749 | 27,373 | 25,520 | 23,846 |
| Tularemia | 157 | 165 | 141 | 196 | 234 | 288 | 275 | 310 |
| Typhoid fever | 419 | 398 | 505 | 528 | 510 | 584 | 425 | 507 |
| Varicella (chickenpox) | 183,990 | 188,396 | 154,089 | 199,081 | 190,894 | 200,766 | 167,423 | 177,462 |
| Yellow fever | | | | ¶ | | | | |

* Cutaneous diphtheria is no longer notifiable nationally after 1979.

[†]Beginning in 1984, data were recorded by date of report to state health departments. Before 1984, data were recorded by onset date.

[§]No cases with paralytic poliomyelitis caused by wild virus have been reported in the United States since 1979.

[¶]Last indigenous case of yellow fever reported in 1911; last imported case reported in 1999.

Note: Data in the *MMWR Summary of Notifiable Disease, United States* might not match data in other CDC surveillance reports because of differences in the timing of reports, the source of the data, and the use of different case definitions.

*Source*: Centers for Disease Control and Prevention. *Summary of Notifiable Diseases, United States, 1999. MMWR* 1999, 48, no. 53. http://www.cdc.gov/mmwr/PDF/wk/mm4853.pdf.

# Table A1.5. Reported Cases of Notifiable Diseases, United States, 1968–1975

| Disease | 1968 | 1969 | 1970 | 1971 | 1972 | 1973 | 1974 | 1975 |
|---|---|---|---|---|---|---|---|---|
| Amebiasis | 3,005 | 2,915 | 2,888 | 2,752 | 2,199 | 2,235 | 2,743 | 2,775 |
| Anthrax | 3 | 4 | 2 | 5 | 2 | 2 | 2 | 2 |
| Aseptic meningitis | 4,494 | 3,672 | 6,480 | 5,176 | 4,634 | 4,846 | 3,197 | 4,475 |
| Botulism | 7 | 16 | 12 | 25 | 22 | 34 | 28 | 20 |
| Brucellosis | 218 | 235 | 213 | 183 | 196 | 202 | 240 | 310 |
| Chancroid | 845 | 1,104 | 1,416 | 1,320 | 1,414 | 1,165 | 945 | 700 |
| Cholera | — | — | — | 1 | — | 1 | — | — |
| Diphtheria | 260 | 241 | 435 | 215 | 152 | 228 | 272 | 307 |
| Encephalitis, primary | 1,781 | 1,613 | 1,580 | 1,524 | 1,059 | 1,613 | 1,164 | 4,064 |
| Postinfectious | 502 | 304 | 370 | 439 | 243 | 354 | 218 | 237 |
| Gonorrhea | 464,543 | 534,872 | 600,072 | 670,268 | 767,215 | 842,621 | 906,121 | 999,937 |
| Granuloma inguinale | 156 | 154 | 124 | 89 | 81 | 62 | 47 | 60 |
| Hansen disease (leprosy) | 123 | 98 | 129 | 131 | 130 | 146 | 118 | 162 |
| Hepatitis A (infectious) | 45,893 | 48,416 | 56,797 | 59,606 | 54,074 | 50,749 | 40,358 | 35,855 |
| Hepatitis B (serum) | 4,829 | 5,909 | 8,310 | 9,556 | 9,402 | 8,451 | 10,631 | 13,121 |
| Hepatitis, unspecified | | | | * | | | | 7,158 |
| Leptospirosis | 69 | 89 | 47 | 62 | 41 | 57 | 8,351 | 93 |
| Lymphogranuloma venereum | 485 | 520 | 612 | 692 | 756 | 408 | 394 | 353 |
| Malaria | 2,317 | 3,102 | 3,051 | 2,375 | 742 | 237 | 293 | 373 |
| Measles | 22,231 | 25,826 | 47,351 | 75,290 | 32,275 | 26,690 | 22,094 | 24,374 |
| Meningococcal disease | 2,623 | 2,951 | 2,505 | 2,262 | 1,323 | 1,378 | 1,346 | 1,478 |
| Mumps | 152,209 | 90,918 | 104,953 | 124,939 | 74,215 | 69,612 | 59,128 | 59,647 |
| Murine typhus fever | 36 | 36 | 27 | 23 | 18 | 32 | 26 | 41 |
| Pertussis (whooping cough) | 4,810 | 3,285 | 4,249 | 3,036 | 3,287 | 1,759 | 2,402 | 1,738 |
| Plague | 3 | 5 | 13 | 2 | 1 | 2 | 8 | 20 |
| Poliomyelitis, total | 53 | 20 | 33 | 21 | 31 | 8 | 7 | 13 |
| Paralytic | 53 | 18 | 31 | 17 | 29 | 7 | 7 | 13 |
| Psittacosis | 43 | 57 | 35 | 32 | 52 | 33 | 164 | 49 |
| Rabies, animal | 3,591 | 3,490 | 3,224 | 4,310 | 4,369 | 3,640 | 3,151 | 2,627 |
| Rabies, human | 1 | 1 | 3 | 2 | 2 | 1 | — | 2 |
| Rheumatic fever, acute | 3,470 | 3,229 | 3,227 | 2,793 | 2,614 | 2,560 | 2,431 | 2,854 |
| Rocky Mountain spotted fever | 298 | 498 | 380 | 432 | 523 | 668 | 754 | 844 |
| Rubella | 49,371 | 57,686 | 56,552 | 45,086 | 25,507 | 27,804 | 11,917 | 16,652 |
| Rubella, congenital syndrome | 14 | 31 | 77 | 68 | 42 | 35 | 45 | 30 |
| Salmonellosis, excluding typhoid fever | 16,514 | 18,419 | 22,096 | 21,928 | 22,151 | 23,818 | 21,980 | 22,612 |
| Shigellosis | 12,180 | 11,946 | 13,845 | 16,143 | 20,207 | 22,642 | 22,600 | 16,584 |
| Streptococcal sore throat and scarlet fever | 435,013 | 450,008 | 433,405 | | | † | | |
| Syphilis, primary and secondary | 19,019 | 19,130 | 21,982 | 23,783 | 24,429 | 24,825 | 25,385 | 25,561 |
| Total, all stages | 96,271 | 92,162 | 91,382 | 95,997 | 91,149 | 87,469 | 83,771 | 80,356 |
| Tetanus | 178 | 192 | 148 | 116 | 128 | 101 | 101 | 102 |
| Trichinosis | 77 | 215 | 109 | 103 | 89 | 102 | 120 | 252 |
| Tuberculosis[§] | 42,623 | 39,120 | 37,137 | 35,217 | 32,882 | 30,998 | 30,122 | 33,989 |
| Tularemia | 186 | 149 | 172 | 187 | 152 | 171 | 144 | 129 |
| Typhoid fever | 395 | 364 | 346 | 407 | 398 | 680 | 437 | 375 |
| Varicella (chickenpox) | | | * | | 164,114 | 182,927 | 141,495 | 154,248 |
| Yellow fever | | | | | ¶ | | | |

* Not previously notifiable nationally.

[†]No longer notifiable nationally.

[§]Case data after 1974 are not comparable with earlier years because of changes in reporting criteria that became effective in 1975.

[¶]Last indigenous case of yellow fever reported in 1911; last imported case reported in 1999.

Note: Data in the *MMWR Summary of Notifiable Disease, United States* might not match data in other CDC surveillance reports because of differences in the timing of reports, the source of the data, and the use of different case definitions.

*Source*: Centers for Disease Control and Prevention. *Summary of Notifiable Diseases, United States, 1999. MMWR* 1999, 48, no. 53. http://www.cdc.gov/mmwr/PDF/wk/mm4853.pdf.

## Table A1.6. Deaths from Selected Notifiable Diseases, United States, 1989–1998

| Cause of Death | ICD* | 1989 | 1990 | 1991 | 1992 | 1993 | 1994 | 1995 | 1996 | 1997 | 1998 |
|---|---|---|---|---|---|---|---|---|---|---|---|
| AIDS† | *042–*044 | 22,082 | 25,188 | 29,555 | 33,566 | 37,267 | 42,114 | 43,115 | 31,130 | 16,516 | 13,426 |
| Anthrax | 022 | — | — | — | — | — | — | — | — | — | — |
| Botulism, foodborne | 005.1 | 2 | 4 | 2 | 1 | — | — | 2 | 1 | 2 | — |
| Brucellosis | 023 | — | — | — | — | 1 | — | 1 | — | 1 | 1 |
| Chancroid | 099.0 | — | — | 1 | — | — | — | — | — | — | — |
| Cholera | 001 | — | 2 | 2 | 2 | — | 1 | — | 2 | — | 1 |
| Diphtheria | 032 | — | 1 | — | 1 | — | — | 1 | — | — | 1 |
| Encephalitis, California serogroup viral | 062.5 | — | — | — | — | — | — | — | 1 | 1 | — |
| Encephalitis, Eastern equine | 062.2 | 1 | 1 | 1 | 1 | 1 | — | 1 | 1 | 2 | 1 |
| Encephalitis, St. Louis | 062.3 | — | 13 | 9 | 2 | 1 | 3 | 6 | — | 1 | — |
| Encephalitis, Western equine | 062.1 | — | — | — | — | — | — | — | — | — | 1 |
| Gonococcal infections | 098 | 4 | 3 | 3 | 4 | 5 | 3 | 3 | 4 | 3 | 4 |
| *Haemophilus influenzae*, invasive disease | 041.5 | 16 | 16 | 17 | 16 | 7 | 5 | 12 | 7 | 7 | 11 |
| Hansen disease (leprosy) | 030 | 4 | 3 | — | 2 | 1 | 3 | 2 | — | 2 | — |
| Hepatitis, viral, infectious (Hep A) | 070.0, 070.1 | 88 | 76 | 71 | 82 | 95 | 97 | 142 | 121 | 127 | 114 |
| Hepatitis, viral, serum (Hep B) | 070.2, 070.3 | 711 | 816 | 912 | 903 | 1,041 | 1,120 | 1,027 | 1,082 | 1,030 | 1,052 |
| Hepatitis, viral, other and unspecified | 070.4–070.9 | 717 | 686 | 857 | 1,016 | 1,353 | 1,844 | 2,231 | 2,577 | 2,900 | 3,630 |
| Malaria | 084 | 11 | 3 | 4 | 8 | 12 | 3 | 8 | 4 | 7 | 6 |
| Measles | 055 | 32 | 64 | 27 | 4 | — | — | 2 | 1 | 2 | — |
| Meningococcal disease | 036 | 273 | 215 | 198 | 201 | 260 | 276 | 273 | 290 | 309 | 234 |
| Mumps | 072 | 3 | 1 | 1 | — | — | — | — | 1 | — | 1 |
| Pertussis (whooping cough) | 033 | 12 | 12 | — | 5 | 7 | 8 | 6 | 4 | 6 | 5 |
| Plague | 020 | — | — | — | 1 | 2 | 2 | 1 | 2 | — | — |
| Poliomyelitis, total | 045.0–045.9 | — | — | 1 | — | — | — | 1 | — | — | — |
| Psittacosis | 073 | 1 | 2 | — | 4 | 1 | — | — | 1 | — | — |
| Rabies, human | 071 | 1 | 1 | 3 | 1 | 1 | 3 | 3 | 3 | 4 | 1 |
| Rubella | 056 | 4 | 8 | 1 | 1 | — | — | 1 | — | — | — |
| Salmonellosis, including paratyphoid fever | 002.1–002.9, 003 | 99 | 80 | 53 | 47 | 52 | 49 | 66 | 58 | 51 | 37 |
| Shigellosis | 004 | 16 | 10 | 10 | 8 | 5 | 13 | 8 | 5 | 5 | 5 |
| Spotted fevers | 082.0 | 10 | 20 | 13 | 13 | 5 | 9 | 8 | 6 | 12 | 3 |
| Syphilis | 090–097 | 105 | 106 | 93 | 91 | 80 | 79 | 65 | 73 | 62 | 45 |
| Tetanus | 037 | 9 | 11 | 11 | 9 | 11 | 9 | 5 | 1 | 4 | 7 |
| Trichinosis | 124 | 1 | — | — | — | — | — | — | — | — | — |
| Tuberculosis (all forms) | 010–018 | 1,970 | 1,810 | 1,713 | 1,705 | 1,631 | 1,478 | 1,336 | 1,202 | 1,166 | 1,112 |
| Typhoid fever | 002.0 | — | 1 | 1 | — | — | 1 | — | 1 | — | — |
| Varicella (chickenpox)§ | 052 | 89 | 120 | 81 | 100 | 100 | 124 | 115 | 81 | 99 | 81 |
| Yellow fever | 060 | — | — | — | — | — | — | — | 1 | — | — |

* *International Classification of Diseases, Ninth Revision, 1975.* Numbers in this column are *ICD-9* categories.

†Acquired immunodeficiency syndrome (AIDS). In 1987, the National Center for Health Statistics introduced categories *042-8044 for classifying and coding human immunodeficiency virus (HIV) infection. The asterisks are not footnote symbols, but indicate that these codes are not part of *ICD-9*.

§Varicella was taken off the nationally notifiable disease list in 1991. Many states continue to report these cases to CDC.

Note: Data in the annual *MMWR Summary of Notifiable Diseases, United States* might not match data in other CDC surveillance reports because of differences in the timing of reports, the source of the data, and the use of different case definitions.

*Source*: Centers for Disease Control and Prevention. *Summary of Notifiable Diseases, United States, 1999. MMWR* 1999, 48, no. 53. http://www.cdc.gov/mmwr/PDF/wk/mm4853.pdf.

## Table A2.1. Reported Cases of Notifiable Diseases,* by Month, United States, 1999

| Disease | Total | Jan. | Feb. | Mar. | Apr. | May | June | July | Aug. | Sept. | Oct. | Nov. | Dec. |
|---|---|---|---|---|---|---|---|---|---|---|---|---|---|
| AIDS[†] | 45,104 | 3,084 | 3,878 | 4,450 | 3,357 | 3,784 | 4,556 | 3,240 | 3,887 | 3,834 | 3,371 | 3,567 | 4,096 |
| Botulism, foodborne | 23 | — | 3 | 1 | 1 | 1 | 4 | 2 | 1 | 3 | 4 | 1 | 2 |
| Infant | 92 | 3 | 7 | 2 | 7 | 13 | 4 | 11 | 4 | 10 | 14 | 8 | 9 |
| Other (includes wound) | 39 | 4 | 1 | 3 | 1 | 1 | 4 | 3 | 5 | 1 | 2 | 4 | 10 |
| Brucellosis | 82 | 3 | 6 | 2 | 4 | 4 | 4 | 10 | 6 | 4 | 4 | 5 | 30 |
| Chancroid[§] | 143 | | 24 | | | 24 | | | 64 | | | 31 | |
| Chlamydia[§¶] | 656,721 | | 153,227 | | | 162,460 | | | 163,475 | | | 177,559 | |
| Cholera | 6 | — | — | — | — | 2 | — | 2 | — | 1 | — | — | 1 |
| Cryptosporidiosis | 2,361 | 55 | 113 | 102 | 146 | 163 | 179 | 198 | 211 | 361 | 342 | 181 | 310 |
| Cyclosporiasis | 56 | — | — | — | 4 | 6 | 5 | 10 | 17 | 5 | 1 | 1 | 7 |
| Diphtheria | 1 | — | — | — | — | — | — | — | — | — | — | — | 1 |
| Ehrlichiosis, human granulocytic | 203 | 1 | 3 | 5 | 10 | 12 | 38 | 33 | 17 | 18 | 9 | 10 | 47 |
| Human monocytic | 99 | 2 | 1 | 2 | 1 | — | 4 | 19 | 14 | 8 | 5 | 6 | 37 |
| Encephalitis, California serogroup viral | 70 | — | — | — | — | — | 1 | 2 | 19 | 14 | 24 | 6 | 4 |
| Eastern equine | 5 | — | — | — | — | — | 1 | 1 | — | 2 | — | — | 1 |
| St. Louis | 4 | — | — | — | — | — | — | — | — | — | 2 | 1 | 1 |
| Western equine | 1 | — | — | — | — | — | — | — | — | — | — | 1 | — |
| *Escherichia coli* 0157:H7 | 4,513 | 78 | 77 | 91 | 88 | 167 | 216 | 493 | 509 | 889 | 532 | 325 | 1,048 |
| Gonorrhea[§] | 360,076 | | 80,692 | | | 84,600 | | | 96,231 | | | 98,553 | |
| *Haemophilus influenzae*, invasive disease | 1,309 | 77 | 109 | 103 | 90 | 121 | 97 | 138 | 75 | 76 | 101 | 83 | 239 |
| Hansen disease (leprosy) | 108 | 6 | 7 | 7 | 4 | 20 | 6 | 8 | 10 | 12 | 13 | 4 | 11 |
| Hantavirus pulmonary syndrome** | 33 | 1 | 3 | 5 | 5 | 5 | 6 | 3 | 1 | 2 | 1 | — | 1 |
| Hemolytic uremic syndrome, postdiarrheal | 181 | 3 | 5 | 4 | 2 | 9 | 14 | 19 | 21 | 14 | 16 | 12 | 62 |
| Hepatitis A | 17,047 | 1,060 | 1,446 | 1,316 | 1,365 | 1,635 | 1,184 | 1,426 | 1,194 | 1,385 | 1,537 | 1,298 | 2,201 |
| Hepatitis B | 7,694 | 337 | 418 | 604 | 573 | 747 | 610 | 679 | 601 | 558 | 605 | 536 | 1,426 |
| Hepatitis C; non-A, non-B | 3,111 | 114 | 174 | 170 | 216 | 295 | 257 | 337 | 197 | 253 | 350 | 270 | 478 |
| Legionellosis | 1,108 | 48 | 87 | 66 | 64 | 68 | 78 | 98 | 76 | 106 | 142 | 91 | 184 |
| Lyme disease | 16,273 | 253 | 332 | 375 | 433 | 752 | 1,306 | 3,394 | 2,291 | 2,026 | 1,960 | 1,249 | 1,902 |
| Malaria | 1,666 | 79 | 101 | 81 | 70 | 117 | 117 | 184 | 159 | 141 | 170 | 100 | 347 |
| Measles | 100 | 12 | 6 | 8 | 14 | 15 | 2 | 6 | 3 | 4 | 15 | 7 | 8 |
| Meningococcal disease | 2,501 | 156 | 233 | 300 | 216 | 266 | 189 | 205 | 125 | 135 | 189 | 122 | 365 |
| Mumps | 387 | 22 | 36 | 42 | 25 | 38 | 28 | 39 | 16 | 22 | 38 | 24 | 57 |
| Pertussis (whooping cough) | 7,288 | 305 | 322 | 625 | 651 | 495 | 422 | 527 | 548 | 628 | 730 | 630 | 1,405 |
| Plague | 9 | — | — | — | — | — | 2 | — | 1 | 3 | — | 2 | 1 |
| Psittacosis | 16 | 3 | 1 | 2 | 3 | — | — | 1 | 1 | — | 2 | 1 | 2 |
| Rabies, animal | 6,730 | 298 | 421 | 479 | 540 | 746 | 505 | 661 | 590 | 660 | 753 | 474 | 603 |
| Rocky Mountain spotted fever | 579 | 10 | 9 | 7 | 13 | 30 | 53 | 125 | 118 | 67 | 59 | 43 | 45 |
| Rubella, congenital syndrome | 9 | — | — | 1 | 1 | — | 2 | — | — | 1 | 3 | 1 | — |
| Rubella | 267 | — | 2 | 5 | 17 | 46 | 72 | 35 | 39 | 15 | 6 | 3 | 27 |
| Salmonellosis | 40,596 | 1,702 | 1,814 | 1,788 | 2,009 | 3,173 | 3,253 | 5,222 | 4,177 | 4,152 | 5,024 | 3,259 | 5,023 |
| Shigellosis | 17,521 | 930 | 942 | 858 | 809 | 1,383 | 1,293 | 1,757 | 1,720 | 1,850 | 2,051 | 1,487 | 2,441 |
| Streptococcal disease, invasive, group A | 2,382 | 107 | 169 | 211 | 218 | 294 | 154 | 219 | 113 | 119 | 184 | 171 | 423 |
| *Streptococcus pneumoniae*, drug-resistant, invasive disease | 4,618 | 114 | 194 | 315 | 281 | 734 | 211 | 333 | 194 | 136 | 250 | 211 | 1,645 |
| Streptococcal toxic-shock syndrome | 61 | 1 | 8 | 12 | 8 | 11 | 4 | 2 | — | 1 | 3 | 1 | 10 |
| Syphilis, congenital (age <1 yr)[§] | 556 | | 156 | | | 124 | | | 142 | | | 134 | |
| Primary and secondary[§] | 6,657 | | 1,561 | | | 1,600 | | | 1,778 | | | 1,718 | |
| Total (all stages)[§] | 35,628 | | 9,184 | | | 8,956 | | | 8,487 | | | 9,001 | |
| Tetanus | 40 | 3 | 2 | 2 | 2 | 4 | 1 | 2 | 4 | 6 | 4 | 3 | 7 |
| Toxic-shock syndrome | 113 | 8 | 12 | 8 | 7 | 10 | 7 | 10 | 10 | 3 | 12 | 8 | 18 |
| Trichinosis | 12 | 3 | — | 1 | 2 | 1 | 1 | — | 1 | — | — | — | 3 |
| Tuberculosis[††] | 17,531 | 613 | 952 | 1,376 | 1,529 | 1,197 | 1,662 | 1,602 | 1,507 | 1,399 | 1,454 | 1,160 | 3,080 |
| Typhoid fever | 346 | 12 | 21 | 34 | 25 | 26 | 24 | 42 | 25 | 35 | 34 | 24 | 44 |
| Varicella (chickenpox) | 46,016 | 4,404 | 4,598 | 5,435 | 3,592 | 6,949 | 2,664 | 1,070 | 2,498 | 980 | 3,036 | 3,303 | 7,487 |
| Yellow fever | 1 | — | — | — | — | — | — | — | — | — | — | 1 | — |

* No cases of anthrax, paralytic poliomyelitis, or human rabies were reported in 1999.

[†]Total number of acquired immunodeficiency syndrome (AIDS) cases reported to the Division of HIV/AIDS Prevention—Surveillance and Epidemiology, National center for HIV, STD, and TB Prevention (NCHSTP), through December 31, 1999.

[§]Totals reported to the Division of Sexually Transmitted Diseases Prevention, NCHSTP, as of August 8, 2000.

[¶]chlamydia refers to genital infections caused by *C. trachomatis.*

** Totals reported to the National Center for Infectious Diseases as of June 30, 2000.

[††]Totals reported to the Division of Tuberculosis Elimination, NCHSTP, as of May 3, 2000.

*Source*: Centers for Disease Control and Prevention. *Summary of Notifiable Diseases, United States, 1999. MMWR* 1999, 48, no. 53. http://www.cdc.gov/mmwr/PDF/wk/mm4853.pdf.

## Table A2.2. Reported Cases of Notifiable Diseases,* by Geographic Division and Area, United States, 1999

| Area | Total resident population (in thousands) | AIDS† | Botulism | | | Brucellosis | Chancroid¶ |
|---|---|---|---|---|---|---|---|
| | | | Foodborne | Infant | Other§ | | |
| **United States** | **272,692** | **45,104**** | **23** | **92** | **39** | **82** | **143** |
| **New England** | **13,496** | **2,293** | **—** | **1** | **1** | **3** | **2** |
| Maine | 1,253 | 80 | — | — | — | — | — |
| N.H. | 1,201 | 46 | — | 1 | — | — | NN |
| Vt. | 594 | 20 | — | — | — | — | NN |
| Mass. | 6,175 | 1,454 | — | — | 1 | 2 | 1 |
| R.I. | 991 | 107 | — | — | — | — | 1 |
| Conn. | 3,282 | 586 | — | — | — | 1 | — |
| **Mid. Atlantic** | **38,334** | **11,713** | **1** | **24** | **—** | **2** | **39** |
| Upstate N.Y. | 10,827 | 1,690 | 1 | — | — | 2 | — |
| N.Y. City | 7,370 | 6,013 | — | 1 | — | — | 39 |
| N.J. | 8,143 | 2,043 | — | 14 | — | — | — |
| Pa. | 11,994 | 1,967 | — | 9 | — | — | — |
| **E.N. Central** | **44,442** | **3,268** | **1** | **2** | **—** | **14** | **4** |
| Ohio | 11,257 | 547 | — | 1 | — | — | — |
| Ind. | 5,943 | 363 | 1 | — | — | 1 | — |
| Ill. | 12,128 | 1,557 | — | — | — | 10 | NN |
| Mich. | 9,864 | 649 | — | — | — | 2 | — |
| Wis. | 5,250 | 152 | — | 1 | — | 1 | 4 |
| **W.N. Central** | **18,800** | **1,069** | **1** | **5** | **1** | **7** | **1** |
| Minn. | 4,776 | 190 | — | — | — | — | 1 |
| Iowa | 2,869 | 87 | 1 | NN | — | 6 | — |
| Mo. | 5,468 | 531 | — | 2 | — | 1 | — |
| N. Dak. | 634 | 7 | — | 1 | 1 | — | NN |
| S. Dak. | 733 | 16 | — | 1 | — | — | — |
| Nebr. | 1,666 | 67 | — | 1 | — | — | — |
| Kans. | 2,654 | 171 | — | — | — | — | — |
| **S. Atlantic** | **49,561** | **12,460** | **4** | **10** | **—** | **3** | **62** |
| Del. | 754 | 186 | — | — | — | — | — |
| Md. | 5,172 | 1,525 | — | 3 | — | — | — |
| D.C. | 519 | 838 | — | — | — | — | — |
| Va. | 6,873 | 943 | — | 3 | — | — | 3 |
| W. Va. | 1,807 | 69 | — | — | — | — | — |
| N.C. | 7,651 | 794 | — | 2 | — | — | 7 |
| S.C. | 3,886 | 959 | — | — | — | NN | 48 |
| Ga. | 7,788 | 1,678 | — | 2 | — | — | 1 |
| Fla. | 15,111 | 5,468 | 4 | — | — | 3 | 3 |
| **E.S. Central** | **16,584** | **1,933** | **2** | **5** | **—** | **2** | **1** |
| Ky. | 3,961 | 277 | — | 3 | — | — | — |
| Tenn. | 5,484 | 759 | 2 | 2 | — | — | — |
| Ala. | 4,370 | 476 | — | — | — | 2 | 1 |
| Miss. | 2,769 | 421 | — | — | — | — | — |
| **W.S. Central** | **30,325** | **4,377** | **—** | **6** | **—** | **25** | **25** |
| Ark. | 2,551 | 194 | — | — | — | 2 | — |
| La. | 4,372 | 854 | — | 1 | — | — | 9 |
| Okla. | 3,358 | 148 | — | 1 | — | — | — |
| Tex. | 20,044 | 3,181 | — | 4 | — | 23 | 16 |
| **Mountain** | **17,128** | **1,742** | **—** | **10** | **1** | **6** | **1** |
| Mont. | 883 | 13 | — | 1 | — | — | — |
| Idaho | 1,252 | 25 | — | 1 | — | — | — |
| Wyo. | 480 | 15 | — | — | — | — | 1 |
| Colo. | 4,056 | 319 | — | 2 | 1 | 4 | — |
| N. Mex. | 1,740 | 93 | — | 1 | — | 1 | — |
| Ariz. | 4,778 | 880 | — | — | — | 1 | — |
| Utah | 2,130 | 155 | — | 4 | — | — | — |
| Nev. | 1,809 | 242 | — | 1 | — | — | — |
| **Pacific** | **44,022** | **6,145** | **14** | **29** | **36** | **20** | **8** |
| Wash. | 5,756 | 360 | 7 | — | — | — | — |
| Oreg. | 3,316 | 225 | — | 3 | 1 | — | 1 |
| Calif. | 33,145 | 5,445 | 4 | 26 | 35 | 18 | 7 |
| Alaska | 620 | 15 | 3 | — | — | — | — |
| Hawaii | 1,185 | 100 | — | — | — | 2 | NN |
| Guam | 149 | 10 | — | — | — | — | — |
| P.R. | 3,890 | 1,247 | — | — | — | — | 1 |
| V.I. | 118 | 39 | NN | NN | NA | NN | — |
| American Samoa | 62 | — | NA | NA | NA | NA | NA |
| C.N.M.I. | 67 | — | NA | NA | NA | NA | NA |

* No cases of anthrax were reported in 1999.

†Total number of acquired immunodeficiency syndrome (AIDS) cases reported to the Division of HIV/AIDS Prevention—Surveillance and Epidemiology, National center for HIV, STD, and TB Prevention (NCHSTP), through December 31, 1999.

§Includes cases reported as wound or unspecified botulism.

¶Totals reported to the Division of Sexually Transmitted Diseases Prevention, NCHSTP, as of August 8, 2000.

** Total includes 104 cases among persons with unknown state of residence.

*Source:* Centers for Disease Control and Prevention. Summary of Notifiable Diseases, United States, 1999. *MMWR* 1999, 48, no. 53. http://www.cde.gov/mmwr/PDF/wk/mm4853.pdf.

## Table A2.2. *(Continued)*

| Area | Chlamydia* | Cholera | Cryptosporidiosis | Cyclosporiasis | Diphtheria | Ehrlichiosis | |
|---|---|---|---|---|---|---|---|
| | | | | | | Human granulocytic | Human monocytic |
| **United States** | **656,721** | **6** | **2,361** | **56** | **1** | **203** | **99** |
| **New England** | **21,224** | **—** | **186** | **7** | **—** | **90** | **—** |
| Maine | 1,220 | — | 31 | — | — | — | — |
| N.H. | 976 | — | 20 | — | — | 1 | — |
| Vt. | 485 | — | 36 | NN | — | NN | NN |
| Mass. | 8,776 | — | 71 | 7 | — | 9 | — |
| R.I. | 2,345 | — | 6 | — | — | 7 | — |
| Conn. | 7,422 | — | 22 | — | — | 73 | — |
| **Mid. Atlantic** | **66,209** | **1** | **629** | **18** | **—** | **87** | **—** |
| Upstate N.Y. | NN | — | 192 | — | — | 75 | — |
| N.Y. City | 26,766 | — | 260 | 18 | — | 2 | — |
| N.J. | 12,424 | 1 | 54 | — | — | — | — |
| Pa. | 27,019 | — | 123 | — | — | 10 | — |
| **E.N. Central** | **111,571** | **—** | **256** | **1** | **—** | **—** | **—** |
| Ohio | 29,398 | — | 67 | 1 | — | — | — |
| Ind. | 11,734 | — | 47 | NN | — | NN | NN |
| Ill. | 32,870 | — | 90 | — | — | NN | NN |
| Mich. | 23,107 | — | 52 | — | — | - | — |
| Wis. | 14,462 | — | NN | NN | — | NN | NN |
| **W.N. Central** | **38,516** | **—** | **217** | **—** | **—** | **4** | **53** |
| Minn. | 7,450 | — | 91 | — | — | — | — |
| Iowa | 5,511 | — | 56 | — | — | — | — |
| Mo. | 13,355 | — | 26 | — | — | 3 | 53 |
| N. Dak. | 947 | — | 20 | — | — | — | — |
| S. Dak. | 1,544 | — | 7 | — | — | — | — |
| Nebr. | 3,616 | — | 15 | — | — | — | — |
| Kans. | 6,093 | — | 2 | — | — | 1 | — |
| **S. Atlantic** | **134,306** | **1** | **452** | **28** | **—** | **—** | **21** |
| Del. | 2,761 | — | 1 | — | — | — | — |
| Md. | 13,568 | — | 17 | NN | — | NN | NN |
| D.C. | NN | — | 7 | 5 | — | NN | NN |
| Va. | 13,735 | — | 30 | — | — | — | — |
| W. Va. | 1,820 | — | 3 | 3 | — | — | — |
| N.C. | 21,812 | — | 35 | — | — | — | 12 |
| S.C. | 18,499 | — | — | — | — | — | — |
| Ga. | 30,368 | 1 | 170 | 10 | — | — | 1 |
| Fla. | 31,743 | — | 189 | 10 | — | — | 8 |
| **E.S. Central** | **45,514** | **—** | **48** | **—** | **—** | **21** | **—** |
| Ky. | 7,378 | — | 7 | — | — | — | — |
| Tenn. | 14,216 | — | 13 | — | — | 21 | — |
| Ala. | 12,375 | — | 16 | — | — | NN | NN |
| Miss. | 11,545 | — | 12 | — | — | NN | NN |
| **W.S. Central** | **93,653** | **—** | **95** | **—** | **—** | **—** | **23** |
| Ark. | 5,865 | — | 2 | — | — | — | 22 |
| La. | 16,635 | — | 24 | — | — | NN | NN |
| Okla. | 8,195 | — | NN | NN | — | NN | NN |
| Tex. | 62,958 | — | 69 | — | — | — | 1 |
| **Mountain** | **37,430** | **2** | **101** | **2** | **—** | **—** | **1** |
| Mont. | 1,584 | — | 13 | — | — | NN | NN |
| Idaho | 1,778 | — | NN | NN | — | NN | NN |
| Wyo. | 787 | — | 1 | — | — | — | — |
| Colo. | 10,848 | — | 14 | 2 | — | — | — |
| N. Mex. | 5,017 | — | 44 | — | — | NN | NN |
| Ariz. | 12,111 | 2 | 16 | — | — | — | — |
| Utah | 2,219 | — | 4 | — | — | — | 1 |
| Nev. | 3,086 | — | 9 | — | — | NN | NN |
| **Pacific** | **108,298** | **2** | **377** | **—** | **1** | **1** | **1** |
| Wash. | 11,964 | — | NN | — | 1 | NN | NN |
| Oreg. | 6,127 | — | 98 | — | — | NN | NN |
| Calif. | 85,156 | 1 | 279 | — | — | 1 | 1 |
| Alaska | 1,886 | — | — | — | — | NN | NN |
| Hawaii | 3,165 | 1 | — | — | — | NN | NN |
| Guam | 497 | — | — | — | — | — | — |
| P.R. | 1,445 | — | — | — | — | — | — |
| V.I. | 136 | NA | NA | NA | NA | NA | NA |
| American Samoa | NA | NA | NA | NA | NA | NA | NA |
| C.N.M.I. | NA | NA | NA | NA | NA | NA | NA |

* Chlamydia refers to genital infections caused by *C. trachomatis.* Totals reported to the Division of Sexually Transmitted Diseases Prevention, NCHSTP, as of August 8, 2000.

## Table A2.2. *(Continued)*

| Area | Encephalitis: California serogroup viral | Encephalitis: Eastern equine | Encephalitis: St. Louis | Encephalitis: Western equine | *Escherichia coli* O157:H7: NETSS* | *Escherichia coli* O157:H7: PHLIS† | Gonorrhea§ |
|---|---|---|---|---|---|---|---|
| **United States** | **70** | **5** | **4** | **1** | **4,513** | **2,809** | **360,076** |
| **New England** | **—** | **—** | **—** | **—** | **404** | **366** | **6,625** |
| Maine | — | — | — | — | 40 | NA | 83 |
| N.H. | — | — | — | — | 36 | 34 | 115 |
| Vt. | — | — | — | — | 32 | 21 | 52 |
| Mass. | — | — | — | — | 177 | 188 | 2,453 |
| R.I. | — | — | — | — | 27 | 26 | 601 |
| Conn. | — | — | — | — | 92 | 97 | 3,321 |
| **Mid. Atlantic** | **—** | **—** | **—** | **—** | **1,034** | **239** | **40,973** |
| Upstate N.Y. | — | — | — | — | 939 | 18 | 7,616 |
| N.Y. City | — | — | — | — | 17 | 18 | 12,210 |
| N.J. | — | — | — | — | 78 | 144 | 7,852 |
| Pa. | — | — | — | — | NN | 59 | 13,295 |
| **E.N. Central** | **31** | **—** | **—** | **—** | **994** | **532** | **70,056** |
| Ohio | 14 | — | — | — | 262 | 219 | 18,141 |
| Ind. | — | — | — | — | 107 | 67 | 6,092 |
| Ill. | 3 | — | — | — | 498 | 92 | 23,254 |
| Mich. | 1 | — | — | — | 127 | 85 | 15,907 |
| Wis. | 13 | — | — | — | NN | 69 | 6,662 |
| **W.N. Central** | **6** | **—** | **—** | **1** | **595** | **550** | **16,793** |
| Minn. | 6 | — | — | 1 | 175 | 187 | 2,830 |
| Iowa | — | — | — | — | 114 | 82 | 1,365 |
| Mo. | — | — | — | — | 47 | 71 | 8,187 |
| N. Dak. | — | — | — | — | 19 | 19 | 83 |
| S. Dak. | — | — | — | — | 47 | 62 | 192 |
| Nebr. | — | — | — | — | 159 | 113 | 1,471 |
| Kans. | — | — | — | — | 34 | 16 | 2,665 |
| **S. Atlantic** | **26** | **3** | **4** | **—** | **357** | **190** | **104,262** |
| Del. | — | — | — | — | 6 | 3 | 1,662 |
| Md. | — | NN | — | — | 43 | 4 | 10,430 |
| D.C. | — | — | — | — | 1 | NA | 3,536 |
| Va. | — | — | — | — | 79 | 63 | 9,402 |
| W. Va. | 16 | — | — | — | 16 | 11 | 584 |
| N.C. | 10 | — | — | — | 74 | 53 | 19,428 |
| S.C. | — | — | — | — | 22 | 14 | 15,037 |
| Ga. | — | — | — | — | 43 | 3 | 21,244 |
| Fla. | — | 3 | 4 | — | 73 | 39 | 22,939 |
| **E.S. Central** | **7** | **—** | **—** | **—** | **142** | **106** | **36,014** |
| Ky. | 1 | — | — | — | 50 | 35 | 3,349 |
| Tenn. | 6 | — | — | — | 55 | 45 | 11,366 |
| Ala. | — | — | — | — | 28 | 21 | 10,888 |
| Miss. | — | — | — | — | 9 | 5 | 10,411 |
| **W.S. Central** | **—** | **2** | **—** | **—** | **174** | **174** | **53,346** |
| Ark. | — | — | — | — | 15 | 14 | 3,226 |
| La. | — | 2 | — | — | 14 | 15 | 13,189 |
| Okla. | — | — | — | — | 40 | 30 | 4,021 |
| Tex. | — | — | — | — | 105 | 115 | 32,910 |
| **Mountain** | **—** | **—** | **—** | **—** | **346** | **245** | **9,535** |
| Mont. | — | — | — | — | 25 | NA | 53 |
| Idaho | — | — | — | — | 78 | 43 | 89 |
| Wyo. | — | — | — | — | 17 | 17 | 43 |
| Colo. | — | — | — | — | 115 | 89 | 2,526 |
| N. Mex. | — | — | — | — | 13 | 7 | 974 |
| Ariz. | — | — | — | — | 37 | 24 | 4,293 |
| Utah | — | — | — | — | 36 | 50 | 254 |
| Nev. | — | — | — | — | 25 | 15 | 1,303 |
| **Pacific** | **—** | **—** | **—** | **—** | **467** | **407** | **22,472** |
| Wash. | NN | NN | — | — | 186 | 185 | 2,132 |
| Oreg. | NN | NN | NN | NN | 68 | 69 | 903 |
| Calif. | — | — | — | — | 197 | 140 | 18,672 |
| Alaska | NN | NN | NN | NN | 1 | 1 | 302 |
| Hawaii | — | — | — | NN | 15 | 12 | 463 |
| Guam | — | — | — | — | NN | NA | 59 |
| P.R. | — | — | — | — | 9 | NA | 321 |
| V.I. | NA | NA | NA | NA | NA | NA | 51 |
| American Samoa | NA | NA | NA | NA | NN | NA | NA |
| C.N.M.I. | NA | NA | NA | NA | NN | NA | NA |

* National Electronic Telecommunications System for Surveillance.

†Public Health Laboratory Information System. Totals reported to the National Center for Infectious Diseases as of July 18, 2000.

§Totals reported to the Division of Sexually Transmitted Diseases Prevention, NCHSTP, as of August 8, 2000.

## Table A2.2. *(Continued)*

| Area | *Haemophilus influenzae,* invasive disease | Hansen disease (leprosy) | Hantavirus pulmonary syndrome* | Hemolytic uremic syndrome, postdiarrheal | Hepatitis A | Hepatitis B | Hepatitis C; non-A, non-B | Legionellosis |
|---|---|---|---|---|---|---|---|---|
| **United States** | **1,309** | **108** | **33** | **181** | **17,047** | **7,694** | **3,111** | **1,108** |
| **New England** | **117** | **1** | **—** | **12** | **373** | **153** | **16** | **91** |
| Maine | 8 | — | — | — | 27 | 3 | 2 | 3 |
| N.H. | 19 | — | — | — | 18 | 17 | NN | 10 |
| Vt. | 6 | NN | — | 1 | 24 | 5 | 7 | 15 |
| Mass. | 41 | 1 | — | — | 142 | 44 | 4 | 27 |
| R.I. | 9 | — | — | 1 | 35 | 43 | 3 | 20 |
| Conn. | 34 | — | — | 10 | 127 | 41 | — | 16 |
| **Mid. Atlantic** | **210** | **12** | **2** | **38** | **1,211** | **922** | **136** | **273** |
| Upstate N.Y. | 86 | — | — | 25 | 293 | 200 | 68 | 74 |
| N.Y. City | 57 | 9 | — | 7 | 403 | 293 | — | 44 |
| N.J. | 59 | 2 | — | 6 | 151 | 138 | — | 24 |
| Pa. | 8 | 1 | 2 | — | 364 | 291 | 68 | 131 |
| **E.N. Central** | **212** | **2** | **1** | **12** | **2,940** | **913** | **893** | **279** |
| Ohio | 63 | 2 | — | 12 | 655 | 95 | 4 | 85 |
| Ind. | 32 | NN | 1 | NN | 105 | 77 | 3 | 52 |
| Ill. | 89 | — | NN | NN | 849 | 202 | 48 | 33 |
| Mich. | 20 | — | — | — | 1,253 | 509 | 822 | 64 |
| Wis. | 8 | — | — | NN | 78 | 30 | 16 | 45 |
| **W.N. Central** | **92** | **1** | **4** | **23** | **1,133** | **393** | **344** | **71** |
| Minn. | 57 | — | — | 13 | 128 | 80 | 25 | 18 |
| Iowa | 2 | — | 2 | — | 161 | 44 | — | 17 |
| Mo. | 14 | — | — | 6 | 712 | 227 | 315 | 22 |
| N. Dak. | 2 | NN | — | — | 3 | 2 | 1 | 2 |
| S. Dak. | 4 | — | — | 4 | 10 | 1 | — | 6 |
| Nebr. | 5 | — | NN | NN | 53 | 22 | 3 | 6 |
| Kans. | 8 | 1 | 2 | — | 66 | 17 | — | — |
| **S. Atlantic** | **289** | **4** | **—** | **25** | **2,151** | **1,412** | **184** | **165** |
| Del. | 1 | — | — | — | 2 | 1 | — | 21 |
| Md. | 71 | 1 | NN | NN | 306 | 148 | 22 | 37 |
| D.C. | 5 | — | — | — | 59 | 25 | 1 | 5 |
| Va. | 24 | — | NN | 3 | 185 | 106 | 11 | 41 |
| W. Va. | 8 | — | — | — | 47 | 29 | 21 | NN |
| N.C. | 36 | — | NN | 10 | 167 | 224 | 33 | 15 |
| S.C. | 6 | — | — | — | 48 | 64 | 22 | 12 |
| Ga. | 80 | NN | — | 4 | 482 | 230 | 4 | 5 |
| Fla. | 58 | 3 | — | 8 | 855 | 585 | 70 | 29 |
| **E.S. Central** | **72** | **—** | **—** | **10** | **404** | **473** | **348** | **53** |
| Ky. | 9 | — | — | NN | 67 | 50 | 28 | 22 |
| Tenn. | 40 | — | — | 8 | 147 | 207 | 123 | 24 |
| Ala. | 18 | — | NN | 2 | 62 | 86 | 1 | 5 |
| Miss. | 5 | — | NN | — | 128 | 130 | 196 | 2 |
| **W.S. Central** | **68** | **24** | **1** | **19** | **3,343** | **1,319** | **713** | **41** |
| Ark. | 2 | — | — | — | 81 | 98 | 31 | 1 |
| La. | 15 | 3 | — | — | 213 | 172 | 302 | 11 |
| Okla. | 47 | 1 | — | 1 | 533 | 185 | 18 | 7 |
| Tex. | 4 | 20 | 1 | 18 | 2,516 | 864 | 362 | 22 |
| **Mountain** | **117** | **3** | **14** | **9** | **1,258** | **614** | **237** | **49** |
| Mont. | 3 | — | 2 | — | 18 | 21 | 5 | — |
| Idaho | 2 | — | 2 | 2 | 47 | 29 | 8 | 3 |
| Wyo. | 1 | — | 1 | 1 | 9 | 14 | 88 | — |
| Colo. | 15 | 1 | 2 | 2 | 219 | 99 | 37 | 14 |
| N. Mex. | 19 | — | 4 | 1 | 55 | 215 | 34 | 1 |
| Ariz. | 63 | — | 2 | NN | 700 | 138 | 49 | 7 |
| Utah | 10 | — | — | 1 | 64 | 39 | 6 | 18 |
| Nev. | 4 | 2 | 1 | 2 | 146 | 59 | 10 | 6 |
| **Pacific** | **132** | **61** | **11** | **33** | **4,234** | **1,495** | **240** | **86** |
| Wash. | 9 | 1 | 5 | NN | 505 | 111 | 24 | 22 |
| Oreg. | 45 | 2 | NN | 4 | 251 | 116 | 23 | NN |
| Calif. | 54 | 35 | 6 | 29 | 3,439 | 1,234 | 193 | 62 |
| Alaska | 9 | 1 | — | — | 15 | 18 | — | 1 |
| Hawaii | 15 | 22 | — | — | 24 | 16 | — | 1 |
| Guam | — | 1 | — | — | 1 | 4 | 2 | — |
| P.R. | 2 | 5 | — | — | 417 | 307 | — | — |
| V.I. | NA | NA | — | NA | NA | NA | NA | NA |
| American Samoa | NA | NA | — | NA | NA | NA | NA | NA |
| C.N.M.I. | NA | NA | - | NA | NA | NA | NA | NA |

* Totals reported to the National Center for Infectious Diseases as of June 30, 2000.

## Table A2.2. *(Continued)*

| Area | Lyme disease | Malaria | Measles | | Meningo-coccal disease | Mumps | Pertussis | Plague |
|---|---|---|---|---|---|---|---|---|
| | | | Indigenous | Imported* | | | | |
| **United States** | **16,273** | **1,666** | **66** | **34** | **2,501** | **387** | **7,288** | **9** |
| **New England** | **4,642** | **70** | **5** | **6** | **115** | **9** | **978** | **—** |
| Maine | 41 | 3 | — | — | 5 | — | 33 | — |
| N.H. | 27 | 2 | — | 1 | 13 | 2 | 116 | — |
| Vt. | 26 | 5 | — | — | 5 | 1 | 96 | — |
| Mass. | 787 | 22 | 4 | 4 | 66 | 4 | 649 | — |
| R.I. | 546 | 8 | — | — | 9 | 2 | 49 | — |
| Conn. | 3,215 | 30 | 1 | 1 | 17 | — | 35 | — |
| **Mid. Atlantic** | **8,902** | **431** | **—** | **5** | **237** | **46** | **1,319** | **—** |
| Upstate N.Y. | 4,266 | 78 | — | 2 | 80 | 14 | 1,020 | — |
| N.Y. City | 136 | 251 | — | 3 | 57 | 12 | 61 | — |
| N.J. | 1,719 | 57 | — | — | 52 | 1 | 19 | — |
| Pa. | 2,781 | 45 | — | — | 48 | 19 | 219 | — |
| **E.N. Central** | **586** | **169** | **5** | **5** | **423** | **56** | **743** | **—** |
| Ohio | 47 | 18 | — | — | 134 | 21 | 322 | — |
| Ind. | 21 | 22 | 1 | 1 | 76 | 5 | 90 | — |
| Ill. | 17 | 77 | — | 2 | 111 | 16 | 140 | — |
| Mich. | 11 | 42 | 4 | 2 | 64 | 10 | 74 | — |
| Wis. | 490 | 10 | — | — | 38 | 4 | 117 | — |
| **W.N. Central** | **407** | **104** | **—** | **1** | **243** | **16** | **571** | **—** |
| Minn. | 283 | 71 | — | 1 | 56 | 1 | 281 | — |
| Iowa | 24 | 13 | — | — | 42 | 8 | 111 | — |
| Mo. | 72 | 14 | — | — | 94 | 1 | 75 | — |
| N. Dak. | 1 | — | — | — | 4 | 1 | 31 | — |
| S. Dak. | — | — | — | — | 11 | — | 8 | — |
| Nebr. | 11 | 1 | — | — | 13 | 1 | 9 | — |
| Kans. | 16 | 5 | — | — | 23 | 4 | 56 | — |
| **S. Atlantic** | **1,353** | **395** | **15** | **5** | **446** | **55** | **500** | **—** |
| Del. | 167 | 2 | — | — | 10 | — | 8 | — |
| Md. | 899 | 110 | — | — | 55 | 6 | 124 | — |
| D.C. | 6 | 19 | — | — | 4 | 2 | 1 | — |
| Va. | 122 | 76 | 15 | 3 | 60 | 11 | 65 | — |
| W. Va. | 20 | 4 | — | — | 9 | — | 6 | — |
| N.C. | 74 | 36 | — | — | 49 | 9 | 104 | — |
| S.C. | 6 | 19 | — | — | 48 | 6 | 27 | — |
| Ga. | — | 32 | — | — | 72 | 4 | 52 | — |
| Fla. | 59 | 97 | — | 2 | 139 | 17 | 113 | — |
| **E.S. Central** | **102** | **27** | **2** | **—** | **161** | **12** | **118** | **—** |
| Ky. | 19 | 7 | 2 | — | 35 | — | 49 | — |
| Tenn. | 59 | 9 | — | — | 65 | — | 45 | — |
| Ala. | 20 | 7 | — | — | 38 | 11 | 21 | NN |
| Miss. | 4 | 4 | — | — | 23 | 1 | 3 | — |
| **W.S. Central** | **96** | **128** | **8** | **4** | **260** | **50** | **230** | **—** |
| Ark. | 7 | 3 | 5 | — | 35 | — | 26 | — |
| La. | 9 | 10 | — | — | 70 | 11 | 9 | — |
| Okla. | 8 | 2 | — | — | 40 | 4 | 43 | — |
| Tex. | 72 | 113 | 3 | 4 | 115 | 35 | 152 | — |
| **Mountain** | **17** | **46** | **2** | **—** | **149** | **27** | **829** | **9** |
| Mont. | — | 4 | — | — | 5 | — | 2 | — |
| Idaho | 3 | 3 | — | — | 14 | 4 | 146 | — |
| Wyo. | 3 | 1 | — | — | 5 | — | 2 | — |
| Colo. | 3 | 18 | — | — | 39 | 6 | 313 | 3 |
| N. Mex. | 1 | 4 | — | — | 16 | NN | 155 | 6 |
| Ariz. | 3 | 7 | 1 | — | 45 | 8 | 139 | — |
| Utah | 2 | 4 | — | — | 17 | 4 | 58 | — |
| Nev. | 2 | 5 | 1 | — | 8 | 5 | 14 | — |
| **Pacific** | **168** | **296** | **29** | **8** | **467** | **116** | **2,000** | **—** |
| Wash. | 14 | 43 | 4 | 1 | 93 | 2 | 739 | — |
| Oreg. | 15 | 22 | 12 | — | 76 | NN | 61 | — |
| Calif. | 139 | 218 | 13 | 4 | 280 | 95 | 1,144 | — |
| Alaska | — | 1 | — | — | 8 | 3 | 5 | — |
| Hawaii | NN | 12 | — | 3 | 10 | 16 | 51 | — |
| Guam | — | 1 | 1 | — | 1 | 3 | 2 | — |
| P.R. | — | 3 | 1 | — | 15 | 1 | 14 | — |
| V.I. | NA | NA | NA | NA | NA | NA | NA | NA |
| American Samoa | NA | NA | NA | NA | NA | NA | NA | NA |
| C.N.M.I. | NA | NA | NA | NA | NA | NA | NA | NA |

* Imported cases include only those resulting from importation from other countries.

## Table A2.2. *(Continued)*

| Area | Psittacosis | Rabies, Animal | RMSF[†] | Rubella: Rubella | Rubella: Congenital syndrome | Salmonellosis: NETSS[§] | Salmonellosis: PHLIS[¶] |
|---|---|---|---|---|---|---|---|
| **United States** | **16** | **6,730** | **579** | **267** | **9** | **40,596** | **32,782** |
| **New England** | **—** | **919** | **6** | **7** | **—** | **2,237** | **2,250** |
| Maine | — | 200 | — | — | — | 132 | 104 |
| N.H. | — | 47 | — | — | — | 141 | 137 |
| Vt. | — | 92 | — | — | NN | 93 | 82 |
| Mass. | — | 226 | 2 | 7 | — | 1,208 | 1,229 |
| R.I. | — | 101 | 4 | — | — | 151 | 169 |
| Conn. | NN | 253 | — | — | — | 512 | 529 |
| **Mid. Atlantic** | **4** | **1,305** | **39** | **35** | **2** | **5,634** | **5,280** |
| Upstate N.Y. | 1 | 919 | 14 | 21 | — | 1,516 | 1,363 |
| N.Y. City | 1 | NA | — | 6 | 2 | 1,457 | 1,527 |
| N.J. | 1 | 180 | 7 | 5 | — | 1,199 | 1,119 |
| Pa. | 1 | 206 | 18 | 3 | — | 1,462 | 1,271 |
| **E.N. Central** | **2** | **172** | **32** | **2** | **—** | **5,432** | **4,690** |
| Ohio | 1 | 36 | 8 | — | — | 1,313 | 1,093 |
| Ind. | 1 | 13 | 12 | 1 | — | 572 | 479 |
| Ill. | — | 10 | 7 | 1 | — | 1,600 | 1,568 |
| Mich. | — | 92 | 5 | — | — | 973 | 968 |
| Wis. | — | 21 | — | — | — | 974 | 582 |
| **W.N. Central** | **—** | **746** | **33** | **140** | **—** | **2,349** | **2,410** |
| Minn. | — | 120 | 1 | 5 | — | 626 | 710 |
| Iowa | — | 159 | 1 | 30 | — | 260 | 232 |
| Mo. | — | 31 | 16 | 2 | — | 758 | 881 |
| N. Dak. | — | 147 | — | — | — | 58 | 62 |
| S. Dak. | — | 180 | 4 | — | — | 100 | 118 |
| Nebr. | — | 4 | 9 | 103 | — | 214 | 180 |
| Kans. | — | 105 | 2 | — | — | 333 | 227 |
| **S. Atlantic** | **3** | **2,172** | **279** | **39** | **—** | **9,742** | **6,489** |
| Del. | — | 58 | — | — | — | 179 | 160 |
| Md. | 1 | 394 | 33 | 1 | — | 860 | 888 |
| D.C. | — | — | — | — | — | 76 | NA |
| Va. | — | 581 | 20 | — | — | 1,286 | 1,036 |
| W. Va. | — | 115 | 1 | — | — | 189 | 154 |
| N.C. | 1 | 442 | 152 | 37 | — | 1,331 | 1,311 |
| S.C. | — | 149 | 52 | — | — | 702 | 530 |
| Ga. | — | 247 | 14 | — | — | 1,976 | 1,701 |
| Fla. | 1 | 186 | 7 | 1 | — | 3,143 | 709 |
| **E.S. Central** | **1** | **256** | **99** | **2** | **—** | **2,239** | **1,481** |
| Ky. | — | 35 | 3 | — | — | 419 | 294 |
| Tenn. | — | 95 | 65 | — | — | 593 | 597 |
| Ala. | 1 | 124 | 17 | 2 | — | 605 | 491 |
| Miss. | — | 2 | 14 | — | — | 622 | 99 |
| **W.S. Central** | **—** | **524** | **66** | **22** | **—** | **4,088** | **2,807** |
| Ark. | — | 31 | 25 | 12 | — | 698 | 265 |
| La. | — | — | 2 | — | — | 726 | 617 |
| Okla. | NN | 94 | 29 | 1 | — | 466 | 352 |
| Tex. | NN | 399 | 10 | 9 | — | 2,198 | 1,573 |
| **Mountain** | **3** | **272** | **19** | **16** | **5** | **3,071** | **2,615** |
| Mont. | — | 64 | 2 | — | — | 86 | 2 |
| Idaho | — | 6 | — | — | — | 135 | 97 |
| Wyo. | 1 | 45 | 5 | — | — | 70 | 59 |
| Colo. | 2 | 51 | 4 | 1 | 1 | 720 | 708 |
| N. Mex. | — | 9 | 1 | — | 1 | 370 | 293 |
| Ariz. | — | 81 | 1 | 13 | 2 | 924 | 820 |
| Utah | — | 8 | 5 | 1 | 1 | 566 | 587 |
| Nev. | — | 8 | 1 | 1 | — | 200 | 49 |
| **Pacific** | **3** | **364** | **6** | **4** | **2** | **5,804** | **4,760** |
| Wash. | — | — | 3 | — | — | 792 | 848 |
| Oreg. | — | 4 | 2 | — | — | 426 | 477 |
| Calif. | 3 | 351 | 1 | 4 | 2 | 4,193 | 3,111 |
| Alaska | — | 9 | NN | — | NN | 55 | 35 |
| Hawaii | — | — | NN | — | — | 338 | 289 |
| Guam | — | — | — | — | — | 37 | NA |
| P.R. | — | 74 | — | 2 | — | 715 | NA |
| V.I. | NA | NA | NA | NA | NA | NA | NA |
| American Samoa | NA | NA | NA | NA | NA | NA | NA |
| C.N.M.I. | NA | NA | NA | NA | NA | NA | NA |

* No cases of paralytic poliomyelitis or human rabies were reported in 1999.

[†]Rocky Mountain spotted fever.

[§]National Electronic Telecommunications System for Surveillance.

[¶]Public Health laboratory Information System. Totals reported to the National Center for Infectious Diseases as of May 4, 2000.

## Table A2.2. *(Continued)*

| Area | Shigellosis NETSS* | Shigellosis PHLIS† | Streptococcal disease, invasive, group A | *Streptococcus pneumoniae*, drug resistant | Streptococcal toxic-shock syndrome | Syphilis§ Congenital (age <1 yr) | Syphilis§ Primary & secondary |
|---|---|---|---|---|---|---|---|
| **United States** | **17,521** | **10,084** | **2,382** | **4,618** | **61** | **556** | **6,657** |
| **New England** | **885** | **851** | **81** | **14** | **1** | **2** | **60** |
| Maine | 5 | — | 9 | — | — | — | — |
| N.H. | 19 | 17 | 17 | NN | — | 1 | 1 |
| Vt. | 7 | 4 | 14 | 14 | 1 | — | 3 |
| Mass. | 748 | 731 | 26 | NN | — | — | 37 |
| R.I. | 37 | 29 | 15 | — | — | — | 3 |
| Conn. | 69 | 70 | — | — | NN | 1 | 16 |
| **Mid. Atlantic** | **1,188** | **750** | **410** | **152** | **4** | **96** | **302** |
| Upstate N.Y. | 314 | 84 | 245 | 150 | NN | 2 | 20 |
| N.Y. City | 353 | 247 | 118 | NA | — | 41 | 130 |
| N.J. | 297 | 236 | 29 | — | 3 | 46 | 68 |
| Pa. | 224 | 183 | 18 | 2 | 1 | 7 | 84 |
| **E.N. Central** | **3,300** | **1,853** | **638** | **197** | **43** | **93** | **1,254** |
| Ohio | 422 | 150 | 149 | — | 14 | 6 | 92 |
| Ind. | 368 | 118 | 37 | 197 | 2 | 7 | 450 |
| Ill. | 1,330 | 1,018 | 246 | NN | 27 | 53 | 422 |
| Mich. | 535 | 489 | 206 | NN | — | 20 | 249 |
| Wis. | 645 | 78 | NN | NN | NN | 7 | 41 |
| **W.N. Central** | **1,246** | **806** | **252** | **626** | **3** | **10** | **135** |
| Minn. | 254 | 254 | 182 | 609 | — | — | 10 |
| Iowa | 74 | 62 | — | NN | — | — | 9 |
| Mo. | 721 | 353 | 45 | — | — | 9 | 96 |
| N. Dak. | 3 | 2 | 8 | 5 | — | — | — |
| S. Dak. | 18 | 10 | 11 | 3 | — | 1 | — |
| Nebr. | 87 | 68 | — | — | — | — | 6 |
| Kans. | 89 | 57 | 6 | 9 | 3 | — | 14 |
| **S. Atlantic** | **2,702** | **534** | **334** | **1,708** | **4** | **115** | **2,102** |
| Del. | 15 | 11 | — | 10 | — | — | 10 |
| Md. | 162 | 58 | NN | NN | NN | 27 | 343 |
| D.C. | 53 | NA | 11 | 45 | NN | — | 45 |
| Va. | 136 | 66 | 36 | NN | — | 3 | 153 |
| W. Va. | 9 | 5 | 27 | 31 | — | — | 5 |
| N.C. | 211 | 93 | 48 | NN | — | 19 | 464 |
| S.C. | 122 | 64 | 5 | 356 | — | 19 | 269 |
| Ga. | 284 | 83 | 112 | 555 | — | 15 | 430 |
| Fla. | 1,710 | 154 | 95 | 711 | 4 | 32 | 383 |
| **E.S. Central** | **1,223** | **699** | **85** | **318** | **5** | **25** | **1,138** |
| Ky. | 235 | 149 | 26 | — | — | — | 101 |
| Tenn. | 691 | 476 | 59 | 318 | 5 | 7 | 641 |
| Ala. | 117 | 63 | — | — | — | 6 | 202 |
| Miss. | 180 | 11 | NN | NN | NN | 12 | 194 |
| **W.S. Central** | **3,143** | **1,212** | **243** | **1,558** | **—** | **102** | **1,053** |
| Ark. | 76 | 27 | 8 | 30 | — | 14 | 87 |
| La. | 226 | 137 | 1 | 116 | NN | 12 | 306 |
| Okla. | 560 | 171 | NN | NN | NN | 8 | 187 |
| Tex. | 2,281 | 877 | 234 | 1,412 | — | 68 | 473 |
| **Mountain** | **1,164** | **773** | **311** | **44** | **1** | **25** | **241** |
| Mont. | 10 | — | — | — | NN | — | 1 |
| Idaho | 28 | 12 | 7 | NN | — | — | 1 |
| Wyo. | 3 | 1 | 2 | 8 | — | — | — |
| Colo. | 205 | 164 | — | 6 | — | 1 | 8 |
| N. Mex. | 152 | 109 | 41 | 20 | — | — | 12 |
| Ariz. | 602 | 413 | 260 | — | — | 24 | 212 |
| Utah | 66 | 68 | NN | NN | 1 | — | 2 |
| Nev. | 98 | 6 | 1 | 10 | — | — | 5 |
| **Pacific** | **2,670** | **2,606** | **28** | **1** | **—** | **88** | **372** |
| Wash. | 172 | 116 | NN | NN | — | — | 77 |
| Oreg. | 95 | 91 | NN | NN | NN | — | 8 |
| Calif. | 2,364 | 2,358 | NN | — | NN | 88 | 283 |
| Alaska | 4 | 5 | — | — | — | — | 1 |
| Hawaii | 35 | 36 | 28 | 1 | — | — | 3 |
| Guam | 19 | NA | 3 | — | — | — | 2 |
| P.R. | 141 | NA | — | — | — | 17 | 146 |
| V.I. | NA | NA | NA | NA | NN | — | 1 |
| American Samoa | NA | NA | NA | NA | NA | NA | NA |
| C.N.M.I. | NA | NA | NA | NA | NA | NA | NA |

* National Electronic Telecommunications System for Surveillance.

†Public Health Laboratory Information System. Totals reported to the National Center for Infectious Diseases as of April 17, 2000.

§Totals reported to the Division of Sexually Transmitted Diseases Prevention, NCHSTP, as of August 8, 2000.

## Table A2.2. *(Continued)*

| Area | Syphilis* All stages | Tetanus | Toxic-shock syndrome | Trichinosis | Tuberculosis† | Typhoid fever | Varicella§ (chickenpox) | Yellow fever |
|---|---|---|---|---|---|---|---|---|
| **United States** | **35,628** | **40** | **113** | **12** | **17,531** | **346** | **46,016** | **1** |
| **New England** | **587** | **—** | **7** | **1** | **489** | **28** | **497** | **—** |
| Maine | 1 | — | 2 | — | 23 | — | 45 | — |
| N.H. | 17 | — | 2 | — | 19 | — | NN | NN |
| Vt. | 3 | — | — | — | 3 | 1 | NN | — |
| Mass. | 385 | — | 3 | — | 270 | 17 | 427 | — |
| R.I. | 55 | — | — | — | 53 | 3 | 25 | — |
| Conn. | 126 | — | NN | 1 | 121 | 7 | NN | — |
| **Mid. Atlantic** | **5,826** | **5** | **13** | **3** | **2,862** | **100** | **—** | **—** |
| Upstate N.Y. | 357 | 4 | 6 | 3 | 377 | 15 | NN | — |
| N.Y. City | 3,737 | — | 2 | — | 1,460 | 49 | NN | — |
| N.J. | 800 | — | — | — | 571 | 35 | NN | — |
| Pa. | 932 | 1 | 5 | — | 454 | 1 | NN | — |
| **E.N. Central** | **4,101** | **4** | **35** | **3** | **1,753** | **41** | **28,004** | **—** |
| Ohio | 364 | 2 | 4 | — | 317 | 4 | 1,307 | — |
| Ind. | 802 | 2 | 2 | — | 150 | 6 | NN | — |
| Ill. | 1,967 | — | 5 | 2 | 825 | 17 | 13,846 | — |
| Mich. | 778 | — | 17 | — | 351 | 14 | 12,260 | — |
| Wis. | 190 | — | 7 | 1 | 110 | — | 591 | — |
| **W.N. Central** | **625** | **3** | **13** | **1** | **582** | **3** | **5,297** | **—** |
| Minn. | 71 | 1 | 2 | — | 201 | 1 | NN | — |
| Iowa | 37 | — | 4 | — | 58 | 1 | NN | — |
| Mo. | 395 | 1 | 3 | — | 208 | — | 5,291 | — |
| N. Dak. | — | — | — | — | 7 | — | 5 | — |
| S. Dak. | 3 | — | — | — | 21 | — | NN | — |
| Nebr. | 24 | — | 2 | — | 18 | — | 1 | — |
| Kans. | 95 | 1 | 2 | 1 | 69 | 1 | NN | — |
| **S. Atlantic** | **10,220** | **5** | **8** | **1** | **3,518** | **57** | **3,565** | **—** |
| Del. | 72 | — | — | — | 34 | 2 | 5 | — |
| Md. | 1,385 | — | NN | — | 294 | 9 | NN | NN |
| D.C. | 458 | — | — | — | 70 | — | 75 | — |
| Va. | 722 | — | — | — | 334 | 11 | 1,490 | — |
| W. Va. | 15 | — | — | — | 41 | — | 1,995 | — |
| N.C. | 1,713 | 2 | 1 | — | 488 | 3 | NN | — |
| S.C. | 925 | — | 2 | — | 315 | 3 | NN | — |
| Ga. | 1,973 | — | 2 | — | 665 | 5 | NN | — |
| Fla. | 2,957 | 3 | 3 | 1 | 1,277 | 24 | NN | — |
| **E.S. Central** | **3,960** | **—** | **7** | **—** | **1,120** | **2** | **584** | **—** |
| Ky. | 302 | — | 3 | NN | 209 | 1 | NN | — |
| Tenn. | 1,734 | — | 4 | — | 382 | 1 | 584 | — |
| Ala. | 1,018 | — | — | — | 314 | — | NN | — |
| Miss. | 906 | — | NN | — | 215 | — | NN | — |
| **W.S. Central** | **6,024** | **6** | **2** | **—** | **2,395** | **24** | **7,646** | **—** |
| Ark. | 364 | — | — | NN | 181 | 1 | NN | — |
| La. | 1,423 | — | — | — | 357 | — | 173 | — |
| Okla. | 538 | — | 2 | NN | 208 | — | NN | — |
| Tex. | 3,699 | 6 | NN | — | 1,649 | 23 | 7,473 | — |
| **Mountain** | **1,161** | **—** | **4** | **1** | **580** | **7** | **423** | **—** |
| Mont. | 3 | — | — | — | 14 | — | NN | — |
| Idaho | 13 | — | — | — | 16 | — | NN | — |
| Wyo. | — | — | 1 | — | 3 | — | NN | — |
| Colo. | 91 | — | — | 1 | 88 | 2 | NN | — |
| N. Mex. | 80 | — | 2 | — | 64 | — | NN | — |
| Ariz. | 833 | — | — | — | 262 | 2 | 245 | — |
| Utah | 49 | — | 1 | — | 40 | 2 | 136 | — |
| Nev. | 92 | — | — | — | 93 | 1 | 42 | NN |
| **Pacific** | **3,124** | **17** | **24** | **2** | **4,232** | **84** | **—** | **1** |
| Wash. | 204 | — | 5 | — | 258 | 8 | NN | — |
| Oreg. | 37 | 1 | NN | — | 123 | 5 | NN | — |
| Calif. | 2,859 | 16 | 19 | 2 | 3,606 | 71 | NN | 1 |
| Alaska | 13 | — | NN | — | 61 | — | NN | — |
| Hawaii | 11 | — | NN | — | 184 | — | NN | — |
| Guam | 12 | — | — | — | 69 | — | 210 | — |
| P.R. | 1,457 | 2 | — | — | 200 | — | 5,019 | — |
| V.I. | 13 | NA | NA | NA | NA | NA | NA | NA |
| American Samoa | NA | NA | NA | NA | 4 | NA | NA | NA |
| C.N.M.I. | NA | NA | NA | NA | 66 | NA | NA | NA |

* Totals reported to the Division of Sexually Transmitted Diseases Prevention, NCHSTP, as of August 8, 2000.

†Totals reported to the Division of Tuberculosis Elimination, NCHSTP, as of May 3, 2000.

§Although not nationally notifiable, reporting is recommended by the Council for State and Territorial Epidemiologists.

## Table A2.3. Reported Cases and Incidence Rates of Notifiable Diseases,* by Age Group, United States, 1999

| Disease | Total | <1 yrs | | 1–4 yrs | | 5–14 yrs | | 15–24 yrs | | 25–39 yrs | | 40–64 yrs | | ≥65 yrs | | Age not stated |
|---|---|---|---|---|---|---|---|---|---|---|---|---|---|---|---|---|
| | | No. | (Rate) | No. | (Rate) | No. | (Rate) | No. | (Rate) | No. | (Rate) | No. | (Rate) | No. | (Rate) | |
| AIDS† | 45,104 | 88 | (2.31) | 89 | (0.59) | 135 | (0.34) | 1,700 | (4.51) | 23,291 | (38.57) | 19,083 | (23.45) | 718 | (2.08) | — |
| Botulism, foodborne | 23 | 7 | (0.18) | — | (0.00) | — | (—) | 1 | (0.00) | 2 | (0.00) | 10 | (0.01) | 3 | (0.01) | — |
| Infant | 92 | 89 | (2.36) | 1 | (0.01) | 1 | (0.00) | — | (—) | — | (—) | — | (—) | — | (—) | 1 |
| Other (includes wound) | 39 | 1 | (0.03) | — | (0.00) | — | (—) | 1 | (0.00) | 18 | (0.03) | 18 | (0.02) | 1 | (0.00) | — |
| Brucellosis | 82 | 1 | (0.03) | 1 | (0.01) | 12 | (0.03) | 15 | (0.04) | 13 | (0.02) | 29 | (0.04) | 10 | (0.03) | 1 |
| Chlamydia§¶ | 655,335 | NA | (NA) | NA | (NA) | NA | (NA) | 480,195 | (1,273.72) | 138,422 | (229.24) | 13,036 | (16.02) | 899 | (2.60) | 7,004 |
| Cholera | 6 | — | (—) | 1 | (0.01) | 1 | (0.00) | 1 | (0.00) | — | (—) | 1 | (0.00) | 2 | (0.01) | — |
| Cryptosporidiosis | 2,361 | 51 | (1.42) | 432 | (3.03) | 338 | (0.91) | 205 | (0.58) | 710 | (1.24) | 492 | (0.64) | 108 | (0.33) | 25 |
| Cyclosporiasis | 56 | 4 | (0.11) | 3 | (0.02) | 3 | (0.01) | 11 | (0.03) | 6 | (0.01) | 23 | (0.03) | 5 | (0.02) | 1 |
| Diphtheria | 1 | — | (—) | — | (—) | — | (—) | — | (—) | — | (—) | — | (—) | 1 | (0.00) | — |
| Ehrlichiosis, | | | | | | | | | | | | | | | | |
| Human granulocytic | 203 | 1 | (0.03) | 4 | (0.03) | 8 | (0.03) | 10 | (0.03) | 46 | (0.10) | 77 | (0.12) | 56 | (0.21) | 1 |
| Human monocytic | 99 | 2 | (0.07) | — | (—) | 3 | (0.01) | 4 | (0.01) | 16 | (0.03) | 49 | (0.08) | 22 | (0.08) | 3 |
| Encephalitis, California serogroup viral | 70 | 2 | (0.05) | 12 | (0.08) | 46 | (0.12) | 4 | (0.01) | 1 | (0.00) | 3 | (0.00) | 2 | (0.01) | — |
| Eastern equine | 5 | — | (—) | — | (—) | 2 | (0.01) | 1 | (0.00) | — | (—) | 2 | (0.00) | — | (—) | — |
| St. Louis | 4 | — | (—) | — | (—) | — | (—) | — | (—) | 1 | (0.00) | 2 | (0.00) | 1 | (0.00) | — |
| Western equine | 1 | — | (—) | — | (—) | — | (—) | — | (—) | — | (—) | — | (—) | 1 | (0.00) | — |
| *Escherichia coli* O157:H7 | 4,513 | 99 | (2.75) | 792 | (5.56) | 915 | (2.47) | 593 | (1.67) | 609 | (1.07) | 875 | (1.15) | 392 | (1.23) | 238 |
| Gonorrhea¶ | 359,442 | NA | (NA) | NA | (NA) | NA | (NA) | 210,892 | (559.39) | 110,680 | (183.29) | 26,402 | (32.44) | 894 | (2.59) | 3,612 |
| *Haemophilus influenzae,* invasive disease | 1,309 | 149 | (3.91) | 105 | (0.70) | 59 | (0.15) | 57 | (0.15) | 110 | (0.18) | 305 | (0.37) | 504 | (1.46) | 20 |
| Hansen disease (leprosy) | 108 | — | (—) | — | (—) | 2 | (0.01) | 7 | (0.02) | 29 | (0.05) | 29 | (0.04) | 17 | (0.05) | 24 |
| Hantavirus pulmonary syndrome** | 33 | — | (—) | — | (—) | 3 | (0.01) | 3 | (0.01) | 12 | (0.02) | 12 | (0.01) | 3 | (0.01) | — |
| Hemolytic uremic syndrome, postdiarrheal | 181 | 5 | (0.16) | 92 | (0.73) | 42 | (0.13) | 8 | (0.03) | 6 | (0.01) | 11 | (0.02) | 17 | (0.06) | — |
| Hepatitis A | 17,047 | 85 | (2.23) | 888 | (5.88) | 3,546 | (9.00) | 2,768 | (7.34) | 5,246 | (8.69) | 3,503 | (4.30) | 877 | (2.54) | 134 |
| Hepatitis B | 7,694 | 33 | (0.87) | 30 | (0.20) | 73 | (0.19) | 1,311 | (3.48) | 3,375 | (5.59) | 2,395 | (2.94) | 333 | (0.96) | 144 |
| Hepatitis C; non-A, non-B | 3,111 | 29 | (0.76) | 7 | (0.05) | 16 | (0.04) | 182 | (0.48) | 980 | (1.62) | 1,654 | (2.03) | 164 | (0.48) | 79 |
| Legionellosis | 1,108 | 3 | (0.08) | 1 | (0.01) | 5 | (0.01) | 25 | (0.07) | 120 | (0.20) | 503 | (0.63) | 440 | (1.30) | 11 |
| Lyme disease | 16,273 | 33 | (0.87) | 870 | (5.79) | 3,160 | (8.05) | 1,410 | (3.76) | 2,722 | (4.53) | 5,837 | (7.20) | 2,100 | (6.11) | 141 |
| Malaria | 1,666 | 7 | (0.18) | 76 | (0.50) | 155 | (0.39) | 315 | (0.84) | 600 | (0.99) | 438 | (0.54) | 47 | (0.14) | 28 |
| Measles | 100 | 17 | (0.45) | 24 | (0.16) | 21 | (0.05) | 12 | (0.03) | 20 | (0.03) | 5 | (0.01) | — | (—) | 1 |
| Meningococcal disease | 2,501 | 354 | (9.29) | 364 | (2.41) | 322 | (0.82) | 467 | (1.24) | 222 | (0.37) | 379 | (0.47) | 375 | (1.09) | 18 |
| Mumps | 387 | 4 | (0.11) | 61 | (0.41) | 156 | (0.40) | 42 | (0.11) | 62 | (0.10) | 44 | (0.06) | 7 | (0.02) | 11 |
| Pertussis (whooping cough) | 7,288 | 2,168 | (56.87) | 833 | (5.52) | 2,056 | (5.22) | 883 | (2.34) | 579 | (0.96) | 674 | (0.83) | 80 | (0.23) | 15 |
| Plague | 9 | — | (—) | — | (—) | 1 | (0.00) | — | (—) | 1 | (0.00) | 3 | (0.00) | 4 | (0.01) | — |
| Psittacosis | 16 | — | (—) | — | (—) | — | (—) | — | (—) | 2 | (0.00) | 10 | (0.01) | 3 | (0.01) | 1 |
| Rocky Mountain spotted fever | 579 | 1 | (0.03) | 38 | (0.25) | 89 | (0.23) | 57 | (0.15) | 124 | (0.21) | 200 | (0.25) | 66 | (0.19) | 4 |
| Rubella | 267 | 16 | (0.42) | 15 | (0.10) | 4 | (0.01) | 111 | (0.29) | 97 | (0.16) | 20 | (0.02) | 1 | (0.00) | 3 |
| Salmonellosis | 40,596 | 5,163 | (135.44) | 6,682 | (44.27) | 4,963 | (12.59) | 3,472 | (9.21) | 5,505 | (9.12) | 6,280 | (7.72) | 3,580 | (10.37) | 4,951 |
| Shigellosis | 17,521 | 370 | (9.71) | 4,667 | (30.92) | 4,619 | (11.72) | 1,228 | (3.26) | 2,397 | (3.97) | 1,322 | (1.62) | 327 | (0.95) | 2,591 |
| Streptococcal disease, invasive, group A | 2,382 | 102 | (3.49) | 142 | (1.23) | 184 | (0.61) | 132 | (0.46) | 339 | (0.73) | 732 | (1.15) | 726 | (2.64) | 25 |
| *Streptococcus pneumoniae,* drug-resistant, invasive | 4,618 | 715 | (26.81) | 1,232 | (11.66) | 153 | (0.56) | 95 | (0.36) | 363 | (0.87) | 878 | (1.56) | 1,062 | (4.39) | 120 |
| Streptococcal toxic-shock syndrome | 61 | — | (—) | — | (—) | 10 | (0.03) | 6 | (0.02) | 15 | (0.03) | 23 | (0.04) | 7 | (0.03) | — |
| Syphilis | | | | | | | | | | | | | | | | |
| Primary and secondary¶ | 6,650 | NA | (NA) | NA | (NA) | NA | (NA) | 1,410 | (3.74) | 3,239 | (5.36) | 1,793 | (2.20) | 74 | (0.21) | 17 |
| Tetanus | 40 | — | (—) | 1 | (0.01) | 1 | (0.00) | 3 | (0.01) | 14 | (0.02) | 12 | (0.01) | 9 | (0.03) | — |
| Toxic-shock syndrome | 113 | 2 | (0.06) | 2 | (0.02) | 17 | (0.05) | 19 | (0.06) | 35 | (0.07) | 30 | (0.04) | 8 | (0.03) | — |
| Trichinosis | 12 | — | (—) | — | (—) | — | (—) | 4 | (0.01) | 4 | (0.01) | 1 | (0.00) | 3 | (0.01) | — |
| Tuberculosis†† | 17,531 | 98 | (2.57) | 507 | (3.36) | 439 | (1.11) | 1,516 | (4.02) | 4,388 | (7.27) | 6,552 | (8.05) | 4,028 | (11.67) | 3 |
| Typhoid fever | 346 | 1 | (0.03) | 46 | (0.30) | 74 | (0.19) | 73 | (0.19) | 88 | (0.15) | 51 | (0.06) | 12 | (0.03) | 1 |
| Yellow fever | 1 | — | (—) | — | (—) | — | (—) | — | (—) | — | (—) | 1 | (0.00) | — | (—) | — |

* No cases of anthrax, paralytic poliomyelitis, or human rabies were reported in 1999.

†Total number of acquired immunodeficiency syndrome (AIDS) cases reported to the Division of HIV/AIDS Prevention—Surveillance and Epidemiology, National Center for HIV, STD, and TB Prevention (NCHSTP), through December 31, 1999.

§Chlamydia refers to genital infections caused by *C. trachomatis.*

¶Age-related data are collected on aggregate forms different from those used for reported cases. Thus, the total cases reported on this table will differ slightly from others. Cases among persons aged <15 years are not shown because some might not be caused by sexual transmission. However, these cases are included in the totals. Totals reported to the Division of Sexually Transmitted Diseases Prevention, NCHSTP, as of August 8, 2000.

** Totals reported to the National Center for Infectious Diseases as of June 30, 2000.

††Totals reported to the Division of Tuberculosis Elimination, NCHSTP, as of May 3, 2000.

Note: Rates <0.01 after rounding are listed as 0.00.

*Source*: Centers for Disease Control and Prevention. *Summary of Notifiable Diseases, United States, 1999. MMWR* 1999, 48, no. 53. http://www.cdc.gov/mmwr/PDF/wk/mm4853.pdf.

## Table A2.4. Reported Cases and Incidence Rates of Notifiable Diseases,* by Sex, United States, 1999

| Disease | Total | Male No. | Male (Rate) | Female No. | Female (Rate) | Sex not stated |
|---|---|---|---|---|---|---|
| AIDS† | 45,104 | 34,532 | (25.95) | 10,572 | (7.59) | — |
| Botulism, foodborne | 23 | 12 | (0.01) | 11 | (0.01) | — |
| Infant | 92 | 44 | (1.15) | 45 | (1.23) | 3 |
| Other (includes wound) | 39 | 26 | (0.02) | 13 | (0.01) | — |
| Brucellosis | 82 | 58 | (0.04) | 24 | (0.02) | — |
| Chancroid§ | 143 | 91 | (0.07) | 51 | (0.04) | 1 |
| Chlamydia§¶ | 656,721 | NA | (NA) | 534,612 | (400.99) | 2,331 |
| Cholera | 6 | 4 | (0.00) | 2 | (0.00) | — |
| Cryptosporidiosis | 2,361 | 1,419 | (1.13) | 930 | (0.71) | 12 |
| Cyclosporiasis | 56 | 29 | (0.02) | 27 | (0.02) | — |
| Diphtheria | 1 | 1 | (0.00) | — | (—) | — |
| Ehrlichiosis, human granulocytic | 203 | 113 | (0.11) | 90 | (0.08) | — |
| Human monocytic | 99 | 69 | (0.07) | 30 | (0.03) | — |
| Encephalitis, California serogroup viral | 70 | 48 | (0.04) | 22 | (0.02) | — |
| Eastern equine | 5 | 3 | (0.00) | 2 | (0.00) | — |
| St. Louis | 4 | 4 | (0.00) | — | (—) | — |
| Western equine | 1 | 1 | (0.00) | — | (—) | — |
| *Escherichia coli* 0157:H7 | 4,513 | 2,053 | (1.65) | 2,329 | (1.79) | 131 |
| Gonorrhea§ | 360,076 | 179,564 | (134.92) | 179,534 | (128.94) | 978 |
| *Haemophilus influenzae*, invasive disease | 1,309 | 614 | (0.46) | 684 | (0.49) | 11 |
| Hansen disease (leprosy) | 108 | 65 | (0.05) | 21 | (0.02) | 22 |
| Hantavirus pulmonary syndrome** | 33 | 20 | (0.02) | 13 | (0.01) | — |
| Hemolytic uremic syndrome, postdiarrheal | 181 | 73 | (0.07) | 106 | (0.09) | 2 |
| Hepatitis A | 17,047 | 10,286 | (7.73) | 6,653 | (4.78) | 108 |
| Hepatitis B | 7,694 | 4,532 | (3.41) | 3,095 | (2.22) | 67 |
| Hepatitis C; non-A, non-B | 3,111 | 1,889 | (1.42) | 1,179 | (0.85) | 43 |
| Legionellosis | 1,108 | 666 | (0.51) | 436 | (0.32) | 6 |
| Lyme disease | 16,273 | 8,511 | (6.42) | 7,715 | (5.56) | 47 |
| Malaria | 1,666 | 1,063 | (0.80) | 570 | (0.41) | 33 |
| Measles | 100 | 46 | (0.03) | 54 | (0.04) | — |
| Meningococcal disease | 2,501 | 1,223 | (0.92) | 1,254 | (0.90) | 24 |
| Mumps | 387 | 191 | (0.15) | 188 | (0.14) | 8 |
| Pertussis (whooping cough) | 7,288 | 3,341 | (2.51) | 3,931 | (2.82) | 16 |
| Plague | 9 | 4 | (0.00) | 5 | (0.00) | — |
| Psittacosis | 16 | 5 | (0.00) | 11 | (0.01) | — |
| Rocky Mountain spotted fever | 579 | 331 | (0.25) | 245 | (0.18) | 3 |
| Rubella | 267 | 171 | (0.13) | 93 | (0.07) | 3 |
| Salmonellosis | 40,596 | 17,310 | (13.01) | 18,477 | (13.27) | 4,809 |
| Shigellosis | 17,521 | 6,793 | (5.10) | 8,082 | (5.80) | 2,646 |
| Streptococcal disease, invasive, group A | 2,382 | 1,199 | (1.16) | 1,097 | (1.01) | 86 |
| *Streptococcus pneumoniae*, drug-resistant, invasive disease | 4,618 | 2,288 | (2.47) | 1,985 | (2.05) | 345 |
| Streptococcal toxic-shock syndrome | 61 | 27 | (0.03) | 34 | (0.03) | — |
| Syphilis, primary and secondary§ | 6,657 | 3,856 | (2.90) | 2,796 | (2.01) | 5 |
| Tetanus | 40 | 29 | (0.02) | 11 | (0.01) | — |
| Toxic-shock syndrome | 113 | 25 | (0.02) | 88 | (0.07) | — |
| Trichinosis | 12 | 10 | (0.01) | 2 | (0.00) | — |
| Tuberculosis†† | 17,531 | 10,948 | (8.23) | 6,582 | (4.73) | 1 |
| Typhoid fever | 346 | 159 | (0.12) | 180 | (0.13) | 7 |
| Yellow fever | 1 | 1 | (0.00) | — | (—) | — |

* No cases of anthrax, paralytic poliomyelitis, or human rabies were reported in 1999.

†Total number of acquired immunodeficiency syndrome (AIDS) cases reported to the Division of HIV/AIDS Prevention—Surveillance and Epidemiology, National Center for HIV, STD, and TB Prevention (NCHSTP), through December 31, 1999.

§Totals reported to the Division of Sexually Transmitted Diseases Prevention, NCHSTP, as of August 8, 2000.

¶Chlamydia refers to genital infections caused by *C. trachomatis*.

** Totals reported to the National Center for Infectious Diseases as of June 30, 2000.

††Totals reported to the Division of Tuberculosis Elimination, NCHSTP, as of May 3, 2000.

Note: Rates <0.01 after rounding are listed as 0.00.

*Source*: Centers for Disease Control and Prevention. *Summary of Notifiable Diseases, United States, 1999. MMWR* 1999, 48, no. 53. http://www.cdc.gov/mmwr/PDF/wk/mm4853.pdf.

## Table A2.5. Reported Cases and Incidence Rates of Notifiable Diseases* by Race, United States, 1999

| Disease | Total | American Indian or Alaska Native | | Asian or Pacific Islander | | Black | | White | | Other | Race not stated |
|---|---|---|---|---|---|---|---|---|---|---|---|
| | | No. | (Rate) | No. | (Rate) | No. | (Rate) | No. | (Rate) | No. | No. |
| AIDS[†] | 45,104 | 178 | (7.42) | 361 | (3.34) | 21,877 | (62.75) | 14,805 | (6.59) | — | 7,883[§] |
| Botulism, foodborne | 23 | 2 | (0.08) | 2 | (0.02) | — | (—) | 17 | (0.01) | 1 | 1 |
| Infant | 92 | 1 | (2.35) | 3 | (1.65) | 2 | (0.35) | 54 | (1.78) | — | 32 |
| Other (includes wound) | 39 | — | (—) | — | (—) | 3 | (0.01) | 17 | (0.01) | — | 19 |
| Brucellosis | 82 | — | (—) | — | (—) | — | (—) | 47 | (0.02) | 1 | 34 |
| Chlamydia[¶]** | 655,335 | 8,746 | (364.81) | 9,121 | (84.29) | 228,126 | (654.37) | 136,881 | (60.94) | — | 272,461[§] |
| Cholera | 6 | — | (—) | 2 | (0.02) | 1 | (0.00) | — | (—) | — | 3 |
| Cryptosporidiosis | 2,361 | 5 | (0.26) | 31 | (0.30) | 289 | (0.85) | 1,312 | (0.62) | 3 | 721 |
| Cyclosporiasis | 56 | — | (—) | 1 | (0.01) | 6 | (0.02) | 34 | (0.02) | — | 15 |
| Diphtheria | 1 | — | (—) | — | (—) | — | (—) | 1 | (0.00) | — | — |
| Ehrlichiosis, | | | | | | | | | | | |
| Human granulocytic | 203 | 3 | (0.21) | 2 | (0.02) | — | (—) | 134 | (0.08) | — | 64 |
| Human monocytic | 99 | — | (—) | — | (—) | 5 | (0.02) | 66 | (0.04) | — | 28 |
| Encephalitis, California serogroup viral | 70 | 3 | (0.14) | — | (—) | 1 | (0.00) | 61 | (0.03) | — | 5 |
| Eastern equine | 5 | — | (—) | — | (—) | 1 | (0.00) | 4 | (0.00) | — | — |
| St. Louis | 4 | — | (—) | — | (—) | — | (—) | 4 | (0.00) | — | — |
| Western equine | 1 | — | (—) | — | (—) | — | (—) | — | (—) | — | 1 |
| *Escherichia coli* 0157:H7 | 4,513 | 10 | (0.43) | 33 | (0.31) | 97 | (0.29) | 2,265 | (1.08) | 6 | 2,102 |
| Gonorrhea** | 359,442 | 1,719 | (71.70) | 1,662 | (15.36) | 220,581 | (632.72) | 40,896 | (18.21) | — | 94,584 |
| *Haemophilus influenzae*, invasive disease | 1,309 | 33 | (1.38) | 17 | (0.16) | 179 | (0.51) | 767 | (0.34) | 1 | 312 |
| Hansen disease (leprosy) | 108 | — | (—) | 27 | (0.25) | 9 | (0.03) | 26 | (0.01) | — | 46 |
| Hantavirus pulmonary syndrome[††] | 33 | 4 | (0.17) | 1 | (0.01) | — | (—) | 28 | (0.01) | — | — |
| Hemolytic uremic syndrome, postdiarrheal | 181 | — | (—) | 3 | (0.03) | 8 | (0.03) | 134 | (0.07) | 1 | 35 |
| Hepatitis A | 17,047 | 177 | (7.38) | 279 | (2.58) | 1,915 | (5.49) | 9,246 | (4.12) | 58 | 5,372 |
| Hepatitis B | 7,694 | 83 | (3.46) | 431 | (3.98) | 1,540 | (4.42) | 3,075 | (1.37) | 30 | 2,535 |
| Hepatitis C; non-A, non-B | 3,111 | 4 | (0.17) | 4 | (0.04) | 41 | (0.12) | 145 | (0.06) | — | 2,917 |
| Legionellosis | 1,108 | 2 | (0.09) | 6 | (0.06) | 117 | (0.34) | 737 | (0.34) | 8 | 238 |
| Lyme disease | 16,273 | 23 | (0.96) | 86 | (0.85) | 192 | (0.55) | 12,481 | (5.57) | 39 | 3,452 |
| Malaria | 1,666 | 3 | (0.13) | 107 | (0.99) | 706 | (2.03) | 403 | (0.18) | 24 | 423 |
| Measles | 100 | 1 | (0.04) | 15 | (0.14) | 9 | (0.03) | 62 | (0.03) | 2 | 11 |
| Meningococcal disease | 2,501 | 27 | (1.13) | 36 | (0.33) | 372 | (1.07) | 1,547 | (0.69) | 6 | 513 |
| Mumps | 387 | 9 | (0.41) | 26 | (0.24) | 32 | (0.09) | 191 | (0.09) | 3 | 126 |
| Pertussis (whooping cough) | 7,288 | 55 | (2.29) | 109 | (1.01) | 397 | (1.14) | 5,003 | (2.23) | 37 | 1,687 |
| Plague | 9 | 2 | (0.08) | — | (—) | — | (—) | 7 | (0.00) | — | — |
| Psittacosis | 16 | — | (—) | — | (—) | 1 | (0.00) | 11 | (0.01) | — | 4 |
| Rocky Mountain spotted fever | 579 | 9 | (0.39) | 3 | (0.03) | 31 | (0.09) | 449 | (0.20) | — | 87 |
| Rubella | 267 | — | (—) | 3 | (0.03) | 3 | (0.01) | 194 | (0.09) | — | 67 |
| Rubella, congenital syndrome | 9 | — | (—) | 1 | (0.01) | — | (—) | 3 | (0.00) | 1 | 4 |
| Salmonellosis | 40,596 | 264 | (11.01) | 561 | (5.18) | 3,282 | (9.41) | 19,504 | (8.68) | 96 | 16,889 |
| Shigellosis | 17,521 | 220 | (9.18) | 143 | (1.32) | 2,417 | (6.93) | 7,333 | (3.26) | 129 | 7,279 |
| Streptococcal disease, invasive, group A | 2,382 | 56 | (3.57) | 24 | (0.41) | 339 | (1.17) | 1,364 | (0.78) | 2 | 597 |
| *Streptococcus pneumoniae*, drug-resistant, invasive disease | 4,618 | 11 | (0.69) | 24 | (0.29) | 581 | (2.48) | 1,736 | (1.11) | 6 | 2,260 |
| Streptococcal toxic-shock syndrome | 61 | — | (—) | — | (—) | 8 | (0.03) | 48 | (0.03) | — | 5 |
| Syphilis, primary and secondary** | 6,650 | 54 | (2.25) | 41 | (0.38) | 4,854 | (1 3.92) | 1,008 | (0.45) | — | 693[§] |
| Tetanus | 40 | — | (—) | 1 | (0.01) | 3 | (0.01) | 25 | (0.01) | — | 11 |
| Toxic-shock syndrome | 113 | — | (—) | 5 | (0.06) | 3 | (0.01) | 91 | (0.05) | — | 14 |
| Trichinosis | 12 | — | (—) | — | (—) | 1 | (0.00) | 10 | (0.00) | — | 1 |
| Tuberculosis[§§] | 17,531 | 253 | (10.55) | 3,639 | (33.63) | 5,666 | (16.25) | 7,913 | (3.52) | — | 60 |
| Typhoid fever | 346 | — | (—) | 99 | (0.91) | 18 | (0.05) | 65 | (0.03) | 15 | 149 |
| Yellow fever | 1 | — | (—) | — | (—) | — | (—) | 1 | (0.00) | — | — |

* No cases of anthrax, paralytic poliomyelitis, or human rabies were reported in 1999.

[†]Total number of acquired immunodeficiency syndrome (AIDS) cases reported to the Division of HIV/AIDS Prevention—Surveillance and Epidemiology, National Center for HIV, STD, and TB Prevention (NCHSTP), through December 31, 1999.

[§]Includes the following cases originally reported as Hispanic: 7,764 for AIDS; 81,708 for chlamydia; 17,170 for gonorrhea; and 527 for syphilis, primary and secondary.

[¶]Chlamydia refers to genital infections caused by *C. trachomatis.*

** In addition to data collected through the National Electronic Telecommunications System for Surveillance (NETSS), some data concerning ethnicity are collected on aggregate forms different from those used for reported cases. Thus, the total number of cases reported on this table can differ slightly from others. Totals reported to the Division of Sexually Transmitted Diseases Prevention, NCHSTP, as of August 8, 2000.

[††]Totals reported to the National Center for Infectious Diseases as of June 30, 2000.

[§§]Totals reported to the Division of Tuberculosis Elimination, NCHSTP, as of May 3, 2000.

Note: Rates <0.01 after rounding are listed as 0.00.

*Source*: Centers for Disease Control and Prevention. *Summary of Notifiable Diseases, United States, 1999. MMWR* 1999, 48, no. 53. http://www.cdc.gov/mmwr/PDF/wk/mm4853.pdf.

## Table A2.6. Reported Cases and Incidence Rates of Notifiable Diseases,* by Ethnicity, United States, 1999

| Disease | Total | Hispanic No. | Hispanic (Rate) | Non-Hispanic No. | Non-Hispanic (Rate) | Ethnicity not stated |
|---|---|---|---|---|---|---|
| AIDS† | 45,104 | 7,764 | ( 24.78) | 36,682 | ( 15.20) | 658 |
| Botulism, foodborne | 23 | 1 | ( 0.00) | 18 | ( 0.01) | 4 |
| Infant | 92 | 16 | ( 2.22) | 46 | ( 1.48) | 30 |
| Other (includes wound) | 39 | 13 | ( 0.04) | 19 | ( 0.01) | 7 |
| Brucellosis | 82 | 47 | ( 0.15) | 14 | ( 0.01) | 21 |
| Chlamydia§¶ | 655,335 | 81,708 | (260.74) | 365,007 | (151.23) | 208,620 |
| Cholera | 6 | — | ( —) | 4 | ( 0.00) | 2 |
| Cryptosporidiosis | 2,361 | 208 | ( 0.68) | 1,154 | ( 0.51) | 999 |
| Cyclosporiasis | 56 | 5 | ( 0.02) | 29 | ( 0.01) | 22 |
| Diphtheria | 1 | — | ( —) | 1 | ( 0.00) | — |
| Ehrlichiosis | | | | | | |
| Human granulocytic | 203 | 3 | ( 0.01) | 141 | ( 0.08) | 59 |
| Human monocytic | 99 | 3 | ( 0.01) | 67 | ( 0.04) | 29 |
| Encephalitis, California serogroup viral | 70 | — | ( —) | 36 | ( 0.02) | 34 |
| Eastern equine | 5 | — | ( —) | 3 | ( 0.00) | 2 |
| St. Louis | 4 | — | ( —) | 4 | ( 0.00) | — |
| Western equine | 1 | — | ( —) | — | ( 0.00) | 1 |
| *Escherichia coli* 0157:H7 | 4,513 | 110 | ( 0.36) | 1,788 | ( 0.80) | 2,615 |
| Gonorrhea¶ | 359,442 | 17,170 | ( 54.79) | 261,477 | (108.34) | 80,795 |
| *Haemophilus influenzae*, invasive disease | 1,309 | 90 | ( 0.29) | 648 | ( 0.27) | 571 |
| Hansen disease (leprosy) | 108 | 33 | ( 0.11) | 40 | ( 0.02) | 35 |
| Hantavirus pulmonary syndrome** | 33 | 2 | ( 0.01) | 15 | ( 0.01) | 16 |
| Hemolytic uremic syndrome, postdiarrheal | 181 | 18 | ( 0.06) | 117 | ( 0.06) | 46 |
| Hepatitis A | 17,047 | 3,949 | ( 12.60) | 7,243 | ( 3.00) | 5,855 |
| Hepatitis B | 7,694 | 693 | ( 2.21) | 4,030 | ( 1.67) | 2,971 |
| Hepatitis C; non-A, non-B | 3,111 | 23 | ( 0.07) | 111 | ( 0.05) | 2,977 |
| Legionellosis | 1,108 | 25 | ( 0.08) | 591 | ( 0.25) | 492 |
| Lyme disease | 16,273 | 181 | ( 0.58) | 7,613 | ( 3.17) | 8,479 |
| Malaria | 1,666 | 188 | ( 0.60) | 916 | ( 0.38) | 562 |
| Measles | 100 | 11 | ( 0.04) | 84 | ( 0.03) | 5 |
| Meningococcal disease | 2,501 | 227 | ( 0.72) | 1,384 | ( 0.57) | 890 |
| Mumps | 387 | 75 | ( 0.25) | 181 | ( 0.08) | 131 |
| Pertussis (whooping cough) | 7,288 | 935 | ( 2.98) | 4,768 | ( 1.98) | 1,585 |
| Plague | 9 | 1 | ( 0.00) | 7 | ( 0.00) | 1 |
| Psittacosis | 16 | — | ( —) | 7 | ( 0.00) | 9 |
| Rocky Mountain spotted fever | 579 | 7 | ( 0.02) | 378 | ( 0.16) | 194 |
| Rubella | 267 | 183 | ( 0.58) | 53 | ( 0.02) | 31 |
| Rubella, congenital syndrome | 9 | 7 | ( 0.02) | — | ( —) | 2 |
| Salmonellosis | 40,596 | 2,498 | ( 7.97) | 15,684 | ( 6.50) | 22,414 |
| Shigellosis | 17,521 | 2,998 | ( 9.57) | 6,181 | ( 2.56) | 8,342 |
| Streptococcal disease, invasive, group A | 2,382 | 197 | ( 1.00) | 1,135 | ( 0.59) | 1,050 |
| *Streptococcus pneumoniae*, drug-resistant, invasive | 4,618 | 152 | ( 0.57) | 1,636 | ( 1.00) | 2,830 |
| Streptococcal toxic-shock syndrome | 61 | 1 | ( 0.01) | 39 | ( 0.02) | 21 |
| Syphilis, primary and secondary | 6,650 | 527 | ( 1.68) | 5,862 | ( 2.43) | 261 |
| Tetanus | 40 | 14 | ( 0.04) | 22 | ( 0.01) | 4 |
| Toxic-shock syndrome | 113 | 6 | ( 0.02) | 59 | ( 0.03) | 48 |
| Trichinosis | 12 | 1 | ( 0.00) | 10 | ( 0.00) | 1 |
| Tuberculosis†† | 17,531 | 3,875 | ( 12.37) | 13,621 | ( 5.64) | 35 |
| Typhoid fever | 346 | 69 | ( 0.22) | 130 | ( 0.05) | 147 |
| Yellow fever | 1 | — | ( —) | 1 | ( 0.00) | — |

* No cases of anthrax, paralytic poliomyelitis, or human rabies were reported in 1999.

†Total number of acquired immunodeficiency syndrome (AIDS) cases reported to the Division of HIV/AIDS Prevention—Surveillance and Epidemiology, National Center for HIV, STD, and TB Prevention (NCHSTP), through December 31, 1999.

§Chlamydia refers to genital infections caused by *C. trachomatis.*

¶In addition to data collected through the National Electronic Telecommunications System for Surveillance (NETSS), some data concerning ethnicity are collected on aggregate forms different from those used for reported cases. Thus, the total number of cases reported on this table can differ slightly from others. Totals reported to the Division of Sexually Transmitted Diseases Prevention, NCHSTP, as of August 8, 2000.

** Totals reported to the National Center for Infectious Diseases as of June 30, 2000.

††Totals reported to the Division of Tuberculosis Elimination, NCHSTP, as of May 3, 2000.

Note: Rates <0.01 after rounding are listed as 0.00.

*Source*: Centers for Disease Control and Prevention. *Summary of Notifiable Diseases, United States, 1999. MMWR* 1999, 48, no. 53. http://www.cdc.gov/mmwr/PDF/wk/mm4853.pdf.

## Table A3.1. Cholera—Reported Cases, United States and Territories, 1999

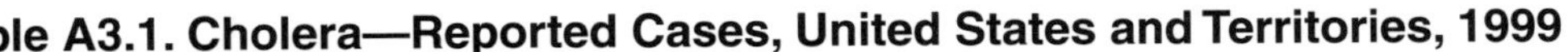

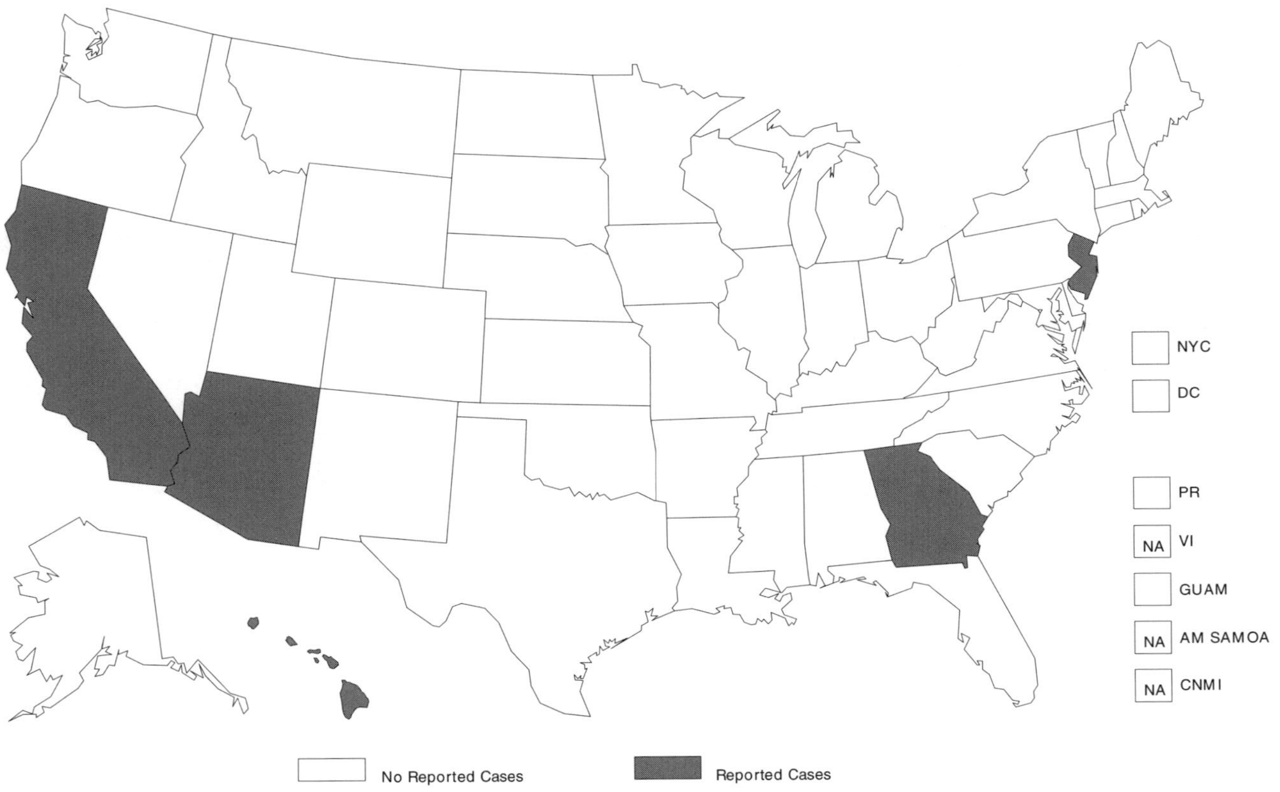

*Source*: Centers for Disease Control and Prevention. *Summary of Notifiable Diseases, United States, 1999. MMWR* 1999, 48, no. 53. http://www.cdc.gov/mmwr/PDF/wk/mm4853.pdf.

## Table A3.2. Diptheria—Reported Cases by Year, United States, 1969–1999

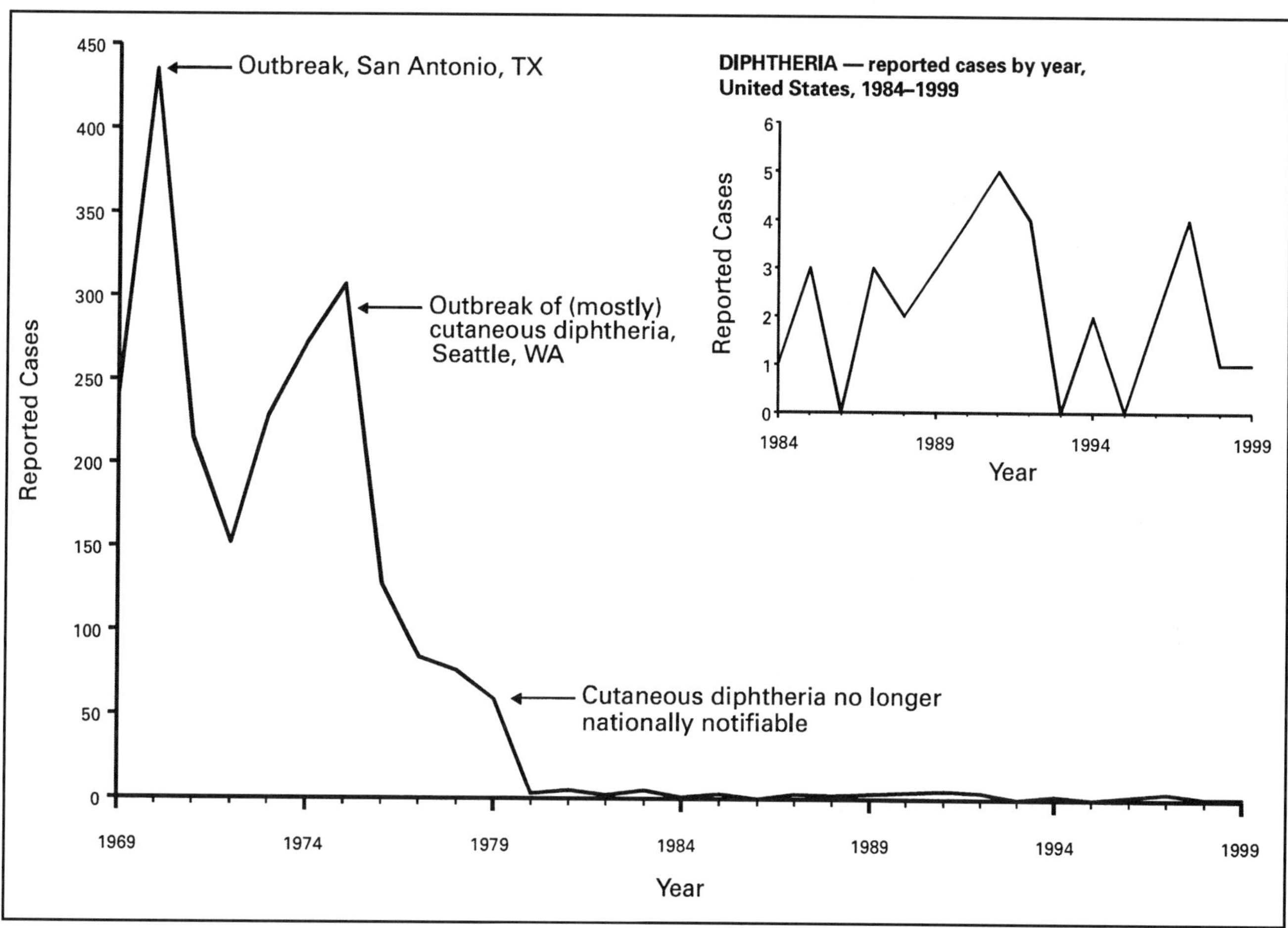


*Source*: Centers for Disease Control and Prevention. *Summary of Notifiable Diseases, United States, 1999. MMWR* 1999, 48, no. 53. http://www.cdc.gov/mmwr/PDF/wk/mm4853.pdf.

**Table A3.3. *Haemophilus Influenzae*, Invasive Disease—Reported Cases per 100,000 Population by Age Group, United States, 1991–1999**

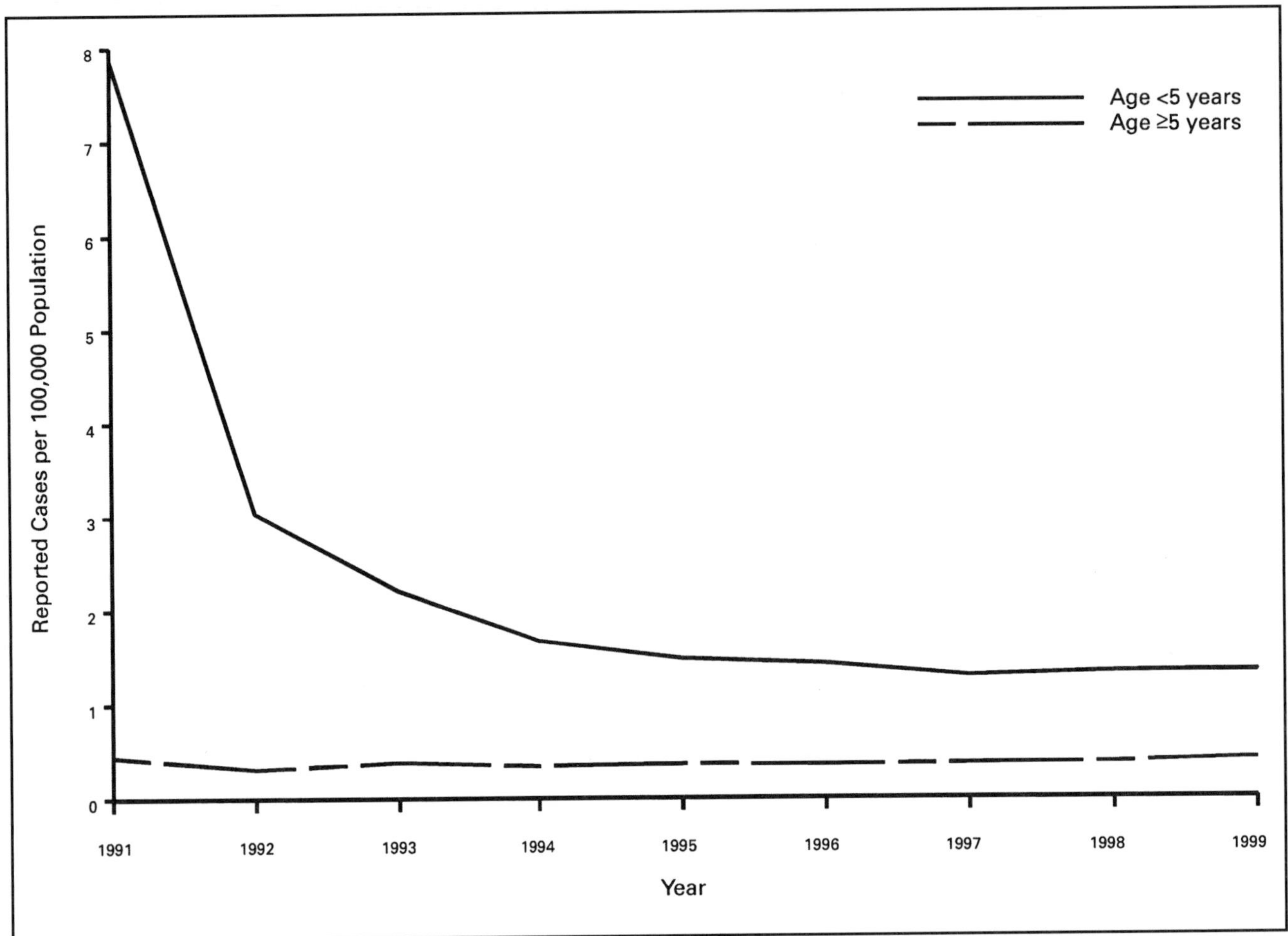


*Source*: Centers for Disease Control and Prevention. *Summary of Notifiable Diseases, United States, 1999. MMWR* 1999, 48, no. 53. http://www.cdc.gov/mmwr/PDF/wk/mm4853.pdf.

**Table A3.4. Hansen Disease (Leprosy)—Reported Cases by Year, United States, 1969–1999**

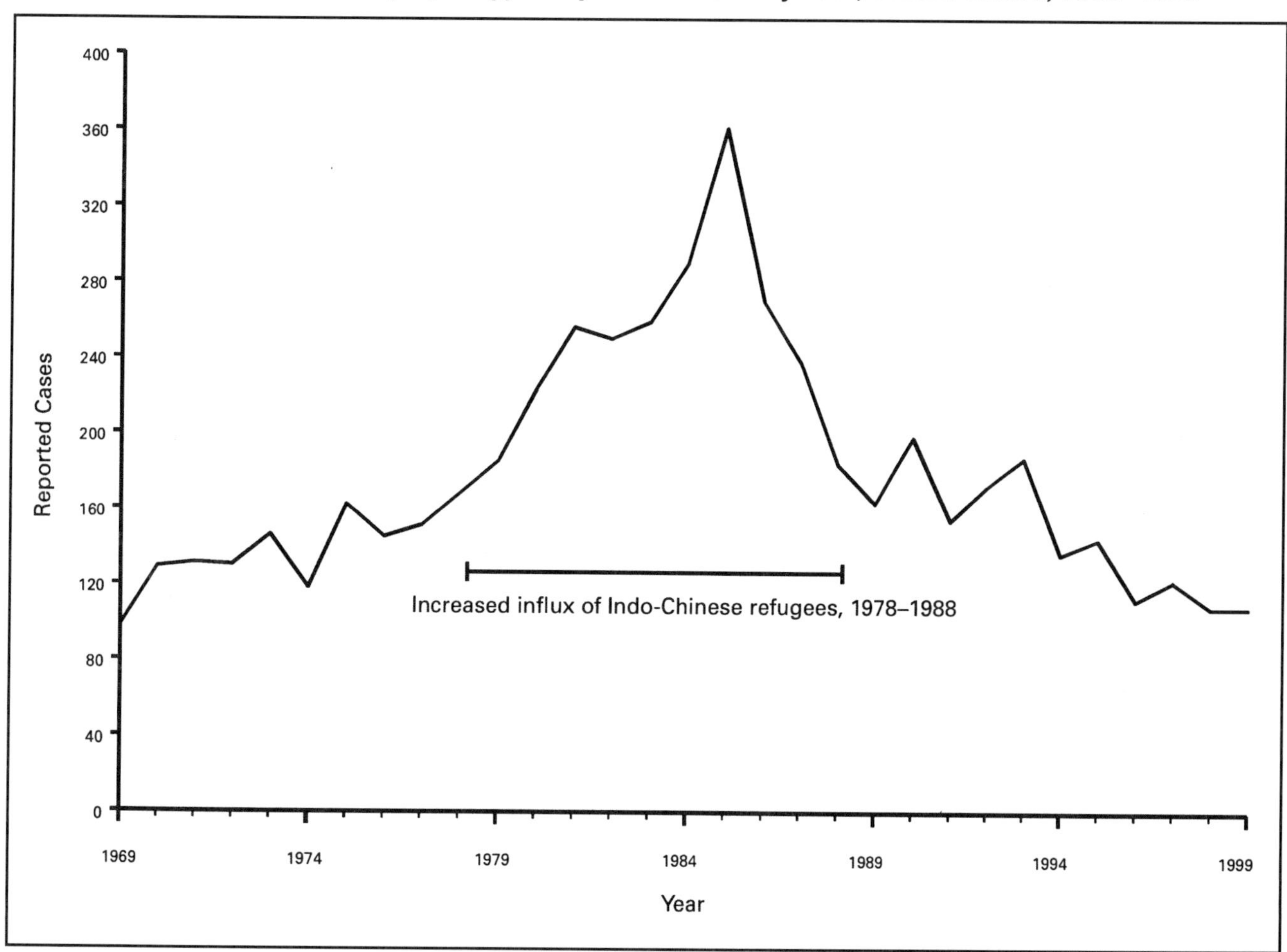


*Source*: Centers for Disease Control and Prevention. *Summary of Notifiable Diseases, United States, 1999. MMWR* 1999, 48, no. 53. http://www.cdc.gov/mmwr/PDF/wk/mm4853.pdf.

## Table A3.5. Hepatitis—Reported Cases per 100,000 Population by Year, United States, 1969–1999

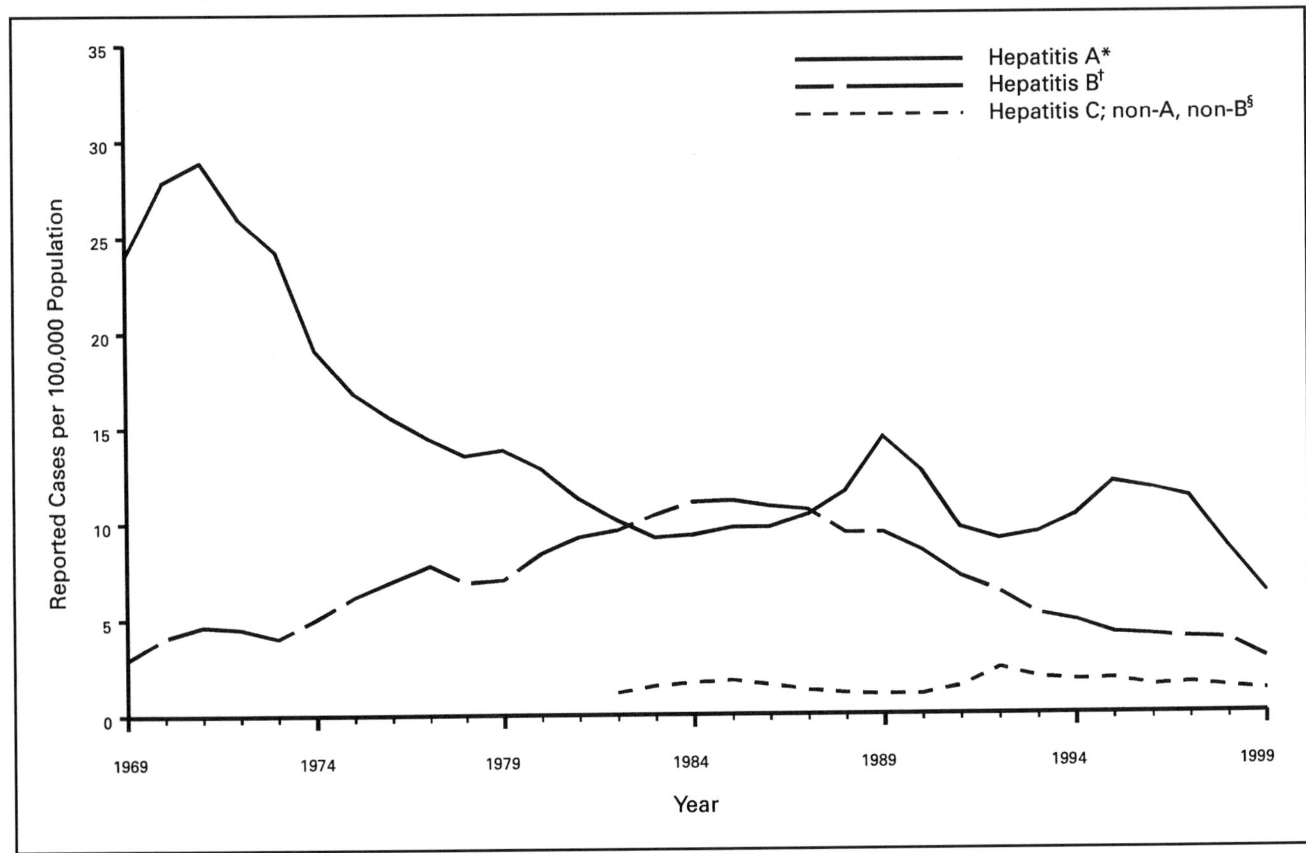


* Hepatitis A vaccine was first licensed in 1995.

†Hepatitis B vaccine was first licensed in 1982.

§An anti-HCV (hepatitis C virus) antibody test first became available in 1990.

*Source*: Centers for Disease Control and Prevention. *Summary of Notifiable Diseases, United States, 1999. MMWR* 1999, 48, no. 53. http://www.cdc.gov/mmwr/PDF/wk/mm4853.pdf.

**Table A3.6. Hepatitis A—Reported Cases per 100,000 Population, United States and Territories, 1999**

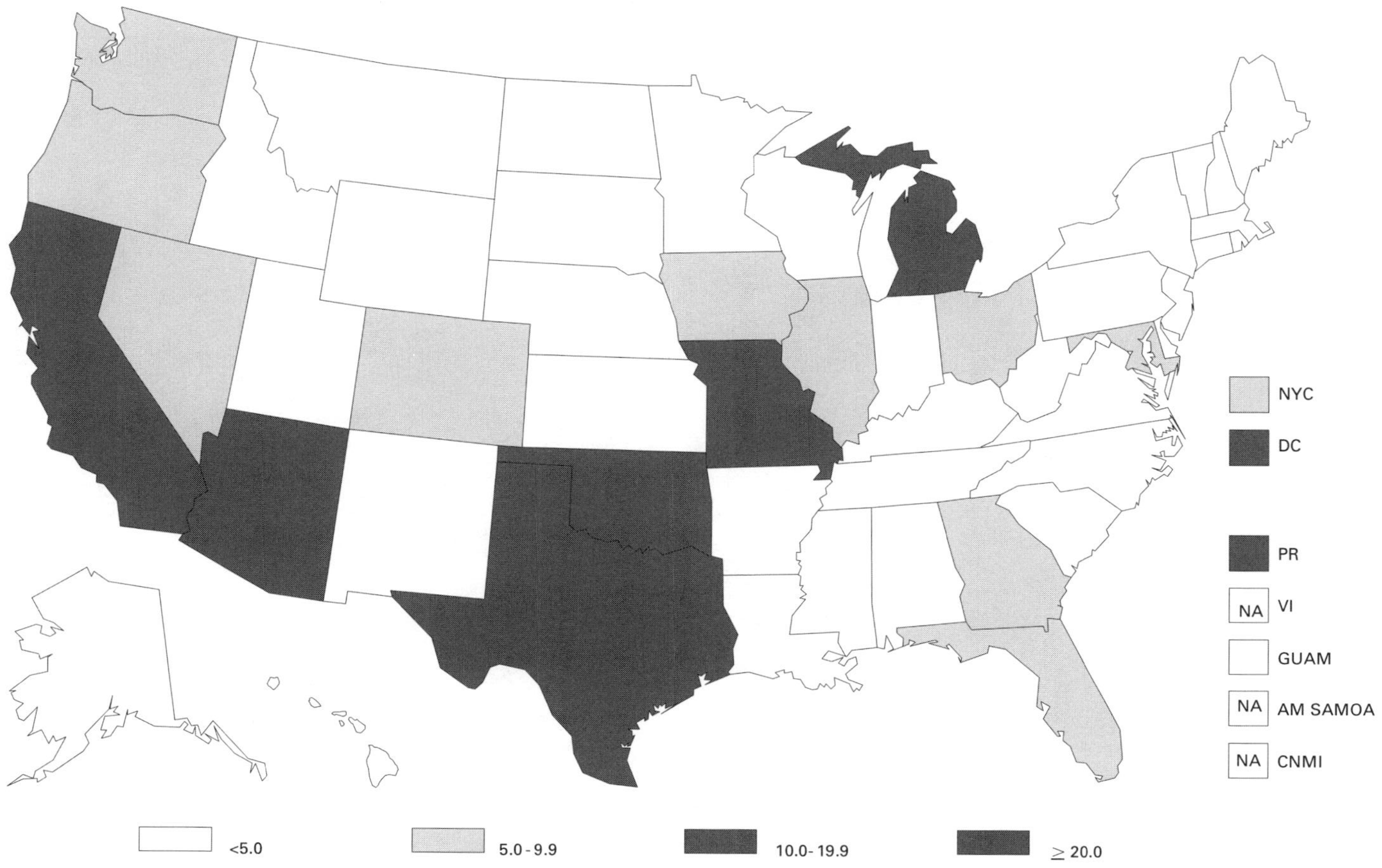

NYC
DC
PR
NA VI
GUAM
NA AM SAMOA
NA CNMI

<5.0
5.0 - 9.9
10.0 - 19.9
≥ 20.0

*Source*: Centers for Disease Control and Prevention. *Summary of Notifiable Diseases, United States, 1999. MMWR* 1999, 48, no. 53. http://www.cdc.gov/mmwr/PDF/wk/mm4853.pdf.

## Table A3.7. Lyme Disease—Reported Cases* by County, United States, 1998

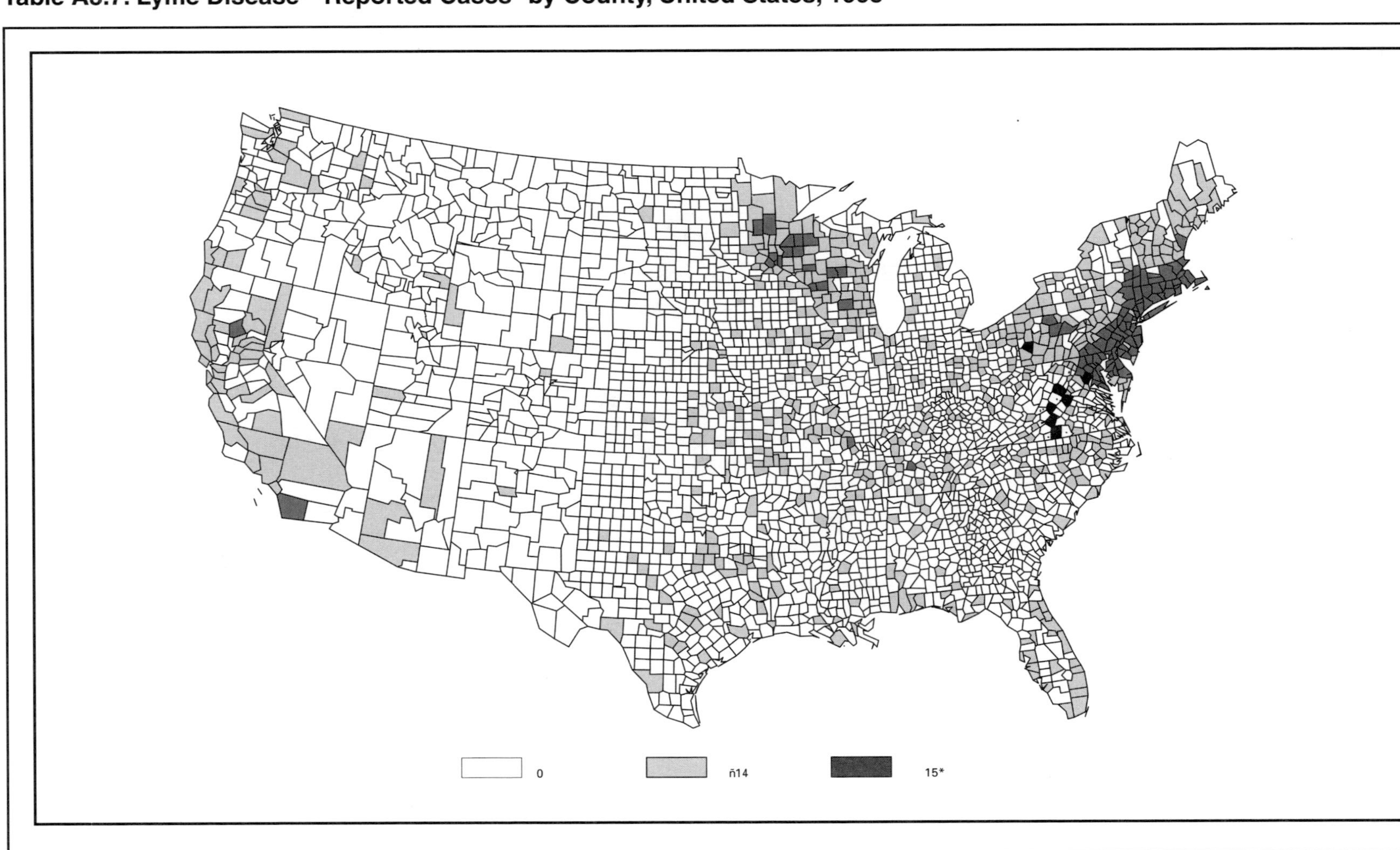


* One case=one dot randomly placed in the patient's county of residence.

In 1998, a total of 16,801 cases of Lyme Disease were reported, the highest number of cases ever reported. In December 1998, a new Lyme disease vaccine was approved by the U.S. Food and Drug Administration. The Advisory Committee on Immunization Practices (ACIP) issued recommendations for the use of this vaccine in June 1999 (*MMWR* 1999; 48[RR-7]).

*Source*: Centers for Disease Control and Prevention. *Summary of Notifiable Diseases, United States, 1999. MMWR* 1999, 48, no. 53. http://www.cdc.gov/mmwr/PDF/wk/mm4853.pdf.

**Table A3.8. Measles (Rubeola)—Reported Cases (Thousands) by Year, United States, 1964–1999**

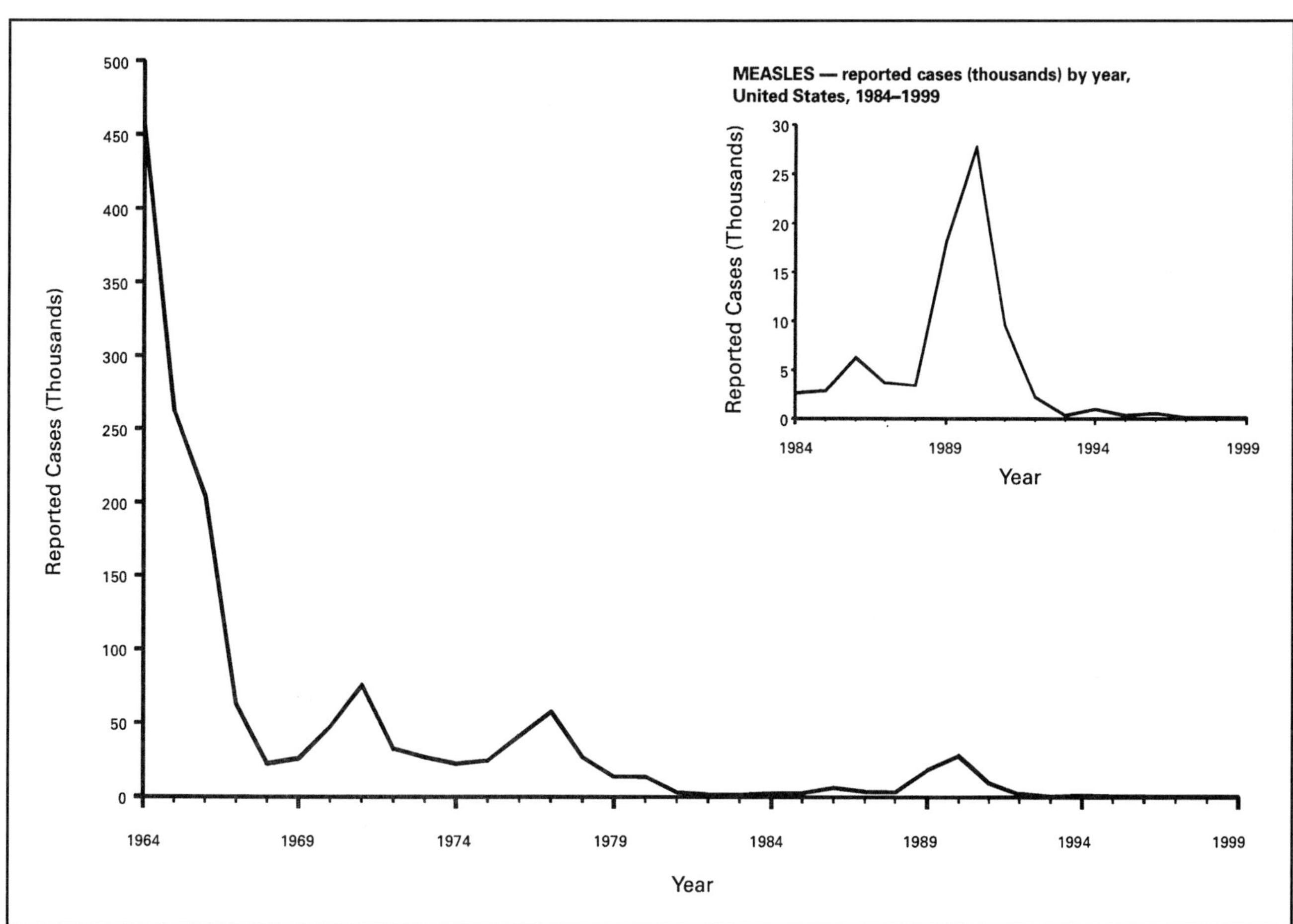


Measles incidence remained at <1 case/1,000,000 population for the third consecutive year; with 100 cases reported in 1999. Of these cases, 66% were imported from outside the United States. Measles is not currently endemic in this country.

*Source*: Centers for Disease Control and Prevention. *Summary of Notifiable Diseases, United States, 1999. MMWR* 1999, 48, no. 53. http://www.cdc.gov/mmwr/PDF/wk/mm4853.pdf.

**Table A3.9. Meningococcal Disease—Reported Cases per 100,000 Population by Year, United States, 1969–1999**

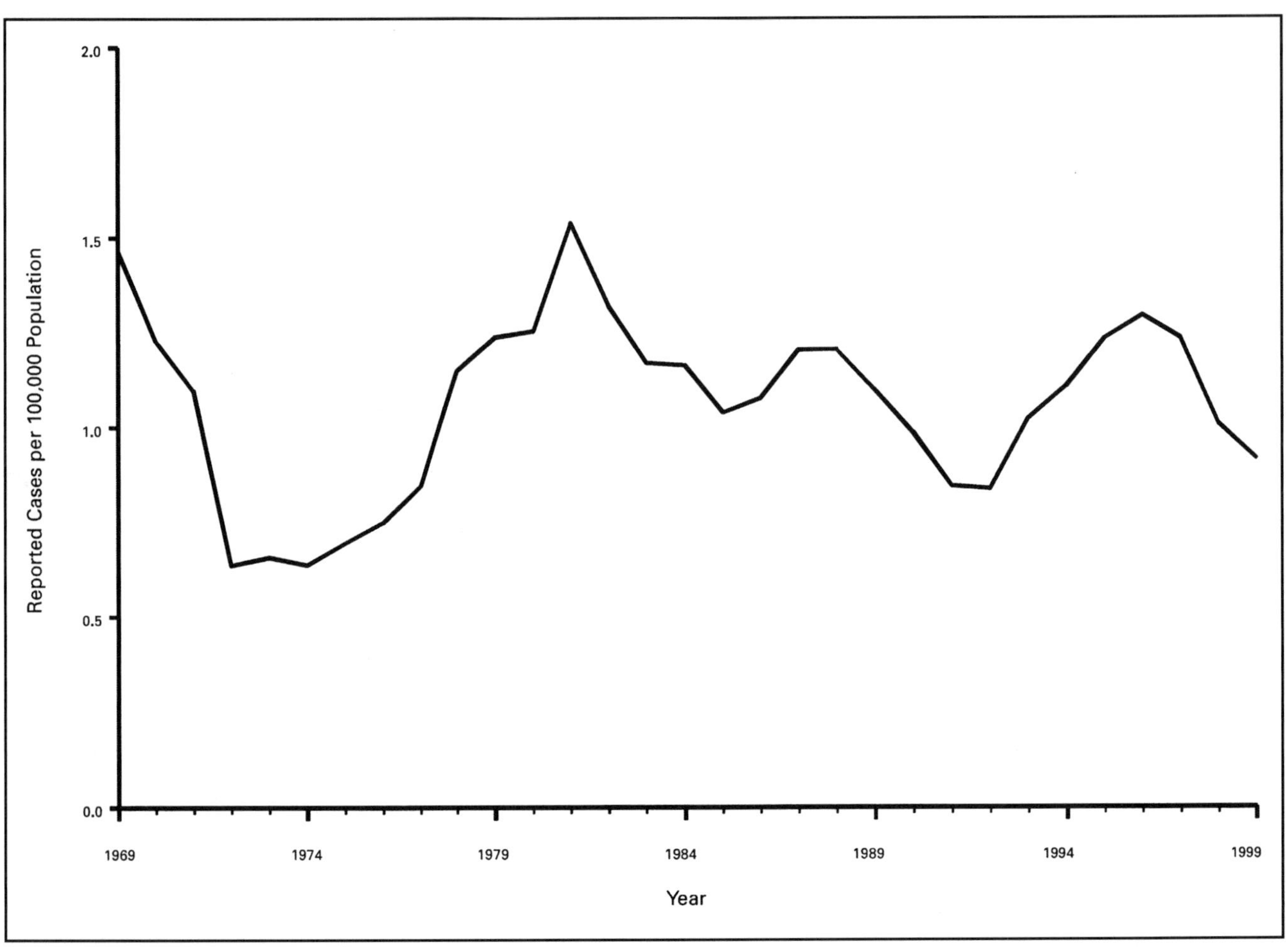


Meningococcal disease rates have remained stable since the 1960s, with 2,501 cases reported in 1999. However, case fatality rates remain high; of the 1,091 patients with outcome reported in 1999, a total of 12.5% died. Serogroup information was reported for 36.7% of cases, with serogroups B, C, and Y each accounting for approximately one-third of these cases.

*Source*: Centers for Disease Control and Prevention. *Summary of Notifiable Diseases, United States, 1999. MMWR* 1999, 48, no. 53. http://www.cdc.gov/mmwr/PDF/wk/mm4853.pdf.

## Table A3.10. Mumps—Reported Cases per 100,000 Population by Year, United States, 1974–1999

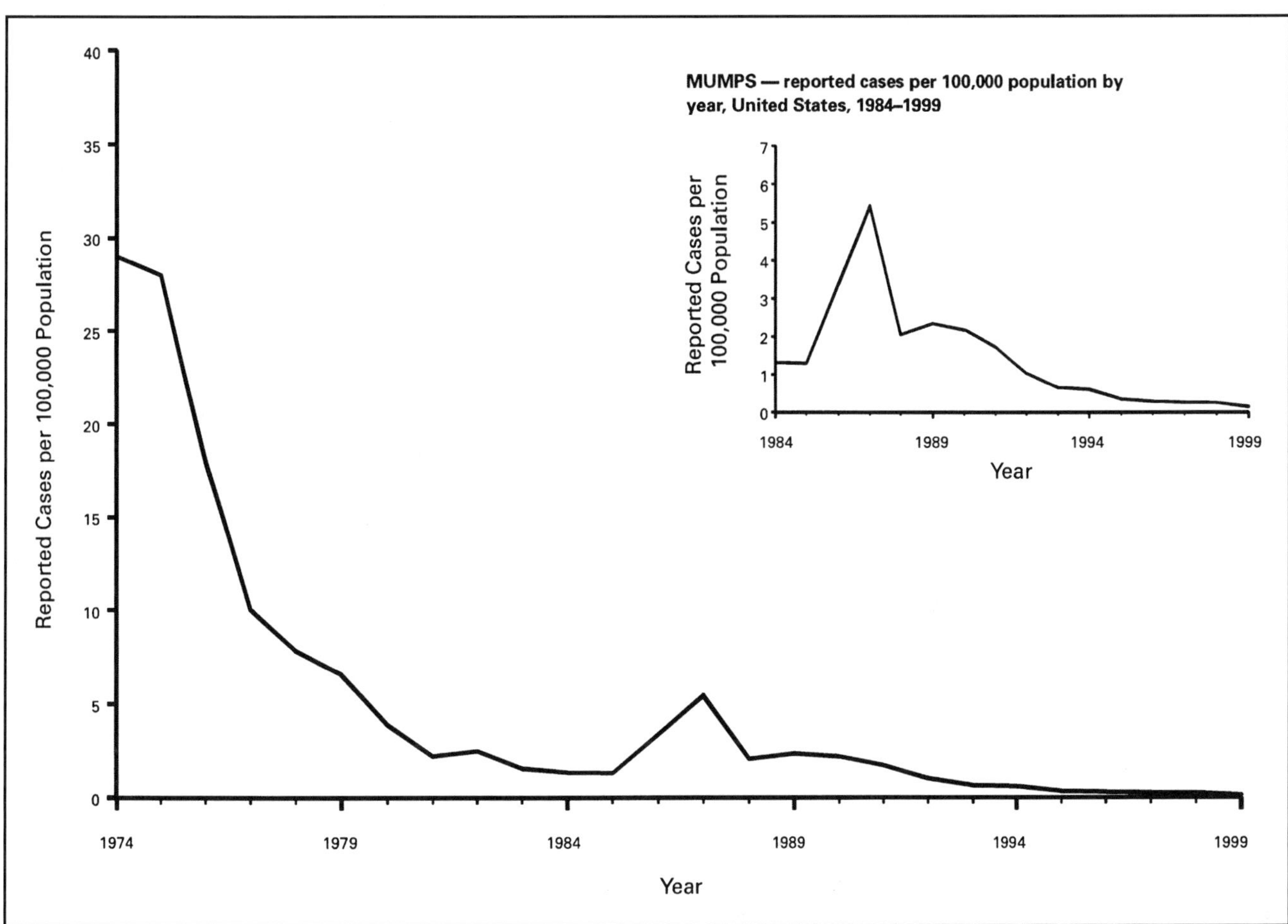


In 1999, a record low of 387 mumps cases were reported, meeting the *Healthy People 2000* objective of 500 cases per year.

*Source*: Centers for Disease Control and Prevention. *Summary of Notifiable Diseases, United States, 1999. MMWR* 1999, 48, no. 53. http://www.cdc.gov/mmwr/PDF/wk/mm4853.pdf.

## Table A3.11. Pertussis (Whooping Cough)—Reported Cases per 100,000 Population by Year, United States, 1969–1999

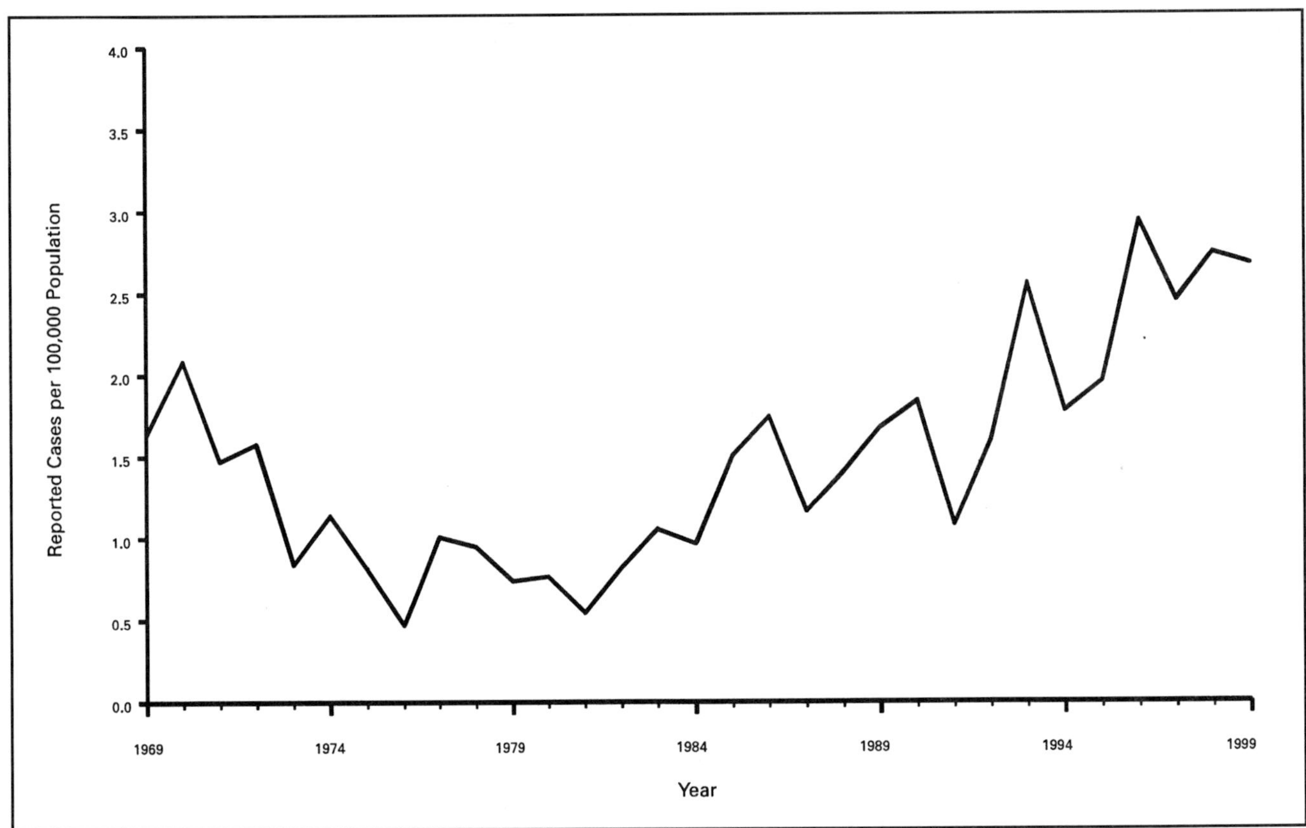


Pertussis epidemics occur every 3-4 years. In 1996, the highest number of pertussis cases (7,796) since 1967 was reported (incidence: 2.9 cases/100,000 population). Since 1993, the number of cases reported after each epidemic year has not returned to the baseline of the pre-epidemic year.

Note: A pertussis vaccine was first licensed in 1949.

*Source*: Centers for Disease Control and Prevention. *Summary of Notifiable Diseases, United States, 1999. MMWR* 1999, 48, no. 53. http://www.cdc.gov/mmwr/PDF/wk/mm4853.pdf.

## Table A3.12. Pertussis (Whooping Cough)—Reported Cases by Age Group, United States, 1999

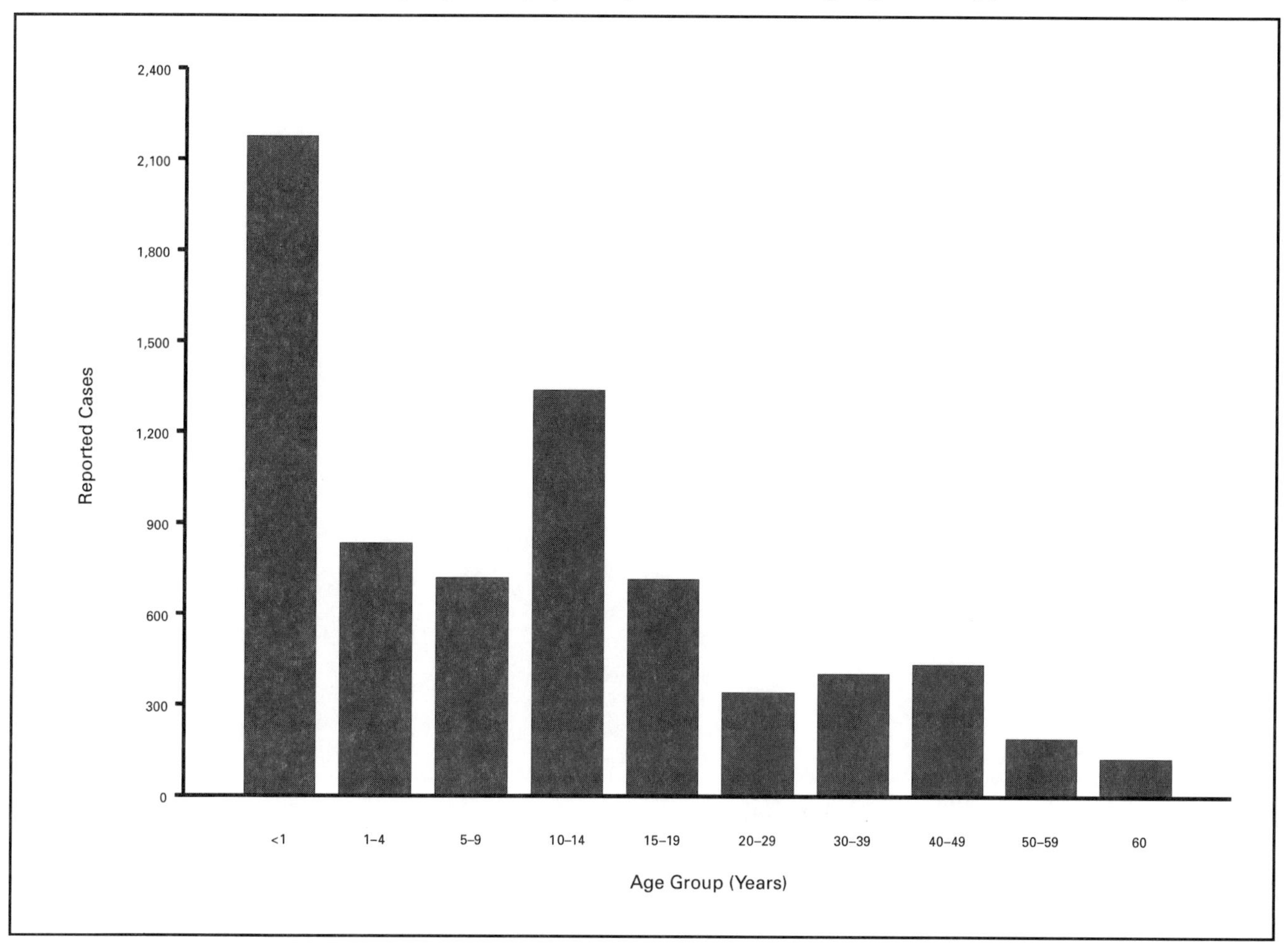


Most reported cases of pertussis continue to occur among children aged <1 year, but cases among adolescents and adults are increasingly reported to CDC. In 1999, a total of 49% of all reported cases occurred among persons aged >10 years. the proportion of reported cases among persons aged >10 years was 24% during 1990–1992, 29% during 1993–1995, and 46% during 1996–1999

*Source*: Centers for Disease Control and Prevention. *Summary of Notifiable Diseases, United States, 1999. MMWR* 1999, 48, no. 53. http://www.cdc.gov/mmwr/PDF/wk/mm4853.pdf.

## Table A3.13. Plague—Among Humans, by Year, United States, 1969–1999

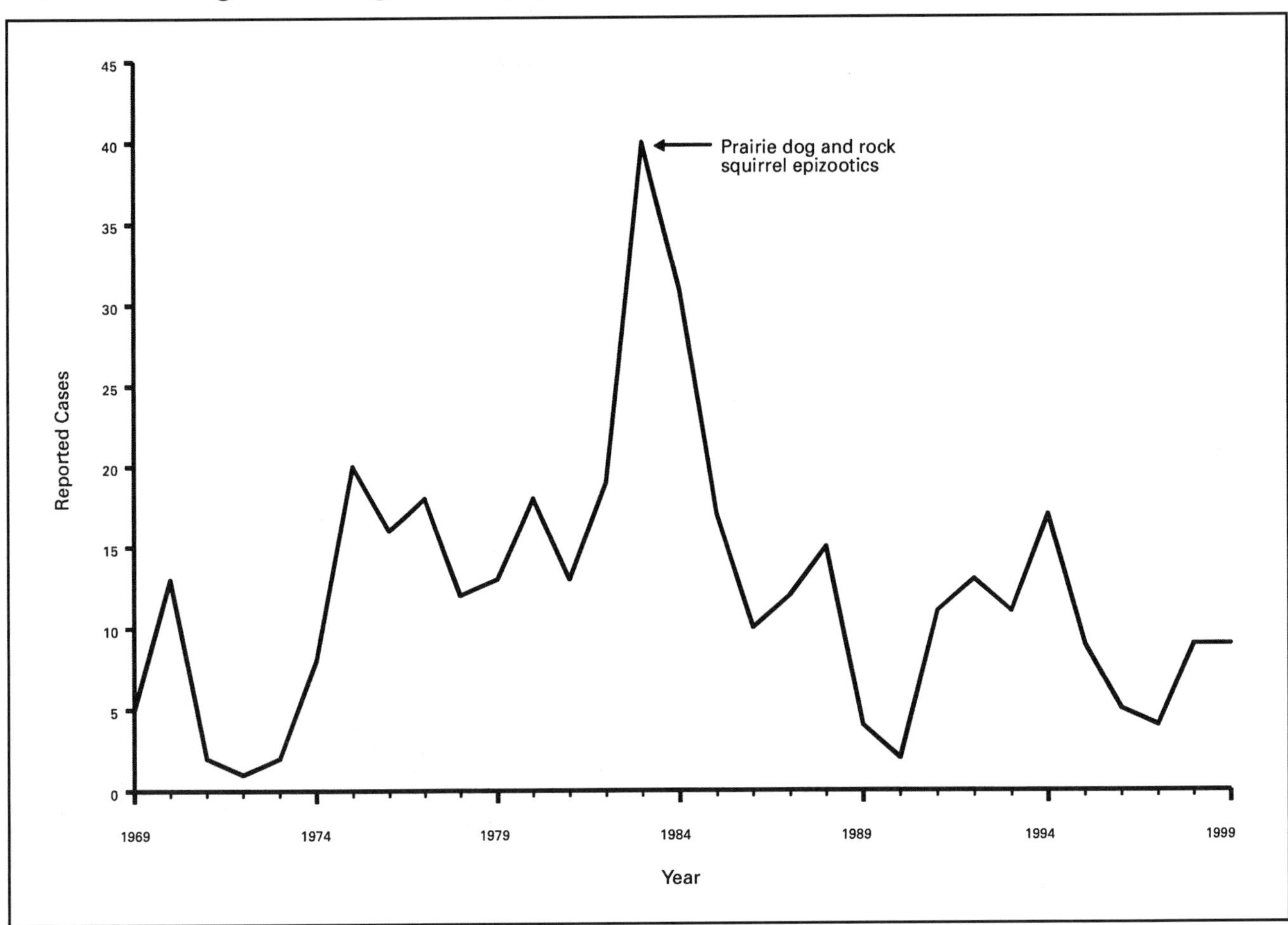


In 1999, nine laboratory-confirmed cases (one fatal) of human plague were identified (three in Colorado and six in New Mexico). All cases were naturally acquired from handling infected animals or being bitten by infectious wild rodent fleas.

*Source*: Centers for Disease Control and Prevention. *Summary of Notifiable Diseases, United States, 1999. MMWR* 1999, 48, no. 53. http://www.cdc.gov/mmwr/PDF/wk/mm4853.pdf.

**Table A3.14. Poliomyelitis (Paralytic)—Reported Cases by Year, United States, 1969–1999**

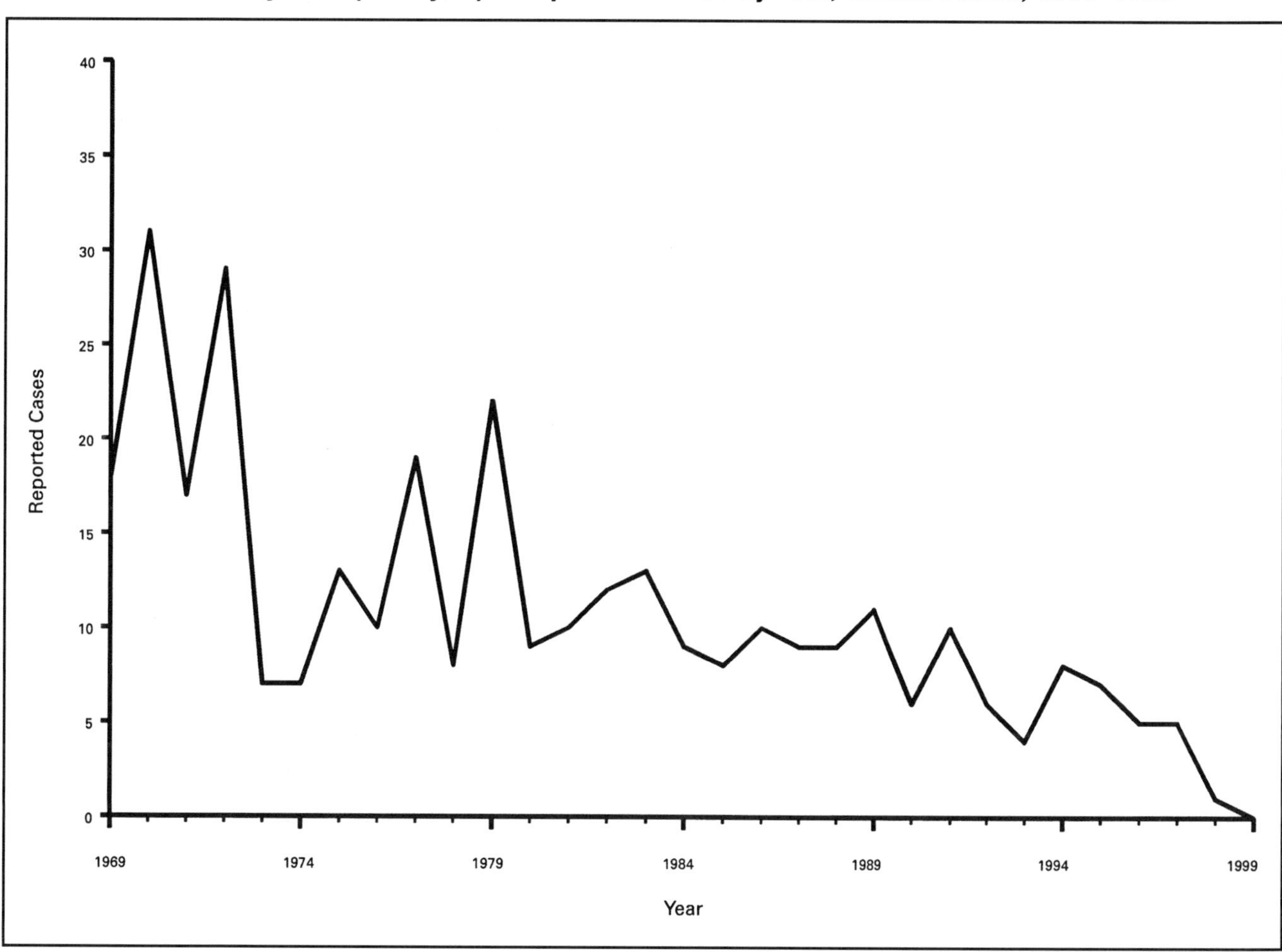


Data suggest a decline in vaccine-associated paralytic polio (VAPP) since the introduction of a sequential immunization schedule with inactivated poliovirus vaccine (IPV) and live, attenuated oral poliovirus vaccine (OPV) in 1997. This trend is expected to continue with the all-IPV schedule initiated in January 2000. Continued monitoring with additional observation time is required to confirm these preliminary findings because of potential delays in reporting.
*Source*: Centers for Disease Control and Prevention. *Summary of Notifiable Diseases, United States, 1999. MMWR* 1999, 48, no. 53. http://www.cdc.gov/mmwr/PDF/wk/mm4853.pdf.

## Table A3.15. Rabies—Reported Wild and Domestic Animals, by Year* United States and Puerto Rico, 1969–1999

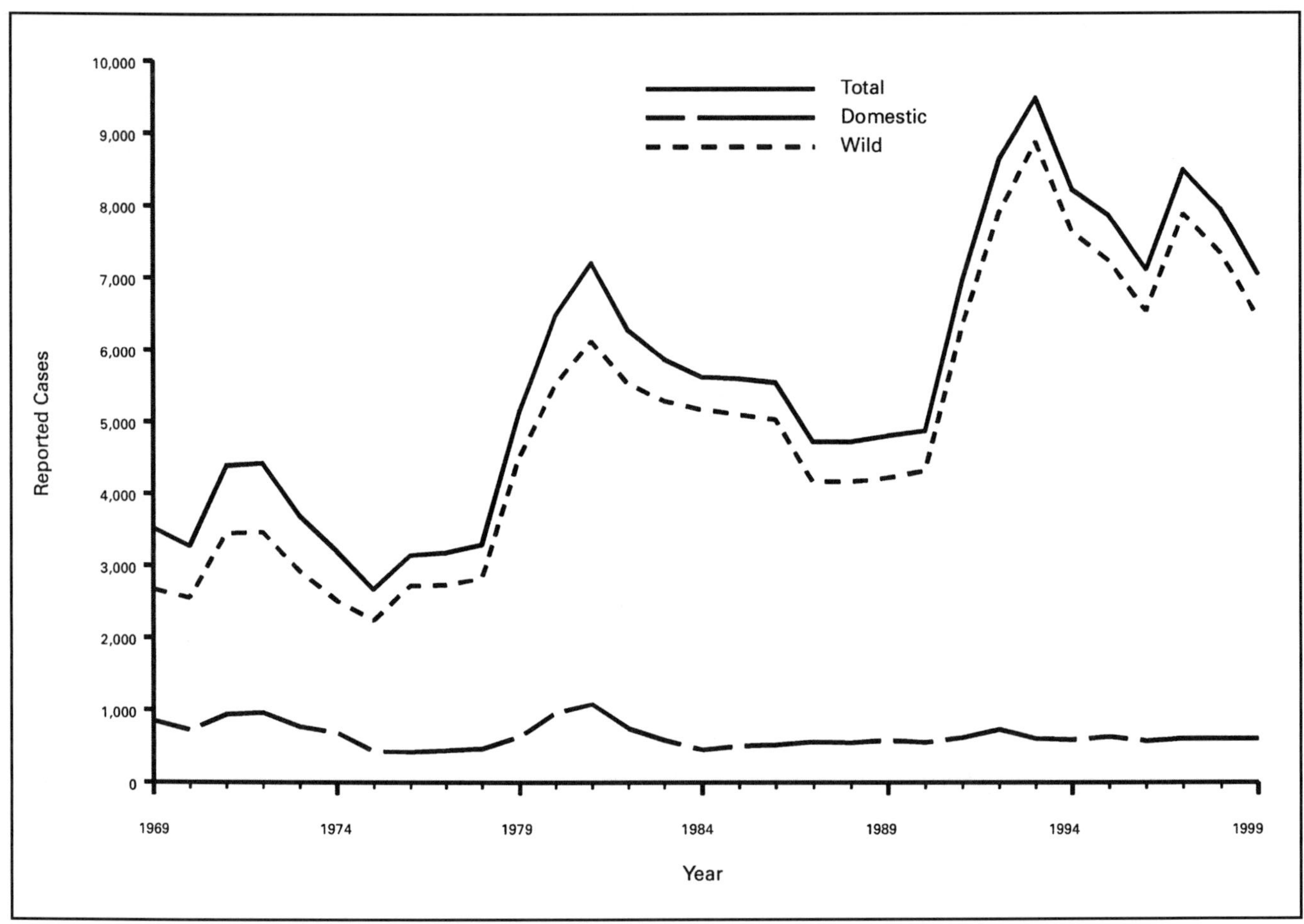


*Data from the National Center for Infectious Diseases.

Periods of resurgence and decline of rabies incidence are primarily the result of cyclic reemergence, mainly among raccoons in the eastern United States. Wildlife populations increase and reach densities sufficient to support epizootic transmission of the disease, resulting in substantial increases in reported cases. As populations are decimated by these epizootics, numbers of reported cases decline until populations again reach levels to support epizootic transmission of the disease.

*Source*: Centers for Disease Control and Prevention. *Summary of Notifiable Diseases, United States, 1999. MMWR* 1999, 48, no. 53. http://www.cdc.gov/mmwr/PDF/wk/mm4853.pdf.

**Table A3.16. Rubella (German Measles)—Reported Cases per 100,000 Population by Year, United States, 1969–1999**

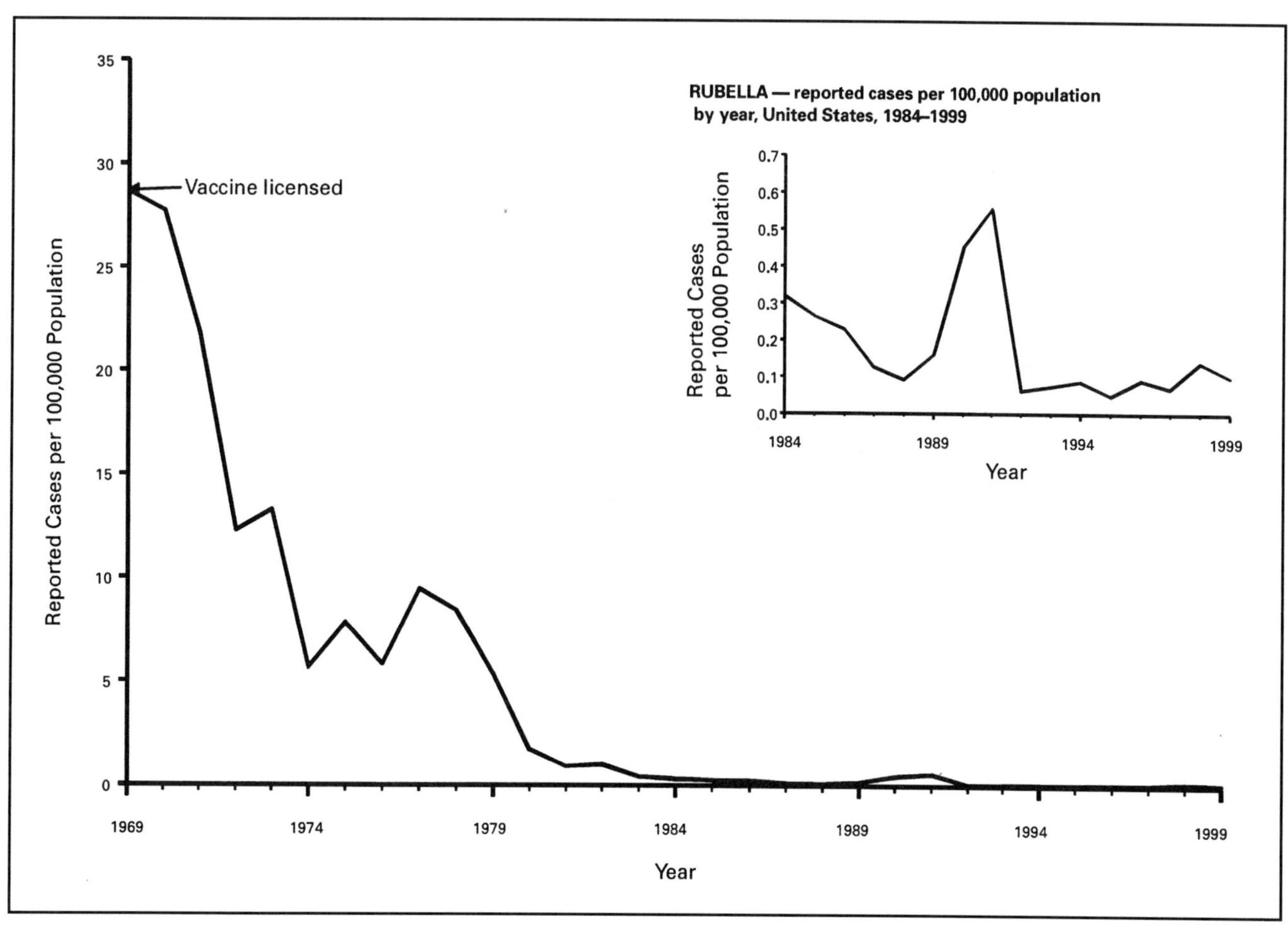


Since 1992, the incidence of rubella has continued to be low. In 1999, approximately 75% of cases occurred among Hispanics aged >15 years.

*Source*: Centers for Disease Control and Prevention. *Summary of Notifiable Diseases, United States, 1999. MMWR* 1999, 48, no. 53. http://www.cdc.gov/mmwr/PDF/wk/mm4853.pdf.

## Table A3.17. Tetanus—Reported Cases by Year, United States, 1969–1999

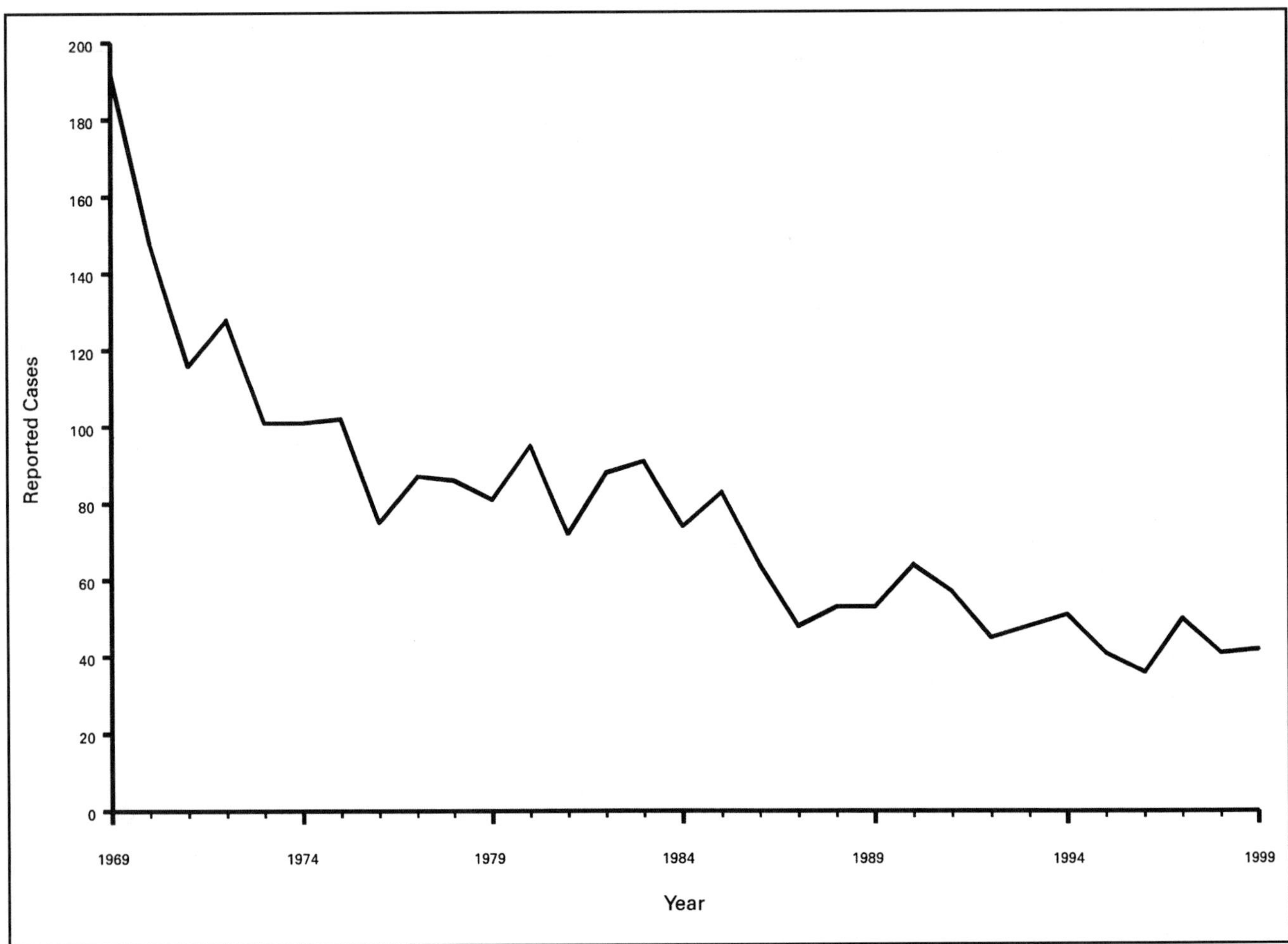


In 1999, a total of 40 cases of tetanus was reported. A shift has occurred in the age distribution of cases, with the percentage of cases among persons aged 25–59 years increasing in the past decade.

*Source*: Centers for Disease Control and Prevention. *Summary of Notifiable Diseases, United States, 1999. MMWR* 1999, 48, no. 53. http://www.cdc.gov/mmwr/PDF/wk/mm4853.pdf.

## Table A3.18. Typhoid Fever—Reported Cases by Year, United States, 1969–1999

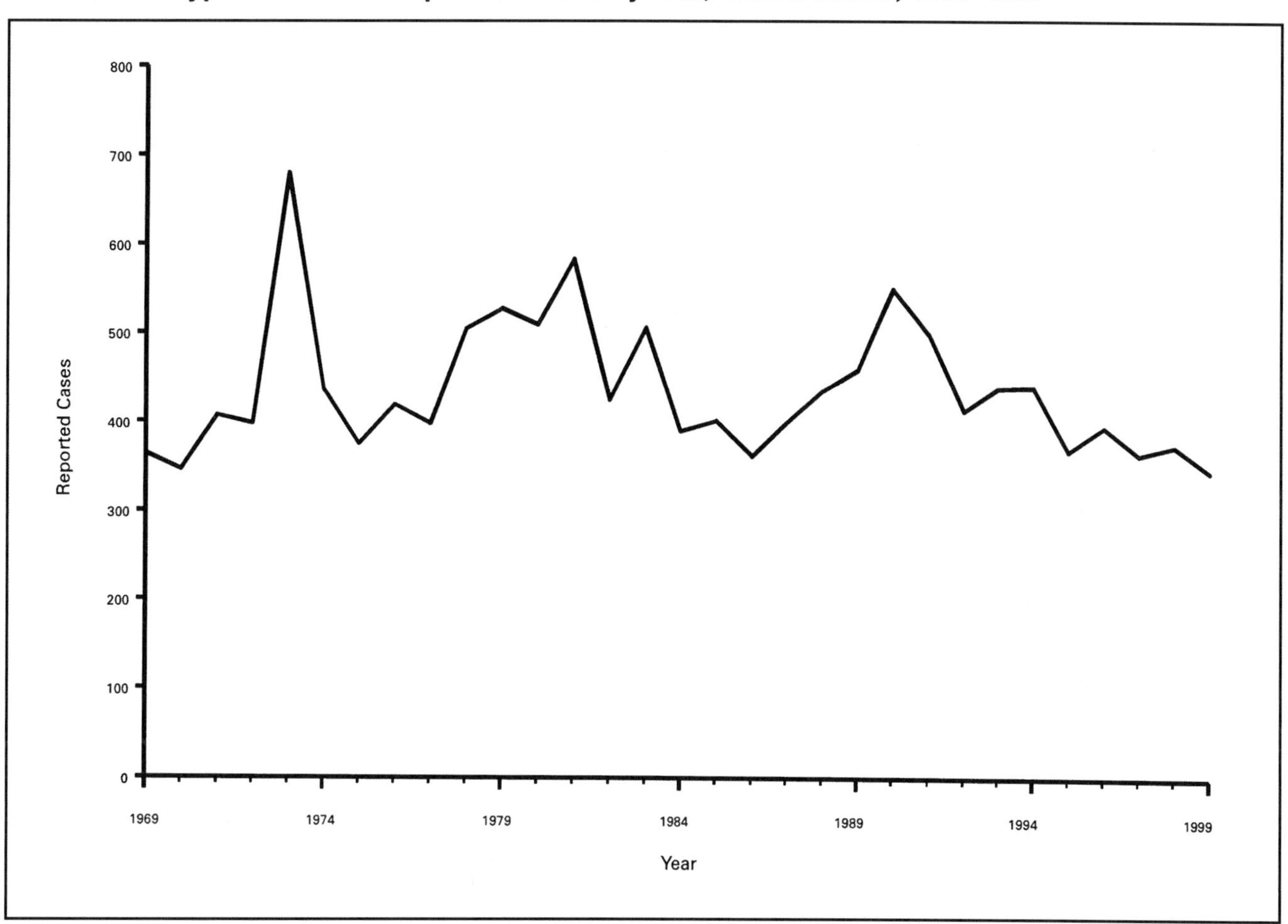


The recent discontinuation of a licensed typhoid fever vaccine and shortages of a second vaccine could cause an increase in preventable cases of typhoid fever among persons traveling internationally.

*Source*: Centers for Disease Control and Prevention. *Summary of Notifiable Diseases, United States, 1999. MMWR* 1999, 48, no. 53. http://www.cdc.gov/mmwr/PDF/wk/mm4853.pdf.

**Table A3.19. Varicella (Chickenpox)—Reported Cases* from Selected U.S. States (n = 7), 1990–1999**

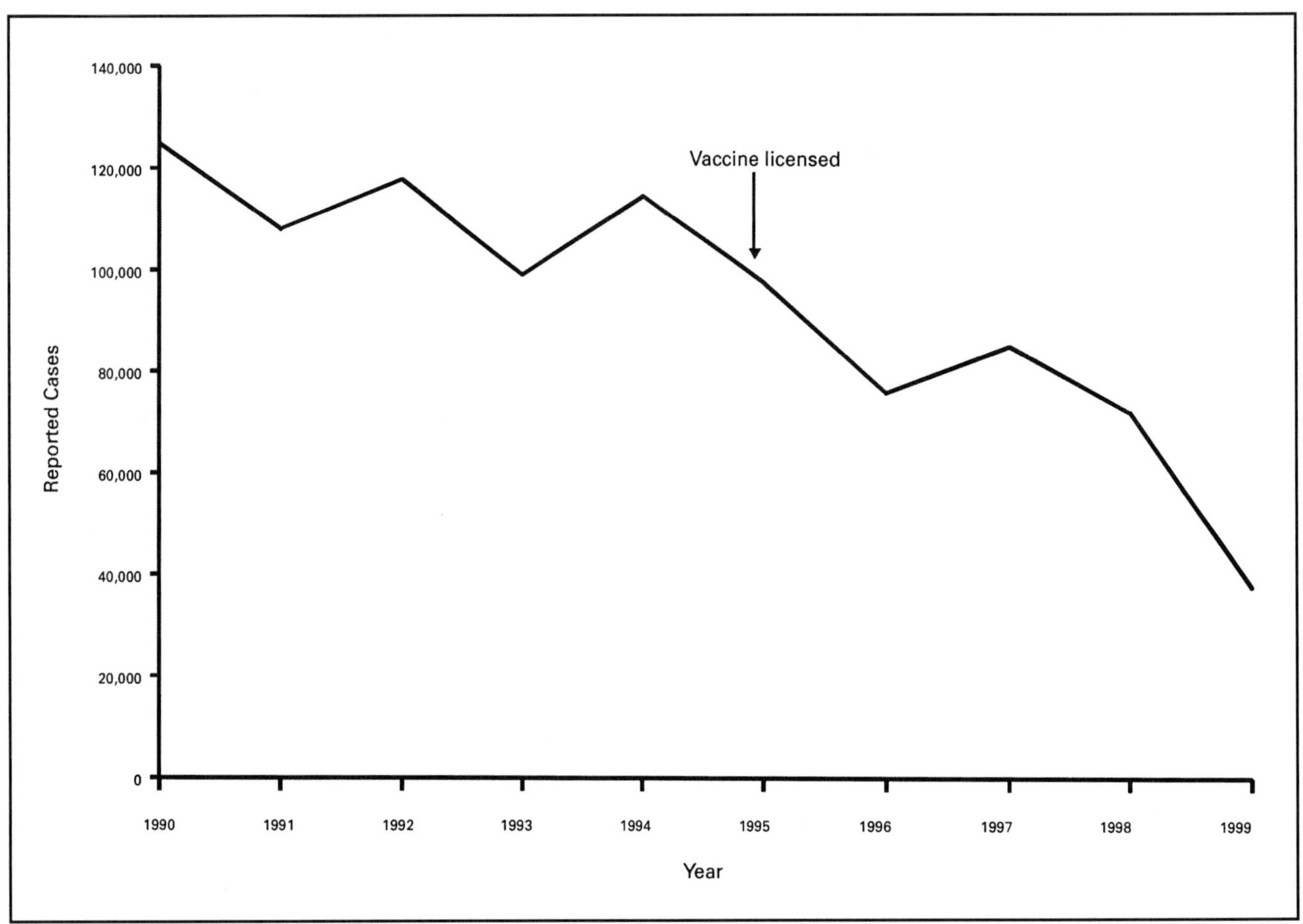


*Illinois, Massachusetts, Michigan, Missouri, Rhode Island, Texas, and West Virginia maintained adequate reporting by reporting cases constituting >5% of their birth cohort during 1990–1995 (National Immunization Program).

*Source*: Centers for Disease Control and Prevention. *Summary of Notifiable Diseases, United States, 1999. MMWR* 1999, 48, no. 53. http://www.cdc.gov/mmwr/PDF/wk/mm4853.pdf.

# B. Human Immunodeficiency Virus (HIV) and Acquired Immunodeficiency Syndrome (AIDS)

## OVERVIEW

Since the first cases of acquired immunodeficiency syndrome (AIDS) were identified in 1981[1] and since the human immunodeficiency virus (HIV) was recognized as the etiologic agent in 1984, great strides have been made in understanding both AIDS and HIV infection, their clinical outcomes, and their epidemiology. Progress has been made on many fronts. Today we have a clear understanding of the principal determinants of HIV transmission and of diverse behavioral and biomedical interventions for combating HIV. Recently introduced therapies have reduced illness, disability, and death due to HIV/AIDS. Some therapeutic agents slow replication of the virus and give hope to people infected with HIV. Other drugs are successful in the treatment and prevention of some opportunistic infections associated with AIDS. New prevention and control strategies have been developed that target the epidemic in minority populations. Still others under development seek to address the challenges presented by the multiplicity of linguistic, cultural, racial, and ethnic groups impacted by HIV/AIDS. Prospects for the availability of a safe and effective HIV vaccine continue to increase. Vaccine development for both infected and uninfected people is a high priority.

Nonetheless, today HIV and AIDS remain multifaceted national and international problems of considerable magnitude. HIV and AIDS continue to constitute growing threats to the health of the United States and will continue to make major demands on health and social service systems for many decades. Currently, HIV/AIDS has been reported in virtually every racial and ethnic population, every age group, and every socioeconomic group in every state and most large cities in the United States.[2] Initially identified on the East and West Coasts among men who have sex with men,[3] the AIDS epidemic is composed of diverse multiple subepidemics (the morbidity that occurs within a portion of the population infected by the epidemic) that vary by region and community. The HIV/AIDS subepidemics not only vary by region and community but also may vary by population, risk behavior, and geography.

In the United States, HIV/AIDS remains a significant cause of illness, disability, and death, despite declines in 1996 and 1997.[4] Estimates of the number of people infected with HIV in the United States range from 800,000 to 900,000.[5] The numbers, as well as the estimates, are staggering—and sobering. As of December 31, 2000, CDC had received reports of 774,467 persons with AIDS in the United States; 448,060 (58%) are known to have died. As persons with AIDS are surviving longer, they are contributing to steady increases in the number of persons living with AIDS. Through December 2000 there were 450,151 persons reported to the CDC as living with HIV infection or with AIDS. These reports include only persons diagnosed with HIV infection in states with integrated HIV/AIDS surveillance systems and persons diagnosed with AIDS in all states and territories. In 1999, CDC estimated 800,000 to 900,000 persons in the United States were living with HIV or AIDS. Note, too, totals of AIDS cases and deaths diagnosed before 1981 and through December 2000 or occurring during this same interval. Through December 2000, a total of 765,559 AIDS cases among adults/adolescents were diagnosed, and a total of 442,882 deaths were reported for this same group. For children under 13 years old, the total number of cases diagnosed through December 2000 was 8,908, and deaths totaled 5,178.[6]

## DEFINITION

Acquired immunodeficiency syndrome (AIDS) is not a single distinct disease, but rather a disorder characterized by a severe suppression of the immune system. This immunodeficiency renders the body susceptible to a variety of normally manageable infections, cancers, and other diseases. It is believed that AIDS is caused by the human immunodeficiency virus (HIV), a virus that infects certain cells throughout the body. Most significantly, HIV infects white blood cells of the immune system, particularly T cells, or more specifically CD4+ cells, the role of which is to help clear disease-causing substances from the body. AIDS is the name given to a late stage of HIV infection in which there is evidence of significant impairment to the immune system. Because the illness is best understood as a continuum from initial infection to, in many cases, death, the term HIV/AIDS is frequently used. At the present time, there are two known versions of HIV, both of which can cause AIDS. HIV-1, which has spread throughout the world, and HIV-2, a far less common and somewhat less harmful version largely restricted to West Africa. In the absence of further clarification, the generic term "HIV" almost universally refers to HIV-1.

## CASE DEFINITION AND CASE CLASSIFICATION

Since the epidemic was first identified in the United States in 1981, population-based AIDS surveillance (i.e., reporting of AIDS cases and their characteristics to public health authorities for epidemiologic analysis) has been used to track the progression of the epidemic. Case definitions, first for acquired immunodeficiency syndrome (AIDS) and later for human immunodeficiency virus (HIV), form the cornerstones of surveillance.

In 1987 the Centers for Disease Control and Prevention published the acquired immunodeficiency syndrome (AIDS) surveillance case definition. The definition included 23 clinical conditions, specifically: candidiasis of bronchi, trachea, or lungs; esophageal candidiasis; invasive cervical cancer; disseminated or extrapulmonary coccidiodomycosis; extrapulmonary cryptococcosis; chronic intestinal cryptosporidiosis (>1 month's duration); cytomegalovirus disease (other than liver, spleen, or nodes); cytomegalovirus retinitis (with loss of vision); HIV-related encephalopathy; herpes simplex (chronic ulcer[s] of >1 month's duration), or bronchitis, pneumonitis, or esophagitis; disseminated or extrapulmonary histoplasmosis; chronic intestinal isosporiasis (>1 month's duration); Kaposi's sarcoma; Burkitt's lymphoma (or equivalent term); immunoblastic lymphoma (or equivalent term); primary lymphoma of the brain; disseminated or extrapulmonary *mycobacterium avium* complex of *M. Kansasii*; pulmonary or extrapulmonary *Mycobacterium tuberculosis; Pneumocystis carinii* pneumonia; recurrent pneumonia; progressive multifocal leukoencephalopathy; recurrent *Salmonella* septicemia; toxoplasmosis of the brain; and wasting syndrome due to HIV.[7]

In 1993 Centers for Disease Control and Prevention expanded the acquired immunodeficiency syndrome (AIDS) surveillance case definition to include all human immunodeficiency virus (HIV)-infected adolescents and adults aged 13 years or older who have either a) CD4+ T-lymphocyte counts of <200 cells/cubic millimeter, b) a CD4+ percentage of <14, or c) any of the following three newly-included clinical conditions: pulmonary tuberculosis, recurrent pneumonia, or invasive cervical cancer; or one of the 23 clinical conditions in the AIDS surveillance case definition published in 1987. This expanded definition requires laboratory confirmation of HIV infection in persons with a CD4+ T-lymphocyte count of <200 cells/cubic millimeter or with one of the 26 clinical conditions. This expanded definition for reporting cases to the CDC became effective January 1, 1993.[8]

The AIDS surveillance case definition for children aged <13 years has not changed and retains the clinical conditions listed in the AIDS surveillance case definition published in 1987. However, definitions for HIV encephalopathy, HIV wasting syndrome, and HIV infection in children have been revised and the 1987 definition has been updated.[9]

With the publication of the expanded AIDS surveillance case definition, CDC also revised the classification system for HIV infection to emphasize the clinical importance of the CD4+ T-lymphocyte count in the categorization of HIV-related clinical conditions. This classification system replaces the system published by CDC in 1986.[10]

Guidelines for national human immunodeficiency virus case surveillance, including monitoring for human immunodeficiency virus infection and AIDS, were published in late 1999[11]—over a decade after the Centers for Disease Control and Prevention published the AIDS surveillance case definition. The guidelines include a history of AIDS and HIV case surveillance and considerations in implementing nationwide HIV case surveillance. The guidelines also include a revised case definition for HIV infection, which applies to any HIV (e.g., HIV-1 or HIV-2) and integrates reporting criteria for HIV infection and AIDS into a single case definition. The revised case definition for HIV infection also incorporates new laboratory tests into the laboratory criteria for HIV case reporting. The 2000 case definition for HIV infection includes HIV nucleic acid (DNA or RNA) detection tests that were not commercially available when the AIDS case definition was revised in 1993. The revised case definition for HIV infection also permits states to report cases to CDC based on the result of any test licensed for diagnosing HIV infection in the United States. Although the reporting criteria generally reflect the recommendations for diagnosing HIV infection, the HIV reporting criteria are for public health surveillance and are not designed for making a diagnosis for an individual patient.

## SYMPTOMS AND PATHOLOGIES

In the very early period following HIV infection, there may be signs of an acute, brief, nonspecific viral infection with fever, malaise, rash, arthralgias, and lymphadenopathy, although most patients do not experience this. Serologic evidence of AIDS then appears. After this infection, the patient may remain an asymptomatic carrier and may remain so for years. The time from infection to clinical diagnosis varies from several years to more than a decade. The time from infection to evidence of antibody formation is about 3 months. In rare cases, persons known to have been infected with the virus and to have developed the disease have not produced antibodies.

As a syndrome rather than a single distinct disease, AIDS encompasses a number of distinct forms of pathology (illness). Most AIDS-related pathologies are caused by cancers or by opportunistic infections by bacteria, viruses, fungi, protozoa, or other microbes that the body cannot combat because HIV has so seriously damaged the immune system. Other AIDS-related pathologies result from the direct infection by HIV of cells in the nervous or digestive systems. Still other medical conditions are the undesirable side effects of the powerful toxic drugs used to combat HIV and its associated illnesses. Some but not all of the pathologies associated with HIV/AIDS are officially recognized as AIDS-defining illnesses; when they occur in a person with HIV, that individual then has a formal diagnosis of AIDS.

## DIAGNOSIS

The presence of antibodies to HIV in the blood is a sign of HIV infection. These antibodies do not destroy the virus, but simply serve as markers of infection. A diagnosis of AIDS is made whenever a person is HIV-positive and has a CD4+ cell count below 200 cells per microliter, when his or her CD4+ cells account for fewer than 14 percent of all lymphocytes, or when that person has been diagnosed with one or more of the AIDS-defining illnesses listed in the expanded AIDS surveillance case definition.

Additional illnesses that are AIDS-defining in children but not adults include multiple, recurrent bacterial infections and lymphoid interstitial pneumonia/pulmonary lymphoid hyperplasia.

## TRANSMISSION

Unlike many other diseases, HIV is not transmitted through routine casual contact, through the air, or through insect bites. Rather, HIV is transmitted by certain specific behaviors involving the exchange of bodily fluids. Sexual activities can transmit HIV when they involve direct contact between the HIV-infected bodily fluids (such as semen, vaginal secretions, and blood) of one person and the mucous membranes (such as in the vagina, rectum, and mouth) of another. Needles used to inject drugs can transmit HIV when they are used by more than one person. Additionally, HIV can be transmitted from person to person through the transfusion of blood and blood products. However, routine screening for HIV of the blood supply has dramatically reduced this mode of transmission, at least in the developed world. HIV can also be transmitted from mother to fetus/baby while it is still in the uterus, during the delivery process, and through breast-feeding. There is strong evidence that the use of antiviral medications during pregnancy can reduce maternal transmission of HIV.

To date, researchers have been able to isolate HIV in virtually every fluid secreted by the body—including tears, saliva, urine, blood, semen, mucus, and vaginal secretions. Nonetheless, HIV remains a virus that is not easily transmitted from one person to another. HIV's ability to successfully leave one person's body and enter another's is highly dependent on secondary factors. These secondary factors, called risk factors, are based on both biological and behavioral characteristics. The biological factors associated with HIV transmission are numerous and complicated. Characteristics on which a determination of the probability of sexual transmission depends include the type of bodily fluid, the concentration of HIV in the fluid, the integrity or relative vulnerability of involved mucous membranes, the duration of exposure, and the strain of virus transmitted. The way in which the fluid enters the body is commonly referred to as the route of transmission and is yet another important biological characteristic that may be associated with HIV transmission. HIV-infected bodily fluids can be swallowed, accepted into the vagina or rectum, or injected directly into the bloodstream. HIV is much more likely to directly enter the body and cause infection through some routes more than others, however.

## TREATMENT

Treatment for HIV/AIDS has three main dimensions: attacking the virus itself, strengthening the immune system, and controlling AIDS-related cancers and opportunistic infections. There have been significant advances in all three types of treatment since the start of the epidemic. To date, there is no proven "cure" for AIDS, in the sense of a single treatment that could eliminate HIV from the human body or reverse the damage done by HIV to the immune system. There is no effective vaccine to prevent new infections.

## SURVEILLANCE

The history of HIV and AIDS surveillance reflects our evolving understanding of both diseases. In the case of each disease, revisions in case definitions have had, and continue to have, dramatic impact on disease surveillance.[12]

**Surveillance of HIV infection** Before 1991, surveillance of HIV infection was not standardized and reporting of HIV infections was based primarily on passive surveillance. Many cases reported before 1991 do not have complete information. Since then, CDC has assisted states in conducting active surveillance of HIV infection using standardized report forms and software. However, collection of demographic and risk information still varies among states.

As of April 2001, 33 states and the U.S. Virgin Islands had implemented confidential reporting of HIV among adults and adolescents as an extension of AIDS surveillance.

CDC advises that HIV infection data should be interpreted with caution:

> HIV surveillance reports may not be representative of all persons infected with HIV since not all infected persons have been tested. Many HIV-reporting states offer anonymous HIV testing and home collection HIV test kits are widely available in the United States. Anonymous test results are not reported to state and local health departments' confidential name-based HIV registries. Therefore, confidential HIV infection reports may not represent all persons testing positive for HIV infection. Furthermore, many factors may influence testing patterns, including the extent that testing is targeted or routinely offered to specific groups and the availability of and access to medical care and testing services. These data provide a minimum estimate of the number of persons known to be HIV infected in states with confidential HIV reporting.[13]

Several factors influence the number of HIV infection cases reported. These include the following: (1) the length of time reporting has been in place in each state; (2) whether or not a given state or states had collected reports of HIV infection prior to initiation of statewide reporting; (3) whether or not a state with confidential HIV infection reporting also reports persons testing positive in that state who are residents of other states; and (4) when HIV infection cases later reported with AIDS are deleted from the HIV infection tables. Completeness of reporting for HIV is estimated to be more than 85% complete.[14] CDC estimates approximately 2% of HIV cases are duplicates based on matching of the national coded surveillance database.[15]

Readers must take three other factors into consideration when interpreting HIV infection data. First, since not all people infected with HIV have received a positive diagnosis, it becomes difficult to calculate a direct measurement of HIV incidence and prevalence. Second, readers should take local practices into account when interpreting the data; the data can be influenced by both the availability of HIV test facilities and the proportion of HIV-infected persons who may defer testing. Finally, states have differing reporting criteria; some states report prevalent HIV cases while others just the new HIV cases. In addition, because persons are counted only once in the HIV/AIDS system, people who are reported as having HIV and AIDS are counted as only AIDS cases.

**Surveillance of AIDS** In 1981, after reports of *Pneumocystis carinii* pneumonia, Kaposi's sarcoma, and other opportunistic infections in young gay men in San Francisco, New York, and Los Angeles, the CDC developed a surveillance for a newly recognized constellation of diseases eventually to be called AIDS. In 1982, the CDC developed a surveillance case definition for this syndrome focusing on the presence of opportunistic infections; it initially received case reports directly from both health care providers and state and local health departments. Once HIV was identified as the causative agent of AIDS and the epidemic became more widespread, state and local health departments assumed responsibility for AIDS surveillance. By 1985, all states and local governments had rules requiring health care providers to report AIDS directly to the state or local health department. These entities then report to the CDC, which in turn produces national surveillance data.

All 50 states, the District of Columbia, U.S. dependencies and possessions, and independent nations in free association with the United States report AIDS cases to CDC using a uniform surveillance case definition and case report form. The original case definition of AIDS was modified in 1985 (*MMWR* 34 (1985): 373–75) and 1987 (*MMWR* 36 no. 1S (1987): 1S–15S). The case definition for adults and adolescents was modified again in 1993 (*MMWR* 41, no. RR-17 (1992): 1–19; see also *MMWR* 44 (1995): 64–67). The revisions incorporated a broader range of AIDS-indicator diseases and conditions and used HIV diagnostic tests to improve the sensitivity and specificity of the definition. The laboratory and diagnostic criteria for the 1987 pediatric case definition (*MMWR* 36 (1987): 225–30, 235) were updated in 1994 (*MMWR* 43, no. RR-12 (1994): 1–19). Effective January 1, 2000, the surveillance case definition for HIV infection was revised to reflect advances in laboratory HIV virologic tests. The definition incorporates the reporting criteria for HIV infection and AIDS into a single case definition for adults and children (*MMWR* 48, no. RR-13 (1999): 29–31).

For persons with laboratory-confirmed HIV infection, the 1987 revision incorporated HIV encephalopathy, wasting syndrome, and other indicator diseases that are diagnosed presumptively. In addition to the 23 clinical conditions in the 1987 definition, the 1993 case definition for adults and adolescents includes HIV-infected persons with CD4+ T-lymphocyte counts of less than 200/uL or a CD4+ percentage of less than 14 and persons diagnosed with pulmonary tuberculosis, recurrent pneumonia, and invasive cervical cancer. For adults, adolescents, and children 18 months of age or older, the 2000 revised HIV surveillance case definition incorporates positive results or reports of a detectable quantity of HIV nucleic acid or plasma HIV RNA.

The pediatric case definition incorporates the revised 1994 pediatric classification system for evidence of HIV infection. Children with their first positive results on Western blot or HIV detection tests before October 1994 were categorized based on the 1987 classification system. Those tested during or after October 1994 are categorized under the revised 1994 pediatric classification system. For children of any age with an AIDS-defining condition that requires evidence of HIV infection, a single positive HIV-detection test is sufficient for a reportable AIDS diagnosis if the diagnosis is confirmed by a physician. For children under 18 months of age, the pediatric HIV reporting criteria reflect diagnostic advances that permit the diagnosis of HIV infection during the first months of life. With HIV nucleic acid detection tests, HIV infection can be detected in nearly all infants aged 1 month and older. The timing of the HIV serologic and HIV nucleic acid detection tests in the definitive and presumptive criteria for HIV infection are based on the recommended practices for diagnosing infection in children aged under 18 months and on evaluation of the performance of those tests for children in this age group.[16]

Although completeness of reporting of diagnosed AIDS cases to state and local health departments varies by geographic region and patient population, studies conducted by state and local health departments indicate that reporting of AIDS cases in most areas of the United States is more than 85% complete.[17] Multiple routes of exposure, opportunistic diseases diagnosed after the initial AIDS case report was submitted to CDC, and vital status may not be determined or reported for all cases. However, among persons reported with AIDS, reporting of deaths is estimated to be more than 90% complete.[18] CDC estimates approximately 3% of AIDS cases are duplicates based on matching of the national coded surveillance database.[19]

As with HIV infection data, AIDS data should also be interpreted with caution. Readers are advised to take several factors into consideration when interpreting AIDS data. First, tabulations of persons living with HIV infection and AIDS include persons whose vital status was reported "alive" as of last update; persons whose vital status is missing or unknown is not included. Tabulations of deaths in persons with AIDS include persons whose vital status was reported "dead" as of last update; persons whose vital status is missing or unknown are not included. Note, too, that states vary in the frequency with which they review the vital status of persons reported with HIV infection and AIDS. In addition, some cases may be lost to follow-up.

Second, estimates of AIDS incidence and deaths are not actual counts of persons reported to the surveillance system. The estimates are adjusted for delays in reporting of cases and deaths and are based on a number of assumptions. The date of death for decedents with a missing date of death was imputed as the date the death was reported to CDC less the estimated median months required to report deaths. The median reporting delay for deaths is 3 months. If AIDS diagnosis occurred after the date was imputed, then the date of AIDS diagnosis was used as the date of death.

Third, there are several cautionary notes for interpreting data pertaining to exposure categories. For surveillance purposes, HIV infection cases and AIDS cases are counted only once in a hierarchy of exposure categories. Persons with more than one reported mode of exposure to HIV are classified in the exposure category listed first in the hierarchy, except for men with both a history of sexual contact with other men and injecting drug use. They make up a separate exposure category. Additionally, adults/adolescents born, or who had sex with someone born, in a country where heterosexual transmission was believed to be the predominant mode of HIV transmission are no longer classified as having heterosexually acquired AIDS. These reports are now classified (in the absence of other risk information that would classify them in another exposure category) as "no risk reported or identified."[20] Children whose mother was born, or whose mother had sex with someone born, in a country where heterosexual transmission was believed to be the predominant mode of HIV transmission are now classified (in the absence of other risk information that would classify them in another exposure category) as "Mother with/at risk for HIV infection: has HIV infection, risk not specified." "No risk reported or identified" (NIR) cases are persons with no reported history of exposure to HIV through any of the routes listed in the hierarchy of exposure categories. Persons who have an exposure mode identified at the time of follow-up are reclassified into the appropriate exposure category. Historically, investigations and follow-up for modes of exposure by state health departments was conducted routinely for persons reported with AIDS and as resources allowed for persons reported with HIV infection. Therefore the percentage of HIV-infected persons with risk not reported or identified is substantially higher than for those reported with AIDS. As of September 2000 the procedures for the investigation of cases reported without risk changed from ascertaining risk for all persons reported to population-based sampling and statistical modeling to estimate risk distributions. Lastly, because recently reported AIDS cases are more likely to be reported as NIR, recent AIDS incidence in some exposure categories will be underestimated unless an adjustment is made.[21]

Fourth, readers are advised of several factors relevant to interpreting trends in AIDS incidence. Note first that because of the temporary distortion caused by the 1993 expansion of the case definition, trends in AIDS incidence were estimated by statistically adjusting cases reported based on the criteria added to the case definition in 1993. By the end of 1996, the temporary distortion caused by reporting prevalent as well as incident cases that met criteria added in 1993 had almost entirely waned. In addition, after the end of 1996, the incidence of AIDS opportunistic infections could no longer be readily estimated because data are not currently available to model the increasing effects of therapy on rate of disease progression. Therefore, from 1996 forward, trends in AIDS incidence will be adjusted for reporting delay, but not for the 1993 expansion of the case definition. These trends represent the incidence of AIDS (1993 criteria) in the population and represent persons newly diagnosed with HIV at the time of AIDS, those identified with HIV who did not seek or receive treatment, and those for whom treatment has failed.

Last, readers are advised to bear in mind that reporting delays (time between diagnosis of HIV infection or AIDS and report to CDC) may vary among exposure, geographic, racial/ethnic, age, and sex categories. Delays have been as long as several years for some AIDS cases. About 40% of all AIDS cases were reported to CDC within 3 months of diagnosis and about 80% were reported within 1 year. Among persons with AIDS, estimates in delay of reporting of death show that approximately 90% of deaths are reported within 1 year. For HIV infection cases diagnosed since implementation of uniform reporting through the HIV/AIDS reporting system on January 1, 1994, about 68% of all HIV infection cases were reported to CDC within 3 months of diagnosis and about 92% were reported within 1 year.

## HEALTHY PEOPLE

When the U.S. Public Health Service first presented quantified 10-year objectives for disease prevention and health promotion in 1980,[22] HIV/AIDS was barely a blip on the screen. With the publication of *Healthy People 2000*, however, the situation had radically changed: today HIV/AIDS is front-and-center in any dialogue about the nation's health and priorities for health promotion and disease prevention. *Healthy People 2000* includes a broad range of objectives relative to HIV infection. Note that the first Health Status Objective in this suite speaks to the confinement of the annual incidence of diagnosed AIDS cases. Risk reduction objectives follow, addressing specific behaviors, including sexual intercourse and intravenous drug use. A final risk reduction objective speaks to efforts to prevent transfusion-associated HIV infection. Services and protection objectives are next; these concern testing for HIV infection; primary care and mental health care provider behavior; HIV/AIDS information and education programs in schools; HIV education in colleges and universities; community outreach to intravenous drug users; the need to increase health care access points (public health clinics and community health centers); and worker protection from exposure to bloodborne infections, including HIV. A final suite of objectives addresses personnel needs, notably the need for training about HIV infection, high-risk behavior, and infection control measures; the need for improved training in human sexual behavior; and the need for improved training in recognizing and responding to drug abuse. Surveillance and data needs are also addressed, as are research needs. Note that as regards HIV, related objectives from other *Healthy People 2000* priority areas can be found in sections addressing alcohol and other drugs, educational and community-based programs, diabetes and chronic disabling conditions, sexually transmitted diseases, clinical prevention services, and surveillance and data systems.

## TABLE OVERVIEW

**B1. Persons Living with HIV/AIDS** This table gives an overview of persons living with HIV and AIDS by state. Researchers should use this data cautiously. Figures within the table are not comparable because states initiated reporting at different dates. Through June 2000, a total of 120,223 persons were reported to be living with HIV infection and a total of 302,075 persons were reported to be living with AIDS. The cumulative total of persons reported to be living with HIV infection and with AIDS was 422,086.

**B2.1–B2.7. HIV Infection** The next cluster of tables presents data on HIV by area, age group, exposure category, and sex. Data for HIV infection in this table as others include only persons with HIV who have not developed AIDS. CDC used the 2000 revised HIV surveillance case definition for classifying adults, adolescents and children 18 months or older. It considered children born before 1994 HIV infected if they met the definition stated in the 1987 pediatric classification system.[23] Beginning October 1994, it began considering children less than 18 months of age infected if they meet an expanded and refined definition.[24] The last table in this suite, B2.7, shows health care workers with documented and possible occupationally acquired HIV/AIDS infection. The figures presented are cases of HIV. Not all workers with HIV developed AIDS.

Of the 21,794 reported infection cases from July 1999 to June 2000, infection by exposure category breaks down as follows: 5,992 (28%) men infected by having sex with men; 2,185 (10%) persons infected by injecting drug use; and 3,835 (18%) persons infected heterosexually. Because of careful screening of the blood supply, very few individuals are now contracting HIV from blood transfusions, blood components, or tissue. Men account for 93,527 and women account for 36,814 of the HIV infection cases reported through June 2000. Among men, blacks and Hispanics account for 43,258 and 7,698 of infection cases respectively; among women, blacks account for 24,922 cases and Hispanics account for 2,583 of cases.

**B 3.1–3.9. AIDS Cases** The focus shifts in the next suite of maps and tables to AIDS cases. B3.1 illustrates the burden of AIDS across the country. Tables B3.2 through B3.9 provide data on AIDS cases by age group, exposure category, sex, and race/ethnicity. The last table breaks down deaths from AIDS by age, sex, and race/ethnicity.

Men accounted for almost 80% of the cumulative AIDS cases reported. While the percentage of individuals who contracted AIDS from homosexual sex and intravenous drug use declined, those who were infected through heterosexual contact increased during the July 1999–June 2000 period.

**B4.1–B4.3. Pediatric HIV and AIDS** This small cluster of tables presents the most current information available on pediatric (under 13 years old) HIV and AIDS. Map B4.1 highlights incidence across the country. B4.2 and B4.3 present data by exposure categories and ethnic group. As is the case in adult reporting, the data on HIV include only persons who have not developed AIDS. Mother with/at risk for HIV infection (941 or 91%) is the most significant exposure category for HIV infection, followed by receipt of blood transfusion, blood components, or tissue (22 or 2%). Pediatric AIDS cases follow the same pattern. Mother with/at risk for HIV infection (195 or 87%) is the largest exposure category for the same period, followed by receipt of blood transfusion, blood components, or tissue (4 or 2%).

**B5.1–5.9. Trends** The final suite of tables presents trends in estimated deaths among persons with AIDS, and in the prevalence of AIDS, that is, in the number of persons who are living with AIDS. The numbers in these tables do not represent actual cases of persons living with AIDS but are point estimates of persons living with AIDS derived by subtracting the estimated cumulative number of deaths in persons with AIDS from the estimated cumulative number of persons with AIDS. Estimated AIDS cases and estimated deaths are adjusted for reporting delays, but not for incomplete reporting. B5.1 graphs the incidence of AIDS from 1988 through 1999. The next three tables (B5.2–B5.4) focus on estimated persons living with AIDS from 1993 through 1999 by region of residence, race/ethnicity, age group, sex, and exposure category. The final five tables (B5.5–B5.9) present data on estimated deaths of persons with AIDS for the same time period and organizational criteria.

The expansion of the AIDS surveillance case definition in 1993 caused a substantial increase in reported cases. During the mid-to-late 1990s, the beneficial impact of newly available therapies slowed the progression from human immunodeficiency virus (HIV) to AIDS and from AIDS to death. Consequently, and during the same period, a decline was seen in the number of new AIDS cases, and an increase was seen in the number of persons living with HIV infection and AIDS. Although this trend continued through 1998, provisional data for 1999 suggest that the number of AIDS cases and deaths might be leveling off. AIDS data reflect a combination of factors, including (1) variation in HIV transmission patterns over a long period, (2) differences in access to and use of testing and treatment among populations who are at risk or infected, and (3) treatment regimens that might be failing because of drug resistance and poor adherence.

## NOTES

1. Centers for Disease Control, "Kaposi's Sarcoma and Pneumocystis Pneumonia among Homosexual Men—New York City and California," *Morbidity and Mortality Weekly Report* 30, no. 25 (1981): 305–8.
2. Centers for Disease Control and Prevention (CDC), *HIV/AIDS Surveillance Report* 10, no. 2 (1998).
3. Centers for Disease Control, "Update on Acquired Immune Deficiency Syndrome (AIDS)—United States," *Morbidity and Mortality Weekly Report* 31, no. 37 (1982): 507–14.
4. Centers for Disease Control and Prevention, "Update: Trends in AIDS Incidence, Deaths, and Prevention—United States, 1996," *Morbidity and Mortality Weekly Report* 46, no. 8 (1997): 166–73; Centers for Disease Control and Prevention, *HIV/AIDS Surveillance Report* 9, no. 2 (1997).
5. Centers for Disease Control and Prevention, "CDC Guidelines for National Human Immunodeficiency Virus Case Surveillance, Including Monitoring for Human Immunodeficiency Virus infection and Acquired Immunodeficiency Syndrome," *Morbidity and Mortality Weekly Report* 48, no. RR-13 (1999).
6. All figures in this paragraph taken from Centers for Disease Control and Prevention, *HIV/AIDS Surveillance Report, 2000* 12, no. 2.
7. Complete information referring to this case definition can be found in Centers for Disease Control and Prevention, "Revised Classification System for HIV Infection and Expanded Surveillance Case Definition for AIDS Among Adolescents and Adults." *MMWR* 41, no. RR-17 (1992). *See also* "Revision of the CDC Surveillance Case Definition for Acquired Immunodeficiency Syndrome." *MMWR* 36 supplement no. 15 (1987): 1–155.
8. *MMWR* 41, (RR-17) (1992); *see also MMWR* 44 (1995): 64–67.
9. See the following for complete information pertaining to this case definition: Centers for Disease Control and Prevention, "Revised Classification System for Human Immunodeficiency Virus Infection in Children Less Than 13 Years of Age," *MMWR* 43, no. RR-12 (1994).
10. See the following for complete information pertaining to this case definition: CDC, "1993 Revised Classification System for HIV Infection and Expanded Surveillance Case Definition for AIDS Among Adolescents and Adults." *MMWR* 41, no. RR-17 (1992).
11. CDC, "Guidelines for National Human Immunodeficiency Virus Case Surveillance, Including Monitoring for Human Immunodeficiency Virus Infection and Acquired Immunodeficiency Syndrome." *MMWR* 48, no. RR-13 (1997).
12. Today, the *Morbidity and Mortality Weekly Report (MMWR)* remains a primary source of information about the epidemiology, surveillance, prevention, care, and treatment of HIV and AIDS. The *HIV/AIDS Surveillance Report* is published semiannually by the Division of HIV/AIDS Prevention—Surveillance and Epidemiology, National Center for HIV, STD, and TB Prevention, Centers for Disease Control and Prevention. The year-end edition contains additional tables and graphs. All data are provisional. The *HIV/AIDS Surveillance Report* is accessible via the Internet at http://www.cdc.gov/hiv. A compilation of notable *MMWR* reports on HIV and AIDS is available at http://www.cdc.gov/ mmwr/hiv_aids20.html.
13. *HIV/AIDS Surveillance Report.* 12, no. 2 (2000): 41.
14. *MMWR* 47 (1998): 309–14.
15. *HIV/AIDS Surveillance Report.* 12, no. 2 (2000): 41.
16. *MMWR* 48, no. RR-13 (1999): 29–31; *MMWR* 47, no. RR-4 (1998).
17. *J Acquir Immune Def Syndr* 5 (1992): 257–64; *Am J Public Health* 82 (1992): 1495–99; *AIDS* 13 (1999): 1109–14.
18. *JAMA* 276 (1996): 126–31.
19. *HIV/AIDS Surveillance Report,* 12, no. 1 (2000): 37.
20. *MMWR* 43 (1994): 155–60.
21. For further discussion, see Centers for Disease Control and Prevention, *HIV/AIDS Surveillance Report, 2000* 12, no. 2 (2000): 43.
22. U.S. Department of Health and Human Services, *Promoting Health/Preventing Disease: Objectives for the Nation* Washington, DC: U.S. Department of Health and Human Services, 1980.
23. *MMWR* 43, no. RR-12 (1994): 1–10.
24. Ibid.

## Table B1. Persons Reported to Be Living with HIV Infection[1] and with AIDS, by Area and Age Group,[2] Reported through December 2000[3]

| Area of residence (Date HIV reporting initiated) | Living with HIV infection[4] | | | Living with AIDS[5] | | | Cumulative totals | | |
|---|---|---|---|---|---|---|---|---|---|
| | Adults/ adolescents | Children <13 years old | Total | Adults/ adolescents | Children <13 years old | Total | Adults/ adolescents | Children <13 years old | Total |
| Alabama (Jan. 1988) | 5,014 | 32 | 5,046 | 3,142 | 17 | 3,159 | 8,156 | 49 | 8,205 |
| Alaska (Feb. 1999) | 29 | – | 29 | 229 | 1 | 230 | 258 | 1 | 259 |
| Arizona (Jan. 1987) | 4,296 | 28 | 4,324 | 3,217 | 9 | 3,226 | 7,513 | 37 | 7,550 |
| Arkansas (July 1989) | 2,001 | 15 | 2,016 | 1,612 | 20 | 1,632 | 3,613 | 35 | 3,648 |
| California | – | – | – | 43,606 | 155 | 43,761 | 43,606 | 155 | 43,761 |
| Colorado (Nov. 1985) | 5,265 | 18 | 5,283 | 2,878 | 1 | 2,879 | 8,143 | 19 | 8,162 |
| Connecticut (July 1992)[6] | – | 74 | 74 | 5,788 | 58 | 5,846 | 5,788 | 132 | 5,920 |
| Delaware | – | – | – | 1,193 | 13 | 1,206 | 1,193 | 13 | 1,206 |
| District of Columbia | – | – | – | 6,389 | 84 | 6,473 | 6,389 | 84 | 6,473 |
| Florida (July 1997) | 18,774 | 165 | 18,939 | 35,195 | 475 | 35,670 | 53,969 | 640 | 54,609 |
| Georgia | – | – | – | 10,206 | 84 | 10,290 | 10,206 | 84 | 10,290 |
| Hawaii | – | – | – | 982 | 5 | 987 | 982 | 5 | 987 |
| Idaho (June 1986) | 321 | 3 | 324 | 223 | – | 223 | 544 | 3 | 547 |
| Illinois | – | – | – | 9,761 | 107 | 9,868 | 9,761 | 107 | 9,868 |
| Indiana (July 1988) | 3,252 | 27 | 3,279 | 2,693 | 13 | 2,706 | 5,945 | 40 | 5,985 |
| Iowa (July 1998) | 354 | 5 | 359 | 573 | 5 | 578 | 927 | 10 | 937 |
| Kansas (July 1999) | 930 | 10 | 940 | 980 | 3 | 983 | 1,910 | 13 | 1,923 |
| Kentucky | – | – | – | 1,619 | 14 | 1,633 | 1,619 | 14 | 1,633 |
| Louisiana (Feb. 1993) | 6,975 | 88 | 7,063 | 5,448 | 49 | 5,497 | 12,423 | 137 | 12,560 |
| Maine | – | – | – | 441 | 5 | 446 | 441 | 5 | 446 |
| Maryland | – | – | – | 9,933 | 129 | 10,062 | 9,933 | 129 | 10,062 |
| Massachusetts | – | – | – | 6,770 | 58 | 6,828 | 6,770 | 58 | 6,828 |
| Michigan (April 1992) | 4,611 | 73 | 4,684 | 4,618 | 23 | 4,641 | 9,229 | 96 | 9,325 |
| Minnesota (Oct. 1985) | 2,552 | 24 | 2,576 | 1,632 | 9 | 1,641 | 4,184 | 33 | 4,217 |
| Mississippi (Aug. 1988) | 4,104 | 38 | 4,142 | 2,102 | 23 | 2,125 | 6,206 | 61 | 6,267 |
| Missouri (Oct. 1987) | 4,159 | 35 | 4,194 | 4,263 | 16 | 4,279 | 8,422 | 51 | 8,473 |
| Montana | – | – | – | 165 | – | 165 | 165 | – | 165 |
| Nebraska (Sept. 1995) | 474 | 5 | 479 | 482 | 4 | 486 | 956 | 9 | 965 |
| Nevada (Feb. 1992) | 2,591 | 21 | 2,612 | 2,084 | 10 | 2,094 | 4,675 | 31 | 4,706 |
| New Hampshire | – | – | – | 478 | 4 | 482 | 478 | 4 | 482 |
| New Jersey (Jan. 1992) | 12,367 | 314 | 12,681 | 14,910 | 185 | 15,095 | 27,277 | 499 | 27,776 |
| New Mexico (Jan. 1998) | 630 | – | 630 | 956 | 6 | 962 | 1,586 | 6 | 1,592 |
| New York | – | – | – | 54,290 | 503 | 54,794 | 54,290 | 503 | 54,794 |
| North Carolina (Feb. 1990) | 9,133 | 93 | 9,226 | 4,511 | 37 | 4,548 | 13,644 | 130 | 13,774 |
| North Dakota (Jan. 1988) | 63 | 1 | 64 | 44 | 1 | 45 | 107 | 2 | 109 |
| Ohio (June 1990) | 5,409 | 54 | 5,463 | 4,487 | 36 | 4,523 | 9,896 | 90 | 9,986 |
| Oklahoma (June 1988) | 2,239 | 11 | 2,250 | 1,574 | 6 | 1,580 | 3,813 | 17 | 3,830 |
| Oregon (Sept. 1988)[6] | – | 13 | 13 | 2,022 | 5 | 2,027 | 2,022 | 18 | 2,040 |
| Pennsylvania | – | – | – | 11,487 | 152 | 11,639 | 11,487 | 152 | 11,639 |
| Rhode Island | – | – | – | 893 | 6 | 899 | 893 | 6 | 899 |
| South Carolina (Feb. 1986) | 6,367 | 82 | 6,449 | 4,696 | 26 | 4,722 | 11,063 | 108 | 11,171 |
| South Dakota (Jan. 1988) | 188 | 1 | 189 | 69 | 1 | 70 | 257 | 2 | 259 |
| Tennessee (Jan. 1992) | 5,624 | 54 | 5,678 | 4,701 | 17 | 4,718 | 10,325 | 71 | 10,396 |
| Texas (Jan. 1999)[6] | 6,640 | 236 | 6,876 | 23,869 | 125 | 23,994 | 30,509 | 361 | 30,870 |
| Utah (April 1989) | 711 | 6 | 717 | 993 | 3 | 996 | 1,704 | 9 | 1,713 |
| Vermont | – | – | – | 194 | 2 | 196 | 194 | 2 | 196 |
| Virginia (July 1989) | 7,611 | 61 | 7,672 | 5,774 | 69 | 5,843 | 13,385 | 130 | 13,515 |
| Washington | – | – | – | 4,083 | 11 | 4,094 | 4,083 | 11 | 4,094 |
| West Virginia (Jan. 1989) | 555 | 4 | 559 | 465 | 4 | 469 | 1,020 | 8 | 1,028 |
| Wisconsin (Nov. 1985) | 2,145 | 17 | 2,162 | 1,549 | 11 | 1,560 | 3,694 | 28 | 3,722 |
| Wyoming (June 1989) | 66 | – | 66 | 75 | 1 | 76 | 141 | 1 | 142 |
| **Subtotal** | **125,450** | **1,608** | **127,058** | **310,344** | **2,601** | **312,946** | **435,794** | **4,210** | **440,004** |
| **U.S. dependencies, possessions, and associated nations** | | | | | | | | | |
| Guam (March 2000) | 41 | 1 | 42 | 24 | – | 24 | 65 | 1 | 66 |
| Pacific Islands, U.S. | – | – | – | 2 | – | 2 | 2 | – | 2 |
| Puerto Rico | – | – | – | 9,204 | 89 | 9,293 | 9,204 | 89 | 9,293 |
| Virgin Isl, U.S.(Dec.1998) | 184 | 2 | 186 | 212 | 7 | 219 | 396 | 9 | 405 |
| Total | 125,675 | 1,611 | 127,286 | 320,161 | 2,703 | 322,865 | 445,836 | 4,314 | 450,151 |

[1]Includes only persons reported with HIV infection who have not developed AIDS.

[2]Age group based on person's age as of December 31, 2000.

[3]Persons reported with vital status "alive" as of the last update. Excludes persons whose vital status is unknown.

[4]Includes only persons reported from areas with confidential HIV reporting. Excludes 2,160 adults/adolescents and 51 children reported from areas with confidential HIV infection reporting whose area of residence is unknown or are residents of other areas.

[5]Includes 375 adults/adolescents and 6 children whose area of residence is unknown, and one person missing age.

[6]Connecticut has confidential HIV infection reporting for pediatric cases only; Oregon has confidential HIV infection reporting for children less than 6 years old. Texas reported only pediatric HIV infection cases from February 1994 until January 1999.

*Source*: Centers for Disease Control and Prevention, U.S. Department of Health and Human Services. National Center for HIV, STD, and TB Prevention. Division of HIV/AIDS Prevention—Surveillance and Epidemiology. *HIV/AIDS Surveillance Report 2000* 12, no. 2, year-end edition. http://www.cdc.gov/hiv/stats/hasr1202.pdf.

## Table B2.1. HIV Infection Cases,[1] by Area and Age Group, Reported through December 2000, from Areas with Confidential HIV Infection Reporting

| Area of residence (Date HIV reporting initiated) | 2000 | Cumulative totals: Adults/ adolescents | Children <13 years old | Total |
|---|---|---|---|---|
| Alabama (Jan. 1988) | 498 | 5,222 | 39 | 5,261 |
| Alaska (Feb. 1999) | 26 | 30 | – | 30 |
| Arizona (Jan. 1987) | 450 | 4,552 | 36 | 4,588 |
| Arkansas (July 1989) | 245 | 2,028 | 22 | 2,050 |
| Colorado (Nov. 1985) | 220 | 5,507 | 29 | 5,536 |
| Connecticut (July 1992)[2] | 2 | – | 104 | 104 |
| Florida (July 1997) | 5,810 | 19,137 | 185 | 19,322 |
| Idaho (June 1986) | 44 | 375 | 4 | 379 |
| Indiana (July 1988) | 319 | 3,447 | 38 | 3,485 |
| Iowa (July 1998) | 119 | 358 | 8 | 366 |
| Kansas (July 1999) | 234 | 954 | 15 | 969 |
| Louisiana (Feb. 1993) | 841 | 7,335 | 116 | 7,451 |
| Michigan (April 1992) | 644 | 5,325 | 107 | 5,432 |
| Minnesota (Oct. 1985) | 227 | 2,700 | 34 | 2,734 |
| Mississippi (Aug. 1988) | 459 | 4,307 | 49 | 4,356 |
| Missouri (Oct. 1987) | 348 | 4,320 | 45 | 4,365 |
| Nebraska (Sept. 1995) | 60 | 497 | 6 | 503 |
| Nevada (Feb. 1992) | 296 | 2,923 | 24 | 2,947 |
| New Jersey (Jan. 1992) | 1,455 | 13,836 | 379 | 14,215 |
| New Mexico (Jan. 1998) | 125 | 645 | 3 | 648 |
| North Carolina (Feb. 1990) | 1,011 | 10,022 | 122 | 10,144 |
| North Dakota (Jan. 1988) | 4 | 71 | 1 | 72 |
| Ohio (June 1990) | 601 | 5,748 | 70 | 5,818 |
| Oklahoma (June 1988) | 297 | 2,355 | 18 | 2,373 |
| Oregon (Sept. 1988)[2] | – | – | 16 | 16 |
| South Carolina (Feb. 1986) | 597 | 6,942 | 107 | 7,049 |
| South Dakota (Jan. 1988) | 21 | 205 | 5 | 210 |
| Tennessee (Jan. 1992) | 846 | 5,798 | 66 | 5,864 |
| Texas (Jan. 1999)[2] | 4,204 | 6,675 | 295 | 6,970 |
| Utah (April 1989) | 65 | 724 | 8 | 732 |
| Virginia (July 1989) | 769 | 8,160 | 78 | 8,238 |
| West Virginia (Jan. 1989) | 68 | 581 | 5 | 586 |
| Wisconsin (Nov. 1985) | 198 | 2,310 | 28 | 2,338 |
| Wyoming (June 1989) | 4 | 72 | – | 72 |
| **Subtotal** | **21,107** | **133,161** | **2,062** | **135,223** |
| **U.S. dependencies, possessions, and associated nations** | | | | |
| Guam (March 2000) | 44 | 47 | 1 | 48 |
| Virgin Islands, U.S (Dec. 1998) | 35 | 190 | 3 | 193 |
| Persons reported from states with confidential HIV reporting who were residents of other states[3] | 518 | 2,479 | 68 | 2,547 |
| **Total** | **21,704** | **135,877** | **2,134** | **138,011** |

[1]Includes only persons reported with HIV infection who have not developed AIDS.

[2]Connecticut has confidential HIV infection reporting for pediatric cases only. Oregon has a confidential HIV infection reporting for children less than 6 years old. Texas reported only pediatric HIV infection cases from February 1994 until January 1999.

[3]Includes 569 persons reported from areas with confidential HIV infection reporting, but whose area of residence is unknown. See Technical Notes.

*Source*: Centers for Disease Control and Prevention, U.S. Department of Health and Human Services. National Center for HIV, STD, and TB Prevention. Division of HIV/AIDS Prevention—Surveillance and Epidemiology. *HIV/AIDS Surveillance Report 2000* 12, no. 2, year-end edition. http://www.cdc.gov/hiv/stats/hasr1202.pdf.

## Table B2.2. HIV Infection Cases[1] in Adolescents and Adults under Age 25, by Sex and Exposure Category, Reported through December 2000, from the 34 Areas with Confidential HIV Infection Reporting[2]

| | 13-19 years old | | | | 20-24 years old | | | |
|---|---|---|---|---|---|---|---|---|
| | 2000 | | Cumulative total | | 2000 | | Cumulative total | |
| **Male exposure category** | **No.** | **(%)** | **No.** | **(%)** | **No.** | **(%)** | **No.** | **(%)** |
| Men who have sex with men | 11 | (46) | 1,246 | (52) | 40 | (49) | 6,691 | (56) |
| Injecting drug use | 1 | (4) | 110 | (5) | 7 | (9) | 674 | (6) |
| Men who have sex with men and inject drugs | 1 | (4) | 115 | (5) | 7 | (9) | 795 | (7) |
| Hemophilia/coagulation disorder | – | – | 106 | (4) | – | – | 85 | (1) |
| Heterosexual contact: | – | – | 164 | (7) | 4 | (5) | 784 | (7) |
| *Sex with injecting drug user* | *–* | | *26* | | *–* | | *108* | |
| *Sex with person with hemophilia* | *–* | | *2* | | *–* | | *–* | |
| *Sex with transfusion recipient with HIV infection* | *–* | | *–* | | *–* | | *7* | |
| *Sex with HIV-infected person, risk not specified* | *–* | | *136* | | *4* | | *669* | |
| Receipt of blood transfusion, blood components, or tissue | – | – | 12 | (0) | – | – | 28 | (0) |
| Risk not reported or identified[3] | 11 | (46) | 659 | (27) | 23 | (28) | 2,894 | (24) |
| Male subtotal | 24 | (100) | 2,412 | (100) | 81 | (100) | 11,951 | (100) |
| **Female exposure category** | | | | | | | | |
| Injecting drug use | 4 | (13) | 232 | (7) | 13 | (19) | 770 | (12) |
| Hemophilia/coagulation disorder | – | – | – | – | – | – | 5 | (0) |
| Heterosexual contact: | 14 | (45) | 1,544 | (49) | 32 | (48) | 2,947 | (46) |
| *Sex with injecting drug user* | *4* | | *257* | | *3* | | *628* | |
| *Sex with bisexual male* | *–* | | *112* | | *2* | | *240* | |
| *Sex with person with hemophilia* | *–* | | *22* | | *–* | | *40* | |
| *Sex with transfusion recipient with HIV infection* | *–* | | *4* | | *–* | | *18* | |
| *Sex with HIV-infected person, risk not specified* | *10* | | *1,149* | | *27* | | *2,021* | |
| Receipt of blood transfusion, blood components, or tissue | – | – | 20 | (1) | – | – | 30 | (0) |
| Risk not reported or identified | 13 | (42) | 1,371 | (43) | 22 | (33) | 2,655 | (41) |
| Female subtotal | 31 | (100) | 3,167 | (100) | 67 | (100) | 6,407 | (100) |
| **Total[4]** | **55** | | **5,580** | | **148** | | **18,360** | |

[1]Includes only persons reported with HIV infection who have not developed AIDS.

[2]See table 3 for areas with confidential HIV infection reporting of adults and adolescents.

[3]For HIV infection cases, "risk not reported or identified" refers primarily to persons whose mode of exposure was not reported and who have not been followed up to determine their mode of exposure, and to a smaller number of persons who are not reported with one of the exposures listed above after follow-up. See Technical Notes.

[4]Includes 3 persons whose sex is unknown.

*Source*: Centers for Disease Control and Prevention, U.S. Department of Health and Human Services. National Center for HIV, STD, and TB Prevention. Division of HIV/AIDS Prevention—Surveillance and Epidemiology. *HIV/AIDS Surveillance Report 2000* 12, no. 2, year-end edition. http://www.cdc.gov/hiv/stats/hasr1202.pdf.

## Table B2.3. HIV Infection Cases,[1] by Age Group, Exposure Category, and Sex, Reported through December 2000, from the 36 Areas with Confidential HIV Infection Reporting[2]

| | Males | | | | Females | | | | Totals[3] | | | |
|---|---|---|---|---|---|---|---|---|---|---|---|---|
| | 2000 | | Cumulative total | | 2000 | | Cumulative total | | 2000 | | Cumulative total | |
| **Adult/adolescent exposure category** | **No.** | **(%)** | **No.** | **(%)** | **No.** | **(%)** | **No.** | **(%)** | **No.** | **(%)** | **No.** | **(%)** |
| Men who have sex with men | 6,302 | (43) | 44,467 | (46) | – | – | – | – | 6,302 | (29) | 44,467 | (33) |
| Injecting drug use | 1,367 | (9) | 13,142 | (13) | 855 | (13) | 7,383 | (19) | 2,223 | (10) | 20,526 | (15) |
| Men who have sex with men and inject drugs | 643 | (4) | 6,042 | (6) | – | – | – | – | 643 | (3) | 6,042 | (4) |
| Hemophilia/coagulation disorder | 23 | (0) | 442 | (0) | 8 | (0) | 28 | (0) | 31 | (0) | 470 | (0) |
| Heterosexual contact: | 1,231 | (8) | 7,105 | (7) | 2,448 | (36) | 15,724 | (41) | 3,680 | (17) | 22,830 | (17) |
| *Sex with injecting drug user* | *218* | | *1,528* | | *422* | | *4,056* | | *640* | | *5,584* | |
| *Sex with bisexual male* | – | | – | | *153* | | *1,171* | | *153* | | *1,171* | |
| *Sex with person with hemophilia* | *2* | | *13* | | *14* | | *129* | | *16* | | *142* | |
| *Sex with transfusion recipient with HIV infection* | *7* | | *82* | | *11* | | *109* | | *18* | | *191* | |
| *Sex with HIV-infected person, risk not specified* | *1,004* | | *5,482* | | *1,848* | | *10,259* | | *2,853* | | *15,742* | |
| Receipt of blood transfusion, blood components, or tissue | 54 | (0) | 401 | (0) | 51 | (1) | 429 | (1) | 105 | (0) | 830 | (1) |
| Other/risk not reported or identified[4] | 5,087 | (35) | 26,113 | (27) | 3,407 | (50) | 14,590 | (38) | 8,496 | (40) | 40,712 | (30) |
| Adult/adolescent subtotal | 14,707 | (100) | 97,712 | (100) | 6,769 | (100) | 38,154 | (100) | 21,480 | (100) | 135,877 | (100) |
| **Pediatric (<13 years old) exposure category** | | | | | | | | | | | | |
| Hemophilia/coagulation disorder | 4 | (4) | 98 | (9) | – | – | 1 | (0) | 4 | (2) | 99 | (5) |
| Mother with/at risk for HIV infection: | 90 | (85) | 878 | (83) | 106 | (90) | 982 | (91) | 196 | (88) | 1,860 | (87) |
| *Injecting drug use* | *21* | | *274* | | *20* | | *271* | | *41* | | *545* | |
| *Sex with injecting drug user* | *9* | | *116* | | *10* | | *140* | | *19* | | *256* | |
| *Sex with bisexual male* | *2* | | *16* | | – | | *16* | | *2* | | *32* | |
| *Sex with person with hemophilia* | – | | *2* | | *2* | | *5* | | *2* | | *7* | |
| *Sex with transfusion recipient with HIV infection* | *1* | | *7* | | – | | *5* | | *1* | | *12* | |
| *Sex with HIV-infected person, risk not specified* | *25* | | *195* | | *40* | | *248* | | *65* | | *443* | |
| *Receipt of blood transfusion, blood components, or tissue* | – | | *10* | | *1* | | *11* | | *1* | | *21* | |
| *Has HIV infection, risk not specified* | *32* | | *258* | | *33* | | *286* | | *65* | | *544* | |
| Receipt of blood transfusion, blood components, or tissue | – | – | 15 | (1) | – | – | 22 | (2) | – | – | 37 | (2) |
| Risk not reported or identified[4] | 12 | (11) | 68 | (6) | 12 | (10) | 70 | (7) | 24 | (11) | 138 | (6) |
| Pediatric subtotal | 106 | (100) | 1,059 | (100) | 118 | (100) | 1,075 | (100) | 224 | (100) | 2,134 | (100) |
| **Total** | **14,813** | | **98,771** | | **6,887** | | **39,229** | | **21,704** | | **138,011** | |

[1]Includes only persons reported with HIV infection who have not developed AIDS.

[2]See table 3 for areas with confidential HIV infection reporting.

[3]Includes 11 persons whose sex is unknown.

[4]For HIV infection cases, "risk not reported or identified" refers primarily to persons whose mode of exposure was not reported and who have not been followed up to determine their mode of exposure, and to a smaller number of persons who are not reported with one of the exposures listed above after follow-up. See Technical Notes.

*Source*: Centers for Disease Control and Prevention, U.S. Department of Health and Human Services. National Center for HIV, STD, and TB Prevention. Division of HIV/AIDS Prevention—Surveillance and Epidemiology. *HIV/AIDS Surveillance Report 2000* 12, no. 2, year-end edition. http://www.cdc.gov/hiv/stats/hasr1202.pdf.

## Table B2.4. HIV Infection Cases,[1] by Sex, Age at Diagnosis and Race/Ethnicity, Reported through December 2000, from the 36 Areas with Confidential HIV Infection Reporting[2]

| Male | White, not Hispanic | | Black, not Hispanic | | Hispanic | | Asian/Pacific Islander | | American Indian/ Alaska Native | | Total[3] | |
|---|---|---|---|---|---|---|---|---|---|---|---|---|
| Age at diagnosis (years) | No. | (%) | No. | (%) | No. | (%) | No. | (%) | No. | (%) | No. | (%) |
| Under 5 | 170 | (0) | 525 | (1) | 89 | (1) | 4 | (1) | 2 | (0) | 794 | (1) |
| 5–12 | 99 | (0) | 117 | (0) | 40 | (0) | 3 | (1) | – | – | 265 | (0) |
| 13–19 | 814 | (2) | 1,398 | (3) | 150 | (2) | 9 | (2) | 17 | (3) | 2,412 | (2) |
| 20–24 | 5,196 | (12) | 5,471 | (12) | 987 | (12) | 57 | (14) | 113 | (18) | 11,951 | (12) |
| 25–29 | 9,278 | (22) | 7,866 | (17) | 1,806 | (21) | 89 | (22) | 156 | (24) | 19,468 | (20) |
| 30–34 | 9,912 | (23) | 9,317 | (21) | 1,978 | (23) | 115 | (28) | 140 | (22) | 21,759 | (22) |
| 35–39 | 7,670 | (18) | 8,404 | (19) | 1,637 | (19) | 52 | (13) | 104 | (16) | 18,125 | (18) |
| 40–44 | 4,547 | (11) | 5,934 | (13) | 917 | (11) | 39 | (10) | 57 | (9) | 11,672 | (12) |
| 45–49 | 2,361 | (6) | 3,273 | (7) | 496 | (6) | 18 | (4) | 25 | (4) | 6,280 | (6) |
| 50–54 | 1,243 | (3) | 1,546 | (3) | 227 | (3) | 10 | (2) | 12 | (2) | 3,092 | (3) |
| 55–59 | 528 | (1) | 797 | (2) | 111 | (1) | 4 | (1) | 8 | (1) | 1,469 | (1) |
| 60–64 | 298 | (1) | 388 | (1) | 63 | (1) | 2 | (0) | 3 | (0) | 765 | (1) |
| 65 or older | 268 | (1) | 376 | (1) | 58 | (1) | 3 | (1) | 2 | (0) | 719 | (1) |
| **Male subtotal** | **42,384** | **(100)** | **45,412** | **(100)** | **8,559** | **(100)** | **405** | **(100)** | **639** | **(100)** | **98,771** | **(100)** |
| **Female** | | | | | | | | | | | | |
| **Age at diagnosis (years)** | | | | | | | | | | | | |
| Under 5 | 163 | (2) | 588 | (2) | 89 | (3) | 5 | (3) | 8 | (3) | 860 | (2) |
| 5–12 | 44 | (0) | 131 | (0) | 32 | (1) | 2 | (1) | 2 | (1) | 215 | (1) |
| 13–19 | 628 | (7) | 2,320 | (9) | 172 | (6) | 7 | (5) | 21 | (9) | 3,167 | (8) |
| 20–24 | 1,561 | (17) | 4,284 | (16) | 428 | (15) | 36 | (25) | 42 | (18) | 6,407 | (16) |
| 25–29 | 1,834 | (20) | 4,985 | (19) | 570 | (20) | 35 | (24) | 38 | (16) | 7,527 | (19) |
| 30–34 | 1,782 | (20) | 4,982 | (19) | 591 | (21) | 23 | (16) | 41 | (18) | 7,500 | (19) |
| 35–39 | 1,412 | (15) | 3,961 | (15) | 396 | (14) | 13 | (9) | 42 | (18) | 5,881 | (15) |
| 40–44 | 775 | (8) | 2,587 | (10) | 249 | (9) | 11 | (8) | 27 | (12) | 3,688 | (9) |
| 45–49 | 467 | (5) | 1,314 | (5) | 167 | (6) | 5 | (3) | 9 | (4) | 1,985 | (5) |
| 50–54 | 208 | (2) | 637 | (2) | 75 | (3) | 2 | (1) | 1 | (0) | 930 | (2) |
| 55–59 | 111 | (1) | 338 | (1) | 49 | (2) | 2 | (1) | – | – | 509 | (1) |
| 60–64 | 50 | (1) | 185 | (1) | 24 | (1) | – | – | 1 | (0) | 260 | (1) |
| 65 or older | 87 | (1) | 192 | (1) | 16 | (1) | 2 | (1) | – | – | 300 | (1) |
| **Female subtotal** | **9,122** | **(100)** | **26,504** | **(100)** | **2,858** | **(100)** | **143** | **(100)** | **232** | **(100)** | **39,229** | **(100)** |
| **Total[4]** | **51,507** | | **71,920** | | **11,417** | | **548** | | **871** | | **138,011** | |

[1]Includes only persons reported with HIV infection who have not developed AIDS.

[2]See table 3 for areas with confidential HIV infection reporting.

[3]Includes 1,372 males, 370 females, and 6 persons of unknown sex whose race/ethnicity is unknown.

[4]Includes 11 persons whose sex is unknown.

*Source*: Centers for Disease Control and Prevention, U.S. Department of Health and Human Services. National Center for HIV, STD, and TB Prevention. Division of HIV/AIDS Prevention—Surveillance and Epidemiology. *HIV/AIDS Surveillance Report 2000* 12, no. 2, year-end edition. http://www.cdc.gov/hiv/stats/hasr1202.pdf.

## Table B2.5. Male Adult/Adolescent HIV Infection Cases,[1] by Exposure Category and Race/Ethnicity, Reported through December 2000, from the 34 Areas with Confidential HIV Infection Reporting[2]

| | White, not Hispanic | | | | Black, not Hispanic | | | | Hispanic | | | |
|---|---|---|---|---|---|---|---|---|---|---|---|---|
| | 2000 | | Cumulative total | | 2000 | | Cumulative total | | 2000 | | Cumulative total | |
| **Exposure category** | **No.** | **(%)** | **No.** | **(%)** | **No.** | **(%)** | **No.** | **(%)** | **No.** | **(%)** | **No.** | **(%)** |
| Men who have sex with men | 3,458 | (60) | 26,135 | (62) | 1,814 | (28) | 14,023 | (31) | 877 | (45) | 3,499 | (42) |
| Injecting drug use | 416 | (7) | 3,557 | (8) | 725 | (11) | 7,876 | (18) | 207 | (11) | 1,552 | (18) |
| Men who have sex with men and inject drugs | 355 | (6) | 3,363 | (8) | 211 | (3) | 2,151 | (5) | 62 | (3) | 413 | (5) |
| Hemophilia/coagulation disorder | 16 | (0) | 334 | (1) | 3 | (0) | 90 | (0) | 4 | (0) | 12 | (0) |
| Heterosexual contact: | 177 | (3) | 1,267 | (3) | 898 | (14) | 5,174 | (12) | 135 | (7) | 578 | (7) |
| *Sex with injecting drug user* | *54* | | *331* | | *132* | | *1,033* | | *30* | | *142* | |
| *Sex with person with hemophilia* | *1* | | *3* | | *1* | | *10* | | – | | – | |
| *Sex with transfusion recipient with HIV infection* | *1* | | *21* | | *5* | | *56* | | *1* | | *3* | |
| *Sex with HIV-infected person, risk not specified* | *121* | | *912* | | *760* | | *4,075* | | *104* | | *433* | |
| Receipt of blood transfusion, blood components, or tissue | 22 | (0) | 185 | (0) | 29 | (0) | 182 | (0) | 2 | (0) | 25 | (0) |
| Risk not reported or identified[3] | 1,298 | (23) | 7,274 | (17) | 2,848 | (44) | 15,274 | (34) | 671 | (34) | 2,351 | (28) |
| **Total** | **5,742** | **(100)** | **42,115** | **(100)** | **6,528** | **(100)** | **44,770** | **(100)** | **1,958** | **(100)** | **8,430** | **(100)** |

| | Asian/Pacific Islander | | | | American Indian/Alaska Native | | | | Cumulative totals[4] | | | |
|---|---|---|---|---|---|---|---|---|---|---|---|---|
| | 2000 | | Cumulative total | | 2000 | | Cumulative total | | 2000 | | Cumulative total | |
| **Exposure category** | **No.** | **(%)** | **No.** | **(%)** | **No.** | **(%)** | **No.** | **(%)** | **No.** | **(%)** | **No.** | **(%)** |
| Men who have sex with men | 49 | (48) | 210 | (53) | 52 | (46) | 327 | (51) | 6,302 | (43) | 44,467 | (46) |
| Injecting drug use | 2 | (2) | 18 | (5) | 12 | (11) | 79 | (12) | 1,367 | (9) | 13,142 | (13) |
| Men who have sex with men and inject drugs | 1 | (1) | 8 | (2) | 10 | (9) | 84 | (13) | 643 | (4) | 6,042 | (6) |
| Hemophilia/coagulation disorder | – | – | 2 | (1) | – | – | 1 | (0) | 23 | (0) | 442 | (0) |
| Heterosexual contact: | 2 | (2) | 23 | (6) | 11 | (10) | 38 | (6) | 1,231 | (8) | 7,105 | (7) |
| *Sex with injecting drug user* | – | | *6* | | *2* | | *13* | | *218* | | *1,528* | |
| *Sex with person with hemophilia* | – | | – | | – | | – | | *2* | | *13* | |
| *Sex with transfusion recipient with HIV infection* | – | | *2* | | – | | – | | *7* | | *82* | |
| *Sex with HIV-infected person, risk not specified* | *2* | | *15* | | *9* | | *25* | | *1,004* | | *5,482* | |
| Receipt of blood transfusion, blood components, or tissue | 1 | (1) | 4 | (1) | – | – | 1 | (0) | 54 | (0) | 401 | (0) |
| Risk not reported or identified | 47 | (46) | 133 | (33) | 28 | (25) | 107 | (17) | 5,087 | (35) | 26,113 | (27) |
| **Total** | **102** | **(100)** | **398** | **(100)** | **113** | **(100)** | **637** | **(100)** | **14,707** | **(100)** | **97,712** | **(100)** |

[1]Includes only persons reported with HIV infection who have not developed AIDS.

[2]See table 3 for areas with confidential HIV infection reporting of adults and adolescents.

[3]For HIV infection cases, "risk not reported or identified" refers primarily to persons whose mode of exposure was not reported and who have not been followed up to determine their mode of exposure, and to a smaller number of persons who are not reported with one of the exposures listed above after follow-up. See Technical Notes.

[4]Includes 1,362 men whose race/ethnicity is unknown.

*Source*: Centers for Disease Control and Prevention, U.S. Department of Health and Human Services. National Center for HIV, STD, and TB Prevention. Division of HIV/AIDS Prevention—Surveillance and Epidemiology. *HIV/AIDS Surveillance Report 2000* 12, no. 2, year-end edition. http://www.cdc.gov/hiv/stats/hasr1202.pdf.

## Table B2.6. Female Adult/Adolescent HIV Infection Cases,[1] by Exposure Category and Race/Ethnicity, Reported through December 2000, from the 34 Areas with Confidential HIV Infection Reporting[2]

| | White, not Hispanic | | | | Black, not Hispanic | | | | Hispanic | | | |
|---|---|---|---|---|---|---|---|---|---|---|---|---|
| | 2000 | | Cumulative total | | 2000 | | Cumulative total | | 2000 | | Cumulative total | |
| **Exposure category** | **No.** | **(%)** | **No.** | **(%)** | **No.** | **(%)** | **No.** | **(%)** | **No.** | **(%)** | **No.** | **(%)** |
| Injecting drug use | 323 | (23) | 2,394 | (27) | 454 | (10) | 4,367 | (17) | 64 | (10) | 520 | (19) |
| Hemophilia/coagulation disorder | 1 | (0) | 12 | (0) | 7 | (0) | 16 | (0) | – | – | – | – |
| Heterosexual contact: | 503 | (36) | 3,808 | (43) | 1,632 | (36) | 10,466 | (41) | 265 | (43) | 1,243 | (45) |
| *Sex with injecting drug user* | *115* | | *1,212* | | *243* | | *2,384* | | *52* | | *398* | |
| *Sex with bisexual male* | *44* | | *399* | | *84* | | *693* | | *20* | | *63* | |
| *Sex with person with hemophilia* | *6* | | *80* | | *7* | | *42* | | – | | *4* | |
| *Sex with transfusion recipient with HIV infection* | *4* | | *36* | | *6* | | *59* | | *1* | | *13* | |
| *Sex with HIV-infected person, risk not specified* | *334* | | *2,081* | | *1,292* | | *7,288* | | *192* | | *765* | |
| Receipt of blood transfusion, blood components, or tissue | 10 | (1) | 138 | (2) | 36 | (1) | 259 | (1) | 4 | (1) | 25 | (1) |
| Risk not reported or identified[3] | 572 | (41) | 2,563 | (29) | 2,440 | (53) | 10,677 | (41) | 279 | (46) | 949 | (35) |
| **Total** | **1,409** | **(100)** | **8,915** | **(100)** | **4,569** | **(100)** | **25,785** | **(100)** | **612** | **(100)** | **2,737** | **(100)** |

| | Asian/Pacific Islander | | | | American Indian/Alaska Native | | | | Cumulative totals[4] | | | |
|---|---|---|---|---|---|---|---|---|---|---|---|---|
| | 2000 | | Cumulative total | | 2000 | | Cumulative total | | 2000 | | Cumulative total | |
| **Exposure category** | **No.** | **(%)** | **No.** | **(%)** | **No.** | **(%)** | **No.** | **(%)** | **No.** | **(%)** | **No.** | **(%)** |
| Injecting drug use | 2 | (6) | 11 | (8) | 11 | (20) | 71 | (32) | 855 | (13) | 7,383 | (19) |
| Hemophilia/coagulation disorder | – | – | – | – | – | – | – | – | 8 | (0) | 28 | (0) |
| Heterosexual contact: | 18 | (51) | 66 | (49) | 21 | (38) | 92 | (41) | 2,448 | (36) | 15,724 | (41) |
| *Sex with injecting drug user* | *2* | | *11* | | *8* | | *42* | | *422* | | *4,056* | |
| *Sex with bisexual male* | *2* | | *3* | | *1* | | *6* | | *153* | | *1,171* | |
| *Sex with person with hemophilia* | – | | – | | *1* | | *2* | | *14* | | *129* | |
| *Sex with transfusion recipient with HIV infection* | – | | – | | – | | *1* | | *11* | | *109* | |
| *Sex with HIV-infected person, risk not specified* | *14* | | *52* | | *11* | | *41* | | *1,848* | | *10,259* | |
| Receipt of blood transfusion, blood components, or tissue | 1 | (3) | 3 | (2) | – | – | 2 | (1) | 51 | (1) | 429 | (1) |
| Risk not reported or identified | 14 | (40) | 56 | (41) | 23 | (42) | 57 | (26) | 3,407 | (50) | 14,590 | (38) |
| **Total** | **35** | **(100)** | **136** | **(100)** | **55** | **(100)** | **222** | **(100)** | **6,769** | **(100)** | **38,154** | **(100)** |

[1]Includes only persons reported with HIV infection who have not developed AIDS.

[2]See table 3 for areas with confidential HIV infection reporting of adults and adolescents.

[3]For HIV infection cases, "risk not reported or identified" refers primarily to persons whose mode of exposure was not reported and who have not been followed up to determine their mode of exposure, and to a smaller number of persons who are not reported with one of the exposures listed above after follow-up. See Technical Notes.

[4]Includes 359 women whose race/ethnicity is unknown.

*Source*: Centers for Disease Control and Prevention, U.S. Department of Health and Human Services. National Center for HIV, STD, and TB Prevention. Division of HIV/AIDS Prevention—Surveillance and Epidemiology. *HIV/AIDS Surveillance Report 2000* 12, no. 2, year-end edition. http://www.cdc.gov/hiv/stats/hasr1202.pdf.

## Table B2.7. Health Care Workers with Documented and Possible Occupationally Acquired AIDS/HIV Infection, by Occupation, Reported through June 2000, United States[1]

| Occupation | Documented occupational transmission[2] No. | Possible occupational transmission[3] No. |
|---|---|---|
| Dental worker, including dentist | — | 6 |
| Embalmer/morgue technician | 1 | 2 |
| Emergency medical technician/paramedic | — | 12 |
| Health aide/attendant | 1 | 15 |
| Housekeeper/maintenance worker | 2 | 13 |
| Laboratory technician, clinical | 16 | 17 |
| Laboratory technician, nonclinical | 3 | — |
| Nurse | 23 | 35 |
| Physician, nonsurgical | 6 | 12 |
| Physician, surgical | — | 6 |
| Respiratory therapist | 1 | 2 |
| Technician, dialysis | 1 | 3 |
| Technician, surgical | 2 | 2 |
| Technician/therapist, other than those listed above | — | 9 |
| Other health care occupations | — | 4 |
| **Total** | **56** | **138** |

[1]Health care workers are defined as those persons, including students and trainees, who have worked in a health care, clinical, or HIV laboratory setting at any time since 1978. See *MMWR* 41 (1992): 823–25.
[2]Health care workers who had documented HIV seroconversion after occupational exposure or had other laboratory evidence of occupational infection: 48 had percutaneous exposure, 5 had mucocutaneous exposure, 2 had both percutaneous and mucocutaneous exposures, and 1 had an unknown route of exposure. Forty-nine health care workers were exposed to blood from an HIV-infected person, to visibly bloody fluid, 3 to an unspecified fluid, and 3 to concentrated virus in a laboratory. Twenty-five of these health care workers developed AIDS.
[3]These health care workers have been investigated and are without identifiable behavioral or transfusion risks; each reported percutaneous or mucocutaneous occupational exposures to blood or body fluids, or laboratory solutions containing HIV, but HIV seroconversion specifically resulting from an occupational exposure was not documented.
*Source*: Centers for Disease Control and Prevention, U.S. Department of Health and Human Services. National Center for HIV, STD, and TB Prevention. Division of HIV/AIDS Prevention—Surveillance and Epidemiology. *HIV/AIDS Surveillance Report 2000* 12, no. 1, mid-year edition. http://www.cdc.gov/hiv/stats/hasr1201.pdf.

**Table B3.1. Acquired Immunodeficiency Syndrome—Reported Cases per 100,000 Population, United States, Guam, Puerto Rico, and U.S. Virgin Islands, 1999**

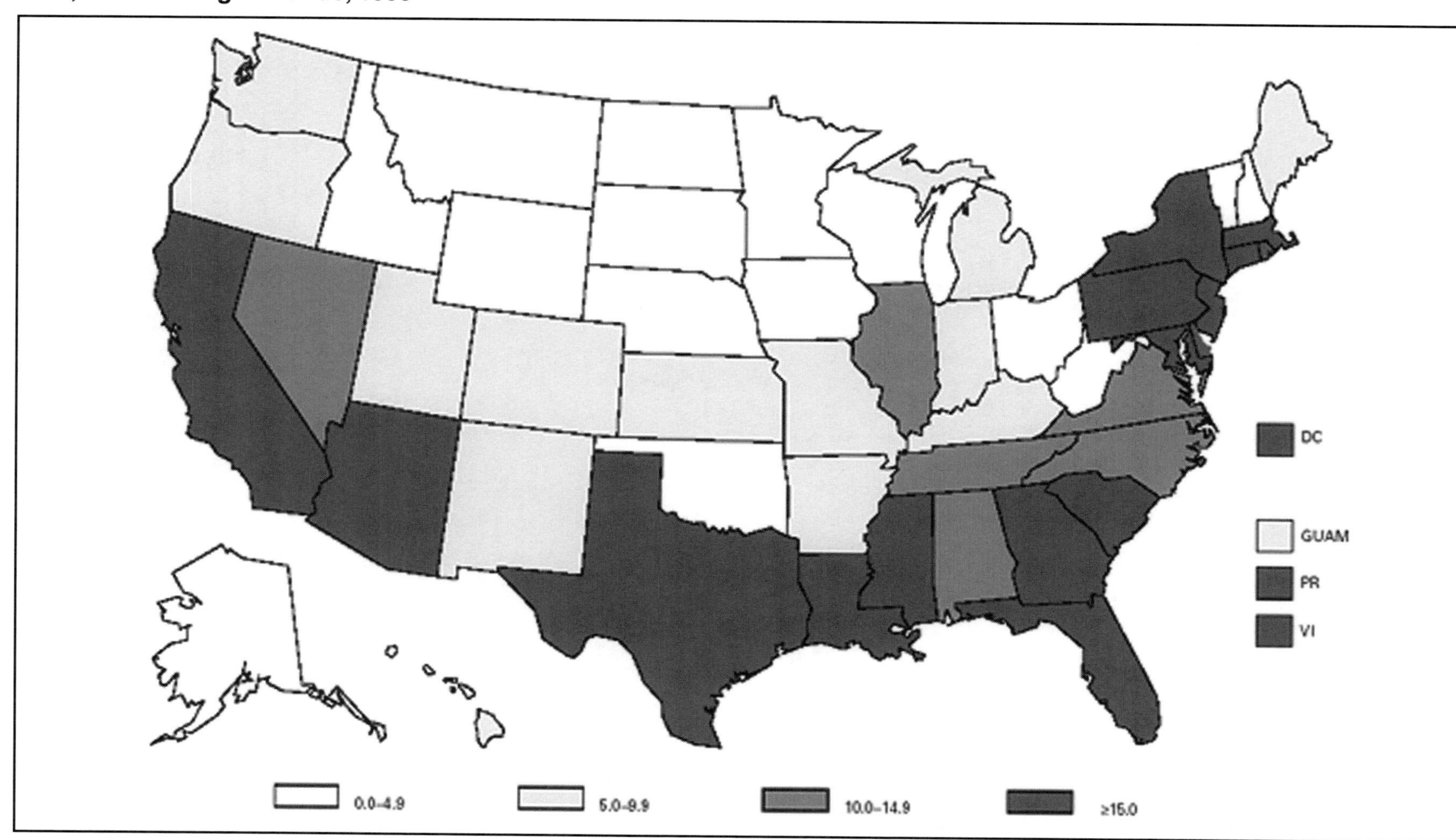


Total number of AIDS cases includes all cases reported to the Division of HIV/AIDS Prevention—Surveillance and Epidemiology, National Center for HIV, STD, and TB Prevention, as of December 31, 1999. Total includes cases among residents in U.S. territories and 104 cases among persons with unknown state of residence.

*Source*: Center for Disease Control and Prevention. U.S. Department of Health and Human Services. *MMWR: Morbidity and Mortality Weekly Review Summary of Notifiable Disease, United States, 1999.* 48, no. 53 (2001). http://www.cdc.gov/mmwr/PDF/wk/mm4853.pdf

## Table B3.2. AIDS Cases and Annual Rates per 100,000 Population, by Area and Age Group, Reported through December 2000, United States

| | 1999 | | 2000 | | Cumulative totals | | |
|---|---|---|---|---|---|---|---|
| Area of residence | No. | Rate | No. | Rate | Adults/ adolescents | Children <13 years old | Total |
| Alabama | 472 | 10.8 | 483 | 10.9 | 6,198 | 72 | 6,270 |
| Alaska | 14 | 2.3 | 22 | 3.5 | 471 | 5 | 476 |
| Arizona | 876 | 18.3 | 460 | 9.0 | 7,404 | 39 | 7,443 |
| Arkansas | 194 | 7.6 | 194 | 7.3 | 2,939 | 38 | 2,977 |
| California | 5,392 | 16.3 | 4,737 | 14.0 | 119,218 | 608 | 119,826 |
| Colorado | 311 | 7.7 | 313 | 7.3 | 6,971 | 29 | 7,000 |
| Connecticut | 584 | 17.8 | 620 | 18.2 | 11,395 | 176 | 11,571 |
| Delaware | 184 | 24.4 | 221 | 28.2 | 2,558 | 22 | 2,580 |
| District of Columbia | 835 | 160.9 | 875 | 153.0 | 12,931 | 171 | 13,102 |
| Florida | 5,421 | 35.9 | 4,976 | 31.1 | 79,014 | 1,402 | 80,416 |
| Georgia | 1,680 | 21.6 | 1,237 | 15.1 | 22,626 | 211 | 22,837 |
| Hawaii | 99 | 8.4 | 115 | 9.5 | 2,445 | 16 | 2,461 |
| Idaho | 25 | 2.0 | 22 | 1.7 | 495 | 2 | 497 |
| Illinois | 1,559 | 12.9 | 1,761 | 14.2 | 24,740 | 269 | 25,009 |
| Indiana | 361 | 6.1 | 389 | 6.4 | 6,108 | 41 | 6,149 |
| Iowa | 85 | 3.0 | 94 | 3.2 | 1,307 | 10 | 1,317 |
| Kansas | 170 | 6.4 | 128 | 4.8 | 2,355 | 13 | 2,368 |
| Kentucky | 277 | 7.0 | 212 | 5.2 | 3,319 | 26 | 3,345 |
| Louisiana | 855 | 19.6 | 679 | 15.2 | 12,520 | 125 | 12,645 |
| Maine | 80 | 6.4 | 40 | 3.1 | 947 | 9 | 956 |
| Maryland | 1,522 | 29.4 | 1,465 | 27.7 | 21,390 | 301 | 21,691 |
| Massachusetts | 1,425 | 23.1 | 1,197 | 18.9 | 16,068 | 206 | 16,274 |
| Michigan | 642 | 6.5 | 767 | 7.7 | 11,215 | 107 | 11,322 |
| Minnesota | 189 | 4.0 | 185 | 3.8 | 3,741 | 23 | 3,764 |
| Mississippi | 419 | 15.1 | 431 | 15.2 | 4,411 | 55 | 4,466 |
| Missouri | 528 | 9.7 | 459 | 8.2 | 9,164 | 57 | 9,221 |
| Montana | 13 | 1.5 | 16 | 1.8 | 323 | 3 | 326 |
| Nebraska | 67 | 4.0 | 79 | 4.6 | 1,086 | 10 | 1,096 |
| Nevada | 242 | 13.4 | 286 | 14.3 | 4,393 | 27 | 4,420 |
| New Hampshire | 47 | 3.9 | 31 | 2.5 | 873 | 9 | 882 |
| New Jersey | 2,037 | 25.0 | 1,929 | 22.9 | 41,392 | 751 | 42,143 |
| New Mexico | 93 | 5.3 | 144 | 7.9 | 2,043 | 8 | 2,051 |
| New York | 7,685 | 42.2 | 6,204 | 32.7 | 139,922 | 2,242 | 142,164 |
| North Carolina | 796 | 10.4 | 696 | 8.6 | 10,320 | 116 | 10,436 |
| North Dakota | 7 | 1.1 | 3 | 0.5 | 105 | 1 | 106 |
| Ohio | 554 | 4.9 | 599 | 5.3 | 11,273 | 121 | 11,394 |
| Oklahoma | 147 | 4.4 | 352 | 10.2 | 3,761 | 26 | 3,787 |
| Oregon | 225 | 6.8 | 210 | 6.1 | 4,782 | 17 | 4,799 |
| Pennsylvania | 1,962 | 16.4 | 1,692 | 13.8 | 24,335 | 325 | 24,660 |
| Rhode Island | 107 | 10.8 | 102 | 9.7 | 2,033 | 21 | 2,054 |
| South Carolina | 956 | 24.6 | 810 | 20.2 | 9,448 | 79 | 9,527 |
| South Dakota | 16 | 2.2 | 8 | 1.1 | 162 | 4 | 166 |
| Tennessee | 755 | 13.8 | 863 | 15.2 | 8,538 | 52 | 8,590 |
| Texas | 3,151 | 15.7 | 2,667 | 12.8 | 53,607 | 380 | 53,987 |
| Utah | 154 | 7.2 | 151 | 6.8 | 1,955 | 21 | 1,976 |
| Vermont | 21 | 3.5 | 38 | 6.2 | 399 | 6 | 405 |
| Virginia | 937 | 13.6 | 891 | 12.6 | 12,919 | 169 | 13,088 |
| Washington | 359 | 6.2 | 515 | 8.7 | 9,468 | 35 | 9,503 |
| West Virginia | 68 | 3.8 | 63 | 3.5 | 1,069 | 9 | 1,078 |
| Wisconsin | 152 | 2.9 | 218 | 4.1 | 3,557 | 29 | 3,586 |
| Wyoming | 15 | 3.1 | 11 | 2.2 | 184 | 2 | 186 |
| **Subtotal** | **44,765** | **16.4** | **40,660** | **14.4** | **739,897** | **8,496** | **748,393** |
| **U.S. dependencies, possessions, and associated nations** | | | | | | | |
| Guam | 10 | 6.6 | 15 | 9.7 | 48 | – | 48 |
| Pacific Islands, U.S. | – | – | – | – | 4 | – | 4 |
| Puerto Rico | 1,244 | 32.0 | 1,349 | 35.4 | 24,495 | 388 | 24,883 |
| Virgin Islands, U.S. | 39 | 32.6 | 34 | 28.1 | 466 | 17 | 483 |
| **Total[1]** | **46,143** | **16.6** | **42,156** | **14.7** | **765,559** | **8,908** | **774,467** |

[1]U.S. totals presented in this report include data from the United States (50 states and the District of Columbia), and from U.S. dependencies, possessions, and independent nations in free association with the United States. See Technical Notes. Totals include 656 persons whose area of residence is unknown.

*Source*: Centers for Disease Control and Prevention, U.S. Department of Health and Human Services. National Center for HIV, STD, and TB Prevention. Division of HIV/AIDS Prevention—Surveillance and Epidemiology. *HIV/AIDS Surveillance Report 2000* 12, no. 2, year-end edition. http://www.cdc.gov/hiv/stats/hasr1202.pdf.

## Table B3.3. AIDS Cases and Annual Rates per 100,000 Population, by Metropolitan Area and Age Group, Reported through December 2000, United States

| Metropolitan area of residence (with 500,000 or more population) | 1999 | | 2000 | | Cumulative totals | | |
|---|---|---|---|---|---|---|---|
| | No. | Rate | No. | Rate | Adults/ adolescents | Children <13 years old | Total |
| Akron, Ohio | 53 | 7.7 | 30 | 4.3 | 586 | 1 | 587 |
| Albany-Schenectady, N.Y. | 79 | 9.1 | 126 | 14.4 | 1,749 | 24 | 1,773 |
| Albuquerque, N.Mex. | 48 | 7.1 | 72 | 10.1 | 1,102 | 2 | 1,104 |
| Allentown, Pa. | 79 | 12.8 | 50 | 7.8 | 829 | 8 | 837 |
| Ann Arbor, Mich. | 27 | 4.8 | 36 | 6.2 | 399 | 9 | 408 |
| Atlanta, Ga. | 1,028 | 26.7 | 707 | 17.2 | 15,763 | 115 | 15,878 |
| Austin, Tex. | 275 | 24.0 | 180 | 14.4 | 3,868 | 25 | 3,893 |
| Bakersfield, Calif. | 90 | 14.0 | 86 | 13.0 | 1,036 | 8 | 1,044 |
| Baltimore, Md. | 1,012 | 40.6 | 973 | 38.1 | 14,306 | 208 | 14,514 |
| Baton Rouge, La. | 189 | 32.6 | 145 | 24.1 | 1,893 | 19 | 1,912 |
| Bergen-Passaic, N.J. | 248 | 18.5 | 211 | 15.4 | 5,386 | 82 | 5,468 |
| Birmingham, Ala. | 137 | 15.0 | 116 | 12.6 | 1,888 | 23 | 1,911 |
| Boston, Mass. | 1,196 | 20.3 | 1,026 | 16.9 | 14,135 | 182 | 14,317 |
| Buffalo, N.Y. | 172 | 15.1 | 83 | 7.1 | 1,814 | 18 | 1,832 |
| Charleston, S.C. | 116 | 21.0 | 116 | 21.1 | 1,551 | 12 | 1,563 |
| Charlotte, N.C. | 162 | 11.4 | 134 | 8.9 | 2,108 | 22 | 2,130 |
| Chicago, Ill. | 1,353 | 16.9 | 1,522 | 18.4 | 21,420 | 238 | 21,658 |
| Cincinnati, Ohio | 60 | 3.7 | 75 | 4.6 | 1,900 | 15 | 1,915 |
| Cleveland, Ohio | 181 | 8.1 | 168 | 7.5 | 3,330 | 42 | 3,372 |
| Colorado Springs, Colo. | 27 | 5.4 | 25 | 4.8 | 451 | 5 | 456 |
| Columbia, S.C. | 281 | 54.4 | 156 | 29.1 | 2,024 | 16 | 2,040 |
| Columbus, Ohio | 87 | 5.8 | 118 | 7.7 | 2,220 | 13 | 2,233 |
| Dallas, Tex. | 626 | 19.1 | 654 | 18.6 | 12,370 | 37 | 12,407 |
| Dayton, Ohio | 47 | 4.9 | 64 | 6.7 | 997 | 17 | 1,014 |
| Denver, Colo. | 231 | 11.7 | 229 | 10.9 | 5,536 | 20 | 5,556 |
| Detroit, Mich. | 417 | 9.3 | 551 | 12.4 | 7,736 | 73 | 7,809 |
| El Paso, Tex. | 91 | 13.0 | 78 | 11.5 | 1,072 | 10 | 1,082 |
| Fort Lauderdale, Fla. | 932 | 60.7 | 861 | 53.0 | 12,700 | 245 | 12,945 |
| Fort Wayne, Ind. | 17 | 3.5 | 25 | 5.0 | 312 | 3 | 315 |
| Fort Worth, Tex. | 133 | 8.2 | 193 | 11.3 | 3,247 | 26 | 3,273 |
| Fresno, Calif. | 65 | 7.4 | 95 | 10.3 | 1,202 | 14 | 1,216 |
| Gary, Ind. | 43 | 6.8 | 62 | 9.8 | 733 | 4 | 737 |
| Grand Rapids, Mich. | 40 | 3.8 | 36 | 3.3 | 761 | 4 | 765 |
| Greensboro, N.C. | 172 | 14.6 | 98 | 7.8 | 1,664 | 21 | 1,685 |
| Greenville, S.C. | 135 | 14.5 | 123 | 12.8 | 1,505 | 6 | 1,511 |
| Harrisburg, Pa. | 74 | 12.0 | 71 | 11.3 | 1,014 | 8 | 1,022 |
| Hartford, Conn. | 178 | 16.0 | 239 | 20.8 | 3,966 | 46 | 4,012 |
| Honolulu, Hawaii | 76 | 8.8 | 84 | 9.6 | 1,786 | 13 | 1,799 |
| Houston, Tex. | 927 | 23.1 | 693 | 16.6 | 18,956 | 160 | 19,116 |
| Indianapolis, Ind. | 183 | 11.9 | 163 | 10.1 | 2,877 | 17 | 2,894 |
| Jacksonville, Fla. | 299 | 28.3 | 289 | 26.3 | 4,419 | 68 | 4,487 |
| Jersey City, N.J. | 249 | 45.0 | 231 | 37.9 | 6,483 | 120 | 6,603 |
| Kansas City, Mo. | 200 | 11.4 | 178 | 10.0 | 3,925 | 15 | 3,940 |
| Knoxville, Tenn. | 46 | 6.8 | 45 | 6.5 | 726 | 6 | 732 |
| Las Vegas, Nev. | 205 | 14.8 | 249 | 15.9 | 3,588 | 26 | 3,614 |
| Little Rock, Ark. | 56 | 10.0 | 54 | 9.2 | 1,043 | 14 | 1,057 |
| Los Angeles, Calif. | 2,050 | 22.0 | 1,667 | 17.5 | 42,020 | 234 | 42,254 |
| Louisville, Ky. | 158 | 15.7 | 93 | 9.1 | 1,630 | 17 | 1,647 |
| McAllen, Tex. | 28 | 5.2 | 42 | 7.4 | 371 | 10 | 381 |
| Memphis, Tenn. | 327 | 29.6 | 327 | 28.8 | 3,164 | 18 | 3,182 |
| Miami, Fla. | 1,414 | 65.0 | 1,306 | 58.0 | 23,672 | 479 | 24,151 |
| Middlesex, N.J. | 113 | 10.0 | 134 | 11.5 | 3,136 | 69 | 3,205 |
| Milwaukee, Wis. | 86 | 5.9 | 136 | 9.1 | 1,962 | 17 | 1,979 |
| Minneapolis-Saint Paul, Minn. | 178 | 6.2 | 170 | 5.7 | 3,333 | 17 | 3,350 |
| Mobile, Ala. | 92 | 17.2 | 99 | 18.3 | 1,191 | 14 | 1,205 |
| Monmouth-Ocean, N.J. | 106 | 9.6 | 130 | 11.5 | 2,816 | 62 | 2,878 |
| Nashville, Tenn. | 230 | 19.6 | 340 | 27.6 | 2,736 | 17 | 2,753 |
| Nassau-Suffolk, N.Y. | 349 | 13.0 | 279 | 10.1 | 6,639 | 110 | 6,749 |
| New Haven, Conn. | 343 | 21.0 | 314 | 18.4 | 6,443 | 124 | 6,567 |
| New Orleans, La. | 415 | 31.8 | 334 | 25.0 | 6,888 | 67 | 6,955 |

## Table B3.3. *(Continued)*

| Metropolitan area of residence (with 500,000 or more population) | 1999 No. | 1999 Rate | 2000 No. | 2000 Rate | Cumulative totals: Adults/ adolescents | Cumulative totals: Children <13 years old | Cumulative totals: Total |
|---|---|---|---|---|---|---|---|
| New York, N.Y. | 6,316 | 72.5 | 5,274 | 56.6 | 118,226 | 2,008 | 120,234 |
| Newark, N.J. | 914 | 46.8 | 802 | 39.4 | 16,792 | 325 | 17,117 |
| Norfolk, Va. | 272 | 17.4 | 284 | 18.1 | 3,742 | 63 | 3,805 |
| Oakland, Calif. | 345 | 14.7 | 266 | 11.1 | 7,996 | 43 | 8,039 |
| Oklahoma City, Okla. | 40 | 3.8 | 202 | 18.6 | 1,772 | 7 | 1,779 |
| Omaha, Nebr. | 44 | 6.3 | 55 | 7.7 | 756 | 3 | 759 |
| Orange County, Calif. | 261 | 9.5 | 288 | 10.1 | 5,610 | 35 | 5,645 |
| Orlando, Fla. | 441 | 28.7 | 374 | 22.7 | 5,956 | 81 | 6,037 |
| Philadelphia, Pa. | 1,652 | 33.4 | 1,386 | 27.2 | 18,864 | 274 | 19,138 |
| Phoenix, Ariz. | 688 | 22.8 | 304 | 9.3 | 5,274 | 25 | 5,299 |
| Pittsburgh, Pa. | 91 | 3.9 | 106 | 4.5 | 2,357 | 17 | 2,374 |
| Portland, Oreg. | 161 | 8.7 | 173 | 9.0 | 3,869 | 8 | 3,877 |
| Providence, R.I. | 98 | 10.8 | 96 | 10.0 | 1,908 | 20 | 1,928 |
| Raleigh-Durham, N.C. | 135 | 12.2 | 148 | 12.5 | 1,996 | 22 | 2,018 |
| Richmond, Va. | 183 | 19.0 | 172 | 17.3 | 2,595 | 28 | 2,623 |
| Riverside-San Bernardino, Calif. | 378 | 11.8 | 404 | 12.4 | 6,904 | 56 | 6,960 |
| Rochester, N.Y. | 180 | 16.7 | 77 | 7.0 | 2,329 | 13 | 2,342 |
| Sacramento, Calif. | 139 | 8.8 | 171 | 10.5 | 3,206 | 24 | 3,230 |
| Saint Louis, Mo. | 304 | 11.8 | 252 | 9.7 | 4,695 | 39 | 4,734 |
| Salt Lake City, Utah | 126 | 9.9 | 134 | 10.0 | 1,697 | 14 | 1,711 |
| San Antonio, Tex. | 202 | 12.9 | 170 | 10.7 | 3,938 | 28 | 3,966 |
| San Diego, Calif. | 547 | 19.4 | 442 | 15.7 | 10,548 | 54 | 10,602 |
| San Francisco, Calif. | 851 | 50.5 | 765 | 44.2 | 27,825 | 45 | 27,870 |
| San Jose, Calif. | 152 | 9.2 | 111 | 6.6 | 3,126 | 14 | 3,140 |
| San Juan, P.R. | 806 | 39.9 | 873 | 44.4 | 15,431 | 242 | 15,673 |
| Sarasota, Fla. | 97 | 17.6 | 131 | 22.2 | 1,450 | 21 | 1,471 |
| Scranton, Pa. | 12 | 2.0 | 19 | 3.0 | 430 | 4 | 434 |
| Seattle, Wash. | 240 | 10.3 | 301 | 12.5 | 6,662 | 20 | 6,682 |
| Springfield, Mass. | 176 | 29.9 | 147 | 24.2 | 1,729 | 24 | 1,753 |
| Stockton, Calif. | 61 | 10.8 | 37 | 6.6 | 757 | 13 | 770 |
| Syracuse, N.Y. | 82 | 11.2 | 91 | 12.4 | 1,301 | 10 | 1,311 |
| Tacoma, Wash. | 49 | 7.1 | 58 | 8.3 | 831 | 9 | 840 |
| Tampa-Saint Petersburg, Fla. | 529 | 23.2 | 470 | 19.6 | 8,334 | 99 | 8,433 |
| Toledo, Ohio | 21 | 3.4 | 32 | 5.2 | 569 | 10 | 579 |
| Tucson, Ariz. | 113 | 14.1 | 81 | 9.6 | 1,516 | 10 | 1,526 |
| Tulsa, Okla. | 70 | 8.9 | 70 | 8.7 | 1,126 | 9 | 1,135 |
| Vallejo, Calif. | 110 | 21.7 | 64 | 12.3 | 1,378 | 11 | 1,389 |
| Ventura, Calif. | 47 | 6.3 | 43 | 5.7 | 815 | 3 | 818 |
| Washington, D.C. | 1,526 | 32.2 | 1,549 | 31.5 | 22,904 | 289 | 23,193 |
| West Palm Beach, Fla. | 458 | 43.6 | 545 | 48.2 | 7,474 | 205 | 7,679 |
| Wichita, Kans. | 63 | 11.5 | 46 | 8.4 | 729 | 2 | 731 |
| Wilmington, Del. | 152 | 26.6 | 174 | 29.7 | 2,041 | 15 | 2,056 |
| Youngstown, Ohio | 47 | 8.0 | 18 | 3.0 | 367 | – | 367 |
| **Metropolitan areas with 500,000 or more population** | **37,410** | **21.5** | **34,096** | **18.9** | **642,202** | **7,557** | **649,759** |
| ***Central counties*** | ***36,503*** | ***23.1*** | ***33,309*** | ***20.4*** | ***629,329*** | ***7,421*** | ***636,750*** |
| ***Outlying counties*** | ***907*** | ***5.7*** | ***787*** | ***4.8*** | ***12,873*** | ***136*** | ***13,009*** |
| **Metropolitan areas with 50,000 to 500,000 population** | **4,879** | **10.2** | **4,614** | **9.4** | **73,792** | **825** | **74,617** |
| ***Central counties*** | ***4,530*** | ***10.7*** | ***4,320*** | ***9.9*** | ***68,915*** | ***751*** | ***69,666*** |
| ***Outlying counties*** | ***349*** | ***6.4*** | ***294*** | ***5.3*** | ***4,877*** | ***74*** | ***4,951*** |
| **Nonmetropolitan areas** | **3,374** | **6.1** | **3,061** | **5.4** | **45,162** | **481** | **45,643** |
| **Total[1]** | **46,143** | **16.6** | **42,156** | **14.7** | **765,559** | **8,908** | **774,467** |

[1]Totals include 4,448 persons whose area of residence is unknown.

*Source*: Centers for Disease Control and Prevention, U.S. Department of Health and Human Services. National Center for HIV, STD, and TB Prevention. Division of HIV/AIDS Prevention—Surveillance and Epidemiology. *HIV/AIDS Surveillance Report 2000* 12, no. 2, year-end edition. http://www.cdc.gov/hiv/stats/hasr1202.pdf.

## Table B3.4. AIDS Cases by Age Group, Exposure Category, and Sex, Reported through December 2000, United States

| | Males | | | | Females | | | | Totals[1] | | | |
|---|---|---|---|---|---|---|---|---|---|---|---|---|
| | 2000 | | Cumulative total | | 2000 | | Cumulative total | | 2000 | | Cumulative total[2] | |
| **Adult/adolescent exposure category** | **No.** | **(%)** | **No.** | **(%)** | **No.** | **(%)** | **No.** | **(%)** | **No.** | **(%)** | **No.** | **(%)** |
| Men who have sex with men | 13,562 | (43) | 355,409 | (56) | – | – | – | – | 13,562 | (32) | 355,409 | (46) |
| Injecting drug use | 5,922 | (19) | 140,536 | (22) | 2,609 | (25) | 52,991 | (41) | 8,531 | (20) | 193,527 | (25) |
| Men who have sex with men and inject drugs | 1,548 | (5) | 48,989 | (8) | – | – | – | – | 1,548 | (4) | 48,989 | (6) |
| Hemophilia/coagulation disorder | 93 | (0) | 4,907 | (1) | 3 | (0) | 283 | (0) | 96 | (0) | 5,190 | (1) |
| Heterosexual contact: | 2,549 | (8) | 29,460 | (5) | 3,981 | (38) | 52,520 | (40) | 6,530 | (16) | 81,981 | (11) |
| *Sex with injecting drug user* | *519* | | *9,225* | | *977* | | *20,610* | | *1,496* | | *29,835* | |
| *Sex with bisexual male* | – | | – | | *175* | | *3,561* | | *175* | | *3,561* | |
| *Sex with person with hemophilia* | *4* | | *64* | | *12* | | *416* | | *16* | | *480* | |
| *Sex with transfusion recipient with HIV infection* | *21* | | *417* | | *23* | | *601* | | *44* | | *1,018* | |
| *Sex with HIV-infected person, risk not specified* | *2,005* | | *19,754* | | *2,794* | | *27,332* | | *4,799* | | *47,087* | |
| Receipt of blood transfusion, blood components, or tissue[3] | 144 | (0) | 4,971 | (1) | 138 | (1) | 3,806 | (3) | 282 | (1) | 8,777 | (1) |
| Other/risk not reported or identified[4] | 7,683 | (24) | 51,179 | (8) | 3,728 | (36) | 20,504 | (16) | 11,411 | (27) | 71,686 | (9) |
| Adult/adolescent subtotal | 31,501 | (100) | 635,451 | (100) | 10,459 | (100) | 130,104 | (100) | 41,960 | (100) | 765,559 | (100) |
| **Pediatric (<13 years old) exposure category** | | | | | | | | | | | | |
| Hemophilia/coagulation disorder | 1 | (1) | 230 | (5) | – | – | 7 | (0) | 1 | (1) | 237 | (3) |
| Mother with/at risk for HIV infection:[4] | 80 | (92) | 4,030 | (88) | 97 | (89) | 4,103 | (95) | 177 | (90) | 8,133 | (91) |
| *Injecting drug use* | *18* | | *1,590* | | *22* | | *1,582* | | *40* | | *3,172* | |
| *Sex with injecting drug user* | *8* | | *757* | | *12* | | *716* | | *20* | | *1,473* | |
| *Sex with bisexual male* | – | | *85* | | *4* | | *91* | | *4* | | *176* | |
| *Sex with person with hemophilia* | – | | *17* | | *1* | | *16* | | *1* | | *33* | |
| *Sex with transfusion recipient with HIV infection* | – | | *11* | | – | | *14* | | – | | *25* | |
| *Sex with HIV-infected person, risk not specified* | *25* | | *610* | | *29* | | *652* | | *54* | | *1,262* | |
| *Receipt of blood transfusion, blood components, or tissue* | *1* | | *74* | | *1* | | *79* | | *2* | | *153* | |
| *Has HIV infection, risk not specified* | *28* | | *886* | | *28* | | *953* | | *56* | | *1,839* | |
| Receipt of blood transfusion, blood components, or tissue[3] | – | – | 241 | (5) | 2 | (2) | 141 | (3) | 2 | (1) | 382 | (4) |
| Other/risk not reported or identified[5] | 6 | (7) | 70 | (2) | 10 | (9) | 86 | (2) | 16 | (8) | 156 | (2) |
| Pediatric subtotal | 87 | (100) | 4,571 | (100) | 109 | (100) | 4,337 | (100) | 196 | (100) | 8,908 | (100) |
| **Total** | **31,588** | | **640,022** | | **10,568** | | **134,441** | | **42,156** | | **774,467** | |

[1]Includes 4 persons whose sex is unknown.

[2]Includes persons known to be infected with human immunodeficiency virus type 2 (HIV-2). See *MMWR* 44 (1995): 603–06.

[3]Forty-one adults/adolescents and 2 children developed AIDS after receiving blood screened negative for HIV antibody. Thirteen additional adults developed AIDS after receiving tissue, organs, or artificial insemination from HIV-infected donors. Four of the 13 received tissue, organs, or artificial insemination from a donor who was negative for HIV antibody at the time of donation. See *N Engl J Med* 326 (1992): 726–32.

[4]Thirty-three adults/adolescents are included in the "other" exposure category who were exposed to HIV-infected blood, body fluids, or concentrated virus in health care, laboratory, or household settings, as supported by seroconversion, epidemiologic, and/or laboratory evidence. See *MMWR* 42 (1993): 329–31, *MMWR* 42 (1993): 948–51, and XI International Conference on AIDS; Vancouver, Canada: July 7–12, 1996;1:179 [abstract Mo.D.1728]. One person was infected following intentional innoculation with HIV-infected blood. Additionally, 180 persons acquired HIV infection perinatally and were diagnosed with AIDS after age 13. These 180 persons are tabulated under the adult/adolescent, not pediatric, exposure category. See Technical Notes.

[5]Includes 3 children who were exposed to HIV-infected blood as supported by seroconversion, epidemiologic, and/or laboratory evidence: 1 child was infected following intentional innoculation with HIV-infected blood and 2 children were exposed to HIV-infected blood in a household setting (see *MMWR* 41 (1992): 228–31 and *N Engl J Med* 329 (1993): 1835–41). Twelve of the children had sexual contact with an adult with or at high risk for HIV infection (see *Pediatrics* 102 (1998): e46).

*Source*: Centers for Disease Control and Prevention, U.S. Department of Health and Human Services. National Center for HIV, STD, and TB Prevention. Division of HIV/AIDS Prevention—Surveillance and Epidemiology. *HIV/AIDS Surveillance Report 2000* 12, no. 2, year-end edition. http://www.cdc.gov/hiv/stats/hasr1202.pdf.

## Table B3.5. AIDS Cases, by Sex, Age at Diagnosis, and Race/Ethnicity, Reported through December 2000, United States

| Male<br>Age at diagnosis (years) | White, not Hispanic No. | (%) | Black, not Hispanic No. | (%) | Hispanic No. | (%) | Asian/Pacific Islander No. | (%) | American Indian/ Alaska Native No. | (%) | Total[1] No. | (%) |
|---|---|---|---|---|---|---|---|---|---|---|---|---|
| Under 5 | 524 | (0) | 2,129 | (1) | 768 | (1) | 17 | (0) | 12 | (1) | 3,454 | (1) |
| 5-12 | 341 | (0) | 475 | (0) | 282 | (0) | 10 | (0) | 6 | (0) | 1,117 | (0) |
| 13-19 | 874 | (0) | 919 | (0) | 523 | (0) | 25 | (1) | 22 | (1) | 2,366 | (0) |
| 20-24 | 7,761 | (3) | 7,160 | (3) | 4,297 | (4) | 174 | (3) | 81 | (4) | 19,499 | (3) |
| 25-29 | 38,283 | (13) | 25,564 | (12) | 16,507 | (14) | 626 | (13) | 334 | (18) | 81,411 | (13) |
| 30-34 | 69,614 | (23) | 44,093 | (21) | 27,268 | (24) | 1,085 | (22) | 497 | (26) | 142,702 | (22) |
| 35-39 | 69,257 | (23) | 48,397 | (23) | 25,680 | (22) | 1,089 | (22) | 425 | (22) | 145,053 | (23) |
| 40-44 | 50,497 | (17) | 38,662 | (18) | 18,124 | (16) | 860 | (17) | 281 | (15) | 108,580 | (17) |
| 45-49 | 30,632 | (10) | 22,833 | (11) | 10,206 | (9) | 529 | (11) | 119 | (6) | 64,411 | (10) |
| 50-54 | 16,650 | (6) | 11,778 | (5) | 5,442 | (5) | 281 | (6) | 54 | (3) | 34,258 | (5) |
| 55-59 | 8,923 | (3) | 6,420 | (3) | 2,989 | (3) | 162 | (3) | 34 | (2) | 18,557 | (3) |
| 60-64 | 4,916 | (2) | 3,510 | (2) | 1,649 | (1) | 69 | (1) | 18 | (1) | 10,174 | (2) |
| 65 or older | 4,051 | (1) | 2,957 | (1) | 1,334 | (1) | 70 | (1) | 14 | (1) | 8,439 | (1) |
| **Male subtotal** | **302,323** | **(100)** | **214,898** | **(100)** | **115,069** | **(100)** | **4,997** | **(100)** | **1,897** | **(100)** | **640,022** | **(100)** |
| **Female**<br>**Age at diagnosis (years)** | | | | | | | | | | | | |
| Under 5 | 496 | (2) | 2,126 | (3) | 763 | (3) | 15 | (2) | 13 | (3) | 3,418 | (3) |
| 5-12 | 187 | (1) | 501 | (1) | 219 | (1) | 9 | (1) | – | – | 919 | (1) |
| 13-19 | 273 | (1) | 1,122 | (1) | 286 | (1) | 8 | (1) | 4 | (1) | 1,695 | (1) |
| 20-24 | 1,671 | (6) | 4,443 | (6) | 1,536 | (6) | 41 | (6) | 34 | (8) | 7,733 | (6) |
| 25-29 | 4,633 | (16) | 11,108 | (14) | 4,157 | (16) | 102 | (14) | 62 | (14) | 20,083 | (15) |
| 30-34 | 6,464 | (22) | 16,777 | (22) | 6,077 | (23) | 136 | (19) | 100 | (23) | 29,608 | (22) |
| 35-39 | 5,812 | (20) | 16,914 | (22) | 5,475 | (21) | 133 | (18) | 85 | (19) | 28,459 | (21) |
| 40-44 | 3,848 | (13) | 11,949 | (15) | 3,613 | (14) | 109 | (15) | 57 | (13) | 19,597 | (15) |
| 45-49 | 2,072 | (7) | 6,079 | (8) | 2,028 | (8) | 72 | (10) | 40 | (9) | 10,313 | (8) |
| 50-54 | 1,183 | (4) | 3,016 | (4) | 1,114 | (4) | 29 | (4) | 20 | (5) | 5,367 | (4) |
| 55-59 | 756 | (3) | 1,649 | (2) | 682 | (3) | 25 | (3) | 15 | (3) | 3,128 | (2) |
| 60-64 | 480 | (2) | 973 | (1) | 363 | (1) | 26 | (4) | 5 | (1) | 1,849 | (1) |
| 65 or older | 959 | (3) | 967 | (1) | 312 | (1) | 26 | (4) | 4 | (1) | 2,272 | (2) |
| **Female subtotal** | **28,834** | **(100)** | **77,624** | **(100)** | **26,625** | **(100)** | **731** | **(100)** | **439** | **(100)** | **134,441** | **(100)** |
| **Total[2]** | **331,160** | | **292,522** | | **141,694** | | **5,728** | | **2,337** | | **774,467** | |

[1]Includes 838 males and 187 females whose race/ethnicity is unknown.

[2]Includes 1 male whose age at diagnosis is unknown, and 4 persons whose sex is unknown.

*Source*: Centers for Disease Control and Prevention, U.S. Department of Health and Human Services. National Center for HIV, STD, and TB Prevention. Division of HIV/AIDS Prevention—Surveillance and Epidemiology. *HIV/AIDS Surveillance Report 2000* 12, no. 2, year-end edition. http://www.cdc.gov/hiv/stats/hasr1202.pdf.

## Table B3.6. Male Adult/Adolescent AIDS Cases, by Exposure Category and Race/Ethnicity, Reported through December 2000, United States

| | White, not Hispanic | | | | Black, not Hispanic | | | | Hispanic | | | |
|---|---|---|---|---|---|---|---|---|---|---|---|---|
| | 2000 | | Cumulative total | | 2000 | | Cumulative total | | 2000 | | Cumulative total | |
| Exposure category | No. | (%) | No. | (%) | No. | (%) | No. | (%) | No. | (%) | No. | (%) |
| Men who have sex with men | 7,097 | (62) | 223,470 | (74) | 3,960 | (30) | 78,651 | (37) | 2,241 | (36) | 48,287 | (42) |
| Injecting drug use | 1,203 | (10) | 28,050 | (9) | 3,040 | (23) | 71,747 | (34) | 1,630 | (26) | 40,025 | (35) |
| Men who have sex with men and inject drugs | 734 | (6) | 24,958 | (8) | 531 | (4) | 15,848 | (7) | 261 | (4) | 7,673 | (7) |
| Hemophilia/coagulation disorder | 71 | (1) | 3,793 | (1) | 11 | (0) | 571 | (0) | 8 | (0) | 437 | (0) |
| Heterosexual contact: | 378 | (3) | 5,586 | (2) | 1,587 | (12) | 16,993 | (8) | 549 | (9) | 6,598 | (6) |
| *Sex with injecting drug user* | *108* | | *1,958* | | *303* | | *5,390* | | *103* | | *1,806* | |
| *Sex with person with hemophilia* | *1* | | *31* | | *2* | | *21* | | *1* | | *11* | |
| *Sex with transfusion recipient with HIV infection* | *6* | | *157* | | *11* | | *161* | | *4* | | *89* | |
| *Sex with HIV-infected person, risk not specified* | *263* | | *3,440* | | *1,271* | | *11,421* | | *441* | | *4,692* | |
| Receipt of blood transfusion, blood components, or tissue | 53 | (0) | 3,173 | (1) | 64 | (0) | 1,077 | (1) | 25 | (0) | 592 | (1) |
| Risk not reported or identified[1] | 1,930 | (17) | 12,428 | (4) | 4,025 | (30) | 27,407 | (13) | 1,571 | (25) | 10,407 | (9) |
| **Total** | **11,466** | **(100)** | **301,458** | **(100)** | **13,218** | **(100)** | **212,294** | **(100)** | **6,285** | **(100)** | **114,019** | **(100)** |

| | Asian/Pacific Islander | | | | American Indian/Alaska Native | | | | Cumulative totals[2] | | | |
|---|---|---|---|---|---|---|---|---|---|---|---|---|
| | 2000 | | Cumulative total | | 2000 | | Cumulative total | | 2000 | | Cumulative total | |
| Exposure category | No. | (%) | No. | (%) | No. | (%) | No. | (%) | No. | (%) | No. | (%) |
| Men who have sex with men | 159 | (53) | 3,562 | (72) | 72 | (53) | 1,067 | (57) | 13,562 | (43) | 355,409 | (56) |
| Injecting drug use | 16 | (5) | 258 | (5) | 22 | (16) | 296 | (16) | 5,922 | (19) | 140,536 | (22) |
| Men who have sex with men and inject drugs | 9 | (3) | 184 | (4) | 11 | (8) | 308 | (16) | 1,548 | (5) | 48,989 | (8) |
| Hemophilia/coagulation disorder | 3 | (1) | 70 | (1) | – | – | 30 | (2) | 93 | (0) | 4,907 | (1) |
| Heterosexual contact: | 26 | (9) | 198 | (4) | 8 | (6) | 54 | (3) | 2,549 | (8) | 29,460 | (5) |
| *Sex with injecting drug user* | *4* | | *51* | | *1* | | *15* | | *519* | | *9,225* | |
| *Sex with person with hemophilia* | – | | *1* | | – | | – | | *4* | | *64* | |
| *Sex with transfusion recipient with HIV infection* | – | | *7* | | – | | *2* | | *21* | | *417* | |
| *Sex with HIV-infected person, risk not specified* | *22* | | *139* | | *7* | | *37* | | *2,005* | | *19,754* | |
| Receipt of blood transfusion, blood components, or tissue | 1 | (0) | 112 | (2) | 1 | (1) | 9 | (0) | 144 | (0) | 4,971 | (1) |
| Risk not reported or identified | 86 | (29) | 586 | (12) | 21 | (16) | 115 | (6) | 7,683 | (24) | 51,179 | (8) |
| **Total** | **300** | **(100)** | **4,970** | **(100)** | **135** | **(100)** | **1,879** | **(100)** | **31,501** | **(100)** | **635,451** | **(100)** |

[1]See Technical Notes.

[2]Includes 831 men whose race/ethnicity is unknown.

*Source*: Centers for Disease Control and Prevention, U.S. Department of Health and Human Services. National Center for HIV, STD, and TB Prevention. Division of HIV/AIDS Prevention—Surveillance and Epidemiology. *HIV/AIDS Surveillance Report 2000* 12, no. 2, year-end edition. http://www.cdc.gov/hiv/stats/hasr1202.pdf.

## Table B3.7. Female Adult/Adolescent AIDS Cases, by Exposure Category and Race/Ethnicity, Reported through December 2000, United States

| Exposure category | White, not Hispanic 2000 No. (%) | White, not Hispanic Cumulative total No. (%) | Black, not Hispanic 2000 No. (%) | Black, not Hispanic Cumulative total No. (%) | Hispanic 2000 No. (%) | Hispanic Cumulative total No. (%) |
|---|---|---|---|---|---|---|
| Injecting drug use | 607 (32) | 11,714 (42) | 1,468 (22) | 30,745 (41) | 502 (27) | 10,171 (40) |
| Hemophilia/coagulation disorder | – – | 105 (0) | 2 (0) | 112 (0) | – – | 55 (0) |
| Heterosexual contact: | 678 (36) | 11,280 (40) | 2,449 (37) | 28,608 (38) | 791 (43) | 12,085 (47) |
| *Sex with injecting drug user* | *229* | *4,551* | *559* | *10,537* | *178* | *5,355* |
| *Sex with bisexual male* | *51* | *1,507* | *86* | *1,407* | *29* | *547* |
| *Sex with person with hemophilia* | *7* | *286* | *4* | *84* | *1* | *39* |
| *Sex with transfusion recipient with HIV infection* | *11* | *312* | *8* | *166* | *3* | *99* |
| *Sex with HIV-infected person, risk not specified* | *380* | *4,624* | *1,792* | *16,414* | *580* | *6,045* |
| Receipt of blood transfusion, blood components, or tissue | 38 (2) | 1,826 (6) | 76 (1) | 1,307 (2) | 18 (1) | 554 (2) |
| Risk not reported or identified[1] | 572 (30) | 3,226 (11) | 2,550 (39) | 14,225 (19) | 544 (29) | 2,778 (11) |
| **Total** | **1,895 (100)** | **28,151 (100)** | **6,545 (100)** | **74,997 (100)** | **1,855 (100)** | **25,643 (100)** |

| Exposure category | Asian/Pacific Islander 2000 No. (%) | Asian/Pacific Islander Cumulative total No. (%) | American Indian/Alaska Native 2000 No. (%) | American Indian/Alaska Native Cumulative total No. (%) | Cumulative totals[2] 2000 No. (%) | Cumulative totals[2] Cumulative total No. (%) |
|---|---|---|---|---|---|---|
| Injecting drug use | 2 (3) | 110 (16) | 28 (41) | 190 (45) | 2,609 (25) | 52,991 (41) |
| Hemophilia/coagulation disorder | – – | 6 (1) | 1 (1) | 3 (1) | 3 (0) | 283 (0) |
| Heterosexual contact: | 33 (43) | 346 (49) | 26 (38) | 157 (37) | 3,981 (38) | 52,520 (40) |
| *Sex with injecting drug user* | *2* | *83* | *9* | *72* | *977* | *20,610* |
| *Sex with bisexual male* | *3* | *71* | *6* | *23* | *175* | *3,561* |
| *Sex with person with hemophilia* | – | *5* | – | *2* | *12* | *416* |
| *Sex with transfusion recipient with HIV infection* | *1* | *20* | – | *3* | *23* | *601* |
| *Sex with HIV-infected person, risk not specified* | *27* | *167* | *11* | *57* | *2,794* | *27,332* |
| Receipt of blood transfusion, blood components, or tissue | 4 (5) | 100 (14) | – – | 14 (3) | 138 (1) | 3,806 (3) |
| Risk not reported or identified | 38 (49) | 145 (21) | 13 (19) | 62 (15) | 3,728 (36) | 20,504 (16) |
| **Total** | **77 (100)** | **707 (100)** | **68 (100)** | **426 (100)** | **10,459 (100)** | **130,104 (100)** |

[1]See Technical Notes.

[2]Includes 179 women whose race/ethnicity is unknown.

*Source*: Centers for Disease Control and Prevention, U.S. Department of Health and Human Services. National Center for HIV, STD, and TB Prevention. Division of HIV/AIDS Prevention—Surveillance and Epidemiology. *HIV/AIDS Surveillance Report 2000* 12, no. 2, year-end edition. http://www.cdc.gov/hiv/stats/hasr1202.pdf.

## Table B3.8. AIDS Cases in Adolescents and Adults under Age 25, by Sex and Exposure Category, Reported through December 2000, United States

| | 13-19 years old | | | | 20-24 years old | | | |
|---|---|---|---|---|---|---|---|---|
| | 2000 | | Cumulative total | | 2000 | | Cumulative total | |
| **Male exposure category** | No. | (%) | No. | (%) | No. | (%) | No. | (%) |
| Men who have sex with men | 48 | (30) | 803 | (34) | 426 | (53) | 11,993 | (62) |
| Injecting drug use | 10 | (6) | 148 | (6) | 83 | (10) | 2,353 | (12) |
| Men who have sex with men and inject drugs | 5 | (3) | 123 | (5) | 28 | (3) | 2,023 | (10) |
| Hemophilia/coagulation disorder | 3 | (2) | 756 | (32) | 19 | (2) | 663 | (3) |
| Heterosexual contact: | 18 | (11) | 107 | (5) | 68 | (8) | 973 | (5) |
| *Sex with injecting drug user* | *2* | | *24* | | *7* | | *283* | |
| *Sex with person with hemophilia* | *1* | | *2* | | – | | *4* | |
| *Sex with transfusion recipient with HIV infection* | – | | – | | *1* | | *15* | |
| *Sex with HIV-infected person, risk not specified* | *15* | | *81* | | *60* | | *671* | |
| Receipt of blood transfusion, blood components, or tissue | 3 | (2) | 95 | (4) | 1 | (0) | 107 | (1) |
| Risk not reported or identified[1] | 71 | (45) | 334 | (14) | 176 | (22) | 1,387 | (7) |
| Male subtotal | 158 | (100) | 2,366 | (100) | 801 | (100) | 19,499 | (100) |
| **Female exposure category** | | | | | | | | |
| Injecting drug use | 12 | (7) | 227 | (13) | 65 | (12) | 2,015 | (26) |
| Hemophilia/coagulation disorder | – | – | 13 | (1) | – | – | 16 | (0) |
| Heterosexual contact: | 73 | (40) | 877 | (52) | 257 | (47) | 4,233 | (55) |
| *Sex with injecting drug user* | *14* | | *285* | | *31* | | *1,565* | |
| *Sex with bisexual male* | *2* | | *46* | | *14* | | *296* | |
| *Sex with person with hemophilia* | – | | *15* | | – | | *54* | |
| *Sex with transfusion recipient with HIV infection* | – | | *2* | | – | | *24* | |
| *Sex with HIV-infected person, risk not specified* | *57* | | *529* | | *212* | | *2,294* | |
| Receipt of blood transfusion, blood components, or tissue | 6 | (3) | 98 | (6) | 3 | (1) | 116 | (2) |
| Risk not reported or identified | 93 | (51) | 480 | (28) | 220 | (40) | 1,353 | (17) |
| Female subtotal | 184 | (100) | 1,695 | (100) | 545 | (100) | 7,733 | (100) |
| **Total** | **342** | | **4,061** | | **1,346** | | **27,232** | |

[1]See Technical Notes.

*Source*: Centers for Disease Control and Prevention, U.S. Department of Health and Human Services. National Center for HIV, STD, and TB Prevention. Division of HIV/AIDS Prevention—Surveillance and Epidemiology. *HIV/AIDS Surveillance Report 2000* 12, no. 2, year-end edition. http://www.cdc.gov/hiv/stats/hasr1202.pdf.

## Table B3.9. Adult/Adolescent AIDS Cases by Single and Multiple Exposure Categories, Reported through December 2000, United States

| Exposure category | AIDS cases No. | (%) |
|---|---|---|
| **Single mode of exposure** | | |
| Men who have sex with men | 339,252 | (44) |
| Injecting drug use | 151,982 | (20) |
| Hemophilia/coagulation disorder | 4,219 | (1) |
| Heterosexual contact | 80,128 | (10) |
| Receipt of transfusion[1] | 8,764 | (1) |
| Receipt of transplant of tissues, organs, or artificial insemination[2] | 13 | (0) |
| Other[3] | 214 | (0) |
| **Single mode of exposure subtotal** | **584,572** | **(76)** |
| **Multiple modes of exposure** | | |
| Men who have sex with men; injecting drug use | 41,390 | (5) |
| Men who have sex with men; hemophilia/coagulation disorder | 192 | (0) |
| Men who have sex with men; heterosexual contact | 12,041 | (2) |
| Men who have sex with men; receipt of transfusion/transplant | 3,537 | (0) |
| Injecting drug use; hemophilia/coagulation disorder | 215 | (0) |
| Injecting drug use; heterosexual contact | 38,321 | (5) |
| Injecting drug use; receipt of transfusion/transplant | 1,728 | (0) |
| Hemophilia/coagulation disorder; heterosexual contact | 124 | (0) |
| Hemophilia/coagulation disorder; receipt of transfusion/transplant | 809 | (0) |
| Heterosexual contact; receipt of transfusion/transplant | 1,853 | (0) |
| Men who have sex with men; injecting drug use; hemophilia/coagulation disorder | 53 | (0) |
| Men who have sex with men; injecting drug use; heterosexual contact | 6,669 | (1) |
| Men who have sex with men; injecting drug use; receipt of transfusion/transplant | 646 | (0) |
| Men who have sex with men; hemophilia/coagulation disorder; heterosexual contact | 25 | (0) |
| Men who have sex with men; hemophilia/coagulation disorder; receipt of transfusion/transplant | 44 | (0) |
| Men who have sex with men; heterosexual contact; receipt of transfusion/transplant | 312 | (0) |
| Injecting drug use; hemophilia/coagulation disorder; heterosexual contact | 90 | (0) |
| Injecting drug use; hemophilia/coagulation disorder; receipt of transfusion/transplant | 38 | (0) |
| Injecting drug use; heterosexual contact; receipt of transfusion/transplant | 1,127 | (0) |
| Hemophilia/coagulation disorder; heterosexual contact; receipt of transfusion/transplant | 38 | (0) |
| Men who have sex with men; injecting drug use; hemophilia/coagulation disorder; heterosexual contact | 17 | (0) |
| Men who have sex with men; injecting drug use; hemophilia/coagulation disorder; receipt of transfusion/transplant | 16 | (0) |
| Men who have sex with men; injecting drug use; heterosexual contact; receipt of transfusion/transplant | 192 | (0) |
| Men who have sex with men; hemophilia/coagulation disorder; heterosexual contact; receipt of transfusion/transplant | 6 | (0) |
| Injecting drug use; hemophilia/coagulation disorder; heterosexual contact; receipt of transfusion/transplant | 26 | (0) |
| Men who have sex with men; injecting drug use; hemophilia/coagulation disorder; heterosexual contact; receipt of transfusion/transplant | 6 | (0) |
| **Multiple modes of exposure subtotal** | **109,515** | **(14)** |
| **Risk not reported or identified[4]** | **71,472** | **(9)** |
| **Total** | **765,559** | **(100)** |

[1]Includes 41 adult/adolescents who developed AIDS after receiving blood screened negative for HIV antibody.

[2]Thirteen adults developed AIDS after receiving tissue, organs, or artificial insemination from HIV-infected donors. Four of the 13 received tissue or organs from a donor who was negative for HIV antibody at the time of donation, See *N Engl J Med* 1992;326:726–32.

[3]"Other" also includes 180 persons who acquired HIV infection perinatally, but were diagnosed with AIDS after age 13. See Technical Notes.

[4]See Technical Notes.

*Source*: Centers for Disease Control and Prevention, U.S. Department of Health and Human Services. National Center for HIV, STD, and TB Prevention. Division of HIV/AIDS Prevention—Surveillance and Epidemiology. *HIV/AIDS Surveillance Report 2000* 12, no. 2, year-end edition. http://www.cdc.gov/hiv/stats/hasr1202.pdf.

**Table B4.1. Acquired Immunodeficiency Syndrome—Reported Pediatric Cases,* United States, Puerto Rico, and U.S. Virgin Islands, 1999**

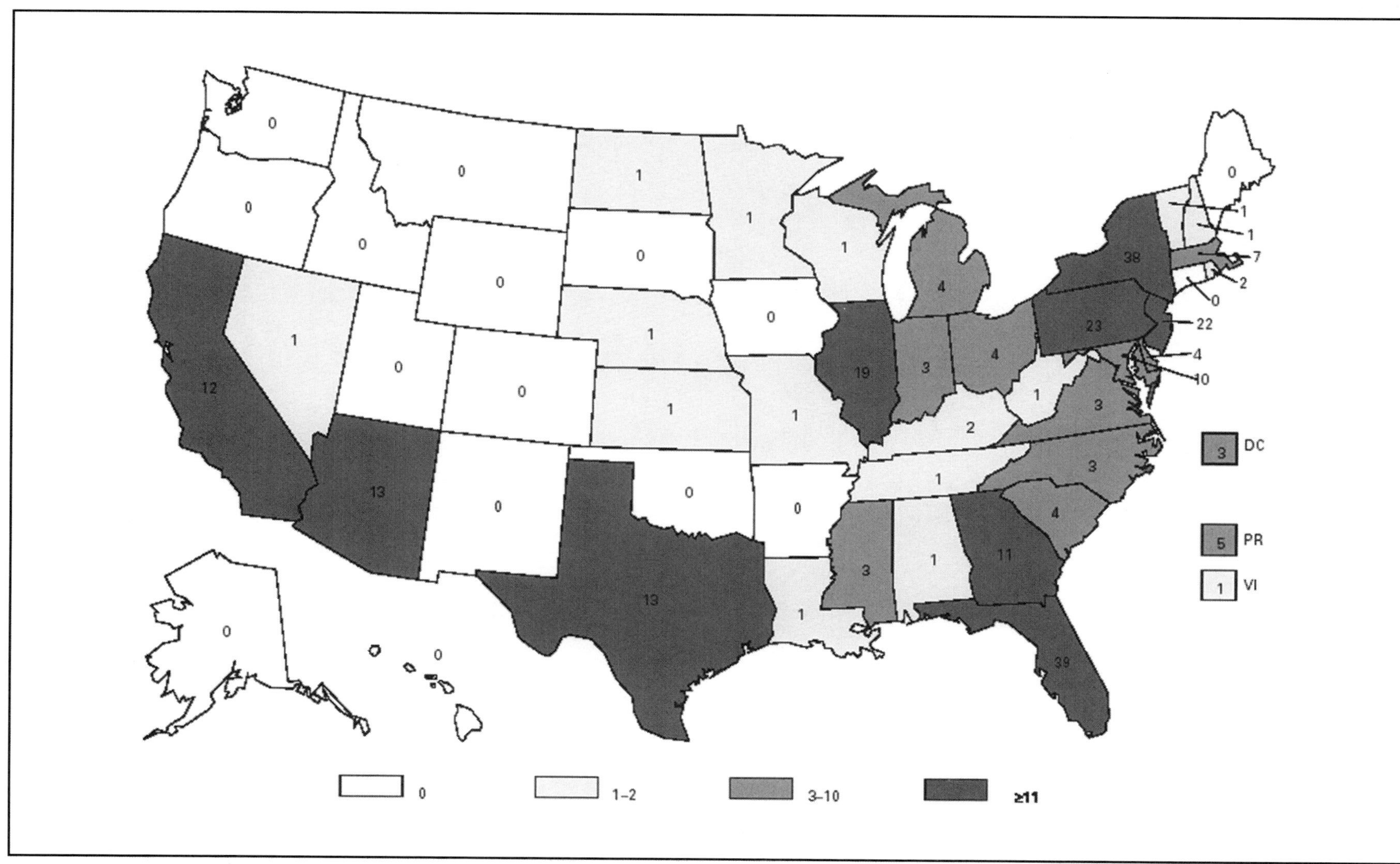


*Children and adolescents aged <13 years.

Trends in AIDS incidence among children continued to decrease with the success of efforts to reduce perinatal (i.e., mother-to-child) human immunodeficiency virus (HIV) transmission. although the number of perinatally acquired AIDS cases declined 43% during 1992-1996, new cases continue to occur disproportionately among young children from racial/ethnic minority populations.

*Source*: Center for Disease Control and Prevention, U.S. Department of Health and Human Services. *MMWR: Morbidity and Mortality Weekly Review Summary of Notifiable Disease, United States, 1999.* 48, no. 53 (2001). http://www.cdc.gov/mmwr/PDF/wk/mm4853.pdf

## Table B4.2. Pediatric HIV Infection Cases,[1] by Exposure Category and Race/Ethnicity, Reported through December 2000, from the 36 Areas with Confidential HIV Infection Reporting[2]

| | White, not Hispanic | | | | Black, not Hispanic | | | | Hispanic | | | |
|---|---|---|---|---|---|---|---|---|---|---|---|---|
| | 2000 | | Cumulative total | | 2000 | | Cumulative total | | 2000 | | Cumulative total | |
| **Exposure category** | **No.** | **(%)** | **No.** | **(%)** | **No.** | **(%)** | **No.** | **(%)** | **No.** | **(%)** | **No.** | **(%)** |
| Hemophilia/coagulation disorder | 4 | (11) | 73 | (15) | – | – | 18 | (1) | – | – | 5 | (2) |
| Mother with/at risk for HIV infection: | 30 | (83) | 362 | (76) | 136 | (91) | 1,250 | (92) | 27 | (87) | 222 | (89) |
| *Injecting drug use* | 5 | | 110 | | 31 | | 369 | | 4 | | 57 | |
| *Sex with injecting drug user* | 6 | | 78 | | 10 | | 136 | | 3 | | 39 | |
| *Sex with bisexual male* | 1 | | 8 | | 1 | | 16 | | – | | 4 | |
| *Sex with person with hemophilia* | 2 | | 5 | | – | | 1 | | – | | – | |
| *Sex with transfusion recipient with HIV infection* | – | | 3 | | – | | 4 | | 1 | | 5 | |
| *Sex with HIV-infected person, risk not specified* | 12 | | 73 | | 40 | | 310 | | 11 | | 55 | |
| *Receipt of blood transfusion, blood components, or tissue* | – | | 8 | | 1 | | 11 | | – | | 2 | |
| *Has HIV infection, risk not specified* | 4 | | 77 | | 53 | | 403 | | 8 | | 60 | |
| Receipt of blood transfusion, blood components, or tissue | – | – | 19 | (4) | – | – | 11 | (1) | – | – | 6 | (2) |
| Risk not reported or identified[3] | 2 | (6) | 22 | (5) | 14 | (9) | 82 | (6) | 4 | (13) | 17 | (7) |
| **Total** | **36** | **(100)** | **476** | **(100)** | **150** | **(100)** | **1,361** | **(100)** | **31** | **(100)** | **250** | **(100)** |

| | Asian/Pacific Islander | | | | American Indian/Alaska Native | | | | Cumulative totals[4] | | | |
|---|---|---|---|---|---|---|---|---|---|---|---|---|
| | 2000 | | Cumulative total | | 2000 | | Cumulative total | | 2000 | | Cumulative total | |
| **Exposure category** | **No.** | **(%)** | **No.** | **(%)** | **No.** | **(%)** | **No.** | **(%)** | **No.** | **(%)** | **No.** | **(%)** |
| Hemophilia/coagulation disorder | – | – | 2 | (14) | – | – | – | – | 4 | (2) | 99 | (5) |
| Mother with/at risk for HIV infection: | 1 | (50) | 8 | (57) | 1 | (50) | 9 | (75) | 196 | (88) | 1,860 | (87) |
| *Injecting drug use* | – | | 2 | | 1 | | 3 | | 41 | | 545 | |
| *Sex with injecting drug user* | – | | – | | – | | 2 | | 19 | | 256 | |
| *Sex with bisexual male* | – | | 2 | | – | | 1 | | 2 | | 32 | |
| *Sex with person with hemophilia* | – | | – | | – | | 1 | | 2 | | 7 | |
| *Sex with transfusion recipient with HIV infection* | – | | – | | – | | – | | 1 | | 12 | |
| *Sex with HIV-infected person, risk not specified* | 1 | | 3 | | – | | – | | 65 | | 443 | |
| *Receipt of blood transfusion, blood components, or tissue* | – | | – | | – | | – | | 1 | | 21 | |
| *Has HIV infection, risk not specified* | – | | 1 | | – | | 2 | | 65 | | 544 | |
| Receipt of blood transfusion, blood components, or tissue | – | – | 1 | (7) | – | – | – | – | – | – | 37 | (2) |
| Risk not reported or identified | 1 | (50) | 3 | (21) | 1 | (50) | 3 | (25) | 24 | (11) | 138 | (6) |
| **Total** | **2** | **(100)** | **14** | **(100)** | **2** | **(100)** | **12** | **(100)** | **224** | **(100)** | **2,134** | **(100)** |

[1]Includes only persons reported with HIV infection who have not developed AIDS.

[2]See table 3 for areas with confidential HIV infection reporting.

[3]For HIV infection cases, "risk not reported or identified" refers primarily to persons whose mode of exposure was not reported and who have not been followed up to determine their mode of exposure, and to a smaller number of persons who are not reported with one of the exposures listed above after follow-up. See Technical Notes.

[4]Includes 21 children whose race/ethnicity is unknown.

*Source*: Centers for Disease Control and Prevention, U.S. Department of Health and Human Services. National Center for HIV, STD, and TB Prevention. Division of HIV/AIDS Prevention—Surveillance and Epidemiology. *HIV/AIDS Surveillance Report 2000* 12, no. 2, year-end edition. http://www.cdc.gov/hiv/stats/hasr1202.pdf.

## Table B4.3. Pediatric AIDS Cases, by Exposure Category and Race/Ethnicity, Reported through December 2000, United States

| | White, not Hispanic | | | | Black, not Hispanic | | | | Hispanic | | | |
|---|---|---|---|---|---|---|---|---|---|---|---|---|
| | 2000 | | Cumulative total | | 2000 | | Cumulative total | | 2000 | | Cumulative total | |
| **Exposure category** | No. | (%) | No. | (%) | No. | (%) | No. | (%) | No. | (%) | No. | (%) |
| Hemophilia/coagulation disorder | – | – | 159 | (10) | – | – | 34 | (1) | – | – | 38 | (2) |
| Mother with/at risk for HIV infection: | 28 | (90) | 1,173 | (76) | 115 | (91) | 5,010 | (96) | 31 | (94) | 1,875 | (92) |
| *Injecting drug use* | *8* | | *486* | | *24* | | *1,915* | | *6* | | *746* | |
| *Sex with injecting drug user* | *5* | | *232* | | *10* | | *735* | | *4* | | *493* | |
| *Sex with bisexual male* | *1* | | *65* | | *1* | | *67* | | *2* | | *41* | |
| *Sex with person with hemophilia* | *1* | | *18* | | – | | *7* | | – | | *8* | |
| *Sex with transfusion recipient with HIV infection* | – | | *8* | | – | | *8* | | – | | *9* | |
| *Sex with HIV-infected person, risk not specified* | *8* | | *149* | | *38* | | *834* | | *8* | | *264* | |
| *Receipt of blood transfusion, blood components, or tissue* | *2* | | *44* | | – | | *74* | | – | | *34* | |
| *Has HIV infection, risk not specified* | *3* | | *171* | | *42* | | *1,370* | | *11* | | *280* | |
| Receipt of blood transfusion, blood components, or tissue | – | – | 189 | (12) | 1 | (1) | 89 | (2) | – | – | 93 | (5) |
| Risk not reported or identified[1] | 3 | (10) | 27 | (2) | 11 | (9) | 98 | (2) | 2 | (6) | 26 | (1) |
| **Total** | **31** | **(100)** | **1,548** | **(100)** | **127** | **(100)** | **5,231** | **(100)** | **33** | **(100)** | **2,032** | **(100)** |

| | Asian/Pacific Islander | | | | American Indian/Alaska Native | | | | Cumulative totals[2] | | | |
|---|---|---|---|---|---|---|---|---|---|---|---|---|
| | 2000 | | Cumulative total | | 2000 | | Cumulative total | | 2000 | | Cumulative total | |
| **Exposure category** | No. | (%) | No. | (%) | No. | (%) | No. | (%) | No. | (%) | No. | (%) |
| Hemophilia/coagulation disorder | – | – | 3 | (6) | – | – | 2 | (6) | 1 | (1) | 237 | (3) |
| Mother with/at risk for HIV infection: | 2 | (67) | 33 | (65) | 1 | (100) | 28 | (90) | 177 | (90) | 8,133 | (91) |
| *Injecting drug use* | *1* | | *6* | | *1* | | *14* | | *40* | | *3,172* | |
| *Sex with injecting drug user* | *1* | | *6* | | – | | *6* | | *20* | | *1,473* | |
| *Sex with bisexual male* | – | | *2* | | – | | – | | *4* | | *176* | |
| *Sex with person with hemophilia* | – | | – | | – | | – | | *1* | | *33* | |
| *Sex with transfusion recipient with HIV infection* | – | | – | | – | | – | | – | | *25* | |
| *Sex with HIV-infected person, risk not specified* | – | | *9* | | – | | *4* | | *54* | | *1,262* | |
| *Receipt of blood transfusion, blood components, or tissue* | – | | *1* | | – | | – | | *2* | | *153* | |
| *Has HIV infection, risk not specified* | – | | *9* | | – | | *4* | | *56* | | *1,839* | |
| Receipt of blood transfusion, blood components, or tissue | 1 | (33) | 11 | (22) | – | – | – | – | 2 | (1) | 382 | (4) |
| Risk not reported or identified | – | – | 4 | (8) | – | – | 1 | (3) | 16 | (8) | 156 | (2) |
| **Total** | **3** | **(100)** | **51** | **(100)** | **1** | **(100)** | **31** | **(100)** | **196** | **(100)** | **8,908** | **(100)** |

[1]See table 5, footnote 5 and Technical Notes.

[2]Includes 15 children whose race/ethnicity is unknown.

*Source*: Centers for Disease Control and Prevention, U.S. Department of Health and Human Services. National Center for HIV, STD, and TB Prevention. Division of HIV/AIDS Prevention—Surveillance and Epidemiology. *HIV/AIDS Surveillance Report 2000* 12, no. 2, year-end edition. http://www.cdc.gov/hiv/stats/hasr1202.pdf.

## Table B5.1. Acquired Immunodeficiency Syndrome—Reported Cases, by Quarter, United States, 1988–1999

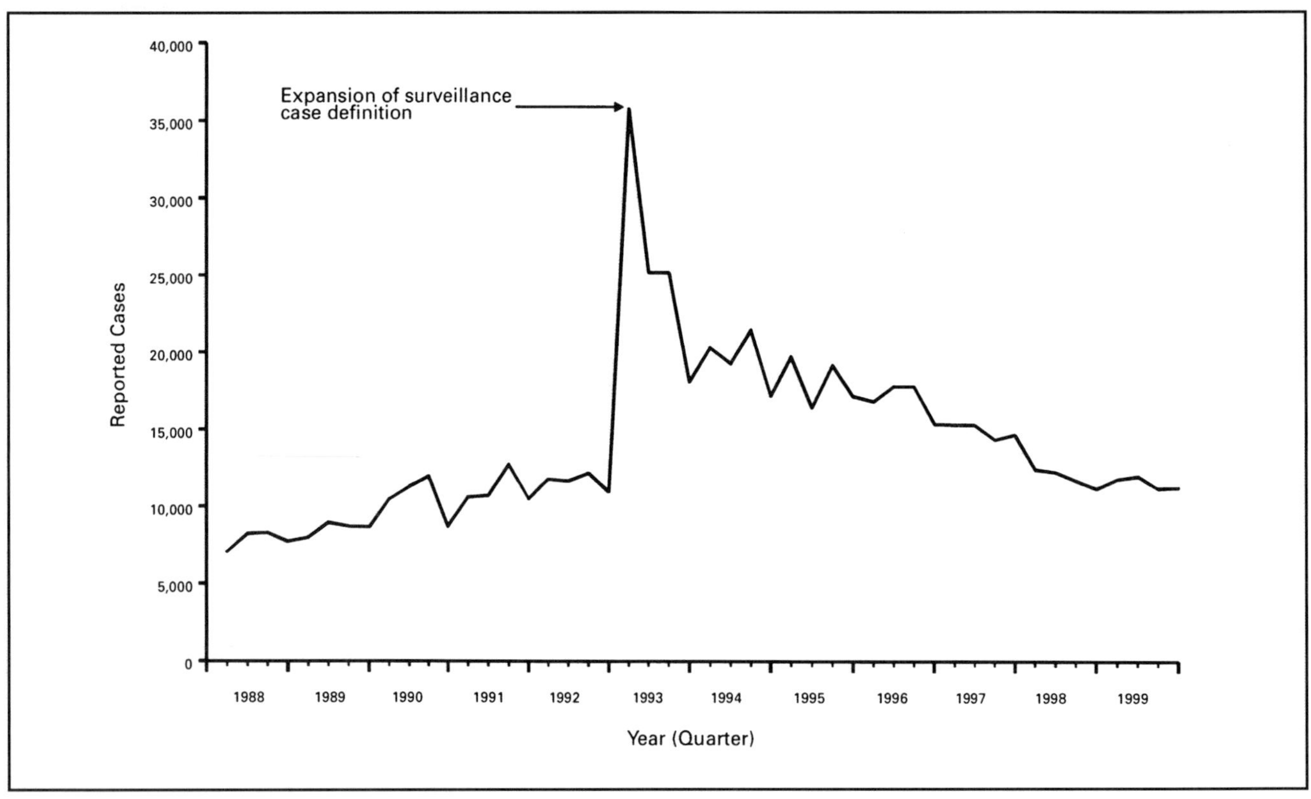


*Includes Guam, Puerto Rico, the U.S. Pacific Islands, and the U.S. Virgin Islands.

Total number of AIDS cases includes all cases reported to the Division of HIV/AIDS Prevention—Surveillance and Epidemiology, National Center for HIV, STD, and TB Prevention, as of December 31, 1999. Total includes cases among residents in U.S. territories and 104 cases among persons with unknown state of residence.

*Source*: Center for Disease Control and Prevention, U.S. Department of Health and Human Services. *MMWR: Morbidity and Mortality Weekly Review Summary of Notifiable Disease, United States, 1999.* 48 no. 53 (2001). http://www.cdc.gov/mmwr/PDF/wk/mm4853.pdf

## Table B5.2. Estimated Persons Living with AIDS, by Region of Residence and Year, 1993 through 1999, United States[1]

| Region of residence[2] | Year 1993 | 1994 | 1995 | 1996 | 1997 | 1998 | 1999 |
|---|---|---|---|---|---|---|---|
| Northeast | 51,891 | 59,501 | 66,230 | 73,434 | 81,481 | 88,204 | 95,445 |
| Midwest | 18,441 | 20,342 | 21,832 | 23,759 | 26,219 | 28,283 | 30,540 |
| South | 58,814 | 68,120 | 75,674 | 85,819 | 97,617 | 108,855 | 119,430 |
| West | 39,373 | 42,757 | 45,484 | 49,024 | 53,831 | 58,026 | 62,357 |
| U.S. dependencies, possessions, and associated nations | 5,725 | 6,340 | 6,790 | 7,344 | 8,162 | 8,918 | 9,596 |
| **Total[3]** | **174,244** | **197,060** | **216,010** | **239,382** | **267,311** | **292,286** | **317,368** |

[1]These numbers do not represent adult cases of persons living with AIDS. Rather, these numbers are point estimates of persons living with AIDS derived by subtracting the estimated cumulative number of deaths in persons with AIDS from the estimated cumulative number of persons with AIDS. Estimated AIDS cases and estimated deaths are adjusted for reporting delays, but not for incomplete reporting. Annual estimates are through the most recent year for which reliable estimates are available. See Technical Notes.

[2]See Technical Notes for a list of states or U.S. dependencies, possessions, and associated nations which comprise each region of residence.

[3]Because column totals were calculated independently of the values for the subpopulations, the values in each column may not sum to the column total.

*Source*: Centers for Disease Control and Prevention, U.S. Department of Health and Human Services. National Center for HIV, STD, and TB Prevention. Division of HIV/AIDS Prevention—Surveillance and Epidemiology. *HIV/AIDS Surveillance Report 2000* 12, no. 2, year-end edition. http://www.cdc.gov/hiv/stats/hasr1202.pdf.

## Table B5.3. Estimated Persons Living with AIDS, by Sex, Exposure Category, and Year, 1993 through 1999, United States[1]

| Male adult/adolescent exposure category | Year | | | | | | |
|---|---|---|---|---|---|---|---|
| | 1993 | 1994 | 1995 | 1996 | 1997 | 1998 | 1999 |
| Men who have sex with men | 86,443 | 94,694 | 100,938 | 110,272 | 121,981 | 132,441 | 143,108 |
| Injecting drug use | 34,400 | 40,046 | 44,345 | 48,763 | 53,812 | 58,118 | 62,418 |
| Men who have sex with men and inject drugs | 13,854 | 14,884 | 15,687 | 16,453 | 17,698 | 18,682 | 19,553 |
| Hemophilia/coagulation disorder | 1,620 | 1,699 | 1,729 | 1,740 | 1,788 | 1,825 | 1,853 |
| Heterosexual contact | 6,109 | 7,903 | 9,760 | 12,174 | 14,907 | 17,627 | 20,495 |
| Receipt of blood transfusion, blood components, or tissue | 893 | 914 | 963 | 1,035 | 1,140 | 1,253 | 1,375 |
| Risk not reported or identified | 989 | 940 | 937 | 974 | 1,023 | 1,080 | 1,151 |
| Male subtotal | 144,309 | 161,081 | 174,361 | 191,410 | 212,348 | 231,022 | 249,951 |
| **Female adult/adolescent exposure category** | | | | | | | |
| Injecting drug use | 13,844 | 16,244 | 18,352 | 20,357 | 22,661 | 24,457 | 26,122 |
| Hemophilia/coagulation disorder | 92 | 108 | 137 | 164 | 201 | 229 | 248 |
| Heterosexual contact | 11,822 | 15,131 | 18,478 | 22,566 | 26,974 | 31,187 | 35,445 |
| Receipt of blood transfusion, blood components, or tissue | 755 | 843 | 888 | 980 | 1,088 | 1,203 | 1,318 |
| Risk not reported or identified | 373 | 376 | 379 | 416 | 463 | 504 | 548 |
| Female subtotal | 26,886 | 32,702 | 38,234 | 44,484 | 51,386 | 57,578 | 63,682 |
| **Pediatric (<13 years old) exposure category** | 3,049 | 3,277 | 3,415 | 3,487 | 3,577 | 3,682 | 3,732 |
| **Total[2]** | **174,244** | **197,060** | **216,010** | **239,382** | **267,311** | **292,286** | **317,368** |

[1]These numbers do not represent adult cases of persons living with AIDS. Rather, these numbers are point estimates of persons living with AIDS derived by subtracting the estimated cumulative number of deaths in persons with AIDS from the estimated cumulative number of persons with AIDS. Estimated AIDS cases and estimated deaths are adjusted for reporting delays, but not for incomplete reporting. Annual estimates are through the most recent year for which reliable estimates are available. See Technical Notes.

[2]Because column totals were calculated independently of the values for the subpopulations, the values in each column may not sum to the column total.

*Source*: Centers for Disease Control and Prevention, U.S. Department of Health and Human Services. National Center for HIV, STD, and TB Prevention. Division of HIV/AIDS Prevention—Surveillance and Epidemiology. *HIV/AIDS Surveillance Report 2000* 12, no. 2, year-end edition. http://www.cdc.gov/hiv/stats/hasr1202.pdf.

## Table B5.4. Estimated Persons Living with AIDS, by Race/Ethnicity and Year, 1993 through 1999, United States[1]

| Race/ethnicity | Year | | | | | | |
|---|---|---|---|---|---|---|---|
| | 1993 | 1994 | 1995 | 1996 | 1997 | 1998 | 1999 |
| White, not Hispanic | 80,320 | 86,417 | 91,302 | 98,119 | 106,734 | 114,079 | 121,485 |
| Black, not Hispanic | 60,655 | 71,818 | 81,152 | 92,167 | 105,142 | 117,110 | 128,941 |
| Hispanic | 31,198 | 36,448 | 40,891 | 46,016 | 51,927 | 57,201 | 62,573 |
| Asian/Pacific Islander | 1,292 | 1,457 | 1,613 | 1,854 | 2,082 | 2,304 | 2,579 |
| American Indian/Alaska Native | 573 | 668 | 723 | 804 | 888 | 966 | 1,068 |
| **Total[2]** | **174,244** | **197,060** | **216,010** | **239,382** | **267,311** | **292,286** | **317,368** |

[1]These numbers do not represent adult cases of persons living with AIDS. Rather, these numbers are point estimates of persons living with AIDS derived by subtracting the estimated cumulative number of deaths in persons with AIDS from the estimated cumulative number of persons with AIDS. Estimated AIDS cases and estimated deaths are adjusted for reporting delays, but not for incomplete reporting. Annual estimates are through the most recent year for which reliable estimates are available. See Technical Notes.

[2]Totals include estimates of persons whose race/ethnicity is unknown. Because column totals were calculated independently of the values for the subpopulations, the values in each column may not sum to the column total.

*Source*: Centers for Disease Control and Prevention, U.S. Department of Health and Human Services. National Center for HIV, STD, and TB Prevention. Division of HIV/AIDS Prevention—Surveillance and Epidemiology. *HIV/AIDS Surveillance Report 2000* 12, no. 2, year-end edition. http://www.cdc.gov/hiv/stats/hasr1202.pdf.

## Table B5.5. AIDS Cases and Deaths, by Year and Age Group, through December 2000, United States[1]

| | Adults/adolescents | | Children <13 years old | |
|---|---|---|---|---|
| Year | Cases diagnosed during interval | Deaths occurring during interval | Cases diagnosed during interval | Deaths occurring during interval |
| Before 1981 | 92 | 29 | 8 | 1 |
| 1981 | 321 | 122 | 16 | 8 |
| 1982 | 1,168 | 452 | 31 | 13 |
| 1983 | 3,075 | 1,480 | 77 | 30 |
| 1984 | 6,243 | 3,470 | 121 | 52 |
| 1985 | 11,783 | 6,872 | 250 | 119 |
| 1986 | 19,040 | 11,988 | 339 | 167 |
| 1987 | 28,586 | 16,167 | 506 | 294 |
| 1988 | 35,481 | 20,883 | 618 | 321 |
| 1989 | 42,744 | 27,639 | 730 | 372 |
| 1990 | 48,697 | 31,382 | 814 | 400 |
| 1991 | 59,706 | 36,635 | 813 | 398 |
| 1992 | 78,646 | 41,197 | 949 | 426 |
| 1993 | 78,948 | 44,914 | 923 | 542 |
| 1994 | 72,174 | 49,548 | 814 | 586 |
| 1995 | 69,098 | 50,260 | 676 | 538 |
| 1996 | 60,216 | 37,049 | 500 | 426 |
| 1997 | 48,467 | 21,188 | 300 | 211 |
| 1998 | 40,567 | 17,186 | 217 | 118 |
| 1999 | 36,575 | 15,147 | 150 | 107 |
| 2000 | 23,932 | 8,867 | 56 | 44 |
| **Total[2]** | **765,559** | **442,882** | **8,908** | **5,178** |

[1]Persons whose vital status is unknown are included in counts of diagnosed cases, but excluded from counts of deaths. Reported deaths are not necessary caused by HIV-related disease.
[2]Death totals include 407 adults/adolescents and 5 children known to have died, but whose dates of death are unknown.
*Source*: Centers for Disease Control and Prevention, U.S. Department of Health and Human Services. National Center for HIV, STD, and TB Prevention. Division of HIV/AIDS Prevention—Surveillance and Epidemiology. *HIV/AIDS Surveillance Report 2000* 12, no. 2, year-end edition. http://www.cdc.gov/hiv/stats/hasr1202.pdf.

## Table B5.6. Estimated Deaths of Persons with AIDS, by Region of Residence and Year of Death, 1993 through 1999, United States[1]

| | Year of death | | | | | | |
|---|---|---|---|---|---|---|---|
| Region of residence[2] | 1993 | 1994 | 1995 | 1996 | 1997 | 1998 | 1999 |
| Northeast | 14,044 | 15,855 | 15,849 | 11,590 | 6,746 | 5,110 | 5,064 |
| Midwest | 4,802 | 5,220 | 5,457 | 4,061 | 2,309 | 1,904 | 1,662 |
| South | 14,743 | 16,494 | 17,344 | 13,642 | 8,327 | 7,252 | 6,832 |
| West | 10,339 | 10,847 | 10,540 | 7,158 | 3,716 | 3,175 | 2,524 |
| U.S. dependencies, possessions, and associated nations | 1,566 | 1,756 | 1,687 | 1,532 | 972 | 768 | 686 |
| **Total[3]** | **45,494** | **50,172** | **50,877** | **37,983** | **22,070** | **18,210** | **16,767** |

[1]These numbers do not represent actual deaths of persons with AIDS. Rather, these numbers are point estimates adjusted for delays in the reporting of deaths, but not for incomplete reporting of deaths. Annual estimates are through the most recent year for which reliable estimates are available. See Technical Notes.
[2]See Technical Notes for a list of states or U.S. dependencies, possessions, and associated nations which comprise each region of residence.
[3]Because column totals were calculated independently of the values for the subpopulations, the values in each column may not sum to the column total.
*Source*: Centers for Disease Control and Prevention, U.S. Department of Health and Human Services. National Center for HIV, STD, and TB Prevention. Division of HIV/AIDS Prevention—Surveillance and Epidemiology. *HIV/AIDS Surveillance Report 2000* 12, no. 2, year-end edition. http://www.cdc.gov/hiv/stats/hasr1202.pdf.

## Table B5.7. Estimated Deaths of Persons with AIDS, by Race/Ethnicity and Year of Death, 1993 through 1999, United States[1]

| | Year of death | | | | | | |
|---|---|---|---|---|---|---|---|
| **Race/ethnicity** | **1993** | **1994** | **1995** | **1996** | **1997** | **1998** | **1999** |
| White, not Hispanic | 21,780 | 22,722 | 22,093 | 14,656 | 7,347 | 5,979 | 5,084 |
| Black, not Hispanic | 15,521 | 17,970 | 19,051 | 15,956 | 10,364 | 8,742 | 8,453 |
| Hispanic | 7,748 | 8,889 | 9,131 | 6,925 | 4,099 | 3,278 | 3,042 |
| Asian/Pacific Islander | 307 | 408 | 367 | 292 | 153 | 124 | 111 |
| American Indian/Alaska Native | 135 | 154 | 195 | 133 | 93 | 75 | 63 |
| **Total[2]** | **45,494** | **50,172** | **50,877** | **37,983** | **22,070** | **18,210** | **16,767** |

[1]These numbers do not represent actual deaths of persons with AIDS. Rather, these numbers are point estimates adjusted for delays in the reporting of deaths, but not for incomplete reporting of deaths. Annual estimates are through the most recent year for which reliable estimates are available. See Technical Notes.
[2]Totals include estimates of persons whose race/ethnicity is unknown. Because column totals were calculated independently of the values for the subpopulations, the values in each column may not sum to the column total.
*Source*: Centers for Disease Control and Prevention, U.S. Department of Health and Human Services. National Center for HIV, STD, and TB Prevention. Division of HIV/AIDS Prevention—Surveillance and Epidemiology. *HIV/AIDS Surveillance Report 2000* 12, no. 2, year-end edition. http://www.cdc.gov/hiv/stats/hasr1202.pdf.

## Table B5.8. Estimated Deaths of Persons with AIDS, by Age Group, Sex, Exposure Category, and Year of Death, 1993 through 1999, United States[1]

| | Year of death | | | | | | |
|---|---|---|---|---|---|---|---|
| **Male adult/adolescent exposure category** | **1993** | **1994** | **1995** | **1996** | **1997** | **1998** | **1999** |
| Men who have sex with men | 23,904 | 25,398 | 24,914 | 16,847 | 8,695 | 6,983 | 6,069 |
| Injecting drug use | 9,298 | 10,387 | 10,786 | 8,527 | 5,369 | 4,416 | 4,041 |
| Men who have sex with men and inject drugs | 3,184 | 3,503 | 3,436 | 2,585 | 1,445 | 1,242 | 1,124 |
| Hemophilia/coagulation disorder | 356 | 348 | 331 | 248 | 137 | 115 | 98 |
| Heterosexual contact | 1,591 | 2,010 | 2,388 | 2,108 | 1,473 | 1,214 | 1,230 |
| Receipt of blood transfusion, blood components, or tissue | 314 | 307 | 262 | 216 | 107 | 83 | 70 |
| Risk not reported or identified | 170 | 147 | 102 | 68 | 45 | 29 | 27 |
| Male subtotal | **38,818** | **42,100** | **42,220** | **30,601** | **17,271** | **14,081** | **12,660** |
| **Female adult/adolescent exposure category** | | | | | | | |
| Injecting drug use | 3,144 | 3,699 | 3,812 | 3,279 | 2,146 | 1,891 | 1,891 |
| Hemophilia/coagulation disorder | 17 | 27 | 30 | 30 | 21 | 15 | 16 |
| Heterosexual contact | 2,656 | 3,478 | 3,988 | 3,434 | 2,301 | 2,008 | 1,989 |
| Receipt of blood transfusion, blood components, or tissue | 239 | 225 | 234 | 174 | 94 | 74 | 73 |
| Risk not reported or identified | 76 | 56 | 56 | 33 | 20 | 15 | 19 |
| Female subtotal | 6,132 | 7,486 | 8,119 | 6,950 | 4,582 | 4,004 | 3,989 |
| **Pediatric (<13 years old) exposure category** | 544 | 586 | 539 | 433 | 218 | 124 | 119 |
| **Total[2]** | **45,494** | **50,172** | **50,877** | **37,983** | **22,070** | **18,210** | **16,767** |

[1]These numbers do not represent actual deaths of persons with AIDS. Rather, these numbers are point estimates adjusted for delays in the reporting of deaths, but not for incomplete reporting of deaths. Annual estimates are through the most recent year for which reliable estimates are available. See Technical Notes.
[2]Because column totals were calculated independently of the values for the subpopulations, the values in each column may not sum to the column total.
*Source*: Centers for Disease Control and Prevention, U.S. Department of Health and Human Services. National Center for HIV, STD, and TB Prevention. Division of HIV/AIDS Prevention—Surveillance and Epidemiology. *HIV/AIDS Surveillance Report 2000* 12, no. 2, year-end edition. http://www.cdc.gov/hiv/stats/hasr1202.pdf.

# Table B5.9. Deaths in Persons with AIDS by Race/Ethnicity, Age at Death, and Sex, Occurring in 1998 and 1999; and Cumulative Totals Reported through December 2000, United States[1]

| Race/ethnicity and age at death[2] | Males | | | Females | | | Both sexes[3] | | |
|---|---|---|---|---|---|---|---|---|---|
| | 1998 | 1999 | Cumulative total | 1998 | 1999 | Cumulative total | 1998 | 1999 | Cumulative total |
| **White, not Hispanic** | | | | | | | | | |
| Under 15 | 6 | 7 | 568 | 6 | 4 | 422 | 12 | 11 | 990 |
| 15-24 | 33 | 19 | 2,541 | 11 | 12 | 480 | 44 | 31 | 3,021 |
| 25-34 | 869 | 598 | 54,902 | 156 | 132 | 4,692 | 1,025 | 730 | 59,594 |
| 35-44 | 2,202 | 1,710 | 81,121 | 288 | 281 | 5,213 | 2,490 | 1,991 | 86,335 |
| 45-54 | 1,328 | 1,169 | 37,252 | 127 | 141 | 2,052 | 1,455 | 1,310 | 39,304 |
| 55 or older | 561 | 475 | 15,732 | 62 | 51 | 1,751 | 623 | 526 | 17,483 |
| All ages | 4,999 | 3,978 | 192,276 | 650 | 621 | 14,632 | 5,649 | 4,599 | 206,909 |
| **Black, not Hispanic** | | | | | | | | | |
| Under 15 | 30 | 37 | 1,444 | 48 | 28 | 1,424 | 78 | 65 | 2,868 |
| 15-24 | 70 | 51 | 2,459 | 87 | 76 | 1,447 | 157 | 127 | 3,906 |
| 25-34 | 1,073 | 859 | 33,731 | 648 | 548 | 11,968 | 1,721 | 1,407 | 45,699 |
| 35-44 | 2,324 | 2,156 | 50,579 | 1,014 | 993 | 15,121 | 3,338 | 3,149 | 65,700 |
| 45-54 | 1,605 | 1,561 | 22,923 | 510 | 507 | 5,465 | 2,115 | 2,068 | 28,388 |
| 55 or older | 699 | 690 | 9,768 | 214 | 215 | 2,406 | 913 | 905 | 12,174 |
| All ages | 5,801 | 5,354 | 121,030 | 2,521 | 2,367 | 37,862 | 8,322 | 7,721 | 158,892 |
| **Hispanic** | | | | | | | | | |
| Under 15 | 10 | 10 | 632 | 9 | 14 | 583 | 19 | 24 | 1,215 |
| 15-24 | 31 | 18 | 1,342 | 12 | 17 | 486 | 43 | 35 | 1,828 |
| 25-34 | 509 | 416 | 20,387 | 179 | 148 | 4,580 | 688 | 564 | 24,967 |
| 35-44 | 1,059 | 900 | 26,518 | 276 | 277 | 5,013 | 1,335 | 1,177 | 31,531 |
| 45-54 | 576 | 502 | 10,859 | 127 | 154 | 1,846 | 703 | 656 | 12,705 |
| 55 or older | 276 | 261 | 4,514 | 68 | 46 | 874 | 344 | 307 | 5,388 |
| All ages | 2,461 | 2,107 | 64,305 | 671 | 656 | 13,393 | 3,132 | 2,763 | 77,698 |
| **Asian/Pacific Islander** | | | | | | | | | |
| Under 15 | – | – | 19 | – | 1 | 16 | – | 1 | 35 |
| 15-24 | 1 | 2 | 37 | – | 1 | 6 | 1 | 3 | 43 |
| 25-34 | 28 | 12 | 720 | 6 | 5 | 82 | 34 | 17 | 802 |
| 35-44 | 39 | 42 | 1,141 | 8 | 1 | 104 | 47 | 43 | 1,245 |
| 45-54 | 18 | 21 | 551 | 3 | 7 | 67 | 21 | 28 | 618 |
| 55 or older | 11 | 7 | 254 | 4 | 2 | 54 | 15 | 9 | 308 |
| All ages | 97 | 84 | 2,724 | 21 | 17 | 331 | 118 | 101 | 3,055 |
| **American Indian/Alaska Native** | | | | | | | | | |
| Under 15 | – | – | 12 | – | – | 8 | – | – | 20 |
| 15-24 | – | – | 26 | – | – | 3 | – | – | 29 |
| 25-34 | 20 | 12 | 388 | 6 | 3 | 74 | 26 | 15 | 462 |
| 35-44 | 21 | 17 | 405 | 8 | 7 | 73 | 29 | 24 | 478 |
| 45-54 | 9 | 12 | 137 | 1 | 1 | 29 | 10 | 13 | 166 |
| 55 or older | 6 | 2 | 46 | – | 3 | 13 | 6 | 5 | 59 |
| All ages | 56 | 43 | 1,017 | 15 | 14 | 200 | 71 | 57 | 1,217 |
| **All racial/ethnic groups** | | | | | | | | | |
| Under 15 | 46 | 54 | 2,677 | 63 | 47 | 2,454 | 109 | 101 | 5,131 |
| 15-24 | 135 | 90 | 6,410 | 110 | 106 | 2,424 | 245 | 196 | 8,834 |
| 25-34 | 2,501 | 1,899 | 110,187 | 995 | 836 | 21,402 | 3,496 | 2,735 | 131,589 |
| 35-44 | 5,651 | 4,831 | 159,883 | 1,595 | 1,561 | 25,537 | 7,246 | 6,392 | 185,421 |
| 45-54 | 3,539 | 3,268 | 71,770 | 768 | 810 | 9,464 | 4,307 | 4,078 | 81,234 |
| 55 or older | 1,553 | 1,435 | 30,338 | 348 | 317 | 5,101 | 1,901 | 1,752 | 35,439 |
| All ages | 13,425 | 11,577 | 381,611 | 3,879 | 3,677 | 66,448 | 17,304 | 15,254 | 448,060 |

[1]Data tabulations for 1998 and 1999 are based on date of death occurrence. Data for deaths occurring in 2000 are incomplete and not tabulated separately, but are included in the cumulative totals. Tabulations for 1998 and 1999 may increase as additional deaths are reported to CDC.

[2]Data tabulated under "all ages" include 412 persons whose age at death is unknown. Data tabulated under "all racial/ethnic groups" include 289 persons whose race/ethnicity is unknown.

[3]Includes 1 person whose sex is unknown.

*Source*: Centers for Disease Control and Prevention, U.S. Department of Health and Human Services. National Center for HIV, STD, and TB Prevention. Division of HIV/AIDS Prevention—Surveillance and Epidemiology. *HIV/AIDS Surveillance Report 2000* 12, no. 2, year-end edition. http://www.cdc.gov/hiv/stats/hasr1202.pdf.

# C. Malaria

## OVERVIEW

An acute and sometimes chronic disorder caused by the presence of protozoan parasites within the red blood cells, malaria remains one of the most widespread and fatal diseases in the world.

Today, although malaria infection remains a devastating global problem, with an estimated 300–500 million cases occurring annually,[1] its incidence and effect in most Western nations, including the United States, is dramatically less than its incidence and effect in malaria-prone countries, such as those in Africa, Asia, and Central and South America. However, in previous years, malaria was also endemic throughout much of the continental United States; an estimated 600,000 cases occurred during 1914.[2] During the late 1940s, a combination of improved socioeconomic conditions, water management, vector-control efforts, and case management was successful at interrupting malaria transmission in the United States.

Despite the fact that its incidence and impact in the United States are vastly different than the incidence and impact of other infectious diseases, malaria remains on the list of nationally notifiable diseases. Public health concern about malaria remains understandably high. Indeed, for over 60 years, malaria case surveillance has been maintained in the United States for two primary reasons—to detect locally acquired cases that could indicate the reintroduction of transmission and to monitor patterns of antimalarial drug resistance seen among U.S. travelers. Surveillance is also conducted to guide malaria prevention recommendations for travelers abroad.

## CASE DEFINITION

There are four main forms of human malaria. In humans, the causative agents are four species of *plasmodium protozoa* (single-celled parasites), including vivax, falciparum, malariae, and ovale.

*Plasmodium vivax* (*p.vivax*) is perhaps the most prevalent of the four and is the species most frequently encountered in temperate zones. *P. vivax* is a tertian malaria since its cyclic paroxysms occur every 48 hours. *Plasmodium falciparum* (*p. falciparum*) is a malignant malaria, and its cyclic paroxysms occur every 36 to 48 hours. It ranks second in prevalence and is chiefly a tropical species. Clinically, *P. falciparum* infections are the most serious of the four, but it tends to run a shorter course without relapses. *Plasmodium malariae (p. malariae)* is a quartan malaria and its cyclic paroxysms occur every 72 hours. *Plasmodium malariae* ranks third in prevalence, but has a widespread distribution. *Plasmodium ovale* (*p. ovale*) is ovale malaria, and its cyclic paroxysms occur every 48 hours. *P. ovale* is the rarest of the four types of malaria found in humans and is more restricted in distribution. It is common in the West African countries of Ghana, Liberia, and Nigeria and in other nearby areas.

Cerebral malaria is *falciparum* malaria in which the brain is infected due to the tendency of parasites to agglutinate or adhere, resulting in clogging of the capillaries, which leads to coma or sometimes sudden death. Caused by *Plasmodium malariae*, quartan is malaria with short and less severe paroxysms; sporulation, or the production of spores, occurs each 72 hours, causing seizures every 4 days. Quotidian malaria is characterized by paroxysms that occur with daily periodicity due to 24-hour sporulation of two groups of *P. vivax*; other symptoms include abrupt rise and fall of temperature. Tertian malaria is characterized by the occurrence of sporulation each 48 hours. Symptoms are more common during the day. Paroxysms are divided into chill, fever, and sweating stages. The cold stage usually is 10 to 15 minutes but may last an hour or more. The febrile stage varies from 4 to 6 hours. Benign tertian malaria is caused by *Plasmodium vivax*, malignant tertian malaria by *Plasmodium falciparum*.

## SYMPTOMS AND PATHOLOGIES

The signs and symptoms of malaria might be vague, but fever is generally present. Other symptoms include headache, chills, increased sweating, back pain, myalgia, diarrhea, nausea, vomiting, and cough. Untreated *Plasmodium falciparum* infection can lead to coma, renal failure, pulmonary edema, and death. Physicians consider the diagnosis of malaria for any person who has these symptoms and who has traveled to an area in which malaria is endemic. They also consider malaria in the differential diagnosis of persons who have a fever of unknown origin, regardless of their travel history. Asymptomatic parasitemia can occur among persons who have been long-term residents of areas in which malaria is endemic. *P. vivax* and *P. ovale* have dormant forms that may initiate a relapse. *P. falciparum* and *P. malariae* have no such dormant forms.

## DIAGNOSIS

Diagnosis is made by identification of the parasites in the blood by a simple blood test.

## TRANSMISSION

Malaria is transmitted to the human by the bite of an infected female anopheles mosquito. The mosquito becomes infected by ingesting the blood of a human infected with malaria.

Most malaria infections in the United States occur among persons who have traveled to areas with ongoing transmission. In addition to the mosquitoborne transmission of malaria in an area where malaria occurs regularly (indigenous malaria), malaria may also be acquired from an imported case in an area where malaria does not occur regularly (introduced malaria). Additionally, malaria may be acquired through artificial means, such as blood transfusion or use of shared syringes (induced malaria). Relapsing malaria occurs when there are renewed manifestations of malarial infection that are separated from previous manifestations of the same infection by an interval greater than the usual periodicity of the paroxysms. Last, note cryptic malaria, an isolated malaria case that cannot be linked epidemiologically to additional cases. Note that malaria cases are classified according to the following World Health Organization categories: autochthonous, imported, induced, relapsing, and cryptic. Autochthonous cases include both indigenous and introduced malaria.

## TREATMENT

Treatment for malaria should be initiated immediately after the diagnosis has been confirmed by a positive blood smear. Treatment for malaria is determined on the basis of the infecting *Plasmodium* species, the probable geographic origin of the parasite, the parasite density, and the patient's clinical status. Chloroquine phosphate is prescribed in all types of malaria except those due to drug-resistant *Plasmodium falciparum*. In drug-resistant *P. falciparum*, treatment with combinations of quinine, pyrimethamine, and a sulfonamide is indicated. Malaria due to other species is treated with both chloroquine and primaquine. Severe malaria due to *P. falciparum* with evidence of cerebral involvement may be treated with continuous infusion of quinidine gluconate and exchange transfusion.

## SURVEILLANCE

Health care providers and/or laboratory staff report confirmed malaria cases to local and/or state health departments, which investigate the cases and report their findings to CDC through the National Malaria Surveillance System (NMSS). CDC staff review all reports at the time of receipt and request additional information if necessary. Health care providers also telephone reports directly to CDC, usually when assistance with diagnosis or treatment is requested.

Data regarding malaria cases are also reported to the National Notifiable Diseases Surveillance System (NNDSS) described earlier in this *Handbook*. NMSS receives more clinical and epidemiological data regarding each case than does NNDSS. Consequently, data on numbers of reported cases may differ between systems. The NNDSS and NMSS surveillance systems are currently assessing the feasibility of developing an integrated approach for electronically reporting malaria case data from the states and territories to CDC. The objectives of this effort are to decrease reporting burden in the states, to streamline the reporting of data to CDC, and to achieve more consistency in the format of data reported to CDC.

## TABLE OVERVIEW

**C1.1–C1.2. General Surveillance Data** C1.1 graphs malaria cases in the United States from 1968 to 1998; C1.2 breaks down annual figures by type of person ill. CDC received reports of 1,392 cases of malaria with onset of symptoms during 1996 among persons in the United States or one of its territories. This number represents an increase of 19.3% from the 1,167 cases reported for 1995.[3] During 1997, CDC received reports of 1,544 malaria cases that had onset of symptoms among persons in the United States and its territories, representing a 10.9% increase from the 1,392 cases reported for 1996. This incidence is the largest number of reported cases since 1980. In 1997, a total of 698 cases occurred in U.S. civilians compared with 618 cases reported for 1996. This incidence represents the largest number of U.S. civilian cases reported since 1968. The number of cases in foreign civilians decreased from 636 in 1996 to 592 in 1997. Cases among U.S. military personnel also decreased from 32 in 1996 to 28 in 1997. Note that a case was defined as symptomatic or asymptomatic illness that occurs in the United States in a person who has microscopically confirmed malaria parasitemia, regardless of whether the person had previous attacks of malaria while in other countries. A subsequent attack of malaria occurring in a person is counted as an additional case if the demonstrated *Plasmodium* species differs from the initially identified species.

**C2. Data by *Plasmodium* Species** The infecting species of *Plasmodium* was identified in 1,288 (92.5%) of the cases reported in 1996 and in 1,410 (91.3%) of the cases reported in 1997. *P. vivax* and *P. falciparum* were identified in 47.4% and 37.4% of infected persons in 1996 and in 48.9% and 36.7% of infected persons in 1997.

**C3.1–C3.2. Area of Acquisition** Among 1,410 cases in which both the region of acquisition and the infecting species were known in 1997, 465 (76.6%) of infections acquired in Africa were attributed to *P. falciparum*; 75 (12.4%) were attributed to *P. vivax*. The converse was true of infections acquired in Asia and the Americas: 432 (89.6%) and 175 (69.7%) were attributed to *P. vivax*, and only 39 (8.1%) and 50 (19.9%) were attributed to *P. falciparum*, respectively. Note the contrast with 1996: Among 1,244 cases in which both the region of acquisition and the infecting species were known, 431 (80.3%) of infections acquired in Africa were attributed to *P. falciparum*, whereas 41 (7.6%) were attributed to *P. vivax*. Note too that in 1996 the converse was also then true of malaria infections acquired in Asia and the Americas: 353 (83.6%) and 160 (81.5%) were attributed to *P. vivax*, and only 45 (10.7%) and 196 (13.7%) were attributed to *P. falciparum*, respectively.

Of all reported cases, 99% (n = 1,381) were reported as imported in 1996. In 1997, approximately 98% (n = 1,522) of all cases were classified as imported. In 1996, of the 1,337 imported cases in which the region of acquisition was known, most, 43.7% (n = 585), were acquired in Africa, whereas 33.1% (n = 442) and 20.0% (n = 267) were acquired in Asia and in the Americas. Note comparisons to 1997: Of the 1,507 imported cases in which the region of acquisition was known, most, 46.2% (n = 697), were acquired in Africa, whereas 33.1% (n = 499) and 16.2% (n = 245) were acquired in Asia and the Americas. The number of reported malaria cases acquired in Africa increased by 19.1% (n = 697) compared with 1996, and cases acquired in Asia increased by 12.9% (n = 499) compared with 1996. Cases from the Americas decreased by 6.0% (n = 251) in 1997 compared with 1996.

**C4.1–C4.2. Imported Malaria Cases by Interval between Arrival in the United States and Onset of Illness** Of those persons who became ill with malaria after arriving in the United States, both the interval between the date of arrival in the United States and onset of illness and the identification of the infecting *Plasmodium* species were known for 1,091 (71.7%) of the imported cases of malaria in 1997. Symptoms began after arrival in the United States for 1,022 (93.7%) of these cases. Clinical malaria developed within 1 month after arrival in 344 (77.6%) of the 443 *P. falciparum* cases and in 124 (21.3%) of the *P. vivax* cases. Only 27 (2.6%) of the 1,022 persons became ill more than 1 year after returning to the United States. An additional 69 persons reported becoming ill before arriving in the United States.

A total of 1,287 imported malaria cases were reported among civilians in 1997. Of these, 695 (54.0%) cases occurred among U.S. residents, and 592 (46.0%) occurred among residents of other countries.

**C.5. Purpose of Travel** The purpose of travel to malarious areas was reported for 469 (67.5%) of the 695 U.S. civilians with imported malaria in 1997. Of the cases in U.S. civilians, the largest percentage (22.6%) of case-patients traveled to visit friends or relatives in malarious areas; the second and third largest percentages, 11.5% and 10.9% respectively, traveled to tour and to do missionary work.

## NOTES

1. *MMWR* 50, no. SS-1 (March 30, 2001):2.
2. Pan American Health Organization, *Report for Registration of Malaria Eradication from United States of America*. Washington, DC: Pan American Health Organization, 1969.
3. Center for Disease Control and Prevention, U.S. Department of Health and Human Services. *MMWR: Morbidity and Mortality Weekly Review, CDC Surveillance Summaries, Malaria Surveillance, United States, 1995* 48, no. SS-1 (1999). http://www.cdc.gov/mmwr/PDF/ss/ss4801.pdf.

**Table C1.1. Malaria—Reported Cases per 100,000 Population, by Year, United States, 1968–1998**

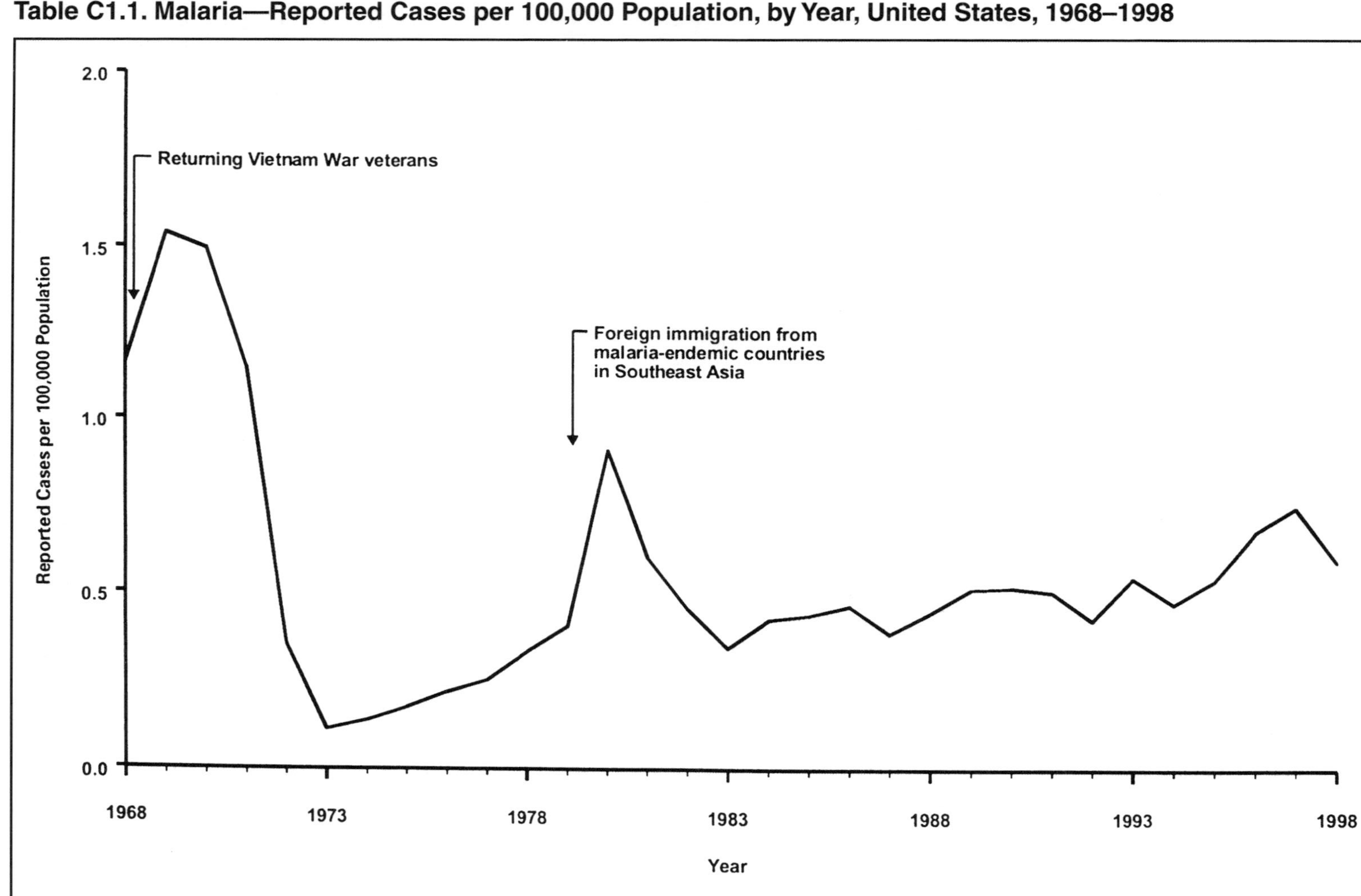


The increasing number of imported malaria cases in the preceding decade is probably related to several factors, including a) increased foreign travel to and from malaria-endemic areas, some of which have higher rates of malaria transmission; b) inadequate chemoprophylaxis used by travelers; and c) increasing antimalarial drug resistance.

*Source*: Centers for Disease Control and Prevention. "Summary of Notifiable Diseases, United States," 1999. *MMWR: Morbidity and Mortality Weekly Report* 48, no. 53 (1999). http://www.cdc.gov/mmwr/PDF/wk/mm4853.pdf

## Table C1.2. Number of Malaria Cases* in U.S. and Foreign Civilians and U.S. Military Personnel—United States, 1968–1997

| Year | U.S. military personnel | U.S. civilians | Foreign civilians | Unknown | Total |
|---|---|---|---|---|---|
| 1968 | 2,567 | 82 | 49 | 0 | **2,698** |
| 1969 | 3,914 | 90 | 47 | 11 | **4,062** |
| 1970 | 4,096 | 90 | 44 | 17 | **4,247** |
| 1971 | 2,975 | 79 | 69 | 57 | **3,180** |
| 1972 | 454 | 106 | 54 | 0 | **614** |
| 1973 | 41 | 103 | 78 | 0 | **222** |
| 1974 | 21 | 158 | 144 | 0 | **323** |
| 1975 | 17 | 199 | 232 | 0 | **448** |
| 1976 | 5 | 178 | 227 | 5 | **415** |
| 1977 | 11 | 233 | 237 | 0 | **481** |
| 1978 | 31 | 270 | 315 | 0 | **616** |
| 1979 | 11 | 229 | 634 | 3 | **877** |
| 1980 | 26 | 303 | 1,534 | 1 | **1,864** |
| 1981 | 21 | 273 | 809 | 0 | **1,103** |
| 1982 | 8 | 348 | 574 | 0 | **930** |
| 1983 | 10 | 325 | 468 | 0 | **803** |
| 1984 | 24 | 360 | 632 | 0 | **1,016** |
| 1985 | 31 | 446 | 568 | 0 | **1,045** |
| 1986 | 35 | 410 | 646 | 0 | **1,091** |
| 1987 | 23 | 421 | 488 | 0 | **932** |
| 1988 | 33 | 550 | 440 | 0 | **1,023** |
| 1989 | 35 | 591 | 476 | 0 | **1,102** |
| 1990 | 36 | 558 | 504 | 0 | **1,098** |
| 1991 | 22 | 585 | 439 | 0 | **1,046** |
| 1992 | 29 | 394 | 481 | 6 | **910** |
| 1993 | 278 | 519 | 453 | 25 | **1,275** |
| 1994 | 38 | 524 | 370 | 82 | **1,014** |
| 1995 | 12 | 599 | 461 | 95 | **1,167** |
| 1996 | 32 | 618 | 636 | 106 | **1,392** |
| 1997 | 28 | 698 | 592 | 226 | **1,544** |

*A case was defined as symptomatic or asymptomatic illness that occurs in the United States in a person who has microscopically confirmed malaria parasitemia, regardless of whether the person had previous attacks of malaria while in other countries. A subsequent attack of malaria occurring in a person is counted as an additional case if the demonstrated *Plasmodium* species differs from the initially identified species. A subsequent attack of malaria occurring in a person while in the United States could indicate a relapsing infection or treatment failure resulting from drug resistance if the demonstrated *Plasmodium* species is the same species identified previously.

*Source*: Centers for Disease Control and Prevention, United States Department for Health and Human Services. Epidemiology Program Office. CDC Surveillance Summaries. "Malaria Surveillance—United States, 1996" and "Malaria Surveillance—United States, 1997." *MMWR: Morbidity and Mortality Weekly Report* 50, no. SS-1 (2001). http://www.cdc.gov/mmwr/PDF/ss/ss5001.pdf.

## Table C2. Number of Malaria Cases, by *Plasmodium* Species—United States, 1996 and 1997

| *Plasmodium* species | 1996 No. | 1996 (%) | 1997 No. | 1997 (%) |
|---|---|---|---|---|
| *P. vivax* | 660 | (47.4) | 755 | (48.9) |
| *P. falciparum* | 521 | (37.4) | 567 | (36.7) |
| *P. malariae* | 75 | (5.4) | 48 | (3.1) |
| *P. ovale* | 28 | (2.0) | 31 | (2.0) |
| Undetermined | 104 | (7.5) | 134 | (8.7) |
| Mixed | 4 | (0.3) | 9 | (0.6) |
| **Total** | **1,392** | **(100.0)** | **1,544** | **(100.0)** |

*Source*: Centers for Disease Control and Prevention, United States Department for Health and Human Services. Epidemiology Program Office. CDC Surveillance Summaries. "Malaria Surveillance—United States, 1996" and "Malaria Surveillance—United States, 1997." *MMWR: Morbidity and Mortality Weekly Report* 50, no. SS-1 (2001). http://www.cdc.gov/mmwr/PDF/ss/ss5001.pdf.

**Table C3.1. Number of Malaria Cases, by *Plasmodium* Species and Area of Acquisition—United States, 1996**

| Area of acquisition | *Plasmodium* species | | | | | | |
|---|---|---|---|---|---|---|---|
| | *P. vivax* | *P. falciparum* | *P. malariae* | *P. ovale* | Unknown | Mixed | Total |
| **AFRICA** | 41 | 431 | 37 | 26 | 48 | 2 | **585** |
| Angola | 0 | 3 | 0 | 0 | 0 | 0 | **3** |
| Benin | 0 | 2 | 0 | 0 | 0 | 0 | **2** |
| Cameroon | 2 | 6 | 1 | 0 | 3 | 0 | **12** |
| Chad | 0 | 1 | 0 | 0 | 1 | 0 | **2** |
| Central African Republic | 0 | 1 | 0 | 0 | 0 | 0 | **1** |
| Comoros | 1 | 0 | 0 | 0 | 0 | 0 | **1** |
| Congo | 0 | 1 | 0 | 0 | 0 | 0 | **1** |
| Côte d'Ivoire | 0 | 21 | 1 | 2 | 3 | 0 | **27** |
| Democratic Republic of the Congo (Zaire) | 2 | 7 | 1 | 1 | 0 | 0 | **11** |
| Equatorial Guinea | 1 | 1 | 0 | 0 | 0 | 0 | **2** |
| Ethiopia | 7 | 2 | 1 | 1 | 0 | 0 | **11** |
| Gabon | 0 | 1 | 0 | 0 | 0 | 0 | **1** |
| Gambia | 0 | 1 | 0 | 0 | 0 | 0 | **1** |
| Ghana | 3 | 70 | 3 | 0 | 5 | 0 | **81** |
| Guinea | 0 | 13 | 0 | 2 | 0 | 0 | **15** |
| Kenya | 5 | 19 | 3 | 4 | 3 | 0 | **34** |
| Liberia | 0 | 22 | 3 | 1 | 3 | 0 | **29** |
| Madagascar | 1 | 0 | 0 | 0 | 0 | 0 | **1** |
| Malawi | 0 | 1 | 0 | 0 | 0 | 0 | **1** |
| Mali | 0 | 4 | 0 | 1 | 0 | 0 | **5** |
| Mauritania | 1 | 0 | 0 | 0 | 0 | 0 | **1** |
| Morocco | 0 | 0 | 0 | 0 | 1 | 0 | **1** |
| Mozambique | 0 | 1 | 0 | 0 | 0 | 1 | **2** |
| Niger | 0 | 1 | 0 | 0 | 0 | 0 | **1** |
| Nigeria | 9 | 143 | 13 | 3 | 15 | 1 | **184** |
| São Tomé | 0 | 0 | 0 | 0 | 1 | 0 | **1** |
| Senegal | 0 | 9 | 0 | 0 | 1 | 0 | **10** |
| Sierra Leone | 0 | 11 | 1 | 1 | 1 | 0 | **14** |
| Somali Republic | 1 | 4 | 0 | 0 | 0 | 0 | **5** |
| South Africa | 0 | 6 | 0 | 0 | 0 | 0 | **6** |
| Sudan | 1 | 2 | 1 | 0 | 1 | 0 | **5** |
| Swaziland | 0 | 0 | 1 | 0 | 0 | 0 | **1** |
| Tanzania | 0 | 4 | 0 | 1 | 0 | 0 | **5** |
| Togo | 0 | 2 | 0 | 0 | 0 | 0 | **2** |
| Uganda | 0 | 3 | 0 | 0 | 1 | 0 | **4** |
| Zambia | 0 | 2 | 0 | 0 | 0 | 0 | **2** |
| Zimbabwe | 0 | 3 | 0 | 0 | 0 | 0 | **3** |
| East Africa, Unspecified | 2 | 10 | 2 | 0 | 0 | 0 | **14** |
| West Africa, Unspecified | 0 | 26 | 2 | 2 | 4 | 0 | **34** |
| South Africa, Unspecified | 0 | 3 | 1 | 0 | 0 | 0 | **4** |
| Africa, Unspecified | 5 | 25 | 3 | 7 | 5 | 0 | **45** |
| **ASIA** | 353 | 45 | 22 | 1 | 20 | 1 | **442** |
| Afghanistan | 1 | 0 | 0 | 0 | 0 | 0 | **1** |
| Bangladesh | 1 | 0 | 0 | 0 | 0 | 0 | **1** |
| Cambodia | 0 | 0 | 0 | 0 | 1 | 0 | **1** |
| China | 0 | 1 | 0 | 0 | 0 | 0 | **1** |
| India | 282 | 21 | 18 | 0 | 14 | 0 | **335** |

## Table C3.1. *(Continued)*

| Area of acquisition | *Plasmodium species* P. vivax | P. falciparum | P. malariae | P. ovale | Unknown | Mixed | Total |
|---|---|---|---|---|---|---|---|
| Indonesia | 12 | 8 | 0 | 0 | 1 | 0 | **21** |
| Iran | 1 | 0 | 0 | 0 | 0 | 0 | **1** |
| Iraq | 1 | 0 | 0 | 0 | 0 | 0 | **1** |
| Korea | 1 | 0 | 0 | 0 | 0 | 0 | **1** |
| Laos | 1 | 3 | 0 | 0 | 0 | 0 | **4** |
| Middle East | 1 | 0 | 0 | 0 | 0 | 0 | **1** |
| Myanmar | 0 | 1 | 0 | 0 | 0 | 0 | **1** |
| Nepal | 1 | 0 | 0 | 0 | 0 | 0 | **1** |
| Pakistan | 33 | 4 | 3 | 0 | 3 | 0 | **43** |
| Philippines | 2 | 2 | 0 | 1 | 0 | 0 | **5** |
| Thailand | 0 | 2 | 0 | 0 | 0 | 0 | **2** |
| Viet Nam | 0 | 1 | 1 | 0 | 1 | 1 | **4** |
| Yemen | 2 | 1 | 0 | 0 | 0 | 0 | **3** |
| Asia, Unspecified | 11 | 1 | 0 | 0 | 0 | 0 | **12** |
| Southeast Asia, Unspecified | 3 | 0 | 0 | 0 | 0 | 0 | **3** |
| **CENTRAL AMERICA AND CARIBBEAN** | 112 | 30 | 9 | 0 | 16 | 0 | **217** |
| Belize | 8 | 0 | 0 | 0 | 1 | 0 | **9** |
| Costa Rica | 5 | 2 | 0 | 0 | 0 | 0 | **7** |
| Dominican Republic | 1 | 0 | 0 | 0 | 0 | 0 | **1** |
| El Salvador | 5 | 0 | 0 | 0 | 0 | 0 | **5** |
| Guatemala | 16 | 1 | 2 | 0 | 1 | 0 | **20** |
| Haiti | 4 | 17 | 1 | 0 | 4 | 0 | **26** |
| Honduras | 77 | 4 | 5 | 0 | 6 | 0 | **92** |
| Nicaragua | 24 | 4 | 1 | 0 | 2 | 0 | **31** |
| Panama | 0 | 0 | 0 | 0 | 1 | 0 | **1** |
| Central America, Unspecified | 21 | 2 | 0 | 0 | 1 | 0 | **24** |
| Caribbean, Unspecified | 1 | 0 | 0 | 0 | 0 | 0 | **1** |
| **NORTH AMERICA** | 26 | 2 | 1 | 1 | 0 | 0 | **30** |
| United States | 8 | 2 | 0 | 1 | 0 | 0 | **11** |
| Mexico | 18 | 0 | 1 | 0 | 0 | 0 | **19** |
| **SOUTH AMERICA** | 22 | 4 | 1 | 0 | 2 | 1 | **30** |
| Bolivia | 1 | 0 | 0 | 0 | 0 | 0 | **1** |
| Brazil | 0 | 1 | 0 | 0 | 0 | 0 | **1** |
| Colombia | 0 | 0 | 0 | 0 | 1 | 0 | **1** |
| Ecuador | 3 | 0 | 0 | 0 | 1 | 0 | **4** |
| French Guiana | 0 | 1 | 0 | 0 | 0 | 0 | **1** |
| Guyana | 5 | 1 | 0 | 0 | 0 | 1 | **7** |
| Peru | 10 | 0 | 1 | 0 | 0 | 0 | **11** |
| Surinam | 1 | 1 | 0 | 0 | 0 | 0 | **2** |
| South America, Unspecified | 2 | 0 | 0 | 0 | 0 | 0 | **2** |
| **America, Unspecified** | 1 | 0 | 0 | 0 | 0 | 0 | 1 |
| **OCEANIA** | 31 | 2 | 3 | 0 | 7 | 0 | **43** |
| Papua New Guinea | 27 | 2 | 3 | 0 | 7 | 0 | **39** |
| Solomon Islands | 2 | 0 | 0 | 0 | 0 | 0 | **2** |
| Oceania, Unspecified | 2 | 0 | 0 | 0 | 0 | 0 | **2** |
| **Unknown** | 24 | 7 | 2 | 0 | 11 | 0 | **44** |
| **Total** | **660** | **521** | **75** | **28** | **104** | **4** | **1,392** |

*Source*: Centers for Disease Control and Prevention, United States Department for Health and Human Services. Epidemiology Program Office. CDC Surveillance Summaries. "Malaria Surveillance—United States, 1996" and "Malaria Surveillance—United States, 1997." *MMWR: Morbidity and Mortality Weekly Report* 50, no. SS-1 (2001). http://www.cdc.gov/mmwr/PDF/ss/ss5001.pdf.

## Table C3.2. Number of Malaria Cases, by *Plasmodium* Species and Area of Acquisition—United States, 1997

| Area of acquisition | *Plasmodium* species | | | | | | Total |
|---|---|---|---|---|---|---|---|
| | *P. vivax* | *P. falciparum* | *P. malariae* | *P. ovale* | Unknown | Mixed | |
| **AFRICA** | 75 | 465 | 34 | 30 | 90 | 3 | **697** |
| Angola | 0 | 2 | 0 | 1 | 0 | 0 | **3** |
| Benin | 1 | 1 | 0 | 1 | 0 | 0 | **3** |
| Cameroon | 0 | 15 | 1 | 1 | 5 | 1 | **23** |
| Central African Republic | 1 | 0 | 0 | 0 | 1 | 0 | **2** |
| Congo | 1 | 0 | 0 | 0 | 1 | 0 | **3** |
| Côte d'Ivoire | 0 | 15 | 1 | 1 | 7 | 0 | **24** |
| Democratic Republic of the Congo (Zaire) | 1 | 4 | 0 | 0 | 1 | 0 | **6** |
| Ethiopia | 9 | 1 | 0 | 0 | 0 | 0 | **10** |
| Gabon | 0 | 0 | 0 | 0 | 1 | 0 | **1** |
| Gambia | 1 | 4 | 0 | 0 | 0 | 0 | **5** |
| Ghana | 4 | 88 | 8 | 1 | 8 | 0 | **109** |
| Guinea | 0 | 9 | 0 | 0 | 0 | 0 | **9** |
| Kenya | 12 | 21 | 2 | 2 | 9 | 0 | **46** |
| Liberia | 3 | 25 | 2 | 0 | 3 | 0 | **33** |
| Madagascar | 8 | 1 | 0 | 1 | 1 | 0 | **11** |
| Malawi | 2 | 3 | 0 | 0 | 1 | 0 | **6** |
| Mali | 0 | 9 | 0 | 0 | 3 | 0 | **12** |
| Mauritania | 0 | 0 | 0 | 0 | 1 | 0 | **1** |
| Mozambique | 1 | 2 | 0 | 0 | 2 | 0 | **5** |
| Nigeria | 7 | 152 | 7 | 10 | 23 | 1 | **200** |
| Rwanda | 0 | 3 | 0 | 0 | 0 | 0 | **3** |
| Senegal | 0 | 7 | 1 | 1 | 1 | 0 | **10** |
| Sierra Leone | 0 | 13 | 2 | 1 | 1 | 0 | **17** |
| Somali Republic | 2 | 0 | 0 | 1 | 1 | 0 | **4** |
| South Africa | 1 | 3 | 1 | 0 | 1 | 0 | **6** |
| Sudan | 3 | 5 | 0 | 0 | 0 | 0 | **8** |
| Tanzania | 2 | 3 | 3 | 2 | 3 | 0 | **13** |
| Togo | 0 | 1 | 0 | 1 | 0 | 0 | **2** |
| Uganda | 1 | 8 | 0 | 1 | 3 | 0 | **13** |
| Zambia | 0 | 2 | 1 | 0 | 1 | 0 | **4** |
| Zimbabwe | 0 | 7 | 0 | 1 | 2 | 0 | **10** |
| East Africa, Unspecified | 5 | 6 | 0 | 0 | 0 | 0 | **11** |
| West Africa, Unspecified | 3 | 26 | 0 | 2 | 1 | 0 | **32** |
| Central Africa, Unspecified | 0 | 0 | 1 | 0 | 0 | 0 | **1** |
| South Africa, Unspecified | 0 | 1 | 0 | 1 | 0 | 0 | **2** |
| Africa, Unspecified | 7 | 27 | 4 | 1 | 9 | 1 | **49** |
| **ASIA** | 432 | 39 | 8 | 1 | 17 | 2 | **499** |
| Afghanistan | 3 | 0 | 0 | 0 | 0 | 0 | **3** |
| Burma | 1 | 0 | 0 | 0 | 1 | 0 | **2** |
| Cambodia | 1 | 0 | 0 | 0 | 0 | 0 | **1** |
| China | 1 | 0 | 0 | 0 | 0 | 0 | **1** |
| India | 371 | 18 | 7 | 1 | 11 | 2 | **410** |
| Indonesia | 11 | 6 | 1 | 0 | 1 | 0 | **19** |
| Iraq | 3 | 1 | 0 | 0 | 0 | 0 | **4** |
| Korea | 3 | 0 | 0 | 0 | 0 | 0 | **3** |

## Table C3.2. *(Continued)*

| Area of acquisition | *Plasmodium* species *P. vivax* | *P. falciparum* | *P. malariae* | *P. ovale* | Unknown | Mixed | Total |
|---|---|---|---|---|---|---|---|
| Laos | 0 | 2 | 0 | 0 | 0 | 0 | **2** |
| Middle East | 4 | 0 | 0 | 0 | 0 | 0 | **4** |
| Pakistan | 11 | 1 | 0 | 0 | 1 | 0 | **13** |
| Philippines | 4 | 0 | 0 | 0 | 1 | 0 | **5** |
| Sri Lanka | 3 | 1 | 0 | 0 | 0 | 0 | **4** |
| Thailand | 1 | 3 | 0 | 0 | 0 | 0 | **4** |
| Viet Nam | 1 | 0 | 0 | 0 | 0 | 0 | **1** |
| Yemen | 1 | 2 | 0 | 0 | 0 | 0 | **3** |
| Asia, Unspecified | 6 | 3 | 0 | 0 | 0 | 0 | **9** |
| Southeast Asia, Unspecified | 7 | 2 | 0 | 0 | 2 | 0 | **11** |
| **CENTRAL AMERICA AND CARIBBEAN** | 143 | 41 | 4 | 0 | 16 | 2 | **206** |
| Belize | 8 | 1 | 0 | 0 | 0 | 0 | **9** |
| Costa Rica | 2 | 1 | 0 | 0 | 0 | 0 | **3** |
| El Salvador | 10 | 1 | 0 | 0 | 0 | 0 | **11** |
| Guatemala | 16 | 0 | 0 | 0 | 2 | 0 | **18** |
| Haiti | 1 | 27 | 1 | 0 | 5 | 0 | **34** |
| Honduras | 69 | 6 | 2 | 0 | 7 | 2 | **86** |
| Nicaragua | 23 | 3 | 1 | 0 | 1 | 0 | **28** |
| Panama | 1 | 0 | 0 | 0 | 1 | 0 | **2** |
| Trinidad-Tobago | 1 | 0 | 0 | 0 | 0 | 0 | **1** |
| Central America, Unspecified | 12 | 2 | 0 | 0 | 0 | 0 | **14** |
| **NORTH AMERICA** | 13 | 1 | 1 | 0 | 0 | 0 | **15** |
| United States | 4 | 1 | 0 | 0 | 0 | 0 | **5** |
| Mexico | 9 | 0 | 1 | 0 | 0 | 0 | **10** |
| **SOUTH AMERICA** | 19 | 8 | 0 | 0 | 2 | 1 | **30** |
| Brazil | 4 | 0 | 0 | 0 | 0 | 0 | **4** |
| Colombia | 1 | 1 | 0 | 0 | 0 | 0 | **2** |
| Ecuador | 1 | 1 | 0 | 0 | 0 | 0 | **2** |
| Guyana | 6 | 4 | 0 | 0 | 2 | 0 | **12** |
| Peru | 4 | 1 | 0 | 0 | 0 | 1 | **6** |
| Surinam | 1 | 0 | 0 | 0 | 0 | 0 | **1** |
| Venezuela | 1 | 0 | 0 | 0 | 0 | 0 | **1** |
| South America, Unspecified | 1 | 1 | 0 | 0 | 0 | 0 | **2** |
| **OCEANIA** | 37 | 4 | 0 | 0 | 4 | 1 | **46** |
| Papua New Guinea | 34 | 4 | 0 | 0 | 4 | 1 | **43** |
| Solomon Islands | 3 | 0 | 0 | 0 | 0 | 0 | **3** |
| **EUROPE/NEWLY INDEPENDENT STATES** | 1 | 0 | 0 | 0 | 0 | 0 | **1** |
| Armenia | 1 | 0 | 0 | 0 | 0 | 0 | **1** |
| Unknown | 28 | 7 | 1 | 0 | 0 | 0 | **36** |
| **Total** | **754** | **567** | **48** | **31** | **134** | **9** | **1,544** |

*Source*: Centers for Disease Control and Prevention, United States Department for Health and Human Services. Epidemiology Program Office. CDC Surveillance Summaries. "Malaria Surveillance—United States, 1996" and "Malaria Surveillance—United States, 1997." *MMWR: Morbidity and Mortality Weekly Report* 50, no. SS-1 (2001). http://www.cdc.gov/mmwr/PDF/ss/ss5001.pdf.

## Table C4.1. Number of Imported Malaria Cases, by *Plasmodium* species and by Interval between Date of Arrival in the Country and Onset of Illness—United States, 1997

| Interval | *Plasmodium* species | | | | | | | | | | Total | |
|---|---|---|---|---|---|---|---|---|---|---|---|---|
| | *P. vivax* | | *P. falciparum* | | *P. malariae* | | *P. ovale* | | Mixed | | | |
| (days) | No. | (%) | No. | (%) | No. | (%) | No. | (%) | No. | (%) | No. | (%) |
| <0* | 20 | ( 3.4) | 46 | ( 10.4) | 1 | ( 2.6) | 1 | ( 4.3) | 1 | ( 20.0) | **69** | **( 6.3)** |
| 0–29 | 124 | ( 21.3) | 344 | ( 77.7) | 18 | ( 47.4) | 6 | ( 26.1) | 2 | ( 40.0) | **494** | **( 45.3)** |
| 30–89 | 134 | ( 23.0) | 35 | ( 7.9) | 8 | ( 21.0) | 6 | ( 26.1) | 2 | ( 40.0) | **185** | **( 16.9)** |
| 90–179 | 132 | ( 22.7) | 10 | ( 2.2) | 9 | ( 23.7) | 6 | ( 26.1) | 0 | ( 0.0) | **157** | **( 14.4)** |
| 180–364 | 146 | ( 25.1) | 7 | ( 1.6) | 2 | ( 5.3) | 4 | ( 17.4) | 0 | ( 0.0) | **159** | **( 14.6)** |
| ≥365 | 26 | ( 4.5) | 1 | ( 0.2) | 0 | ( 0.0) | 0 | ( 0.0) | 0 | ( 0.0) | **27** | **( 2.5)** |
| **Total** | **582** | **(100.0)** | **443** | **(100.0)** | **38** | **(100.0)** | **23** | **(100.0)** | **5** | **(100.0)** | **1,091** | **(100.0)** |

*Case-patients had onset of illness before arriving in the United States.

*Source*: U.S. Department of Health and Human Services. Centers for Disease Control and Prevention. Epidemiology Program Office. CDC Surveillance Summaries, *Malaria Surveillance—United States, 1996 Malaria Surveillance—United States 1997*, March 30, 2001 MMWR: Morbidity and Mortality Weekly Report 50, no. SS-1 (2001). http://www.cdc.gov/mmwr/PDF/ss/ss5001.pdf

## Table C4.2. Number of Imported Malaria Cases in U.S. and Foreign Civilians, by Region of Acquisition—United States, 1997

| Region of acquisition | U.S. civilians No. | U.S. civilians (%) | Foreign civilians No. | Foreign civilians (%) | Total No. | Total (%) |
|---|---|---|---|---|---|---|
| Africa | 353 | ( 50.8) | 209 | ( 35.3) | **562** | **( 43.7)** |
| Asia, Unknown* | 148 | ( 21.3) | 295 | ( 49.8) | **443** | **( 34.4)** |
| Central America and Caribbean | 109 | ( 15.7) | 69 | ( 11.7) | **178** | **( 13.8)** |
| Europe/Newly Independent States | 1 | ( 0.1) | 0 | ( 0.0) | **1** | **( 0.1)** |
| North America | 1 | ( 0.1) | 5 | ( 0.8) | **6** | **( 0.5)** |
| Oceania | 41 | ( 5.9) | 4 | ( 0.7) | **45** | **( 3.5)** |
| South America | 22 | ( 3.2) | 6 | ( 1.0) | **28** | **( 2.2)** |
| Unknown† | 20 | ( 2.9) | 4 | ( 0.7) | **24** | **( 1.9)** |
| **Total** | **695** | **(100.0)** | **592** | **(100.0)** | **1,287** | **(100.1)** |

*Country unknown.

†Region of acquisition unknown.

*Source*: Centers for Disease Control and Prevention, United States Department for Health and Human Services. Epidemiology Program Office. CDC Surveillance Summaries. "Malaria Surveillance—United States, 1996" and "Malaria Surveillance—United States, 1997." *MMWR: Morbidity and Mortality Weekly Report* 50, no. SS-1 (2001). http://www.cdc.gov/mmwr/PDF/ss/ss5001.pdf.

**Table C5. Number of Imported Malaria Cases in U.S. Civilians, by Purpose of Travel at the Time of Acquisition—United States, 1997**

| Category | Imported cases | |
|---|---|---|
| | No. | (%) |
| Other | 226 | ( 32.5) |
| Teacher/Student | 63 | ( 9.1) |
| Visit of a friend or relative | 157 | ( 22.6) |
| Tourist | 80 | ( 11.5) |
| Missionary or dependent | 76 | ( 10.9) |
| Business representative | 65 | ( 9.4) |
| Peace Corps volunteer | 14 | ( 2.0) |
| Sailor/Air crew | 4 | ( 0.6) |
| Refugee/Immigrant | 10 | ( 1.4) |
| **Total** | **695** | **(100.0)** |

*Source*: Centers for Disease Control and Prevention, United States Department for Health and Human Services. Epidemiology Program Office. CDC Surveillance Summaries. "Malaria Surveillance—United States, 1996" and "Malaria Surveillance—United States, 1997." *MMWR: Morbidity and Mortality Weekly Report* 50, no. SS-1 (2001). http://www.cdc.gov/mmwr/PDF/ss/ss5001.pdf.

# D. Sexually Transmitted Diseases

## OVERVIEW

Sexually transmitted diseases (STDs) are any of a group of diseases, affecting both men and women, that are characteristically transmitted by sexual contact from person to person during any kind of heterosexual or homesexual activity. More than 25 diseases are spread primarily through sexual activity, and the trends for each disease vary considerably, but together these infections comprise a significant public health problem. The latest estimates indicate that there are 15 million new STD cases in the United States each year.[1] Approximately one-fourth of these new infections are in teenagers. While some STDs, such as syphilis, have been brought to all-time lows, others like chlamydia, genital herpes, and gonorrhea, continue to resurge and spread throughout the population.

Because there is no single STD epidemic, but rather multiple epidemics, discussions about trends and distribution generally focus on specific STDs. The focus of this chapter is on the most common STDs in the United States, that is, chancroid, chlamydia, genital herpes simplex virus infections, gonorrhoea, human papillomavirus, hepatitis B, nonspecific urethritis, syphilis, and trichomonal and other vaginal infections. The majority of the tables and figures show trends and distribution of the three diseases for which federally funded control programs exist, that is, chlamydia, gonorrhoea, and syphilis.

## TRANSMISSION

Although each STD presents unique diagnostic, therapeutic, and prevention challenges, all STDs share a common mode of transmission. As the "sexually transmitted disease" implies, all of these diseases can be transmitted by sexual intercourse, but some can be transmitted through close intimate contact that does not result in sexual intercourse. In general, populations at risk for one STD are at risk for others, and the presence of one infection may influence the acquisition and course of another.

Viruses, bacteria, parasites, or tiny insects can cause STDs. Organisms that cause most STDs live best in a warm, moist environment like the linings of the genitals or throat; outside of the body most die in less than a minute or two. The organisms that cause these diseases (except for cards and scabies) generally enter the body through the mucous membranes, that is, the warm, moist surfaces of the genitals and the mouth. Viral STDs include herpes, hepatitis, venereal warts, and *Molluscum contagiosum*. The most common bacterial infections include syphilis, gonorrhoea, chlamydia, gardnerella, shigellosis, and chancroid. Other diseases, caused by fungi and various parasites, include candidiasis, trichomoniasis, amebiasis, scabies, and *Pediculosis pubis*, as well as some disease whose status as an STD is being debated. Although HIV can be transmitted sexually, it is typically categorized separately from STDs both in terms of medicine and public policy.

All STDs are preventable. Reducing the risk of contracting one requires taking certain precautions. Effective treatments for most STDs do exist, and the diseases are not always fatal. At the minimum, these diseases cause discomfort. Left untreated, some STDs can causes serious long-term health problems.

## THE DISEASES

Because each STD presents unique diagnostic, therapeutic, and prevention challenges, general information is presented separately for each STD.

**Chancroid** A highly infectious nonsyphiltic venereal ulcer, chancroid is caused by *Haemophilus ducreyi*, a gram-negative bacteria. It begins with pustule or ulcer, characterized by multiple, abrupt edges, rough floor, yellow exudate, and purulent secretion. The sores are painful, tend to merge into large patches of damaged tissue, and are often accompanied by abscess in the groin. Indeed, rapid progress often occurs, and the penis, urethra, vulva, or anus may be affected. If left untreated, they can spread to new locations. Generally, a scar remains after the pustule or ulcer has been treated.

Within the arena of lumps, bumps and sores, it is important to distinguish chancroid sores from chancre sores. If it is a chancre sore, a diagnosis of syphilis can generally be expected. Chancre sores themselves are painless and will disappear on their own in 3 to 8 weeks, but if untreated, the underlying syphilis infection will remain to ravage the body in later years. Of the two kinds of sores, chancre sores are the more insidious ones: easy to ignore, yet ultimately life-threatening.

Types of chancroid include transient (not lasting, of brief duration), phagendenic (the telltale sign is a sloughing ulcer that spreads rapidly), giant, and serpiginous (creeping from one part to another). Ulcers appear within 2 to 7 days after infection. Chancroid is associated with human immunodeficiency virus (HIV); the open sores on the genitals facilitate HIV transmission.

Physicians unfamiliar with the disease often misdiagnose chanroid as genital herpes or syphilis. Since a precise diagnosis requires a culture with a substance that is not readily available, many physicians or clinics are unable to make a definitive diagnosis. They therefore start by ruling out genital herpes and syphilis through tests for those infections. If the tests come back negative, they then diagnose chancroid.

**Chlamydia** Chlamydia is caused by the bacterium *Chlamydia trachomatis*. It is transmitted during vaginal or anal sex with someone who has the infection. It can also be passed by a hand moistened with infected secretions to the eye and from mother to baby during delivery. It is possible but unlikely for women to pass chlamydia to the throat during the performance of oral sex on an infected man.

Because approximately 75% of women and 50% of men have no symptoms, most people infected with chlamydia are not aware of their infections and therefore may not seek health care. When diagnosed, chlamydia can be easily treated and cured. Untreated, chlamydia can causes severe, costly reproductive and other health problems for women, including pelvic inflammatory disease (PID), which is the critical link to infertility, and potentially fatal tubal pregnancy. Up to 40% of women with untreated chlamydia will develop PID. Undiagnosed PID caused by chlamydia is common. Of those with PID, 20% will become infertile, 18% will experience debilitating, chronic pelvic pain; and 9% will have a life-threatening tubal pregnancy. Tubal pregnancy is the leading cause of first-trimester, pregnancy-related deaths in American women. Chlamydia may also result in adverse outcomes of pregnancy, including neonatal conjunctivitis and pneumonia. In addition, recent research has shown that women infected with chlamydia have a threefold to fivefold increased risk of acquiring HIV, if exposed. Pregnant women if infected with chlamydial infection can pass the infection to their infants during delivery, resulting in neonatal ophthalmia and pneumonia.

Chlamydia is also common among young men, who are seldom offered screening. Untreated chlamydia in men typically causes urethral infection, but may also result in complications such as swollen and tender testicles.

The most common symptom among women is increased vaginal discharge, which usually develops 7 to 14 days after exposure to the chlamydia bacterium. Painful urination, unusual vaginal bleeding, bleeding after sex, and low abdominal pain are other signs. The cervix may or may not appear inflamed upon examination.

Men will usually have a burning sensation upon urination and a urethral discharge that appears 1 to 3 weeks after exposure. Symptoms may be similar to those of gonorrhoea but are usually milder. The incubation period is also generally longer—at least 7 days. About 10% of men have no symptoms, even though they can still transmit the disease.

**Genital *Herpes Simplex* Virus Infections** Genital herpes is an infectious disease caused by the *Herpes simplex* viruses type 1 (HSV-1) and type 2 (HSV-2), which enter the body through the skin and mucous membrances of the mouth and genitals and travel along the nerve endings to the base of the spine. There the virus sets up permanent residence, feeding off nutrients produced by the body cells. Cold sores or fever blisters on the lips, face, and mouth usually characterize HSV-1, while HSV-2 most often involves sores in the genital area. While HSV-1 is usually found above the waist and HSV-2 below, there is some crossover, primarily due to the increases in oral-genital sex.

HSV-1 and HSV-2 can be found and released from the sores that the viruses cause, but they also are released between episodes from skin that does not appear to be broken or to have a sore. HSV-1 causes infections of the mouth and lips, so-called "fever blisters." A person can get HSV-1 by coming into contact with the saliva of an infected person. HSV-1 infection of the genitals almost always is caused by oral-genital sexual contact with a person who has the oral HSV-1 infection. A person almost always gets HSV-2 infection during sexual contact with someone who has a genital

HSV-2 infection. Genital herpes often is transmitted by people who are unaware that they are infected or by people who do not recognize that their infection can be transmitted even when they have no symptoms. Most transmission occurs when people are symptomatic.

Herpes is characterized by thin-walled vesicles that tend to recur in the same area of the skin, usually at a site where the mucous membrane joins the skin; however, they may be limited to the gingiva, oropharynx, or conjunctiva. In newborn infants, meningoencephalitis or a panvisceral infection may occur.

Most of the time, HSV-1 and HSV-2 are inactive, or "silent," and cause no symptoms, but some infected people have "outbreaks" of blisters and ulcers. Once infected with HSV, people remain infected for life. Symptoms usually occur 2 to 20 days after infection, although most people may not have symptoms or may not be aware of them until much later. An outbreak of herpes usually begins with a tingling or itching sensation of the skin in the genital area. This is called the prodromal or early stage of symptoms period and may occur several hours to several days before the sores erupt, or it may not occur at all. Women may also experience burning sensations, pains in their legs, buttocks, or genitals, and/or a feeling of pressure in the area. Sores then appear, starting as one or more red bumps and changing to watery blisters within a day or two. Within a few days, the blisters rupture, leaving shallow ulcers that may ooze, weep, or bleed. Usually, after 3 or 4 days a scab forms and the sores heal themselves without treatment. While the sores are active, other symptoms may include painful urination, a dull ache or a sharp burning pain in the entire genital area, pain in the legs, the urge to urinate frequently, vaginal discharge, and/or a painful inflammation of the vulva. During the first outbreak, women may also experience fever, headache, and swelling of the lymph nodes in the groin.

Most people diagnosed with a first episode of genital herpes can expect to have several symptomatic recurrences a year (typically four or five). These recurrences are most noticeable within the first year following the first episode. Typically, the second outbreak will appear weeks or months after the first, but it almost is less severe and shorter than the first episode. Although the infection can stay in the body indefinitely, the number of outbreaks tends to go down over a period of years.

Men may experience pain in the testicles during the *prodromal* period, followed by sores that usually appear on the head and shaft of the penis but can also appear on the scrotum, perineum, buttocks, anus, and thighs. Men can also have sores without knowing it, usually because they are hidden inside the urethra. There may also be a watery discharge from the urethra.

HSV-2 usually produces only mild symptoms or signs or no symptoms at all. However, HSV-2 can cause recurrent painful genital sores in many adults, and HSV-2 infection can be severe in people with suppressed immune systems. Regardless of severity of symptoms, genital herpes frequently causes psychological distress in people who know they are infected. In addition, HSV-2 can cause potentially fatal infections in infants if the mother is shedding virus at the time of delivery. It is important that women avoid contracting herpes during pregnancy, because a first episode during pregnancy causes a greater risk of transmission to the newborn. If a woman has active genital herpes at delivery, a cesarean delivery is usually performed. Infection of an infant from a woman with HSV-2 infection is rare.

In the United States, HSV-2 may play a major role in the heterosexual spread of HIV. Herpes can make people more susceptible to HIV infection, and it can make HIV-infected individuals more infectious.

**Gonorrhea** Caused by infection by the gonococcus *Neisseria gonorrhoeae*, gonorrhea is a specific, contagious, catarrhal inflammation of the genital mucous membrane of either sex. The disease also may affect other structures of the body such as the heart, conjunctiva, oral mucosa, rectum, or joints. In the female the parts involved may be the urethra, vulva, vulvovaginal glands, vagina, endocervix, Skene's glans, Bartholin's glans, or fallopian tubes.

Gonorrhea is transmitted through genital, genital-oral (which exposes the throat), and genital-anal sex. Touching the eye with a hand that is moist with infected discharge will transmit the infection to the eye. A mother can pass it to her children during birth. Rarely, very young children can contract gonorrhea by using towels contaminated with fresh discharge. More frequently, children with gonorrhea are found to have been sexually abused. Gonorrhea has also been transmitted to women through semen used for donor insemination.

The disease is more likely to persist and spread in women than in men. Untreated gonorrhea can lead to serious and painful infection of the pelvic area, pelvic inflammatory disease (PID) which can lead to sterility. A less common complication is proctitis, inflammation of the rectum. If the eyes become infected by gonococcal discharge (gonococcal conjunctivitis), blindness can occur. Disseminated gonococcal infection (DGI), rare but serious, occurs when bacteria travel through the bloodstream, causing infection of the heart valves or arthritic meningitis. Gonorrhea can be treated and cured with antibiotics at any stage to prevent further damage, but damage already done usually cannot be repaired.

In men, symptoms include yellow mucopurulent discharge from the penis resulting from inflammation of the urethra that may become deep-seated and affect the prostate; slow, difficult, and painful urination; and sometimes-painful induration of the penis. Some men may have no symptoms.

In females, gonorrhea may be asymptomatic; even when symptoms are present, they may not cause enough discomfort for the patient to seek medical care. Symptoms usually appear anywhere from 2 days to 3 weeks after exposure and include one or more of the following: urethral or vaginal discharge, painful or frequent urination, lower abdominal pain, tenderness in the area of Bartholin's and Skene's glands, and acute pelvic inflammatory disease. If the disease spreads to the uterus and fallopian tubes, symptoms may also include pain on one or both sides of the lower abdomen, vomiting, fever, and/or irregular menstrual periods. The more severe the infection, the more severe the pain and other symptoms are likely to be. These symptoms may indicate PID. Pharyngeal gonorrhea may be accompanied by no symptoms, sore throat, or swollen glands. Symptoms of DGI include a rash, chills, fever, and pain in the joints and tendons of wrists and fingers. As the disease progresses, sores may appear on the hands, fingers, feet, and toes.

**Human Papillomavirus** Human papillomavirus (HPV) causes genital warts and is similar to the type of virus that causes common skin warts. Over 20 types of HPV cause invisible infections, warts, or flat lesions in the genital area. HPV usually spreads during sexual intercourse with an infected partner.

Symptoms of genital warts usually appear from 3 weeks to 8 months after exposure. During the presymptomatic period (as well as while they are present), warts are the most contagious. In men, warts occur on the head of the penis (often under the foreskin), on the shaft of the penis, or occasionally on the scrotum.

**Nonspecific Urethritis** Nonspecific urethritis is inflammation and irritation of the urethra that in the past was not directly attributable to a specific organism. About half of the cases of nonspecific urethritis are due to *Chlamydia trachomatis*. Nonspecific urethritis can be either posterior—inflammation of the membranous and prostatic portions of the urethra—or specific—urethritis due to a specific organism, usually gonococcus.

**Syphilis** An infectious, chronic, venereal disease characterized by lesions that may involve any organ or tissue, syphilis facilitates the transmission of HIV and may be particularly important in contributing to HIV transmission in those parts of the United States where rates of both infections are high. Syphilis is caused by *Treponema pallidum*, a small, spiral-shaped bacterium called a spirochete that is transmitted by direct contact between humans, contact with freshly contaminated material, transfusion of infected blood or plasma, or in utero by passage of the organism from mother to fetus (congenital syphilis). Syphilis spreads via open sores or rashes containing bacteria that can penetrate the mucous membranes of the genitals, mouth, and anus as well as broken skin on other parts of the body. Transmission of the organism occurs during vaginal, anal, or oral sex.

Depending on how long a pregnant woman has been infected, she has a high chance of having a stillbirth (syphilitic stillbirth) or of giving birth to a baby who dies shortly after birth. If not treated immediately, an infected baby may be born without the symptoms but could develop them within a few weeks. The signs and symptoms can be very serious. Untreated babies may become developmentally delayed, have seizures, or die.

Syphilis has often been called "the great eliminator" because so many of the signs and symptoms are indistinguishable from those of other diseases. Syphilis usually exhibits dermal manifestations, relapses are frequent, and it may exist without symptoms. Untreated early syphilis during pregnancy results in perinatal death in up to 40% of cases and, if acquired during the 4 years preceding pregnancy, may lead to infection of the fetus in over 70% of cases.[2] Congenital syphilis can be fatal for the developing baby. If the baby survives, deafness, anemia, and permanent damage to the bones, liver, and teeth are all possibilities. Sometimes these symptoms do not appear until the child is a teenager. In general, if a woman has had syphilis for more than 4 years, chances are low that the baby will be infected. If she has been infected more recently, especially during her pregnancy, congenital syphilis is likely. Note that the reaction to treatment, the Jarisch-Herxheimer reaction, may induce early labor or cause fetal distress. It is generally considered more important to get treatment than to avoid this possibility.

Once the bacteria have entered the body, the disease may go through four stages, depending on when a person is treated. Symptoms vary depending on the stage—primary, secondary, and latent or late.

The time between infection with syphilis and the start of the first symptom can range from 10 to 90 days (average 21 days). The primary stage of syphilis is usually marked by the appearance of a single sore, called a chancre, but there may be multiple sores. The chancre is usually firm, round, small, and painless. It appears on the spot where syphilis entered the body. The chancre lasts 3–6 weeks, and it will heal on its own, usually in 1–5 weeks, but the bacteria, still in the body, increase and spread. At the primary stage, the chancre is very infectious. If adequate treatment is not administered, the infection progresses to the secondary stage. Note that sometimes the chancre never develops or is hidden, giving no evidence of the disease.

Occurring anywere from 1 week to 6 months later, the secondary stage starts when one or more areas of the skin break into a rash that usually does not itch. Rashes can appear as the chancre is fading or can be delayed for weeks. The rash often appears as rough, red or reddish-brown spots both on the palms of the hands and on the bottoms of the feet. The rash also may appear on other parts of the body with different characteristics, some of which resemble other diseases. Sometimes the rashes are so faint that they are not noticed. Even without treatment, rashes clear up on their own. In addition to rashes, second-stage symptoms can include fever, swollen lymph glands, sore throat, patchy hair loss, headaches, weight loss, muscle aches, and tiredness. A person can easily pass the disease to sex partners when primary- or secondary-stage signs or symptoms are present. The secondary stage usually lasts weeks or months but symptons can come and go for several months.

A stage of infection caused by *T. pallidum* in which organisms persist in the body of the infected person without causing symptoms or signs, latent syphilis may last 10 to 20 years. During this time the bacteria may be invading the inner organs and may begin to damage these organs including the brain, nerves, eyes, heart, blood vessels, liver, bones, and joints. This internal damage may show up many years later in the late or tertiary stage of syphilis. Late-stage signs and symptoms include not being able to coordinate muscle movements, paralysis, numbness, gradual blindness, and dementia. The damage may be serious enough to cause death. The disease is not infectious after the first few years of the latent stage (when no symptoms of second stage are present).

**Trichomonal and Other Vaginal Infections** *T. vaginalis* is a microscopic parasite found worldwide. Infection with trichomonas is called trichomoniasis. Trichomoniasis is spread through sexual activity. Infection is more common in women who have had multiple sexual partners. A common misbelief is that a toilet seat can spread infection; this isn't likely, since the parasite cannot live long in the environment or on objects. Most women who develop symptoms do so within 6 months of being infected. Signs and symptoms of infection among women range from having no symptoms (asymptomatic) to very symptomatic. Typical symptoms include foul-smelling or frothy green discharge from the vagina, vaginal itching, or redness. Other symptoms can include painful sexual intercourse, lower abdominal discomfort, and the urge to urinate. Most men with this infection do not have symptoms. When symptoms are present, they most commonly are discharge from the urethra, the urge to urinate, and a burning sensation with urination.

## SURVEILLANCE

**General Overview** STD surveillance information is compiled from several sources of data. These include case reports from STD project areas; prevalence data from the Regional Infertility Prevention Projects; the U.S. Job Corps, the Jail STD Prevalence Monitoring Projects; the U.S. Army; and the Indian Health Service, as well as national sample surveys implemented by federal and private organizations. The Gonococcal Isolate Surveillance Project (GISP) also provides sentinel surveillance of gonococcal antimicrobial resistance.[3]

STD control programs and health departments in the 50 states, the District of Columbia, selected cities, U.S. dependencies and possessions, and independent nations in free association with the United States comprise the backbone of STD surveillance.

In January 2000, CDC released provisional objectives for *Healthy People 2010* (HP2010).[4] The provisional year 2010 rate objectives for STDs are: primary and secondary syphilis—0.2 cases per 100,000 persons; congenital syphilis—1 case per 100,000 live births; and gonorrhea—19 cases per 100,000 persons. An additional provisional target established in the HP2010 objectives is to reduce the *Chlamydia trachomatis* test positivity to 3% among females aged 15 to 24 years who attend family planning and STD clinics and among males aged 15 to 24 who attend STD clinics.

Discussion of case definitions, reporting practices and sources, and limitations of data for STDs that have federally funded control programs follows. These diseases are chlamydia, gonorrhea, and syphilis. Note that for these three diseases, as with all STDs, the number of cases reported to CDC is less than the actual number of cases occurring among the U.S. population. Note, too, that more is known about the frequency and trends of some STDs than others, since many of the diseases are difficult to track.

Although most areas generally adhere to the case definitions for STDs found in Case Definitions for Infectious Conditions under Public Health Surveillance (*MMWR* 46 (1997) (RR-10):1–56), there are differences between individual areas in case definitions as well as in the policies and systems for collecting surveillance data. Comparisons of case numbers and rates between areas should thus be interpreted with caution. However, since case definitions and surveillance activities within a given area remain relatively stable, trends should be minimally affected. Note too that in many areas, the reporting from publicly supported institutions (e.g., STD clinics) is often more complete than from other sources (e.g., private practitioners). Thus, the trends depicted may not be representative of all segments of the population. Military cases are not reported as a separate category.

*Chlamydia* The expansion of chlamydia screening activities, use of increasingly sensitive diagnostic tests, an increased emphasis on case reporting from providers and laboratories, and improvements in the information systems for reporting led to an increase in reported chlamydial infections during the 1990s. However, as recently as 1999, CDC reports that many women who are at risk for this infection are still not being tested, reflecting the lack of awareness among some health care providers and the limited resources available to support screening. Chlamydia screening and reporting are likely to expand further in response to the recently implemented Health Plan Employer Data and Information Set (HEDIS) measure for chlamydia screening of sexually active women 15 to 25 years of age who are provided care through managed care organizations.[5]

In 1999, New York was the only state that did not yet have laws or policies for uniform reporting of *Chlamydia trachomatis* cases. Chlamydia cases for New York were exclusively based on cases reported by New York City. Trends in many areas were more representative of increases in reporting of cases rather than actual trends in disease. Cases and rates of chlamydia reported in gender-specific tables are underestimated because of some reported cases with unknown gender.

While case reporting of chlamydial infections is improving, it remains incomplete in many areas of the country. A combination of factors limits the documentation of the incidence and prevalence of genital chlamydial infection. These include variable compliance with public health laws and regulations that require health care providers and laboratories to report cases to local health authorities; large numbers of asymptomatic persons who can be identified only through screening; limited resources to support screening activities; and incomplete management systems for collecting, maintaining, and analyzing case reporting and prevalence data. Thus, for most areas, the number of chlamydia cases reported to CDC by state health departments reflects many factors, only one of which is number of infections in the population. CDC's position is that despite problems with underreporting, it is important to publish the data to emphasize the large numbers of cases of chlamydia being detected in the United States. It is expected that as areas develop chlamydia prevention and control programs, including surveillance systems to monitor trends, the data should improve and become more representative of true trends in disease.

*Gonorrhea* In 1994, Georgia reported gonorrhea cases to CDC for only part of a year. Therefore, Georgia cases and population were excluded from gonorrhea figures and tables for 1994.

*Syphilis* Cases of unknown duration, neurosyphilis, and late syphilis with clinical manifestations have been counted with late and late latent syphilis. In 1988, the CDC introduced a new surveillance case definition for congenital syphilis. The new case definition has greater sensitivity than the former definition. In addition, many areas greatly enhanced active case finding for congenital syphilis during this time. For this reason, the number of reported cases increased dramatically during 1989–1991. Note that a period of transition during which trends cannot be clearly interpreted resulted; however, all reporting areas had implemented the new case definition for reporting all cases of congenital syphilis after January 1, 1992. Therefore, the reliability of trends is expected to have stabilized after this date.

In addition to changing the case definition, CDC introduced a new data collection form in 1990. Beginning with 1995, the data collected on this form are used for reporting congenital syphilis reported cases and associated rates. This form is used to collect individual case information, which allows more thorough analysis of cases. For the purposes of these tables, if either the race or the ethnicity question was answered, the case was included. Congenital syphilis cases have been reported by state and city of residence of the mother for 1995 through 1999.

## HEALTHY PEOPLE

Until the 1980s, only five venereal diseases were regularly monitored in the United States. Since the mid 1980s, however, the spectrum of sexually transmitted diseases increased dramatically in both complexity and scope. By the time *Healthy People 2000* was published, more than 50 organisms and syndromes had been recognized:[6] Gonorrhea, chlamydia, syphilis, congenital syphilis, genital herpes and genital warts, pelvic inflammatory disease, and hepatitis B are the focus of the *Healthy People 2000* objectives relative to sexually transmitted diseases. Other objectives in this section focus on adolescent postponement of sexual intercourse, condom use, clinic services for HIV and other sexually transmitted diseases, sexually transmitted disease education in schools, correct management of sexually transmitted disease cases, clinician counseling to prevent sexually transmitted diseases, and partner notification of exposure to sexually transmitted disease.

## TABLE OVERVIEW

**D1. *Healthy People 2000*** Selected tables and figures identify goals that reflect progress toward some of the *Healthy People 2000* (HP2000) national health status objectives for STDs.[7] The original HP2000 health status objectives were developed in 1989 and revised in 1995.[8] The year 2000 objectives for STDs were revised as follows: primary and secondary syphilis—10 cases per 100,000 persons to 4 cases per 100,000 persons; congenital syphilis—50 cases per 100,000 live births to 40 cases per live births; and gonorrhea—225 cases per 100,000 persons to 100 cases per 100,000 persons. These objectives are used as reference in text as well as in accompanying tables and figures.

**D2.1–D2.2 Summary Data** D2.1 reports cases of STDs by gender and reporting source for 1999. D2.2 offers historical data showing cases reported by state health departments and rates per 100,000 civilian population in the United States for syphilis (all stages, primary and secondary, early latent, late and late latent, and congenital), chlamydia, gonorrhea, chancroid, granuloma inguinale, and lympho-granuloma Venereum, spanning 1941–1999.

Infections due to *Chlamydia trachomatis* are the most commonly reported notifiable disease in the United States. They are the most prevalent of all STDs and, since 1994, have comprised the largest proportion of all STDs reported to the CDC. In 1999, 659,441 cases of infection with genital *Chlamydia trachomatis* were reported to CDC. This case count corresponds to a rate of 254.1 cases per 100,000 persons, an increase of 8.5% compared with the rate of 234.2 in 1998.

Following a 72% decline in the reported rate of gonorrhea from 1975 to 1997, in 1999 the gonorrhea rate increased for the second year in a row. The gonorrhea rate for 1999 (133.2 cases per 100,000 persons) was 1.2% higher than the 1998 rate (131.6 cases per 100,000 persons) and 9.2% higher than the rate reported in 1997 (122.0 per 100,000 persons). The 1999 rate for gonorrhea exceeds the *Healthy People 2000* (HP2000) objective of 100 cases per 100,000 persons.

The 6,657 cases of primary and secondary syphilis reported in 1999 were the fewest cases reported in the United States since 1957. The primary and secondary syphilis rate of 2.5 per 100,000 persons (the lowest since national reporting began in 1941) is below the HP2000 objective of 4 cases per 100,000 persons, but remains substantially above the goal for syphilis elimination of 0.4 cases per 100,000 persons (about 1,000 cases per year). The number of primary and secondary syphilis cases reported in 1999 was 5.4% lower than the 7,035 cases reported in 1998. However, this decline was substantially less than the reductions of approximately 20% per year since the last major syphilis epidemic peaked in 1990.

Between 1998 and 1999, the national rate of congenital syphilis decreased from 0.3 to 0.2 per 100,000 population or 838 cases to 556 cases. In 1999, only one state had a reported rate of congenital syphilis that exceeded the HP2000 objective of 40 cases per 100,000 live births.

**D3.1–D3.7 Chlamydia** This cluster of tables shows trends and distribution of chlamydia by age, gender, race/ethnicity, and location. Documentation of the incidence and prevalence of chlamydia is lacking for 1941–1983. Case reporting begins in 1984, with 7,594 cases of chlamydia reported. In 1999, 49 states and the District of Columbia had regulations requiring the reporting of chlamydia cases to CDC. For the state of New York, only cases identified in New York City were reported. In 1999, a total of 659,441 reported cases of *Chlamydia trachomatis* were reported. This case count corresponds to a rate of 254.1 cases per 100,000 persons, an increase of 8.5% compared with the rate of 234.2 in 1998.

For women, the highest age-specific reported rates of chlamydia in 1999 occurred among 15–19-year-olds (2,483.8 per 100,000 females) and 20–24-year-olds (2,187.1 per 100,000 females). Age-specific reported rates among men, while substantially higher than the rates in women of similar ages, were also highest in these age groups.

In 1999, the overall reported rate of chlamydial infection among women (404.5 cases per 100,000 females) was four times the reported rate among men (94.7 cases per 100,000 males). This reflects the large number of women screened for the disease. The lower rates among men suggest that many of the sex partners of women with chlamydia are not diagnosed or reported. However, with the advent of new, highly sensitive nucleic acid amplification tests that can be performed on urine, symptomatic and asymptomatic men are increasingly being diagnosed with chlamydial infection. From 1995 to 1999, the reported chlamydial infection rate in males increased by 64.1% (from 57.7 to 94.7 cases per 100,000) compared with a 27.9% increase in women over this period (from 316.3 to 404.5 cases per 100,000). From 1987 through 1999, the reported rates of chlamydial infection increased from 50.8 to 254.1 cases per 100,000 persons. The continuing increase in reported cases likely represents the further expansion of screening for this infection and also increased use of nucleic acid amplification tests, which are more sensitive than other types of screening tests. For the years 1996–1999, the chlamydia case rate in the southern region of the United States (203.9, 230.1, 268.4, and 289.4 cases per 100,000 persons respectively) was higher than in any other region of the country. The higher rates in this region reflect an expansion of screening activities in the South in addition to the high burden of disease in this region.

**D4.1–D4.10. Gonorrhea** In 1999, 360,076 cases of gonorrhea were reported in the United States. The reported rate of gonococcal infections in the United States (133.2 cases per 100,000 persons) increased by 1.2% compared with the rate reported in 1998 (131.6 cases per 100,000 persons) and 9.2% compared with 1997 (122.0 cases per 100,000). Prior to this increase, in the period from 1977 to 1997, the national gonorrhea rate had been declining following the implementation of the national gonorrhea control program in the mid-1970s. Expansion of screening programs, increased use of new diagnostic tests with improved sensitivity, improvements in surveillance systems, and a true increase in morbidity in some geographic areas and segments of the population are cited as possible reasons for this trend.[9]

In 1999, 26 states and three outlying areas reported gonorrhea rates below the *Healthy People 2000* (HP2000) national objective of 100 cases per 100,000 persons. Eight states and one outlying area had reported rates below the provisional *Healthy People 2010* (HP2010) objective of 19 cases per 100,000 persons.[10] The gonorrhea rates in all four census regions of the United States either increased or stayed approximately constant between 1998 and 1999. All regions, however, had experienced declining rates from 1995 through 1997. As in previous reporting years, the South had the highest rate in 1999 (202.9 cases per 100,000 persons) among the four regions of the country.

There is no meaningful change in the reported gonorrhea rate among women between 1998 and 1999 (130.0 and 129.9 cases per 100,000 females respectively). The gonorrhea rate in men, however, increased by 2.5% from 132.7 to 136.0 cases per 100,000 males from 1998 to 1999. Between 1998 and 1999, the reported gonorrhea rates among 15–19-year-old adolescents decreased from 547.0 to 534.0 cases per 100,000 persons. For 20–24-year-old young adults, the reported rate increased from 605.2 to 614.7 cases per 100,000 persons between 1998 and 1999. Among women in 1999, 15–19-year-olds had the highest reported rate of gonorrhea, while among men, 20–24-year-olds had the highest rate.

Changes in the reported 1999 gonorrhea rates, relative to those reported in 1998, differed depending on racial/ethnic group. For example, the rates among Hispanics and Asian/Pacific Islanders were 4% and 6% higher respectively in 1999 than the corresponding group-specific rates in 1998. The 1999 rate among American Indians/Alaska Natives, however, was 7% lower than the rate reported in 1998. Rates among non-Hispanic whites and blacks were similar in 1998 and 1999.

**D5.1–D5.20. Syphilis** The rate of primary and secondary syphilis is at its lowest reported in the United States since reporting began in 1941. Although syphilis has declined in all regions of the United States and in all racial/ethnic groups, rates remain disproportionately high in the South and among non-Hispanic blacks. Focal outbreaks continue to occur, including recent outbreaks among men who have sex with men. This unprecedented low rate and the concentration of the majority of syphilis cases in a small number of geographic areas have led to the development of the National Plan to Eliminate Syphilis in the United States, announced by the Surgeon General David Satcher in October 1999.[11] The rate of primary and secondary syphilis in the United States declined by 88% from 1990 through 1999. Although the 5.4% decline in the number of primary and secondary syphilis cases reported in 1999 is less than the declines of approximately 20% per year since the last major syphilis epidemic peaked in 1990, it is hypothesized that this smaller decline at least partially reflects improved case finding and reporting resulting from the national syphilis elimination effort.[12] In 1999, 6,657 cases of primary and secondary syphilis were reported to CDC, a decline of 5.4% compared with 1998, when 7,035 cases were reported. The number of primary and secondary syphilis cases reported in 1999 is the lowest yearly number of cases reported since 1957. The reported rate of primary and secondary syphilis in the United States in 1999 (2.5 cases per 100,000) was slightly below the rate reported in 1998 (2.6 cases per 100,000). The 1999 rate is below the *Healthy People 2000* (HP2000) national objective of 4.0 cases per 100,000 persons as it has been since 1997. The current reported rate in the United States exceeds the new *Healthy People 2010* (HP2010) provisional objective of 0.2 cases per 100,000 persons.[13]

Since the peak rate in 1990, the rate of early latent syphilis has exceeded the rate of primary and secondary syphilis. There were approximately 0.9 reported cases of early latent syphilis for every reported case of primary and secondary syphilis in the 5 years preceding 1990 and 1.8 reported cases of early latent syphilis for every reported case of primary and secondary syphilis in 1999.

Since the peak rate in 1993, the rate of late and latent syphilis has exceeded the rate of primary and secondary syphilis. There were approximately 0.6 reported cases of late latent syphilis for every reported case of primary and secondary syphilis in the 5 years preceding 1993 and 2.5 reported cases of late and latent syphilis for every reported case of primary and secondary syphilis in 1999.

In 1999, primary and secondary syphilis rates in 39 states and three outlying areas were below the HP2000 national objective of 4.0 cases per 100,000 persons. Twelve states reported 1999 rates equal to or below the HP2010 provisional objective of 0.2 cases per 100,000 persons. Fourteen states and two outlying areas reported five or fewer cases of primary and secondary syphilis in 1999.

In 1999, the reported rate of primary and secondary syphilis among men (2.9 cases per 100,000 males) was 1.5 times greater than the rate among women (2.0 cases per 100,000 females). The male-to-female ratio of primary and secondary syphilis rates was greater in 1999, as compared to the ratio in 1998, for 16 (59%) of the 26 states and the District of Columbia that reported 25 or more cases in 1998. The male-to-female rate ratio has increased since 1995 in all ethnic groups except American Indian/Alaska Natives. The change in the male-to-female rate ratio was most notable in Hispanics. The primary and secondary rate for 1999 in the southern region of the United States (4.5 cases per 100,000 persons) was higher than the rate reported in any other region of the country. In 1999, the rate of primary and secondary syphilis reported in African Americans (15.2 cases per 100,000 persons) was 30.4 times greater than the rate reported in whites (0.5 cases per 100,000 persons. This differential was substantially less than in 1995, when the rate of primary and secondary syphilis among African Americans was 56.1 times greater than the rate reported among whites. During the period from 1995 to 1998, the rates of primary and secondary syphilis within racial and ethnic groups have generally declined. These group specific rates remained relatively constant between 1998 and 1999 with the exception of the rate among non-Hispanic blacks, which decreased 10% in 1999 from the 1998 figure.

Between 1998 and 1999, the overall rate of congenital syphilis decreased by 34% in the United States from 21.6 to 14.3 cases per 100,000 live births. In 1999, only one state or outlying area (New Jersey) had a reported rate of congenital syphilis that exceeded the HP2000 objective of 40 cases per 100,000 live births. Twenty-eight states and one outlying area had reported congenital syphilis rates in 1999 that exceeded the HP2010 provisional objective of 1 case per 100,000 live births.[14] Among the 24 states and outlying areas with five or more reported cases of congenital syphilis in 1999, 18 had rates that decreased from the 1998 value. Eleven of these states and Puerto Rico had decreases of 30% or more between the 1998 and 1999 reported rates. Congenital syphilis persists in the United States because of the substantial number of women who do not receive syphilis serologic testing during pregnancy or who receive this testing too late in their pregnancy. This lack of screening is often related to a lack of prenatal care or late prenatal care.[15]

**D6.1–D6.7. Chancroid, Genital Herpes Simplex Virus, Human Papillomavirus, Non-Gonococcal Urethritis, and Trichomonal and Other Vaginal Infections** This cluster opens with data on chancroid by state (D6.1) and city (D6.2). Since 1987, reported cases of chancroid have declined steadily. In 1999, a total of 143 cases of chancroid were reported from the United States. Only 16 states and one outlying area reported one or more cases of chancroid in 1999, and three of these states (New York, South Carolina, and Texas) accounted for nearly 72% of the 143 reported cases. Although the decline in reported chancroid cases most likely reflects a decline in the incidence of this disease, these data should be interpreted in view of the fact that *Haemophilus ducreyi*, the causative organism of chancroid, is difficult to culture; as a result, this condition may be substantially underdiagnosed.[16]

Data on genital herpes simplex virus infections is presented in D6.3. Shown are trends in initial visits to physicians' offices in the United States, 1966–1999; data are compared to the Healthy People year 2000 objective. Data on genital herpes simplex virus type 2

(HSV-2) seroprevalence among the non-institutionalized U.S. population are available from the National Health and Nutrition Examination Survey (NHANES). Results are presented in D6.4. In NHANES III (1988–1994), HSV-2 seroprevalence among persons at least 12 years of age was 21.9%. The HSV-2 seroprevalence in NHANES III was 30% higher than the age-adjusted HSV-2 seroprevalence from NHANES II (1976–1980). Increases in HSV-2 seroprevalence between NHANES II and NHANES III were concentrated in younger age groups. There were statistically significant increases overall in the three youngest age groups, including persons aged 12–39 years.[17]

Comprehensive surveillance data for human papillomavirus, non-gonococcal urethritis, and trichomoniasis are not available. Ongoing trend data are limited to estimates of trends in physician's office practices provided by the National Disease and Therapeutic Index (D6.5–D6.7).

## NOTES

1. W. Cates et al. "Estimates of the Incidence and Prevalence of Sexually Transmitted Diseases in the United States." *Sexually Transmitted Diseases* 26, suppl. (1999): S2–S7.
2. N.R. Ingraham. "The Value of Penicillin Alone in the Prevention and Treatment of Congenital Syphilis." *Acta Dermato Venereologica* 31, suppl. 24, (1951): 60.
3. A sentinel system of 26 STD clinics and five regional laboratories located throughout the United States.
4. Ibid.
5. National Committee for Quality Assurance (NCQA) *HEDIS 2000: Technical Specifications.* Washington, DC: National Committee for Quality Assurance, 1999: 68–70, 285–86.
6. K.K. Holmes, P.A. Mardh, P.F. Sparling, P.J. Wiesner, W. Cates, Jr., S.M. Lemon, and W.E. Stamm, eds., *Sexually Transmitted Diseases*, 2d ed. New York: McGraw-Hill, 1990.
7. U.S. Department of Health and Human Services. *Healthy People 2000: Midcourse Review and 1995 Revisions*. Washington, DC: U.S. Government Printing Office, 1995.
8. *Healthy People 2010* was released in 2000. U.S. Department of Health and Human Services. *Healthy People 2010* (conference edition, in 2 volumes). Washington, DC: U.S. Government Printing, Office, 2000.
9. *MMWR: Morbidity and Morality Weekly Report* 48 (2001): x.
10. U.S. Department of Health and Human Services. *Healthy People 2010.*
11. Centers for Disease Control and Prevention. *The National Plan to Eliminate Syphillis from the United States.* Division of STD Prevention, National Center for HIV, STD, and TB Prevention, 1999.
12. Division of STD Prevention. *Sexually Transmitted Disease Surveillance, 1999.* Department of Health and Human Services, Atlanta: Centers for Disease Control and Prevention (CDC), September 2000.
13. U.S. Department of Health and Human Services. *Healthy People 2010*: Understanding and Improving Health and Objectives for Improving Health. 2nd ed. 2 vols. Washington, DC: U.S. Government Printing Office, November 2000.
14. U.S. Department of Health and Human Services. *Healthy People 2010.*
15. K.L. Southwick, H.M. Guidry, M.M. Weldon, K.J. Mert, S.M. Bermin, and W.C. Levine. "An Epidemic of Congenital Syphilis in Jefferson County, Texas, 1994–1995: Inadequate Prenatal Syphilis Testing after an Outbreak in Adults." *American Journal of Public Health* 89 (1999): 557–560.
16. J.M. Schulte, F.A. Martich, and G.P. Schmid. "Chancroid in the United States, 1981–1990: Evidence for Underreporting of Cases," *MMWR* 41, no. SS-3 (1992): 57–61. K.J. Mertz, D. Trees, W.C. Levine, et al. "Etiology of Genital Ulcers and Prevalence of Human Immunodeficiency Virus Coinfection in 10 U.S. Cities." *Journal of Infectious Diseases* 178 (1998): 1795–98.
17. D.T. Fleming, G.M. McQuillan, R.E. Johnson, et al. "Herpes Simplex Virus Type 2 in the United States, 1976 to 1994." *N Engl J Med* 337 (1997): 1105–11.

## Table D1. Healthy People 2000 Sexually Transmitted Diseases Objective 19.1–19.8 Status

| | Objective | Baseline Year | Baseline | 1995 | 1996 | 1997 | 1998 | 1999 | 2000 |
|---|---|---|---|---|---|---|---|---|---|
| **19.1** | **Gonorrhea (per 100,000 persons)** | 1989 | 300 | 149 | 124 | 123 | 133 | 133 | 100 |
| | a. Black (non-Hispanic) | 1989 | 1,990 | 1,046 | 817 | 802 | 851 | 849 | 650 |
| | b. Adolescents 15-19 years | 1989 | 1,123 | 671 | 544 | 522 | 547 | 534 | 375 |
| | c. Female 15-44 years | 1989 | 501 | 299 | 259 | 252 | 282 | 283 | 175 |
| **19.2** | **Chlamydia prevalence among females 15-24 years** | | | | | | | | |
| | Female 15-19 years | 1988 | 12.2% | 6.7% | 5.4% | — | 6.9%* | 6.6%* | 5% |
| | Female 20-24 years | 1988 | 8.5% | 4.2% | 3.4% | — | 4.4%* | 4.5%* | 5% |
| **19.3** | **Primary and secondary syphilis (per 100,000 persons)** | 1989 | 18.1 | 6.3 | 4.3 | 3.2 | 2.6 | 2.5 | 4 |
| | a. Black | 1989 | 118 | 45 | 30 | 22 | 17 | 15 | 30 |
| **19.4** | **Congenital syphilis (per 100,000 live births)** | 1990 | 91.0 | 47.4 | 33.3 | 27.7 | 21.6 | 14.3 | 40 |
| | a. Black | 1992 | [a]417.8 | 213.2 | 150.5 | 122.4 | 90.3 | 57.9 | 175 |
| | b. Hispanic | 1992 | [a]134.6 | 61.2 | 38.9 | 33.4 | 28.7 | 20.4 | 50 |
| **19.5** | **Annual number of first time consultations**[1] | | | | | | | | |
| | Genital herpes | 1988 | 163,000 | 160,000 | 208,000 | 176,000 | 188,000 | 224,000 | 138,500 |
| | Genital warts | 1988 | 290,000 | 253,000 | 191,000 | 145,000 | 211,000 | 240,000 | 246,500 |
| **19.6** | **Pelvic inflammatory disease** | | | | | | | | |
| | Hospitalizations per 100,000 females 15-44 years | 1988 | 311 | 162 | 164 | 157 | 155 | — | 100 |
| | Initial visits to physicians (number of visits)[1] | 1988 | 430,800 | 262,000 | 286,000 | 261,000 | 234,000 | 251,000 | 290,000 |
| | Hospitalizations per 100,000 females | | | | | | | | |
| | a. Black 15-44 years | 1988 | 655 | 296 | 320 | 281 | 291 | — | 150 |
| | b. Adolescents 15-19 years | 1988 | 342 | 141 | 168 | 186 | 162 | — | 110 |
| **19.7**** | **Sexually transmitted Hepatitis B (number of cases)** | 1987 | 47,593 | [2]29,446 | — | — | — | — | 30,500 |
| **19.8** | **Repeat gonorrhea infection in last 12 months** | 1987 | 20% | 18.4% | 18.5% | 17.0% | 17.5% | 17.2% | 15% |
| | a. Black | 1992 | 21.3% | 20.1% | 19.8% | 18.3% | 18.6% | 19.2% | 17% |

—Data not available.
[a]Baseline has been revised.
[1]As measured by first-time visits to physicians' offices.
[2]Data are provisional.

Note: Data include revisions and, therefore, may differ from data previously published in these reports and other publications.

**Data Sources**

| Objective number | Data Source |
|---|---|
| 19.1,19a-c | Sexually Transmitted Disease Surveillance System, CDC, NCHSTP. |
| 19.2 | Sexually Transmitted Disease Surveillance System, CDC, NCHSTP. |
| 19.3,19.3a | Sexually Transmitted Disease Surveillance System, CDC, NCHSTP. |
| 19.4 | Sexually Transmitted Disease Surveillance System, CDC, NCHSTP. |
| 19.5 | National Disease and Therapeutic Index, IMS America, Ltd. |
| 19.6,19.6a-b | For hospitalizations, National Hospital Discharge Survey, CDC, NCHS. |
| | For number of visits, National Disease and Therapeutic Index, IMS America, Ltd. |
| 19.7** | Viral Hepatitis Surveillance System, CDC, NCID. |
| 19.8 | Gonococcal Isolate Surveillance Project, CDC, NCHSTP. |

*Positivity not adjusted for changes in laboratory test method in 1998-1999 and associated increases in test sensitivity.
**Duplicate Objective.
*Source*: Centers for Disease Control and Prevention, U.S. Department of Health and Human Services. National Center for HIV, STD, and TB Prevention, Division of STD Prevention. *Sexually Transmitted Disease Surveillance 1999* (Atlanta, GA: CDC, 2000). http://www.cdc.gov/nchstp/dstd/Stats_Trends/1999Surveillance/99PDF/Surv99Master.pdf.

## Table D2.1. Reported Cases of Sexually Transmitted Disease by Gender and Reporting Source: United States, 1999

| | *Non-STD Clinic* | | | *STD Clinic* | | | *Total*[†] | | |
|---|---|---|---|---|---|---|---|---|---|
| *Disease** | *Male* | *Female* | *Total* | *Male* | *Female* | *Total* | *Male* | *Female* | *Total* |
| Total *Chlamydia Trachomatis* | 65,297 | 426,550 | 493,829 | 54,773 | 110,410 | 165,545 | 120,094 | 537,003 | 659,441 |
| Chlamydial PID[‡] | NA | 2,555 | 2,558 | NA | 478 | 479 | NA | 3,033 | 3,037 |
| Ophthalmia Neonatorum | 115 | 152 | 267 | 11 | 16 | 28 | 126 | 168 | 295 |
| Total Gonorrhea | 80,506 | 126,471 | 207,803 | 99,038 | 53,051 | 152,241 | 179,564 | 179,534 | 360,076 |
| Gonococcal PID | NA | 2,360 | 2,362 | NA | 1,379 | 1,381 | NA | 3,739 | 3,743 |
| Ophthalmia Neonatorum | 15 | 21 | 36 | 3 | 2 | 5 | 18 | 23 | 41 |
| Total Syphilis | NA | NA | NA | NA | NA | NA | 18,771 | 16,803 | 35,628 |
| Primary | 645 | 215 | 860 | 1,156 | 295 | 1,452 | 1,801 | 510 | 2,312 |
| Secondary | 974 | 1,144 | 2,120 | 1,080 | 1,142 | 2,224 | 2,055 | 2,286 | 4,345 |
| Early Latent | 2,915 | 3,166 | 6,087 | 2,893 | 2,697 | 5,590 | 5,808 | 5,863 | 11,677 |
| Late and Late Latent[+] | 4,884 | 4,766 | 9,657 | 3,947 | 3,129 | 7,081 | 8,831 | 7,895 | 16,738 |
| Neurosyphilis[§] | 227 | 93 | 320 | 16 | 5 | 21 | 243 | 98 | 341 |
| Congenital <1 year[¥] | NR | NR | NR | NR | NR | NR | 276 | 249 | 556 |
| Chancroid | 21 | 25 | 46 | 69 | 26 | 95 | 91 | 51 | 143 |
| Granuloma Inguinale | 1 | 0 | 1 | 14 | 4 | 18 | 15 | 4 | 19 |
| Lymphogranuloma Venereum | 6 | 12 | 18 | 33 | 11 | 44 | 39 | 23 | 62 |
| Genital Herpes[¤] | 858 | 2,515 | 3,389 | 3,605 | 3,154 | 6,763 | 4,463 | 5,669 | 10,149 |
| Other and Nonspecified PID | NA | 1,042 | 1,042 | NA | 1,880 | 1,880 | NA | 2,922 | 2,922 |
| Nonspecific Urethritis in Men | 2,704 | NA | 2,704 | 26,027 | NA | 26,027 | 28,731 | NA | 28,731 |

*NA = Not applicable. NR = No report.

[†]Totals include unknown gender and reporting source.

[††]PID = Pelvic inflammatory disease.

[§]Neurosyphilis cases are not included with Total Syphilis cases but are included in the late and late latent syphilis cases.

+ Cases of unknown duration for syphilis are included in late and late latent syphilis.

¥ Cases of congenital syphilis <1 year of age are obtained using reporting from CDC 73.126. Clinic reporting source is not available from that form.

* Genital herpes data are only available for a limited number of states.

*Source*: Centers for Disease Control and Prevention, U.S. Department of Health and Human Services. National Center for HIV, STD, and TB Prevention, Division of STD Prevention. *Sexually Transmitted Disease Surveillance 1999* (Atlanta, GA: CDC, 2000). http://www.cdc.gov/nchstp/dstd/Stats_Trends/1999Surveillance/99PDF/Surv99Master.pdf.

## Table D2.2. Cases of Sexually Transmitted Diseases Reported by State Health Departments and Rates per 100,000 Civilian Population: United States, 1941–1999

| | Syphilis | | | | | | | | | | | | | | | | | | | |
|---|---|---|---|---|---|---|---|---|---|---|---|---|---|---|---|---|---|---|---|---|
| | All Stages | | Primary and Secondary | | Early Latent | | Late and Late Latent | | Congenital | | Chlamydia* | | Gonorrhea | | Chancroid | | Granuloma Inguinale | | Lympho-granuloma Venereum | |
| Year[1] | Cases | Rate | Cases | Rate | Cases | Rate | Cases | Rate | Cases | Rate[2] | Cases | Rate | Cases | Rate | Cases | Rate | Cases | Rate | Cases | Rate |
| 1941 | 485,560 | 368.2 | 68,231 | 51.7 | 109,018 | 82.6 | 202,984 | 153.9 | 17,600 | 13.4 | NR | . | 193,468 | 146.7 | 3,384 | 2.5 | 639 | 0.4 | 1,381 | 1.0 |
| 1942 | 479,601 | 363.4 | 75,312 | 57.0 | 116,245 | 88.0 | 202,064 | 153.1 | 16,918 | 12.8 | NR | . | 212,403 | 160.9 | 5,477 | 4.1 | 1,278 | 0.9 | 1,888 | 1.4 |
| 1943 | 575,593 | 447.0 | 82,204 | 63.8 | 149,390 | 116.0 | 251,958 | 195.7 | 16,164 | 12.6 | NR | . | 275,070 | 213.6 | 8,354 | 6.4 | 1,748 | 1.3 | 2,593 | 2.0 |
| 1944 | 467,755 | 367.9 | 78,443 | 61.6 | 123,038 | 96.7 | 202,848 | 159.6 | 13,578 | 10.7 | NR | . | 300,676 | 236.5 | 7,878 | 6.1 | 1,759 | 1.3 | 2,858 | 2.2 |
| 1945 | 359,114 | 282.3 | 77,007 | 60.5 | 101,719 | 79.9 | 142,187 | 111.8 | 12,339 | 9.7 | NR | . | 287,181 | 225.8 | 5,515 | 4.3 | 1,857 | 1.4 | 2,631 | 2.0 |
| 1946 | 363,647 | 271.7 | 94,957 | 70.9 | 107,924 | 80.6 | 125,248 | 93.6 | 12,106 | 9.0 | NR | . | 368,020 | 275.0 | 7,091 | 5.2 | 2,232 | 1.6 | 2,603 | 1.9 |
| 1947 | 355,592 | 252.3 | 93,545 | 66.4 | 104,124 | 73.9 | 122,089 | 86.6 | 12,200 | 8.7 | NR | . | 380,666 | 270.0 | 9,515 | 6.7 | 2,330 | 1.7 | 2,526 | 1.8 |
| 1948 | 314,313 | 218.2 | 68,174 | 47.3 | 90,598 | 62.9 | 123,312 | 85.6 | 13,931 | 9.7 | NR | . | 345,501 | 239.8 | 7,661 | 5.3 | 2,469 | 1.7 | 2,429 | 1.7 |
| 1949 | 256,463 | 175.3 | 41,942 | 28.7 | 75,045 | 51.3 | 116,397 | 79.5 | 13,952 | 9.5 | NR | . | 317,950 | 217.3 | 6,707 | 4.6 | 2,402 | 1.6 | 1,925 | 1.3 |
| 1950 | 217,558 | 146.0 | 23,939 | 16.7 | 59,256 | 39.7 | 113,569 | 70.2 | 13,377 | 9.0 | NR | . | 286,746 | 192.5 | 4,977 | 3.3 | 1,783 | 1.2 | 1,427 | 1.0 |
| 1951 | 174,924 | 116.1 | 14,485 | 9.6 | 43,316 | 28.7 | 98,311 | 65.2 | 11,094 | 7.4 | NR | . | 254,470 | 168.9 | 4,233 | 2.8 | 1,352 | 0.9 | 1,300 | 0.9 |
| 1952 | 167,762 | 110.2 | 10,449 | 6.9 | 36,454 | 24.0 | 105,238 | 69.1 | 8,553 | 5.6 | NR | . | 244,957 | 160.8 | 3,738 | 2.5 | 951 | 0.6 | 1,200 | 0.8 |
| 1953 | 148,573 | 95.9 | 8,637 | 5.6 | 28,295 | 18.3 | 98,870 | 63.8 | 7,675 | 5.0 | NR | . | 238,340 | 153.9 | 3,338 | 2.2 | 667 | 0.4 | 983 | 0.6 |
| 1954 | 130,687 | 82.9 | 7,147 | 4.5 | 23,861 | 15.1 | 89,123 | 56.5 | 6,676 | 4.2 | NR | . | 242,050 | 153.5 | 3,003 | 1.9 | 618 | 0.4 | 875 | 0.6 |
| 1955 | 122,392 | 76.2 | 6,454 | 4.0 | 20,054 | 12.5 | 86,526 | 53.8 | 5,354 | 3.3 | NR | . | 236,197 | 147.0 | 2,649 | 1.7 | 490 | 0.3 | 762 | 0.5 |
| 1956 | 130,201 | 78.7 | 6,392 | 3.9 | 19,783 | 12.0 | 95,097 | 57.5 | 5,491 | 3.3 | NR | . | 224,346 | 135.7 | 2,135 | 1.3 | 357 | 0.2 | 500 | 0.3 |
| 1957 | 123,758 | 73.5 | 6,576 | 3.9 | 17,796 | 10.6 | 91,309 | 54.2 | 5,288 | 3.1 | NR | . | 214,496 | 127.4 | 1,637 | 1.0 | 348 | 0.2 | 448 | 0.3 |
| 1958 | 113,884 | 66.4 | 7,176 | 4.2 | 16,556 | 9.7 | 83,027 | 48.4 | 4,866 | 2.8 | NR | . | 232,386 | 135.6 | 1,595 | 0.9 | 314 | 0.2 | 434 | 0.3 |
| 1959 | 120,824 | 69.2 | 9,799 | 5.6 | 17,025 | 9.8 | 86,740 | 49.7 | 5,130 | 2.9 | NR | . | 240,254 | 137.6 | 1,537 | 0.9 | 265 | 0.2 | 604 | 0.3 |
| 1960 | 122,538 | 68.8 | 16,145 | 9.1 | 18,017 | 10.1 | 81,798 | 45.9 | 4,416 | 2.5 | NR | . | 258,933 | 145.4 | 1,680 | 0.9 | 296 | 0.2 | 835 | 0.5 |
| 1961 | 124,658 | 68.8 | 19,851 | 11.0 | 19,486 | 10.8 | 79,304 | 43.8 | 4,163 | 2.3 | NR | . | 264,158 | 145.8 | 1,438 | 0.8 | 241 | 0.1 | 787 | 0.4 |
| 1962 | 126,245 | 68.7 | 21,067 | 11.5 | 19,585 | 10.7 | 79,533 | 43.3 | 4,070 | 2.2 | NR | . | 263,714 | 143.6 | 1,344 | 0.7 | 207 | 0.1 | 590 | 0.3 |
| 1963 | 124,137 | 66.6 | 22,251 | 11.9 | 18,235 | 9.8 | 78,076 | 41.9 | 4,031 | 2.2 | NR | . | 278,289 | 149.2 | 1,220 | 0.7 | 173 | 0.1 | 586 | 0.3 |
| 1964 | 114,325 | 60.4 | 22,969 | 12.1 | 17,781 | 9.4 | 68,629 | 36.3 | 3,516 | 1.9 | NR | . | 300,666 | 159.0 | 1,247 | 0.7 | 135 | 0.1 | 732 | 0.4 |
| 1965 | 112,842 | 58.9 | 23,338 | 12.2 | 17,458 | 9.1 | 67,317 | 35.1 | 3,564 | 1.9 | NR | . | 324,925 | 169.6 | 982 | 0.5 | 155 | 0.1 | 878 | 0.5 |
| 1966 | 105,159 | 54.4 | 21,414 | 11.1 | 15,950 | 8.2 | 63,541 | 32.9 | 3,170 | 1.6 | NR | . | 351,738 | 181.9 | 838 | 0.4 | 148 | 0.1 | 308 | 0.2 |
| 1967 | 102,581 | 52.5 | 21,053 | 10.8 | 15,554 | 8.0 | 61,975 | 31.7 | 2,894 | 1.5 | NR | . | 404,836 | 207.3 | 784 | 0.4 | 154 | 0.1 | 371 | 0.2 |
| 1968 | 96,271 | 48.8 | 19,019 | 9.6 | 15,150 | 7.7 | 58,564 | 29.7 | 2,381 | 1.2 | NR | . | 464,543 | 235.7 | 845 | 0.4 | 156 | 0.1 | 485 | 0.2 |
| 1969 | 92,162 | 46.3 | 19,130 | 9.6 | 15,402 | 7.7 | 54,587 | 27.4 | 2,074 | 1.0 | NR | . | 534,872 | 268.6 | 1,104 | 0.6 | 154 | 0.1 | 520 | 0.3 |
| 1970 | 91,382 | 45.3 | 21,982 | 10.9 | 16,311 | 8.1 | 50,348 | 24.9 | 1,953 | 1.0 | NR | . | 600,072 | 297.2 | 1,416 | 0.7 | 124 | 0.1 | 612 | 0.3 |
| 1971 | 95,997 | 46.9 | 23,783 | 11.6 | 19,417 | 9.5 | 49,993 | 24.4 | 2,052 | 1.0 | NR | . | 670,268 | 327.2 | 1,320 | 0.6 | 89 | 0.0 | 692 | 0.3 |
| 1972 | 91,149 | 43.9 | 24,429 | 11.8 | 20,784 | 10.0 | 43,456 | 20.9 | 1,758 | 0.8 | NR | . | 767,215 | 369.7 | 1,414 | 0.7 | 81 | 0.0 | 756 | 0.4 |
| 1973 | 87,469 | 41.7 | 24,825 | 11.8 | 23,584 | 11.3 | 37,054 | 17.7 | 1,527 | 0.7 | NR | . | 842,621 | 402.0 | 1,165 | 0.6 | 62 | 0.0 | 408 | 0.2 |
| 1974 | 83,771 | 39.6 | 25,385 | 12.0 | 25,124 | 11.9 | 31,854 | 15.1 | 1,138 | 0.5 | NR | . | 906,121 | 428.2 | 945 | 0.4 | 47 | 0.0 | 394 | 0.2 |
| 1975 | 80,356 | 37.6 | 25,561 | 12.0 | 26,569 | 12.4 | 27,096 | 12.7 | 916 | 0.4 | NR | . | 999,937 | 467.7 | 700 | 0.3 | 60 | 0.0 | 353 | 0.2 |
| 1976 | 71,761 | 33.2 | 23,731 | 11.0 | 25,363 | 11.7 | 21,905 | 10.1 | 626 | 0.3 | NR | . | 1,001,994 | 464.1 | 628 | 0.3 | 71 | 0.0 | 365 | 0.2 |
| 1977 | 64,621 | 29.6 | 20,399 | 9.4 | 21,329 | 9.8 | 22,313 | 10.2 | 463 | 0.2 | NR | . | 1,002,219 | 459.5 | 455 | 0.2 | 75 | 0.0 | 348 | 0.2 |
| 1978 | 64,875 | 29.4 | 21,656 | 9.8 | 19,628 | 8.9 | 23,038 | 10.4 | 434 | 0.2 | NR | . | 1,013,436 | 459.7 | 521 | 0.2 | 72 | 0.0 | 284 | 0.1 |
| 1979 | 67,049 | 30.1 | 24,874 | 11.2 | 20,459 | 9.2 | 21,301 | 9.6 | 332 | 0.1 | NR | . | 1,004,058 | 450.3 | 840 | 0.4 | 76 | 0.0 | 250 | 0.1 |
| 1980 | 68,832 | 30.5 | 27,204 | 12.1 | 20,297 | 9.0 | 20,979 | 9.3 | 277 | 0.1 | NR | . | 1,004,029 | 445.1 | 788 | 0.3 | 51 | 0.0 | 199 | 0.1 |
| 1981 | 72,799 | 32.0 | 31,266 | 13.7 | 21,033 | 9.2 | 20,168 | 8.9 | 287 | 0.1 | NR | . | 990,864 | 435.2 | 850 | 0.4 | 66 | 0.0 | 263 | 0.1 |
| 1982 | 75,579 | 32.9 | 33,613 | 14.6 | 21,894 | 9.5 | 19,799 | 8.6 | 259 | 0.1 | NR | . | 960,633 | 417.9 | 1,392 | 0.6 | 17 | 0.0 | 235 | 0.1 |
| 1983 | 74,637 | 32.1 | 32,698 | 14.1 | 23,738 | 10.2 | 17,896 | 7.7 | 239 | 0.1 | NR | . | 900.435 | 387.6 | 847 | 0.4 | 24 | 0.0 | 335 | 0.1 |
| 1984 | 69,873 | 29.8 | 28,607 | 12.2 | 23,132 | 9.9 | 17,829 | 7.6 | 305 | 0.1 | 7,594 | 6.5 | 878,556 | 374.8 | 665 | 0.3 | 30 | 0.0 | 170 | 0.1 |
| 1985 | 67,563 | 28.5 | 27,131 | 11.5 | 21,689 | 9.2 | 18,414 | 7.8 | 329 | 0.1 | 25,848 | 17.4 | 911,419 | 384.3 | 2,067 | 0.9 | 44 | 0.0 | 226 | 0.1 |

## Table D2.2. *(Continued)*

| | Syphilis | | | | | | | | | | | | | | | | | | | |
|---|---|---|---|---|---|---|---|---|---|---|---|---|---|---|---|---|---|---|---|---|
| | All Stages | | Primary and Secondary | | Early Latent | | Late and Late Latent | | Congenital | | Chlamydia* | | Gonorrhea | | Chancroid | | Granuloma Inguinale | | Lympho-granuloma Venereum | |
| Year[1] | Cases | Rate | Cases | Rate | Cases | Rate | Cases | Rate | Cases | Rate[2] | Cases | Rate | Cases | Rate | Cases | Rate | Cases | Rate | Cases | Rate |
| 1986 | 67,771 | 28.3 | 27,667 | 11.6 | 21,656 | 9.0 | 18,046 | 7.5 | 410 | 0.2 | 58,001 | 35.2 | 892,229 | 372.8 | 3,045 | 1.3 | 48 | 0.0 | 307 | 0.1 |
| 1987 | 87,278 | 35.9 | 35,585 | 14.6 | 28,233 | 11.6 | 22,988 | 9.4 | 480 | 0.2 | 91,913 | 50.8 | 787,532 | 323.6 | 4,986 | 2.0 | 22 | 0.0 | 302 | 0.1 |
| 1988 | 104,546 | 42.5 | 40,474 | 16.5 | 35,968 | 14.6 | 27,363 | 11.1 | 741 | 0.3 | 157,807 | 87.1 | 738,160 | 300.3 | 4,891 | 2.0 | 11 | 0.0 | 194 | 0.1 |
| 1989 | 115,067 | 46.6 | 45,826 | 18.6 | 45,394 | 18.4 | 22,032 | 8.9 | 1,837 | 0.7 | 200,904 | 102.5 | 733,294 | 297.1 | 4,697 | 1.9 | 7 | 0.0 | 182 | 0.1 |
| 1990 | 135,043 | 54.3 | 50,578 | 20.3 | 55,397 | 22.3 | 25,750 | 10.4 | 3,865 | 1.6 | 323,663 | 160.8 | 690,042 | 277.4 | 4,212 | 1.7 | 97 | 0.0 | 277 | 0.1 |
| 1991 | 128,637 | 51.0 | 42,950 | 17.0 | 53,855 | 21.4 | 27,490 | 10.9 | 4,424 | 1.8 | 381,228 | 180.3 | 621,918 | 246.7 | 3,476 | 1.4 | 29 | 0.0 | 471 | 0.2 |
| 1992 | 112,855 | 44.3 | 33,962 | 13.3 | 49,903 | 19.6 | 25,099 | 9.8 | 3,890 | 1.5 | 409,634 | 183.4 | 502,785 | 197.1 | 1,885 | 0.7 | 6 | 0.0 | 289 | 0.1 |
| 1993 | 101,335 | 39.3 | 26,497 | 10.3 | 41,902 | 16.3 | 29,675 | 11.5 | 3,261 | 1.3 | 405,275 | 179.5 | 444,578 | 172.5 | 1,237 | 0.5 | 19 | 0.0 | 286 | 0.1 |
| 1994 | 82,334 | 31.6 | 20,645 | 7.9 | 32,020 | 12.3 | 27,452 | 10.5 | 2,217 | 0.8 | 451,758 | 194.5 | 419,577 | 165.7 | 779 | 0.3 | 3 | 0.0 | 237 | 0.1 |
| 1995 | 69,353 | 26.4 | 16,543 | 6.3 | 26,657 | 10.1 | 24,296 | 9.2 | 1,857 | 0.7 | 478,577 | 190.4 | 392,651 | 149.4 | 607 | 0.2 | 0 | 0.0 | 188 | 0.1 |
| 1996 | 53,218 | 20.1 | 11,388 | 4.3 | 20,187 | 7.6 | 20,364 | 7.7 | 1,279 | 0.5 | 490,615 | 192.9 | 326,805 | 123.2 | 386 | 0.1 | 10 | 0.0 | 72 | 0.0 |
| 1997 | 46,708 | 17.5 | 8,556 | 3.2 | 16,631 | 6.2 | 20,446 | 7.6 | 1,075 | 0.4 | 531,744 | 207.0 | 326,564 | 122.0 | 246 | 0.1 | 8 | 0.0 | 114 | 0.0 |
| 1998 | 38,366 | 14.2 | 7,035 | 2.6 | 12,741 | 4.7 | 17,752 | 6.6 | 838 | 0.3 | 607,752 | 234.2 | 355,728 | 131.6 | 189 | 0.1 | 3 | 0.0 | 86 | 0.0 |
| 1999 | 35,628 | 13.2 | 6,657 | 2.5 | 11,677 | 4.3 | 16,738 | 6.2 | 556 | 0.2 | 659,441 | 254.1 | 360,076 | 133.2 | 143 | 0.1 | 19 | 0.0 | 62 | 0.0 |

*NR = No Report.

[1]For 1941–1946, data were reported for the federal fiscal year ending June 30 of the year indicated. From 1947 to the present, data were reported for the calendar year ending December 31. For 1941–1958, data for Alaska and Hawaii were not included.

For 1941–1994, rates include all cases of congenitally acquired syphilis per 100,000 population. As of 1995, rates of congenital syphilis <1 year of age per 100,000 population are reported. **For rates of congenital syphilis <1 year of age per 100,000 live births see Table 37, 38, and 39.** As of 1995, cases of congenital syphilis < year of age are obtained in hardcopy and electronic format based on case reporting from CDC 73.126.

Note: Adjustments to the number of cases reported from state health departments were made for hardcopy forms and for electronic data submissions through August 4, 2000 (see Appendix). The number of cases and the rates shown here supersede those published in previous reports. Cases and rates shown in this table exclude the outlying areas of Guam, Puerto Rico and Virgin Islands.

*Source*: Centers for Disease Control and Prevention, U.S. Department of Health and Human Services. National Center for HIV, STD, and TB Prevention, Division of STD Prevention. *Sexually Transmitted Disease Surveillance 1999* (Atlanta, GA: CDC, 2000). http://www.cdc.gov/nchstp/dstd/Stats_Trends/1999Surveillance/99PDF/Surv99Master.pdf.

# Table D3.1. Chlamydia—Reported Cases, by Age, Gender, and Race/Ethnicity: United States, 1996–1999

| | Age | Total | | | White, Non-Hispanic | | | Black, Non-Hispanic | | | Hispanic | | | Asian/Pacific Islander | | | American Indian/ Alaska Native | | |
|---|---|---|---|---|---|---|---|---|---|---|---|---|---|---|---|---|---|---|---|
| | Group | Total | Male | Female | Total | Male | Female | Total | Male | Female | Total | Male | Female | Total | Male | Female | Total | Male | Female |
| 1996 | 10-14 | 9,351 | 459 | 8,892 | 2,672 | 89 | 2,583 | 4,862 | 253 | 4,609 | 1,482 | 86 | 1,396 | 122 | 15 | 107 | 213 | 16 | 197 |
| | 15-19 | 151,344 | 16,897 | 134,447 | 52,737 | 4,167 | 48,570 | 68,501 | 9,133 | 59,368 | 24,823 | 2,963 | 21,860 | 1,935 | 213 | 1,722 | 3,348 | 421 | 2,927 |
| | 20-24 | 119,705 | 21,016 | 98,689 | 41,561 | 6,199 | 35,362 | 49,276 | 10,077 | 39,199 | 23,742 | 3,943 | 19,799 | 2,258 | 340 | 1,918 | 2,868 | 457 | 2,411 |
| | 25-29 | 47,092 | 10,432 | 36,660 | 14,943 | 3,135 | 11,808 | 18,606 | 4,745 | 13,861 | 11,171 | 2,108 | 9,063 | 1,118 | 197 | 921 | 1,254 | 247 | 1,007 |
| | 30-34 | 19,730 | 5,181 | 14,549 | 6,020 | 1,590 | 4,430 | 7,630 | 2,335 | 5,295 | 4,873 | 988 | 3,885 | 565 | 123 | 442 | 642 | 145 | 497 |
| | 35-39 | 9,350 | 2,623 | 6,727 | 3,105 | 871 | 2,234 | 3,615 | 1,185 | 2,430 | 2,006 | 454 | 1,552 | 293 | 62 | 231 | 331 | 51 | 280 |
| | 40-44 | 4,079 | 1,272 | 2,807 | 1,368 | 409 | 959 | 1,583 | 568 | 1,015 | 836 | 222 | 614 | 138 | 44 | 94 | 154 | 29 | 125 |
| | 45-54 | 2,596 | 936 | 1,660 | 985 | 359 | 626 | 957 | 419 | 538 | 472 | 122 | 350 | 93 | 24 | 69 | 89 | 12 | 77 |
| | 55-64 | 517 | 237 | 280 | 210 | 88 | 122 | 181 | 104 | 77 | 88 | 33 | 55 | 13 | 5 | 8 | 25 | 7 | 18 |
| | 65+ | 479 | 117 | 362 | 206 | 63 | 143 | 145 | 30 | 115 | 106 | 16 | 90 | 11 | 5 | 6 | 11 | 3 | 8 |
| | TOTAL | 366,836 | 59,787 | 307,049 | 124,735 | 17,169 | 107,566 | 156,305 | 29,090 | 127,215 | 70,170 | 11,093 | 59,077 | 6,615 | 1,033 | 5,582 | 9,011 | 1,402 | 7,609 |
| 1997 | 10-14 | 8,871 | 429 | 8,442 | 2,594 | 70 | 2,524 | 4,382 | 221 | 4,161 | 1,540 | 122 | 1,418 | 119 | 8 | 111 | 236 | 8 | 228 |
| | 15-19 | 154,992 | 18,940 | 136,052 | 52,717 | 4,379 | 48,338 | 69,632 | 10,180 | 59,452 | 27,320 | 3,787 | 23,533 | 2,235 | 277 | 1,958 | 3,088 | 317 | 2,771 |
| | 20-24 | 127,676 | 25,121 | 102,555 | 41,935 | 6,782 | 35,153 | 54,042 | 12,501 | 41,541 | 26,598 | 5,039 | 21,559 | 2,416 | 424 | 1,992 | 2,685 | 375 | 2,310 |
| | 25-29 | 50,374 | 12,566 | 37,808 | 15,188 | 3,381 | 11,807 | 20,357 | 6,122 | 14,235 | 12,433 | 2,646 | 9,787 | 1,202 | 244 | 958 | 1,194 | 173 | 1,021 |
| | 30-34 | 20,698 | 6,260 | 14,438 | 5,910 | 1,658 | 4,252 | 8,157 | 3,068 | 5,089 | 5,441 | 1,287 | 4,154 | 599 | 152 | 447 | 591 | 95 | 496 |
| | 35-39 | 9,597 | 3,246 | 6,351 | 2,948 | 896 | 2,052 | 3,782 | 1,581 | 2,201 | 2,248 | 640 | 1,608 | 328 | 62 | 266 | 291 | 67 | 224 |
| | 40-44 | 4,126 | 1,522 | 2,604 | 1,343 | 454 | 889 | 1,586 | 750 | 836 | 917 | 267 | 650 | 163 | 36 | 127 | 117 | 15 | 102 |
| | 45-54 | 2,602 | 1,114 | 1,488 | 889 | 382 | 507 | 947 | 503 | 444 | 572 | 180 | 392 | 118 | 38 | 80 | 76 | 11 | 65 |
| | 55-64 | 544 | 267 | 277 | 182 | 84 | 98 | 206 | 116 | 90 | 119 | 54 | 65 | 15 | 3 | 12 | 22 | 10 | 12 |
| | 65+ | 1,096 | 260 | 836 | 370 | 73 | 297 | 456 | 122 | 334 | 218 | 56 | 162 | 17 | 5 | 12 | 35 | 4 | 31 |
| | TOTAL | 382,249 | 70,250 | 311,999 | 124,587 | 18,302 | 106,285 | 164,231 | 35,386 | 128,845 | 77,814 | 14,222 | 63,592 | 7,250 | 1,260 | 5,990 | 8,367 | 1,080 | 7,287 |
| 1998 | 10-14 | 11,198 | 617 | 10,581 | 2,975 | 89 | 2,886 | 6,145 | 377 | 5,768 | 1,656 | 127 | 1,529 | 140 | 11 | 129 | 282 | 13 | 269 |
| | 15-19 | 198,781 | 24,299 | 174,482 | 63,955 | 5,285 | 58,670 | 97,036 | 13,870 | 83,166 | 30,894 | 4,319 | 26,575 | 3,024 | 360 | 2,664 | 3,872 | 465 | 3,407 |
| | 20-24 | 164,663 | 31,609 | 133,054 | 51,159 | 8,427 | 42,732 | 76,759 | 16,149 | 60,610 | 30,455 | 5,999 | 24,456 | 3,146 | 535 | 2,611 | 3,144 | 499 | 2,645 |
| | 25-29 | 64,341 | 15,975 | 48,366 | 17,846 | 4,119 | 13,727 | 29,274 | 8,163 | 21,111 | 14,235 | 3,146 | 11,089 | 1,671 | 348 | 1,323 | 1,315 | 199 | 1,116 |
| | 30-34 | 25,601 | 7,719 | 17,882 | 6,773 | 2,119 | 4,654 | 11,343 | 3,857 | 7,486 | 6,048 | 1,497 | 4,551 | 765 | 159 | 606 | 672 | 87 | 585 |
| | 35-39 | 12,586 | 4,378 | 8,208 | 3,489 | 1,145 | 2,344 | 5,650 | 2,305 | 3,345 | 2,636 | 715 | 1,921 | 455 | 133 | 322 | 356 | 80 | 276 |
| | 40-44 | 5,306 | 2,032 | 3,274 | 1,582 | 607 | 975 | 2,361 | 1,096 | 1,265 | 993 | 251 | 742 | 209 | 46 | 163 | 161 | 32 | 129 |
| | 45-54 | 3,185 | 1,345 | 1,840 | 1,032 | 452 | 580 | 1,373 | 702 | 671 | 543 | 137 | 406 | 119 | 42 | 77 | 118 | 12 | 106 |
| | 55-64 | 659 | 304 | 355 | 174 | 83 | 91 | 320 | 174 | 146 | 114 | 33 | 81 | 28 | 8 | 20 | 23 | 6 | 17 |
| | 65+ | 1,045 | 251 | 794 | 306 | 88 | 218 | 553 | 124 | 429 | 150 | 34 | 116 | 24 | 5 | 19 | 12 | 0 | 12 |
| | TOTAL | 489,252 | 89,081 | 400,171 | 149,787 | 22,572 | 127,215 | 231,717 | 47,067 | 184,650 | 88,137 | 16,383 | 71,754 | 9,613 | 1,655 | 7,958 | 9,998 | 1,404 | 8,594 |
| 1999 | 10-14 | 12,545 | 753 | 11,792 | 3,200 | 117 | 3,083 | 7,015 | 449 | 6,566 | 1,899 | 162 | 1,737 | 158 | 12 | 146 | 273 | 13 | 260 |
| | 15-19 | 231,999 | 29,663 | 202,336 | 73,159 | 6,410 | 66,749 | 115,008 | 17,106 | 97,902 | 35,970 | 5,173 | 30,797 | 3,656 | 454 | 3,202 | 4,206 | 520 | 3,686 |
| | 20-24 | 201,482 | 38,948 | 162,534 | 62,178 | 10,762 | 51,416 | 95,429 | 20,130 | 75,299 | 36,552 | 6,919 | 29,633 | 3,947 | 641 | 3,306 | 3,376 | 496 | 2,880 |
| | 25-29 | 77,036 | 19,346 | 57,690 | 20,688 | 4,885 | 15,803 | 35,495 | 9,981 | 25,514 | 17,192 | 3,727 | 13,465 | 2,146 | 489 | 1,657 | 1,515 | 264 | 1,251 |
| | 30-34 | 30,349 | 9,171 | 21,178 | 7,611 | 2,359 | 5,252 | 13,687 | 4,700 | 8,987 | 7,426 | 1,759 | 5,667 | 970 | 216 | 754 | 655 | 137 | 518 |
| | 35-39 | 14,825 | 5,315 | 9,510 | 4,051 | 1,466 | 2,585 | 6,619 | 2,811 | 3,808 | 3,293 | 822 | 2,471 | 493 | 130 | 363 | 369 | 86 | 283 |
| | 40-44 | 6,461 | 2,685 | 3,776 | 1,877 | 799 | 1,078 | 2,855 | 1,408 | 1,447 | 1,282 | 350 | 932 | 266 | 86 | 180 | 181 | 42 | 139 |
| | 45-54 | 3,957 | 1,806 | 2,151 | 1,128 | 536 | 592 | 1,708 | 941 | 767 | 806 | 235 | 571 | 182 | 66 | 116 | 133 | 28 | 105 |
| | 55-64 | 823 | 419 | 404 | 250 | 160 | 90 | 371 | 193 | 178 | 128 | 41 | 87 | 46 | 13 | 33 | 28 | 12 | 16 |
| | 65+ | 777 | 265 | 512 | 268 | 100 | 168 | 294 | 98 | 196 | 124 | 31 | 93 | 32 | 19 | 13 | 59 | 17 | 42 |
| | TOTAL | 582,207 | 108,967 | 473,240 | 174,921 | 27,750 | 147,171 | 279,529 | 58,121 | 221,408 | 105,007 | 19,337 | 85,670 | 11,932 | 2,137 | 9,795 | 10,818 | 1,622 | 9,196 |

Note: These tables should be used only for race/ethnicity and age comparisons, not for overall totals or gender totals. This is because, if age or race/ethnicity was not specified, cases were prorated according to the distribution of cases for which these variables were specified. For the following years the states listed did not report race/ethnicity for most cases and were excluded: 1996 (Colorado, Delaware, Georgia, Maryland, Michigan, New Jersey, New York, Ohio and South Carolina); 1997 (Colorado, Delaware, District of Columbia, Georgia, Maryland, Michigan, Mississippi, New Jersey, New York, Ohio and South Carolina); 1998 (Colorado, District of Columbia, Michigan, New Jersey, New York, Ohio and South Carolina); 1999 (Colorado, District of Columbia, Michigan, New Jersey and New York). Cases and population denominators have been excluded for these states/areas. Differences between total cases from this table and others in the report are due to different reporting forms and above listed exclusions. The 0 to 9 year age group is not shown because some of these may not be due to sexual transmission; however, they are included in the totals.

*Source*: Centers for Disease Control and Prevention, U.S. Department of Health and Human Services. National Center for HIV, STD, and TB Prevention, Division of STD Prevention. *Sexually Transmitted Disease Surveillance 1999* (Atlanta, GA: CDC, 2000). http://www.cdc.gov/nchstp/dstd/Stats_Trends/1999Surveillance/99PDF/Surv99Master.pdf.

## Table D3.2. Chlamydia—Reported Rates per 100,000 Population, by Age, Gender, and Race/Ethnicity: United States, 1996–1999

| Age | Total | | | White, Non-Hispanic | | | Black, Non-Hispanic | | | Hispanic | | | Asian/Pacific Islander | | | American Indian/ Alaska Native | | | |
|---|---|---|---|---|---|---|---|---|---|---|---|---|---|---|---|---|---|---|---|
| Group | Total | Male | Female | Total | Male | Female | Total | Male | Female | Total | Male | Female | Total | Male | Female | Total | Male | Female | |
| 10-14 | 65.6 | 6.3 | 128.0 | 27.8 | 1.8 | 55.3 | 264.6 | 27.1 | 509.6 | 71.8 | 8.1 | 138.8 | 21.7 | 5.2 | 38.9 | 117.3 | 17.4 | 219.5 | |
| 15-19 | 1,080.0 | 233.6 | 1,982.6 | 560.8 | 86.1 | 1,064.5 | 3,720.0 | 975.9 | 6,555.8 | 1,188.0 | 266.6 | 2,235.1 | 373.8 | 81.1 | 674.8 | 2,077.1 | 518.7 | 3,657.9 | |
| 20-24 | 908.3 | 309.8 | 1,542.9 | 475.9 | 139.0 | 827.3 | 3,026.1 | 1,245.8 | 4,783.2 | 1,125.6 | 340.3 | 2,083.1 | 396.8 | 118.9 | 677.8 | 2,062.2 | 651.3 | 3,499.2 | |
| 25-29 | 333.3 | 146.5 | 523.0 | 155.0 | 65.1 | 244.8 | 1,168.1 | 621.3 | 1,671.8 | 526.2 | 180.4 | 949.3 | 174.4 | 64.3 | 275.3 | 917.8 | 354.6 | 1,503.5 | |
| 30-34 | 125.3 | 65.7 | 185.1 | 54.2 | 28.6 | 79.7 | 448.4 | 290.9 | 589.0 | 225.1 | 85.0 | 387.5 | 89.1 | 40.6 | 133.3 | 469.7 | 214.1 | 720.5 | |
| 35-39 | 56.1 | 31.4 | 80.8 | 25.3 | 14.2 | 36.6 | 207.1 | 143.9 | 263.5 | 105.3 | 45.2 | 172.3 | 47.1 | 20.9 | 71.1 | 243.3 | 76.8 | 401.9 | 1996 |
| 40-44 | 26.5 | 16.6 | 36.2 | 11.7 | 7.0 | 16.5 | 103.0 | 78.8 | 124.4 | 54.7 | 28.2 | 82.9 | 23.8 | 16.3 | 30.3 | 125.9 | 49.4 | 196.7 | |
| 45-54 | 10.9 | 8.0 | 13.7 | 5.2 | 3.9 | 6.6 | 46.3 | 44.4 | 47.9 | 23.9 | 12.4 | 35.3 | 11.1 | 6.2 | 15.4 | 50.1 | 14.1 | 83.4 | |
| 55-64 | 3.3 | 3.1 | 3.4 | 1.6 | 1.4 | 1.9 | 13.6 | 18.0 | 10.3 | 7.6 | 6.0 | 9.0 | 2.7 | 2.2 | 3.0 | 23.4 | 14.0 | 31.7 | |
| 65+ | 1.9 | 1.1 | 2.4 | 1.0 | 0.7 | 1.1 | 8.2 | 4.3 | 10.7 | 8.1 | 2.9 | 12.0 | 2.0 | 2.2 | 1.9 | 9.2 | 5.9 | 11.6 | |
| TOTAL | 185.7 | 61.7 | 305.2 | 86.5 | 24.3 | 145.9 | 751.0 | 293.6 | 1,166.7 | 298.8 | 91.4 | 520.4 | 92.1 | 29.9 | 149.9 | 515.9 | 163.3 | 856.4 | |
| 10-14 | 63.0 | 5.9 | 123.0 | 27.4 | 1.4 | 54.8 | 251.6 | 25.0 | 485.5 | 72.8 | 11.3 | 137.6 | 21.0 | 2.8 | 40.0 | 129.4 | 8.7 | 253.5 | |
| 15-19 | 1,098.8 | 260.1 | 1,993.6 | 556.6 | 89.8 | 1,051.7 | 3,955.5 | 1,135.4 | 6,882.5 | 1,260.0 | 328.4 | 2,318.1 | 413.5 | 101.2 | 733.9 | 1,864.3 | 381.7 | 3,355.3 | |
| 20-24 | 987.1 | 376.8 | 1,636.1 | 490.7 | 155.2 | 842.1 | 3,531.9 | 1,640.3 | 5,409.0 | 1,228.0 | 425.0 | 2,199.5 | 435.4 | 152.5 | 719.5 | 1,946.3 | 540.1 | 3,371.4 | |
| 25-29 | 364.8 | 180.4 | 552.4 | 162.0 | 72.2 | 251.7 | 1,358.4 | 849.1 | 1,830.7 | 580.9 | 224.9 | 1,015.8 | 182.4 | 77.7 | 277.7 | 865.0 | 245.0 | 1,514.5 | |
| 30-34 | 137.4 | 83.0 | 192.0 | 56.2 | 31.6 | 80.7 | 518.1 | 412.3 | 613.0 | 246.7 | 108.4 | 408.1 | 93.5 | 50.0 | 132.7 | 443.9 | 143.6 | 740.4 | |
| 35-39 | 58.3 | 39.3 | 77.2 | 24.4 | 14.8 | 34.1 | 228.7 | 202.1 | 252.6 | 113.2 | 61.0 | 171.7 | 51.9 | 20.5 | 80.6 | 213.5 | 100.4 | 322.2 | 1997 |
| 40-44 | 26.4 | 19.6 | 33.2 | 11.4 | 7.7 | 15.1 | 105.4 | 105.8 | 105.0 | 56.6 | 31.9 | 83.2 | 27.1 | 12.8 | 39.7 | 94.0 | 25.1 | 157.8 | |
| 45-54 | 10.6 | 9.3 | 12.0 | 4.6 | 4.0 | 5.2 | 46.4 | 53.9 | 40.0 | 27.2 | 17.1 | 37.2 | 13.3 | 9.3 | 16.8 | 41.6 | 12.5 | 68.4 | |
| 55-64 | 3.4 | 3.5 | 3.3 | 1.4 | 1.4 | 1.5 | 16.2 | 20.9 | 12.5 | 9.9 | 9.5 | 10.3 | 2.9 | 1.3 | 4.3 | 20.2 | 19.6 | 20.7 | |
| 65+ | 4.4 | 2.5 | 5.7 | 1.7 | 0.8 | 2.4 | 27.7 | 18.8 | 33.4 | 16.1 | 9.7 | 20.8 | 3.0 | 2.1 | 3.6 | 28.5 | 7.7 | 43.8 | |
| TOTAL | 194.8 | 72.9 | 312.4 | 87.1 | 26.1 | 145.5 | 832.1 | 375.8 | 1,248.3 | 320.0 | 113.2 | 541.1 | 98.2 | 35.5 | 156.2 | 476.0 | 125.0 | 815.1 | |
| 10-14 | 72.8 | 7.8 | 141.1 | 29.3 | 1.7 | 58.5 | 282.6 | 34.2 | 538.7 | 73.7 | 11.1 | 139.3 | 22.7 | 3.5 | 42.9 | 150.6 | 13.7 | 291.8 | |
| 15-19 | 1,269.0 | 301.4 | 2,295.6 | 618.4 | 99.2 | 1,170.2 | 4,369.9 | 1,227.8 | 7,623.6 | 1,334.8 | 357.6 | 2,401.2 | 494.4 | 116.2 | 882.4 | 2,206.6 | 529.1 | 3,890.0 | |
| 20-24 | 1,162.1 | 436.8 | 1,919.0 | 550.0 | 176.8 | 942.1 | 3,999.9 | 1,698.9 | 6,258.3 | 1,368.6 | 517.5 | 2,294.1 | 541.7 | 185.2 | 894.3 | 2,201.0 | 696.1 | 3,716.6 | |
| 25-29 | 434.7 | 216.3 | 652.2 | 179.8 | 82.9 | 276.8 | 1,560.9 | 910.9 | 2,155.8 | 658.8 | 279.1 | 1,072.6 | 240.1 | 107.6 | 355.3 | 916.3 | 271.5 | 1,589.7 | |
| 30-34 | 160.2 | 97.2 | 222.5 | 61.8 | 38.7 | 84.8 | 582.1 | 422.8 | 722.4 | 271.3 | 128.6 | 427.3 | 108.3 | 48.4 | 160.3 | 499.5 | 129.5 | 868.7 | |
| 35-39 | 70.2 | 49.0 | 91.4 | 27.0 | 17.7 | 36.4 | 272.2 | 236.8 | 303.5 | 126.3 | 66.2 | 190.9 | 64.2 | 39.4 | 86.6 | 253.6 | 115.5 | 388.1 | 1998 |
| 40-44 | 30.6 | 23.6 | 37.6 | 12.3 | 9.4 | 15.2 | 122.0 | 120.8 | 123.1 | 57.7 | 28.6 | 87.8 | 31.2 | 14.6 | 45.9 | 123.2 | 50.7 | 191.1 | |
| 45-54 | 11.7 | 10.1 | 13.2 | 4.9 | 4.3 | 5.4 | 51.7 | 58.0 | 46.4 | 24.1 | 12.4 | 35.5 | 11.9 | 9.1 | 14.4 | 60.8 | 12.9 | 105.0 | |
| 55-64 | 3.7 | 3.6 | 3.8 | 1.2 | 1.2 | 1.2 | 20.1 | 25.1 | 16.2 | 8.8 | 5.5 | 11.8 | 5.0 | 3.1 | 6.6 | 19.9 | 11.1 | 27.6 | |
| 65+ | 3.8 | 2.2 | 5.0 | 1.3 | 0.9 | 1.6 | 27.4 | 15.6 | 35.0 | 10.3 | 5.5 | 13.9 | 3.8 | 1.9 | 5.2 | 9.3 | 0.0 | 16.0 | |
| TOTAL | 227.9 | 84.7 | 365.3 | 96.9 | 29.8 | 161.4 | 937.6 | 400.6 | 1,424.2 | 345.5 | 126.8 | 569.6 | 118.8 | 42.7 | 188.7 | 549.0 | 156.9 | 927.9 | |
| 10-14 | 76.3 | 8.9 | 147.0 | 29.2 | 2.1 | 57.7 | 294.2 | 37.1 | 559.2 | 83.8 | 14.0 | 156.8 | 25.2 | 3.7 | 47.7 | 144.0 | 13.5 | 278.5 | |
| 15-19 | 1,382.8 | 343.7 | 2,483.8 | 653.1 | 111.1 | 1,228.5 | 4,718.9 | 1,381.2 | 8,167.3 | 1,539.8 | 424.4 | 2,756.9 | 585.8 | 143.7 | 1,038.8 | 2,363.5 | 583.3 | 4,150.9 | |
| 20-24 | 1,328.8 | 503.8 | 2,187.1 | 617.0 | 208.7 | 1,044.7 | 4,541.4 | 1,939.6 | 7,080.4 | 1,627.9 | 591.6 | 2,754.4 | 665.0 | 217.2 | 1,107.6 | 2,325.4 | 680.6 | 3,983.2 | |
| 25-29 | 486.3 | 245.1 | 725.9 | 192.4 | 90.9 | 293.8 | 1,728.3 | 1,019.2 | 2,374.8 | 788.7 | 328.0 | 1,290.2 | 302.5 | 148.3 | 436.4 | 1,038.3 | 354.0 | 1,753.6 | |
| 30-34 | 177.8 | 108.2 | 246.5 | 64.3 | 40.0 | 88.5 | 644.9 | 473.9 | 794.9 | 330.3 | 149.9 | 527.4 | 134.6 | 64.5 | 195.6 | 478.4 | 200.2 | 756.2 | |
| 35-39 | 77.5 | 55.7 | 99.0 | 29.1 | 21.0 | 37.3 | 292.0 | 264.9 | 315.9 | 156.5 | 75.5 | 243.4 | 68.2 | 37.8 | 95.7 | 258.5 | 122.1 | 391.3 | 1999 |
| 40-44 | 34.8 | 29.2 | 40.4 | 13.5 | 11.5 | 15.6 | 134.5 | 141.7 | 128.2 | 73.8 | 39.6 | 109.3 | 39.0 | 26.8 | 49.8 | 136.0 | 65.2 | 202.4 | |
| 45-54 | 13.5 | 12.6 | 14.4 | 4.9 | 4.7 | 5.1 | 58.4 | 70.7 | 48.1 | 35.4 | 21.0 | 49.4 | 17.9 | 14.0 | 21.2 | 67.1 | 29.4 | 102.0 | |
| 55-64 | 4.3 | 4.6 | 4.0 | 1.6 | 2.1 | 1.1 | 21.1 | 25.3 | 17.9 | 9.8 | 6.8 | 12.5 | 8.0 | 4.9 | 10.6 | 23.7 | 21.7 | 25.5 | |
| 65+ | 2.7 | 2.2 | 3.0 | 1.1 | 1.0 | 1.2 | 13.1 | 11.1 | 14.4 | 8.4 | 5.0 | 11.0 | 5.0 | 7.1 | 3.5 | 44.7 | 30.5 | 55.0 | |
| TOTAL | 253.5 | 97.0 | 403.4 | 104.9 | 34.0 | 172.9 | 1,030.4 | 451.3 | 1,553.6 | 407.9 | 148.4 | 673.9 | 144.6 | 54.1 | 227.8 | 584.6 | 178.3 | 977.3 | |

Note: These tables should be used only for race/ethnicity and age comparisons, not for overall totals or gender totals. This is because, if age or race/ethnicity was not specified, cases were prorated according to the distribution of cases for which these variables were specified. For the following years the states listed did not report race/ethnicity for most cases and were excluded: 1996 (Colorado, Delaware, Georgia, Maryland, Michigan, New Jersey, New York, Ohio and South Carolina); 1997 (Colorado, Delaware, District of Columbia, Georgia, Maryland, Michigan, Mississippi, New Jersey, New York, Ohio and South Carolina); 1998 (Colorado, District of Columbia, Michigan, New Jersey, New York, Ohio and South Carolina); 1999 (Colorado, District of Columbia, Michigan, New Jersey and New York). Cases and population denominators have been excluded for these states/areas. Differences between total cases from this table and others in the report are due to different reporting forms and above listed exclusions. The 0 to 9 year age group is not shown because some of these may not be due to sexual transmission; however, they are included in the totals.

*Source*: Centers for Disease Control and Prevention, U.S. Department of Health and Human Services. National Center for HIV, STD, and TB Prevention, Division of STD Prevention. *Sexually Transmitted Disease Surveillance 1999* (Atlanta, GA: CDC, 2000). http://www.cdc.gov/nchstp/dstd/Stats_Trends/1999Surveillance/99PDF/Surv99Master.pdf.

## Table D3.3. Chlamydia—Reported Cases and Rates, by State/Area, Ranked according to Rates: United States and Outlying Areas, 1999

| Rank | State/Area | Cases | Rate per 100,000 Population |
|---|---|---|---|
| 1 | South Carolina | 18,499 | 482.3 |
| 2 | Mississippi | 11,545 | 419.5 |
| 3 | Georgia | 30,368 | 397.4 |
| 4 | Louisiana | 16,635 | 380.8 |
| 5 | Delaware | 2,761 | 371.3 |
| 6 | New York[1] | 26,766 | 360.7 |
| 7 | Texas | 62,958 | 318.6 |
| 8 | Guam | 497 | 311.0 |
| 9 | Alaska | 1,886 | 307.2 |
| 10 | North Carolina | 21,812 | 289.0 |
| 11 | New Mexico | 5,017 | 288.8 |
| 12 | Alabama | 12,375 | 284.4 |
| 13 | Wisconsin | 14,462 | 276.9 |
| 14 | Colorado | 10,848 | 273.2 |
| 15 | Illinois | 32,870 | 272.9 |
| 16 | Hawaii | 3,165 | 265.3 |
| 17 | Maryland | 13,568 | 264.2 |
| 18 | Ohio | 29,398 | 262.3 |
| 19 | Tennessee | 14,216 | 261.8 |
| 20 | California | 85,156 | 260.7 |
| 21 | Arizona | 12,111 | 259.4 |
| | **U.S. TOTAL[2]** | **659,441** | **254.1** |
| 22 | Missouri | 13,355 | 245.6 |
| 23 | Oklahoma | 8,195 | 244.9 |
| 24 | Rhode Island | 2,345 | 237.2 |
| 25 | Michigan | 23,107 | 235.4 |
| 26 | Kansas | 6,093 | 231.8 |
| 27 | Arkansas | 5,865 | 231.1 |
| 28 | Connecticut | 7,422 | 226.7 |
| 29 | Pennsylvania | 27,019 | 225.1 |
| 30 | Nebraska | 3,616 | 217.5 |
| 31 | Florida | 31,743 | 212.8 |
| 32 | Washington | 11,964 | 210.3 |
| 33 | South Dakota | 1,544 | 209.2 |
| 34 | Virginia | 13,735 | 202.2 |
| 35 | Indiana | 11,734 | 198.9 |
| 36 | Iowa | 5,511 | 192.5 |
| 37 | Kentucky | 7,378 | 187.4 |
| 38 | Oregon | 6,127 | 186.7 |
| 39 | Montana | 1,584 | 179.9 |
| 40 | Nevada | 3,086 | 176.7 |
| 41 | Wyoming | 787 | 163.6 |
| 42 | Minnesota | 7,450 | 157.7 |
| 43 | New Jersey | 12,424 | 153.1 |
| 44 | North Dakota | 947 | 148.4 |
| 45 | Idaho | 1,778 | 144.7 |
| 46 | Massachusetts | 8,776 | 142.8 |
| 47 | Virgin Islands | 136 | 124.0 |
| 48 | Utah | 2,219 | 105.7 |
| 49 | West Virginia | 1,820 | 100.5 |
| 50 | Maine | 1,220 | 98.1 |
| 51 | New Hampshire | 976 | 82.4 |
| 52 | Vermont | 485 | 82.1 |
| 53 | Puerto Rico | 1,445 | 37.4 |

[1]New York's cases and rate are based on New York City. No cases were reported outside of New York City.

[2]Includes cases reported by Washington, D.C., but exclude outlying areas (Guam, Puerto Rico and Virgin Islands).

*Source*: Centers for Disease Control and Prevention, U.S. Department of Health and Human Services. National Center for HIV, STD, and TB Prevention, Division of STD Prevention. *Sexually Transmitted Disease Surveillance 1999* (Atlanta, GA: CDC, 2000). http://www.cdc.gov/nchstp/dstd/Stats_Trends/1999Surveillance/99PDF/Surv99Master.pdf.

## Table D3.4. Chlamydia—Reported Cases and Rates, by State/Area and Region Listed in Alphabetical Order: United States and Outlying Areas, 1995–1999

| | Cases* | | | | | Rates per 100,000 Population | | | | |
|---|---|---|---|---|---|---|---|---|---|---|
| *State/Area* | *1995* | *1996* | *1997* | *1998* | *1999* | *1995* | *1996* | *1997* | *1998* | *1999* |
| Alabama | 3,188 | 8,306 | 8,704 | 10,065 | 12,375 | 75.0 | 193.7 | 201.5 | 231.3 | 284.4 |
| Alaska | NR | 1,360 | 1,616 | 1,907 | 1,886 | | 224.8 | 265.2 | 310.6 | 307.2 |
| Arizona | 10,061 | 10,692 | 10,783 | 11,489 | 12,111 | 238.5 | 241.1 | 236.7 | 246.1 | 259.4 |
| Arkansas | 680 | 2,111 | 2,503 | 4,123 | 5,865 | 27.4 | 84.2 | 99.2 | 162.4 | 231.1 |
| California | 61,802 | 61,593 | 68,737 | 76,519 | 85,156 | 195.6 | 193.3 | 213.0 | 234.2 | 260.7 |
| Colorado | 6,650 | 7,282 | 7,749 | 9,113 | 10,848 | 177.5 | 190.8 | 199.1 | 229.5 | 273.2 |
| Connecticut | 6,440 | 6,269 | 6,377 | 6,977 | 7,422 | 196.7 | 191.9 | 195.0 | 213.1 | 226.7 |
| Delaware | 2,701 | 2,271 | 2,613 | 2,608 | 2,761 | 376.6 | 313.9 | 357.2 | 350.7 | 371.3 |
| Florida | 22,294 | 24,763 | 26,788 | 24,949 | 31,743 | 157.4 | 171.7 | 182.8 | 167.3 | 212.8 |
| Georgia | 11,193 | 13,555 | 15,911 | 25,250 | 30,368 | 155.4 | 184.8 | 212.5 | 330.4 | 397.4 |
| Hawaii | 2,135 | 1,816 | 1,829 | 2,604 | 3,165 | 179.9 | 153.5 | 154.1 | 218.3 | 265.3 |
| Idaho | 1,739 | 1,524 | 1,709 | 2,035 | 1,778 | 149.5 | 128.3 | 141.2 | 165.6 | 144.7 |
| Illinois | 24,645 | 24,430 | 23,024 | 26,363 | 32,870 | 208.3 | 206.2 | 193.5 | 218.9 | 272.9 |
| Indiana | 9,102 | 10,334 | 9,600 | 10,801 | 11,734 | 156.8 | 177.3 | 163.7 | 183.1 | 198.9 |
| Iowa | 5,089 | 4,165 | 4,907 | 5,174 | 5,511 | 179.1 | 146.2 | 172.0 | 180.8 | 192.5 |
| Kansas | 5,314 | 4,449 | 4,627 | 5,587 | 6,093 | 207.1 | 172.5 | 178.3 | 212.5 | 231.8 |
| Kentucky | 6,904 | 6,805 | 6,332 | 6,441 | 7,378 | 178.9 | 175.3 | 162.0 | 163.6 | 187.4 |
| Louisiana | 9,111 | 11,020 | 11,545 | 15,188 | 16,635 | 209.8 | 253.9 | 265.3 | 347.6 | 380.8 |
| Maine | 1,144 | 967 | 1,066 | 1,073 | 1,220 | 92.2 | 78.1 | 85.8 | 86.2 | 98.1 |
| Maryland | 10,378 | 11,901 | 13,978 | 13,097 | 13,568 | 205.8 | 235.2 | 274.4 | 255.1 | 264.2 |
| Massachusetts | 7,402 | 6,837 | 7,984 | 8,363 | 8,776 | 121.9 | 112.4 | 130.5 | 136.0 | 142.8 |
| Michigan | 21,666 | 19,865 | 21,399 | 22,156 | 23,107 | 226.9 | 204.1 | 218.9 | 225.7 | 235.4 |
| Minnesota | 6,032 | 5,607 | 6,631 | 6,970 | 7,450 | 130.9 | 120.6 | 141.5 | 147.5 | 157.7 |
| Mississippi | 912 | 4,848 | 10,020 | 10,614 | 11,545 | 33.8 | 178.8 | 367.0 | 385.7 | 419.5 |
| Missouri | 12,110 | 11,959 | 12,257 | 12,670 | 13,355 | 227.5 | 223.0 | 226.9 | 233.0 | 245.6 |
| Montana | 1,198 | 1,124 | 1,146 | 1,412 | 1,584 | 137.7 | 128.2 | 130.4 | 160.4 | 179.9 |
| Nebraska | 2,873 | 2,478 | 2,766 | 2,911 | 3,616 | 175.5 | 150.3 | 166.9 | 175.1 | 217.5 |
| Nevada | 3,049 | 2,847 | 2,887 | 3,320 | 3,086 | 199.3 | 177.8 | 172.2 | 190.1 | 176.7 |
| New Hampshire | 898 | 732 | 816 | 960 | 976 | 78.2 | 63.1 | 69.6 | 81.0 | 82.4 |
| New Jersey | 4,056 | 12,273 | 10,339 | 11,686 | 12,424 | 51.0 | 153.4 | 128.4 | 144.0 | 153.1 |
| New Mexico | 4,285 | 4,007 | 4,021 | 3,793 | 5,017 | 254.2 | 234.2 | 232.5 | 218.4 | 288.8 |
| New York[1] | 26,686 | 26,455 | 28,468 | 26,218 | 26,766 | 365.0 | 360.7 | 387.7 | 353.3 | 360.7 |
| North Carolina | 15,780 | 15,078 | 17,108 | 22,197 | 21,812 | 219.3 | 206.3 | 230.4 | 294.1 | 289.0 |
| North Dakota | 1,324 | 1,016 | 902 | 1,036 | 947 | 206.4 | 158.1 | 140.7 | 162.3 | 148.4 |
| Ohio | 29,124 | 20,653 | 22,827 | 27,786 | 29,398 | 261.2 | 185.0 | 204.1 | 247.9 | 262.3 |
| Oklahoma | 5,065 | 7,379 | 7,419 | 9,393 | 8,195 | 154.5 | 223.9 | 223.7 | 280.7 | 244.9 |
| Oregon | 5,465 | 5,457 | 5,270 | 5,855 | 6,127 | 174.0 | 170.7 | 162.5 | 178.4 | 186.7 |
| Pennsylvania | 22,961 | 19,275 | 19,838 | 24,629 | 27,019 | 190.2 | 160.1 | 165.0 | 205.2 | 225.1 |
| Rhode Island | 1,902 | 1,833 | 2,069 | 2,307 | 2,345 | 192.2 | 185.5 | 209.5 | 233.4 | 237.2 |
| South Carolina | 8,591 | 9,391 | 12,511 | 18,510 | 18,499 | 233.9 | 252.7 | 332.7 | 482.5 | 482.3 |
| South Dakota | 1,313 | 1,538 | 1,439 | 1,572 | 1,544 | 180.1 | 208.5 | 195.0 | 213.0 | 209.2 |
| Tennessee | 13,154 | 13,125 | 12,502 | 13,717 | 14,216 | 250.3 | 247.3 | 232.9 | 252.6 | 261.8 |
| Texas | 44,627 | 43,003 | 50,675 | 60,436 | 62,958 | 238.3 | 225.3 | 260.7 | 305.9 | 318.6 |
| Utah | 1,676 | 1,598 | 1,774 | 2,209 | 2,219 | 85.9 | 79.2 | 86.2 | 105.2 | 105.7 |
| Vermont | 462 | 398 | 434 | 413 | 485 | 79.0 | 67.9 | 73.7 | 69.9 | 82.1 |
| Virginia | 12,285 | 11,756 | 11,955 | 13,561 | 13,735 | 185.6 | 176.4 | 177.5 | 199.7 | 202.2 |
| Washington | 9,462 | 9,236 | 9,523 | 10,998 | 11,964 | 174.2 | 167.3 | 169.7 | 193.3 | 210.3 |
| West Virginia | 2,326 | 2,325 | 3,108 | 2,791 | 1,820 | 127.2 | 127.7 | 171.2 | 154.1 | 100.5 |
| Wisconsin | 8,955 | 10,290 | 9,554 | 13,999 | 14,462 | 174.8 | 200.0 | 184.8 | 268.0 | 276.9 |
| Wyoming | 703 | 621 | 635 | 725 | 787 | 146.4 | 129.4 | 132.4 | 150.8 | 163.6 |
| U.S. TOTAL[2] | 478,577 | 490,615 | 531,744 | 607,752 | 659,441 | 190.4 | 192.9 | 207.0 | 234.2 | 254.1 |
| Northeast | 71,951 | 75,039 | 77,391 | 82,626 | 87,433 | 177.0 | 184.4 | 189.7 | 201.7 | 213.4 |
| Midwest | 127,547 | 116,784 | 119,933 | 137,025 | 150,087 | 206.4 | 187.8 | 192.0 | 217.9 | 238.7 |
| South | 170,854 | 189,635 | 216,741 | 256,122 | 276,193 | 185.9 | 203.9 | 230.1 | 268.4 | 289.4 |
| West | 108,225 | 109,157 | 117,679 | 131,979 | 145,728 | 189.9 | 186.6 | 198.1 | 219.0 | 241.8 |
| Guam | 461 | 304 | 368 | 410 | 497 | 308.9 | 199.1 | 235.6 | 256.5 | 311.0 |
| Puerto Rico | 2,305 | 2,481 | 2,123 | 1,685 | 1,445 | 62.4 | 66.7 | 55.5 | 43.7 | 37.4 |
| Virgin Islands | 17 | 11 | 14 | 10 | 136 | 15.5 | 10.0 | 12.8 | 9.1 | 124.0 |
| OUTLYING AREAS | 2,783 | 2,796 | 2,505 | 2,105 | 2,078 | 70.4 | 70.2 | 61.2 | 51.0 | 50.3 |
| TOTAL | 481,360 | 493,411 | 534,249 | 609,857 | 661,519 | 188.6 | 191.0 | 204.7 | 231.3 | 250.9 |

*NR = No report (see Appendix).

[1]New York's cases and rate are based on New York City. No cases were reported outside of New York City.

[2]Includes cases reported by Washington, D.C., and rates exclude population of states that did not report.

*Source*: Centers for Disease Control and Prevention, U.S. Department of Health and Human Services. National Center for HIV, STD, and TB Prevention, Division of STD Prevention. *Sexually Transmitted Disease Surveillance 1999* (Atlanta, GA: CDC, 2000). http://www.cdc.gov/nchstp/dstd/Stats_Trends/1999Surveillance/99PDF/Surv99Master.pdf.

# Table D3.5. Chlamydia—Reported Cases among Women per 100,000 Female Population, United States, 1999

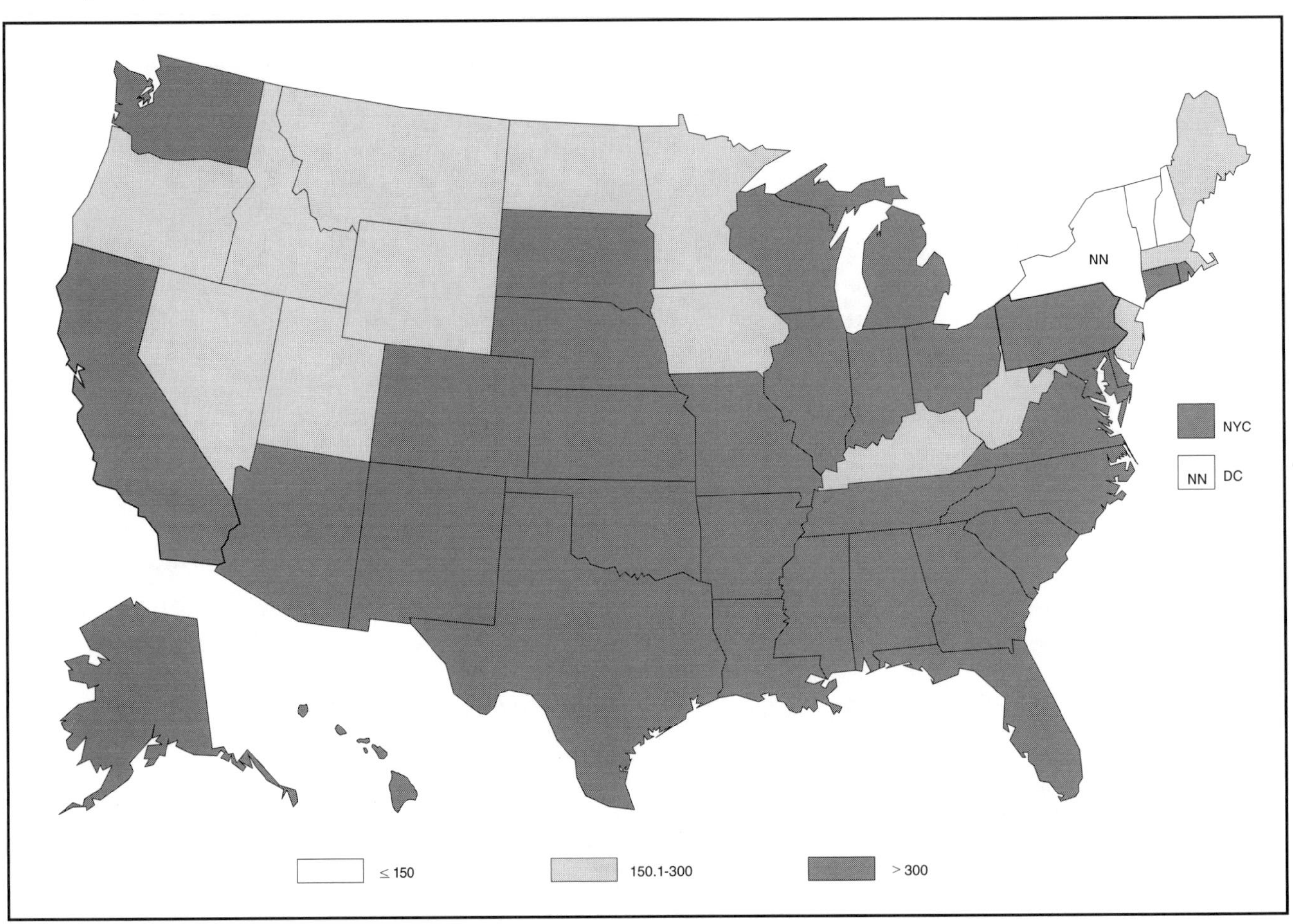


Chlamydia refers to genital infections caused by *Chlamydia trachomatis*. In 1999, the chlamydia rate among women was 400.99 cases/100,000 population. Rates for men are not presented because reporting for men is limited.

*Source*: Center for Disease Control and Prevention. U.S. Department of Health and Human Services. *MMWR: Morbidity and Mortality Weekly Review Summary of Notifiable Disease, United States, 1999* 48 no. 53 (2001). http://www.cdc.gov/mmwr/PDF/wk/mm4853.pdf.

**Table D3.6. Chlamydia—Women—Reported Cases and Rates, by State/Area Listed in Alphabetical Order: United States and Outlying Areas, 1995–1999**

| | Cases* | | | | | Rates per 100,000 Population | | | | |
|---|---|---|---|---|---|---|---|---|---|---|
| State/Area | 1995 | 1996 | 1997 | 1998 | 1999 | 1995 | 1996 | 1997 | 1998 | 1999 |
| Alabama | 2,888 | 7,623 | 7,957 | 9,197 | 11,524 | 130.5 | 342.4 | 354.9 | 406.2 | 509.0 |
| Alaska | NR | 1,071 | 1,291 | 1,479 | 1,456 | | 373.4 | 446.6 | 506.9 | 499.0 |
| Arizona | 8,315 | 8,635 | 8,597 | 9,015 | 9,497 | 389.8 | 385.9 | 374.3 | 382.0 | 402.5 |
| Arkansas | 596 | 1,933 | 2,346 | 3,850 | 4,618 | 46.4 | 149.4 | 180.3 | 293.4 | 351.9 |
| California | 50,314 | 49,158 | 53,536 | 59,747 | 66,334 | 318.6 | 309.1 | 332.4 | 365.6 | 405.9 |
| Colorado | NG | 5,692 | 5,958 | 6,979 | 8,172 | | 295.9 | 303.8 | 348.5 | 408.0 |
| Connecticut | 5,624 | 5,321 | 5,282 | 5,828 | 6,053 | 333.2 | 316.8 | 314.4 | 345.8 | 359.1 |
| Delaware | 2,295 | 1,877 | 2,070 | 2,117 | 2,268 | 623.4 | 506.0 | 551.9 | 554.2 | 593.7 |
| Florida | 18,251 | 20,160 | 21,953 | 20,171 | 26,231 | 249.9 | 271.8 | 291.5 | 262.7 | 341.6 |
| Georgia | 10,263 | 11,744 | 13,927 | 21,156 | 24,685 | 277.4 | 312.3 | 363.1 | 539.2 | 629.1 |
| Hawaii | 1,878 | 1,568 | 1,548 | 2,209 | 2,557 | 320.2 | 267.5 | 262.4 | 371.4 | 429.9 |
| Idaho | 1,370 | 1,177 | 1,336 | 1,553 | 1,308 | 235.1 | 198.1 | 220.8 | 252.3 | 212.5 |
| Illinois | 20,443 | 21,111 | 17,302 | 21,845 | 25,593 | 336.6 | 348.2 | 284.4 | 353.9 | 414.7 |
| Indiana | 7,564 | 8,592 | 7,819 | 8,823 | 9,410 | 253.5 | 287.5 | 260.2 | 291.3 | 310.7 |
| Iowa | 4,210 | 3,443 | 3,900 | 4,077 | 4,208 | 288.4 | 235.9 | 267.0 | 277.6 | 286.5 |
| Kansas | 4,453 | 3,744 | 3,840 | 4,649 | 5,034 | 341.6 | 285.8 | 291.5 | 347.8 | 376.6 |
| Kentucky | 5,995 | 5,604 | 5,128 | 5,126 | 5,891 | 301.4 | 280.8 | 255.3 | 253.0 | 290.7 |
| Louisiana | 7,569 | 9,490 | 9,414 | 12,169 | 13,247 | 335.8 | 422.0 | 417.6 | 536.5 | 584.0 |
| Maine | 1,024 | 829 | 898 | 899 | 991 | 160.7 | 130.8 | 141.4 | 141.0 | 155.4 |
| Maryland | 9,150 | 10,249 | 12,180 | 11,093 | 11,351 | 352.9 | 394.6 | 466.0 | 420.2 | 429.9 |
| Massachusetts | 6,237 | 5,783 | 6,522 | 6,812 | 6,959 | 198.1 | 183.7 | 206.2 | 214.0 | 218.6 |
| Michigan | 18,750 | 16,851 | 18,289 | 18,769 | 18,869 | 382.3 | 337.7 | 365.1 | 372.4 | 374.3 |
| Minnesota | 4,681 | 4,328 | 4,953 | 5,119 | 5,469 | 199.9 | 183.7 | 208.7 | 213.5 | 228.1 |
| Mississippi | 849 | 4,100 | 8,590 | 9,185 | 9,953 | 60.5 | 291.0 | 605.6 | 640.9 | 694.5 |
| Missouri | 10,866 | 10,578 | 10,749 | 11,063 | 11,515 | 395.0 | 382.7 | 386.5 | 394.4 | 410.5 |
| Montana | 995 | 899 | 941 | 1,131 | 1,192 | 227.5 | 204.4 | 213.5 | 255.4 | 269.2 |
| Nebraska | 2,346 | 2,020 | 2,288 | 2,390 | 2,903 | 280.2 | 240.2 | 270.9 | 281.4 | 341.8 |
| Nevada | 2,649 | 2,463 | 2,484 | 2,820 | 2,500 | 352.6 | 313.9 | 302.3 | 328.8 | 291.4 |
| New Hampshire | 725 | 578 | 639 | 726 | 769 | 124.0 | 98.1 | 107.4 | 120.6 | 127.7 |
| New Jersey | 3,902 | 11,463 | 9,641 | 10,735 | 11,123 | 95.2 | 278.2 | 232.6 | 256.6 | 265.8 |
| New Mexico | 3,721 | 3,417 | 3,503 | 3,204 | 4,177 | 435.2 | 394.1 | 399.5 | 363.1 | 473.4 |
| New York[1] | 24,600 | 24,375 | 25,706 | 23,449 | 23,896 | 635.4 | 628.7 | 662.8 | 596.4 | 607.8 |
| North Carolina | 13,589 | 13,072 | 14,553 | 18,646 | 18,416 | 366.8 | 347.9 | 381.5 | 479.8 | 473.9 |
| North Dakota | 1,025 | 714 | 684 | 755 | 680 | 318.6 | 221.9 | 212.9 | 235.5 | 212.1 |
| Ohio | 24,883 | 18,050 | 19,727 | 23,248 | 23,380 | 431.6 | 313.4 | 342.0 | 401.4 | 403.7 |
| Oklahoma | 4,467 | 6,269 | 6,269 | 7,696 | 6,737 | 266.2 | 372.4 | 370.1 | 449.4 | 393.4 |
| Oregon | 4,145 | 4,095 | 3,848 | 4,307 | 4,462 | 260.4 | 253.3 | 234.8 | 259.3 | 268.6 |
| Pennsylvania | 20,290 | 17,227 | 17,257 | 20,878 | 22,470 | 323.5 | 275.9 | 277.0 | 335.0 | 360.6 |
| Rhode Island | 1,598 | 1,600 | 1,738 | 1,779 | 1,769 | 310.8 | 312.0 | 339.4 | 346.5 | 344.6 |
| South Carolina | 6,932 | 7,918 | 11,120 | 16,489 | 16,669 | 364.8 | 412.2 | 572.2 | 829.7 | 838.8 |
| South Dakota | 1,039 | 1,184 | 1,021 | 1,171 | 1,194 | 280.8 | 316.6 | 272.9 | 312.2 | 318.4 |
| Tennessee | 10,517 | 10,004 | 9,605 | 10,552 | 11,084 | 386.5 | 365.0 | 346.4 | 375.5 | 394.4 |
| Texas | 38,517 | 37,240 | 42,750 | 49,940 | 52,071 | 405.9 | 385.6 | 435.0 | 498.7 | 520.0 |
| Utah | 1,316 | 1,229 | 1,357 | 1,616 | 1,618 | 134.2 | 121.4 | 131.3 | 153.0 | 153.2 |
| Vermont | 408 | 336 | 379 | 357 | 414 | 137.2 | 112.9 | 126.9 | 118.9 | 137.8 |
| Virginia | 11,253 | 10,630 | 10,452 | 11,567 | 11,556 | 333.0 | 312.7 | 304.2 | 332.9 | 332.6 |
| Washington | 7,508 | 7,194 | 7,331 | 8,377 | 8,880 | 274.6 | 259.7 | 260.5 | 292.8 | 310.4 |
| West Virginia | 1,961 | 1,894 | 2,590 | 2,340 | 1,585 | 206.9 | 201.1 | 275.8 | 249.3 | 168.9 |
| Wisconsin | 6,860 | 8,170 | 7,459 | 10,846 | 11,225 | 262.9 | 312.5 | 284.2 | 408.2 | 422.5 |
| Wyoming | 560 | 521 | 536 | 595 | 649 | 234.7 | 218.6 | 225.1 | 248.8 | 271.4 |
| U.S. TOTAL[2] | 400,840 | 414,987 | 441,921 | 501,266 | 537,003 | 316.3 | 319.4 | 337.1 | 377.6 | 404.5 |
| Guam | 393 | 260 | 325 | 351 | 432 | 560.3 | 362.3 | 442.6 | 467.3 | 575.1 |
| Puerto Rico | 1,905 | 1,989 | 1,722 | 1,327 | 1,147 | 99.8 | 103.4 | 86.5 | 66.1 | 57.1 |
| Virgin Islands | 9 | 11 | 13 | 10 | 113 | 15.8 | 19.3 | 22.8 | 17.4 | 196.2 |
| OUTLYING AREAS | 2,307 | 2,260 | 2,060 | 1,688 | 1,692 | 113.3 | 110.1 | 97.1 | 78.9 | 79.1 |
| TOTAL | 403,147 | 417,247 | 443,981 | 502,954 | 538,695 | 313.1 | 316.2 | 333.3 | 372.9 | 399.4 |

*NR = No report (see Appendix). NG = Not reported by gender.

[1]New York's cases and rate are based on New York City. No cases were reported outside of New York City.

[2]Includes cases reported by Washington, D.C., and rates exclude population of states that did not report.

Note: Cases and rates underestimated in some areas because of under-reporting or non-reporting by gender.

*Source*: Centers for Disease Control and Prevention, U.S. Department of Health and Human Services. National Center for HIV, STD, and TB Prevention, Division of STD Prevention. *Sexually Transmitted Disease Surveillance 1999* (Atlanta, GA: CDC, 2000). http://www.cdc.gov /nchstp/dstd/Stats_Trends/ 1999Surveillance/99PDF/Surv99Master.pdf.

## Table D3.7. Chlamydia—Men—Reported Cases and Rates, by State/Area Listed in Alphabetical Order: United States and Outlying Areas, 1995–1999

| State/Area | Cases* 1995 | Cases* 1996 | Cases* 1997 | Cases* 1998 | Cases* 1999 | Rates per 100,000 Population 1995 | Rates 1996 | Rates 1997 | Rates 1998 | Rates 1999 |
|---|---|---|---|---|---|---|---|---|---|---|
| Alabama | 285 | 662 | 708 | 844 | 795 | 14.0 | 32.1 | 34.1 | 40.4 | 38.1 |
| Alaska | NR | 289 | 325 | 428 | 430 | | 90.8 | 101.5 | 132.8 | 133.4 |
| Arizona | 1,746 | 2,057 | 2,186 | 2,474 | 2,614 | 83.7 | 93.6 | 96.8 | 107.1 | 113.2 |
| Arkansas | 79 | 178 | 143 | 267 | 1,247 | 6.6 | 14.7 | 11.7 | 21.8 | 101.7 |
| California | 11,248 | 12,157 | 14,875 | 16,525 | 18,236 | 71.2 | 76.2 | 92.0 | 101.2 | 111.7 |
| Colorado | NG | 1,585 | 1,784 | 2,115 | 2,666 | | 83.7 | 92.4 | 107.5 | 135.5 |
| Connecticut | 816 | 948 | 1,095 | 1,149 | 1,369 | 51.4 | 59.7 | 68.9 | 72.3 | 86.2 |
| Delaware | 406 | 394 | 543 | 491 | 493 | 116.3 | 111.8 | 152.3 | 135.8 | 136.3 |
| Florida | 4,043 | 4,603 | 4,835 | 4,363 | 5,384 | 58.9 | 65.7 | 67.9 | 60.3 | 74.4 |
| Georgia | 930 | 1,811 | 1,962 | 3,932 | 5,462 | 26.6 | 50.7 | 53.7 | 105.7 | 146.9 |
| Hawaii | 257 | 248 | 281 | 395 | 583 | 42.8 | 41.6 | 47.1 | 66.0 | 97.5 |
| Idaho | 369 | 347 | 373 | 482 | 446 | 63.6 | 58.5 | 61.6 | 78.6 | 72.7 |
| Illinois | 4,202 | 3,319 | 5,722 | 4,518 | 7,263 | 73.0 | 57.4 | 98.5 | 76.9 | 123.7 |
| Indiana | 1,537 | 1,742 | 1,773 | 1,968 | 2,313 | 54.5 | 61.3 | 62.0 | 68.6 | 80.6 |
| Iowa | 879 | 722 | 1,007 | 1,096 | 1,302 | 63.6 | 52.0 | 72.4 | 78.6 | 93.4 |
| Kansas | 860 | 705 | 787 | 938 | 1,059 | 68.2 | 55.5 | 61.6 | 72.6 | 81.9 |
| Kentucky | 909 | 1,201 | 1,182 | 1,093 | 1,328 | 48.6 | 63.7 | 62.2 | 57.2 | 69.5 |
| Louisiana | 1,542 | 1,530 | 2,131 | 3,019 | 3,388 | 73.8 | 73.1 | 101.6 | 143.7 | 161.3 |
| Maine | 120 | 138 | 168 | 174 | 229 | 19.9 | 22.8 | 27.7 | 28.7 | 37.8 |
| Maryland | 1,228 | 1,652 | 1,798 | 1,973 | 2,196 | 50.1 | 67.1 | 72.5 | 79.1 | 88.0 |
| Massachusetts | 1,165 | 1,054 | 1,462 | 1,551 | 1,817 | 39.8 | 35.9 | 49.5 | 52.3 | 61.3 |
| Michigan | 2,916 | 3,014 | 3,110 | 3,387 | 4,237 | 62.8 | 63.6 | 65.3 | 70.9 | 88.7 |
| Minnesota | 1,351 | 1,279 | 1,678 | 1,851 | 1,981 | 59.6 | 55.8 | 72.6 | 79.5 | 85.1 |
| Mississippi | 63 | 703 | 1,180 | 1,355 | 1,450 | 4.9 | 54.0 | 89.9 | 102.7 | 109.9 |
| Missouri | 1,244 | 1,381 | 1,508 | 1,607 | 1,840 | 48.4 | 53.1 | 57.5 | 61.0 | 69.9 |
| Montana | 203 | 180 | 198 | 281 | 392 | 46.9 | 41.2 | 45.2 | 64.2 | 89.6 |
| Nebraska | 526 | 452 | 473 | 520 | 712 | 65.8 | 56.0 | 58.2 | 63.9 | 87.5 |
| Nevada | 400 | 384 | 403 | 498 | 586 | 51.4 | 47.0 | 47.1 | 56.0 | 65.9 |
| New Hampshire | 173 | 154 | 177 | 234 | 207 | 30.7 | 27.0 | 30.6 | 40.1 | 35.5 |
| New Jersey | 154 | 801 | 689 | 944 | 1,281 | 4.0 | 20.6 | 17.6 | 24.0 | 32.6 |
| New Mexico | 564 | 590 | 518 | 589 | 839 | 67.9 | 69.9 | 60.7 | 68.9 | 98.2 |
| New York[1] | 2,086 | 2,080 | 2,762 | 2,669 | 2,846 | 60.6 | 60.2 | 79.7 | 76.5 | 81.6 |
| North Carolina | 2,191 | 2,006 | 2,555 | 3,551 | 3,396 | 62.8 | 56.5 | 70.8 | 97.0 | 92.8 |
| North Dakota | 299 | 302 | 218 | 281 | 267 | 93.5 | 94.1 | 68.2 | 88.5 | 84.1 |
| Ohio | 4,048 | 2,405 | 2,884 | 4,211 | 5,604 | 75.2 | 44.5 | 53.2 | 77.7 | 103.4 |
| Oklahoma | 598 | 1,110 | 1,150 | 1,697 | 1,458 | 37.4 | 68.9 | 70.8 | 103.8 | 89.2 |
| Oregon | 1,320 | 1,362 | 1,422 | 1,548 | 1,665 | 85.2 | 86.2 | 88.6 | 95.5 | 102.7 |
| Pennsylvania | 2,671 | 2,048 | 2,581 | 3,751 | 4,549 | 46.1 | 35.3 | 44.6 | 65.0 | 78.8 |
| Rhode Island | 304 | 233 | 331 | 528 | 576 | 63.9 | 49.0 | 69.6 | 111.1 | 121.2 |
| South Carolina | 813 | 881 | 1,215 | 1,837 | 1,679 | 45.9 | 49.1 | 66.9 | 99.4 | 90.8 |
| South Dakota | 274 | 354 | 417 | 400 | 348 | 76.3 | 97.4 | 114.6 | 110.2 | 95.8 |
| Tennessee | 2,637 | 3,121 | 2,897 | 3,165 | 3,132 | 104.0 | 121.6 | 111.6 | 120.8 | 119.5 |
| Texas | 6,110 | 5,763 | 7,925 | 10,301 | 10,597 | 66.2 | 61.1 | 82.5 | 105.7 | 108.7 |
| Utah | 360 | 368 | 417 | 593 | 601 | 37.1 | 36.6 | 40.7 | 56.8 | 57.6 |
| Vermont | 54 | 62 | 55 | 56 | 71 | 18.8 | 21.5 | 19.0 | 19.3 | 24.4 |
| Virginia | 989 | 1,109 | 1,379 | 1,988 | 2,177 | 30.5 | 33.9 | 41.8 | 59.9 | 65.6 |
| Washington | 1,954 | 2,042 | 2,192 | 2,621 | 3,084 | 72.5 | 74.3 | 78.4 | 92.7 | 109.0 |
| West Virginia | 359 | 429 | 515 | 448 | 233 | 40.8 | 48.8 | 58.7 | 51.3 | 26.7 |
| Wisconsin | 2,095 | 2,120 | 2,095 | 3,144 | 3,212 | 83.3 | 83.7 | 82.3 | 122.5 | 125.1 |
| Wyoming | 143 | 100 | 99 | 130 | 138 | 59.2 | 41.4 | 41.0 | 53.8 | 57.1 |
| U.S. TOTAL[2] | 69,736 | 74,409 | 88,594 | 104,440 | 120,094 | 57.7 | 59.8 | 70.5 | 82.4 | 94.7 |
| Guam | 68 | 44 | 43 | 59 | 65 | 86.0 | 54.4 | 51.9 | 69.7 | 76.7 |
| Puerto Rico | 400 | 492 | 401 | 358 | 298 | 22.4 | 27.4 | 21.8 | 19.3 | 16.1 |
| Virgin Islands | 8 | NR | 1 | NR | 23 | 15.2 | | 1.9 | | 43.2 |
| OUTLYING AREAS | 476 | 536 | 445 | 417 | 386 | 24.9 | 28.6 | 22.6 | 21.5 | 19.4 |
| TOTAL | 70,212 | 74,945 | 89,039 | 104,857 | 120,480 | 57.2 | 59.3 | 69.7 | 81.5 | 93.6 |

*NR = No report (see Appendix). NG = Not reported by gender.

[1]New York's cases and rate are based on New York City. No cases were reported outside of New York City.

[2]Includes cases reported by Washington, D.C., and rates exclude population of states that did not report.

Note: Cases and rates underestimated in some areas because of under-reporting or non-reporting by gender.

*Source*: Centers for Disease Control and Prevention, U.S. Department of Health and Human Services. National Center for HIV, STD, and TB Prevention, Division of STD Prevention. *Sexually Transmitted Disease Surveillance 1999* (Atlanta, GA: CDC, 2000). http://www.cdc.gov/nchstp/dstd/Stats_Trends/1999Surveillance/99PDF/Surv99Master.pdf.

## Table D4.1. Gonorrhea—Rates by Region: United States, 1981–1999, and the Healthy People Year 2000 Objective

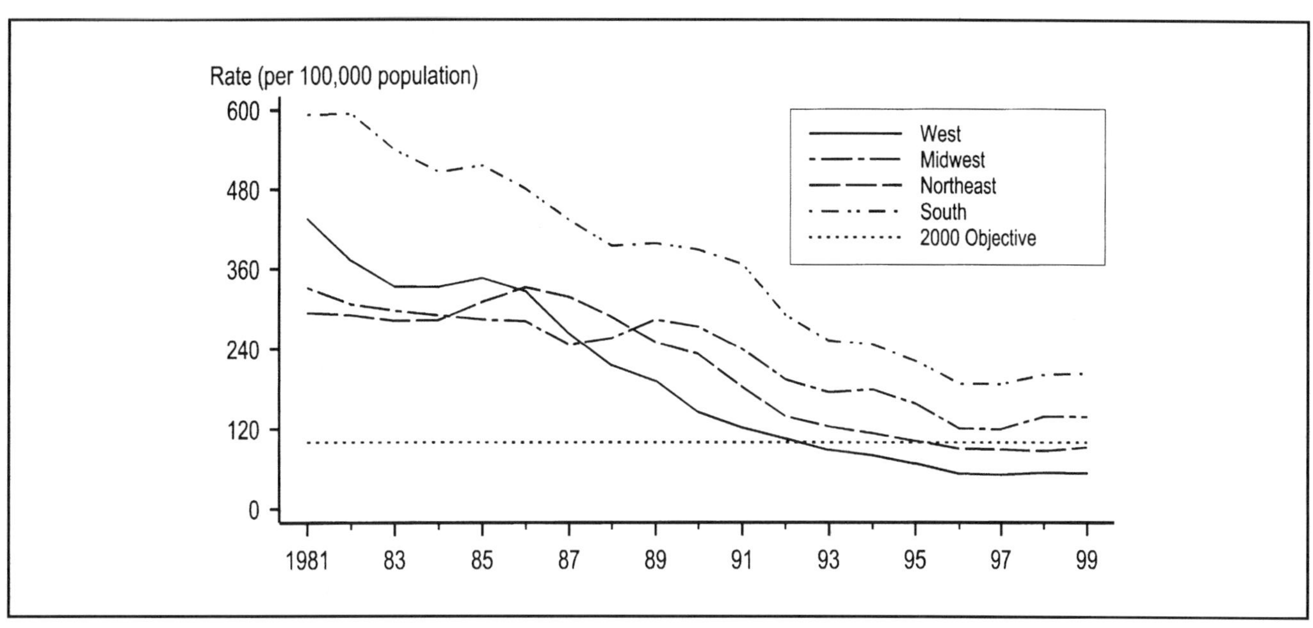


*Source*: Centers for Disease Control and Prevention, U.S. Department of Health and Human Services. National Center for HIV, STD, and TB Prevention, Division of STD Prevention. *Sexually Transmitted Disease Surveillance 1999* (Atlanta, GA: CDC, 2000). http://www.cdc.gov/nchstp/dstd/Stats_Trends/1999Surveillance/99PDF/Surv99Master.pdf.

## Table D4.2. Gonorrhea—Reported Cases per 100,000 Population, United States, 1999

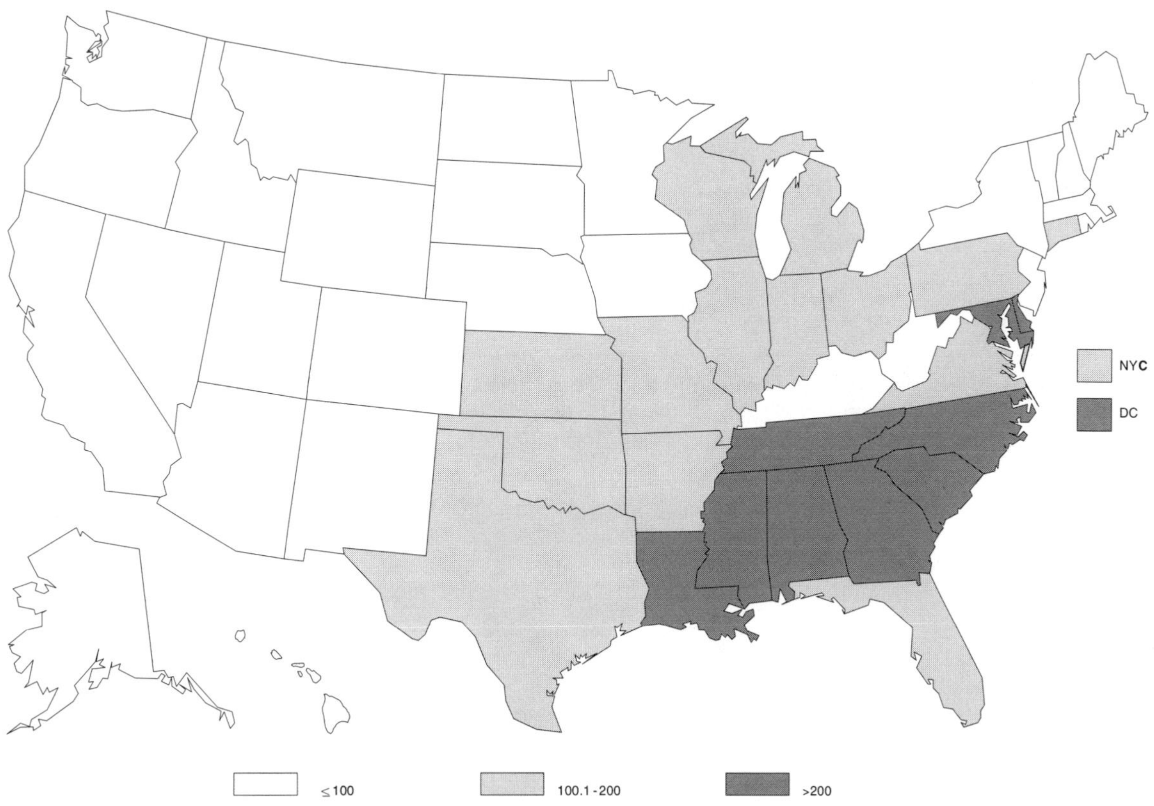

NYC

DC

≤100 100.1-200 >200

In 1999, the overall U.S. rate of gonorrhea was 133.2 cases/100,000 population. Twenty-six states reported gonorrhea rates below the revised *Healthy People 2000* national objective of <100 cases/100,000 population.

*Source*: Center for Disease Control and Prevention. U.S. Department of Health and Human Services. *MMWR: Morbidity and Mortality Weekly Review Summary of Notifiable Disease, United States, 1999* 48 no. 53 (2001). http://www.cdc.gov/mmwr/PDF/wk/mm4853.pdf.

## Table D4.3. Gonorrhea—Reported Cases and Rates, by State/Area, Ranked according to Rates: United States and Outlying Areas, 1999

| Rank | State/Area | Cases | Rate per 100,000 Population |
|---|---|---|---|
| 1 | South Carolina | 15,037 | 392.0 |
| 2 | Mississippi | 10,411 | 378.3 |
| 3 | Louisiana | 13,189 | 301.9 |
| 4 | Georgia | 21,244 | 278.0 |
| 5 | North Carolina | 19,428 | 257.4 |
| 6 | Alabama | 10,888 | 250.2 |
| 7 | Delaware | 1,662 | 223.5 |
| 8 | Tennessee | 11,366 | 209.3 |
| 9 | Maryland | 10,430 | 203.1 |
| 10 | Illinois | 23,254 | 193.1 |
| 11 | Texas | 32,910 | 166.6 |
| 12 | Michigan | 15,907 | 162.0 |
| 13 | Ohio | 18,141 | 161.8 |
| 14 | Florida | 22,939 | 153.8 |
| 15 | Missouri | 8,187 | 150.5 |
| 16 | Virginia | 9,402 | 138.4 |
| | **U.S. TOTAL[1]** | **360,076** | **133.2** |
| 17 | Wisconsin | 6,662 | 127.5 |
| 18 | Arkansas | 3,226 | 127.1 |
| 19 | Oklahoma | 4,021 | 120.1 |
| 20 | Pennsylvania | 13,295 | 110.8 |
| 21 | New York | 19,826 | 109.1 |
| 22 | Indiana | 6,092 | 103.3 |
| 23 | Connecticut | 3,321 | 101.4 |
| 24 | Kansas | 2,665 | 101.4 |
| | **YEAR 2000 OBJECTIVE** | | **100.0** |
| 25 | New Jersey | 7,852 | 96.8 |
| 26 | Arizona | 4,293 | 92.0 |
| 27 | Nebraska | 1,471 | 88.5 |
| 28 | Kentucky | 3,349 | 85.1 |
| 29 | Nevada | 1,303 | 74.6 |
| 30 | Colorado | 2,526 | 63.6 |
| 31 | Rhode Island | 601 | 60.8 |
| 32 | Minnesota | 2,830 | 59.9 |
| 33 | California | 18,672 | 57.2 |
| 34 | New Mexico | 974 | 56.1 |
| 35 | Alaska | 302 | 49.2 |
| 36 | Iowa | 1,365 | 47.7 |
| 37 | Virgin Islands | 51 | 46.5 |
| 38 | Massachusetts | 2,453 | 39.9 |
| 39 | Hawaii | 463 | 38.8 |
| 40 | Washington | 2,132 | 37.5 |
| 41 | Guam | 59 | 36.9 |
| 42 | West Virginia | 584 | 32.2 |
| 43 | Oregon | 903 | 27.5 |
| 44 | South Dakota | 192 | 26.0 |
| 45 | North Dakota | 83 | 13.0 |
| 46 | Utah | 254 | 12.1 |
| 47 | New Hampshire | 115 | 9.7 |
| 48 | Wyoming | 43 | 8.9 |
| 49 | Vermont | 52 | 8.8 |
| 50 | Puerto Rico | 321 | 8.3 |
| 51 | Idaho | 89 | 7.2 |
| 52 | Maine | 83 | 6.7 |
| 53 | Montana | 53 | 6.0 |

[1]Includes cases reported by Washington, D.C., but excludes outlying areas (Guam, Puerto Rico and Virgin Islands).

*Source*: Centers for Disease Control and Prevention, U.S. Department of Health and Human Services. National Center for HIV, STD, and TB Prevention, Division of STD Prevention. *Sexually Transmitted Disease Surveillance 1999* (Atlanta, GA: CDC, 2000). http://www.cdc.gov/nchstp/dstd/Stats_Trends/1999Surveillance/99PDF/Surv99Master.pdf.

## Table D4.4. Gonorrhea—Reported Cases and Rates, by State/Area and Region Listed in Alphabetical Order: United States and Outlying Areas, 1995–1999

| | Cases | | | | | Rates per 100,000 Population | | | | |
|---|---|---|---|---|---|---|---|---|---|---|
| *State/Area* | *1995* | *1996* | *1997* | *1998* | *1999* | *1995* | *1996* | *1997* | *1998* | *1999* |
| Alabama | 14,683 | 13,169 | 12,031 | 12,737 | 10,888 | 345.2 | 307.2 | 278.5 | 292.7 | 250.2 |
| Alaska | 660 | 466 | 391 | 331 | 302 | 109.3 | 77.0 | 64.2 | 53.9 | 49.2 |
| Arizona | 3,844 | 3,709 | 3,802 | 4,213 | 4,293 | 91.1 | 83.6 | 83.5 | 90.2 | 92.0 |
| Arkansas | 5,630 | 5,056 | 4,382 | 3,953 | 3,226 | 226.7 | 201.7 | 173.7 | 155.7 | 127.1 |
| California | 24,606 | 18,674 | 17,979 | 19,590 | 18,672 | 77.9 | 58.6 | 55.7 | 60.0 | 57.2 |
| Colorado | 2,803 | 2,021 | 2,315 | 2,033 | 2,526 | 74.8 | 53.0 | 59.5 | 51.2 | 63.6 |
| Connecticut | 4,055 | 3,388 | 3,154 | 3,177 | 3,321 | 123.8 | 103.7 | 96.5 | 97.0 | 101.4 |
| Delaware | 2,201 | 1,456 | 1,273 | 1,556 | 1,662 | 306.9 | 201.3 | 174.0 | 209.3 | 223.5 |
| Florida | 20,874 | 19,181 | 19,079 | 19,080 | 22,939 | 147.4 | 133.0 | 130.2 | 127.9 | 153.8 |
| Georgia | 21,025 | 19,806 | 18,471 | 20,666 | 21,244 | 292.0 | 270.0 | 246.7 | 270.4 | 278.0 |
| Hawaii | 563 | 497 | 510 | 506 | 463 | 47.4 | 42.0 | 43.0 | 42.4 | 38.8 |
| Idaho | 149 | 98 | 158 | 182 | 89 | 12.8 | 8.3 | 13.1 | 14.8 | 7.2 |
| Illinois | 21,747 | 17,964 | 18,423 | 21,735 | 23,254 | 183.8 | 151.7 | 154.9 | 180.4 | 193.1 |
| Indiana | 8,880 | 6,638 | 6,155 | 6,307 | 6,092 | 153.0 | 113.9 | 105.0 | 106.9 | 103.3 |
| Iowa | 1,723 | 1,145 | 1,311 | 1,616 | 1,365 | 60.6 | 40.2 | 46.0 | 56.5 | 47.7 |
| Kansas | 2,797 | 2,044 | 2,075 | 2,622 | 2,665 | 109.0 | 79.3 | 80.0 | 99.7 | 101.4 |
| Kentucky | 4,751 | 4,229 | 4,027 | 3,813 | 3,349 | 123.1 | 108.9 | 103.0 | 96.9 | 85.1 |
| Louisiana | 9,292 | 9,315 | 10,782 | 12,499 | 13,189 | 214.0 | 214.6 | 247.8 | 286.1 | 301.9 |
| Maine | 94 | 55 | 66 | 67 | 83 | 7.6 | 4.4 | 5.3 | 5.4 | 6.7 |
| Maryland | 12,984 | 11,592 | 11,568 | 11,254 | 10,430 | 257.5 | 229.1 | 227.1 | 219.2 | 203.1 |
| Massachusetts | 2,658 | 2,189 | 2,225 | 2,258 | 2,453 | 43.8 | 36.0 | 36.4 | 36.7 | 39.9 |
| Michigan | 18,220 | 15,130 | 15,736 | 16,359 | 15,907 | 190.8 | 155.5 | 161.0 | 166.6 | 162.0 |
| Minnesota | 2,852 | 2,697 | 2,417 | 2,708 | 2,830 | 61.9 | 58.0 | 51.6 | 57.3 | 59.9 |
| Mississippi | 9,511 | 6,988 | 9,367 | 10,689 | 10,411 | 352.6 | 257.8 | 343.1 | 388.4 | 378.3 |
| Missouri | 11,326 | 8,421 | 7,658 | 9,463 | 8,187 | 212.8 | 157.0 | 141.8 | 174.0 | 150.5 |
| Montana | 65 | 38 | 66 | 55 | 53 | 7.5 | 4.3 | 7.5 | 6.2 | 6.0 |
| Nebraska | 1,133 | 1,164 | 1,210 | 1,204 | 1,471 | 69.2 | 70.6 | 73.0 | 72.4 | 88.5 |
| Nevada | 1,237 | 1,025 | 829 | 1,445 | 1,303 | 80.8 | 64.0 | 49.4 | 82.7 | 74.6 |
| New Hampshire | 118 | 153 | 96 | 91 | 115 | 10.3 | 13.2 | 8.2 | 7.7 | 9.7 |
| New Jersey | 5,783 | 8,721 | 7,566 | 7,858 | 7,852 | 72.8 | 109.0 | 94.0 | 96.8 | 96.8 |
| New Mexico | 1,054 | 890 | 857 | 957 | 974 | 62.5 | 52.0 | 49.5 | 55.1 | 56.1 |
| New York | 25,992 | 20,604 | 22,393 | 19,062 | 19,826 | 143.3 | 113.6 | 123.5 | 104.9 | 109.1 |
| North Carolina | 23,961 | 18,229 | 16,888 | 19,230 | 19,428 | 333.0 | 249.4 | 227.4 | 254.8 | 257.4 |
| North Dakota | 38 | 37 | 68 | 80 | 83 | 5.9 | 5.8 | 10.6 | 12.5 | 13.0 |
| Ohio | 23,176 | 14,946 | 14,961 | 18,275 | 18,141 | 207.8 | 133.9 | 133.7 | 163.0 | 161.8 |
| Oklahoma | 5,077 | 4,897 | 4,760 | 5,243 | 4,021 | 154.9 | 148.6 | 143.5 | 156.7 | 120.1 |
| Oregon | 854 | 887 | 773 | 880 | 903 | 27.2 | 27.8 | 23.8 | 26.8 | 27.5 |
| Pennsylvania | 13,038 | 10,803 | 9,967 | 11,719 | 13,295 | 108.0 | 89.7 | 82.9 | 97.6 | 110.8 |
| Rhode Island | 545 | 486 | 422 | 430 | 601 | 55.1 | 49.2 | 42.7 | 43.5 | 60.8 |
| South Carolina | 12,120 | 11,661 | 11,487 | 11,575 | 15,037 | 330.0 | 313.8 | 305.5 | 301.7 | 392.0 |
| South Dakota | 237 | 176 | 172 | 221 | 192 | 32.5 | 23.9 | 23.3 | 29.9 | 26.0 |
| Tennessee | 13,892 | 11,709 | 11,023 | 11,840 | 11,366 | 264.3 | 220.6 | 205.3 | 218.0 | 209.3 |
| Texas | 30,801 | 23,124 | 26,612 | 32,833 | 32,910 | 164.5 | 121.1 | 136.9 | 166.2 | 166.6 |
| Utah | 306 | 277 | 278 | 236 | 254 | 15.7 | 13.7 | 13.5 | 11.2 | 12.1 |
| Vermont | 69 | 47 | 53 | 38 | 52 | 11.8 | 8.0 | 9.0 | 6.4 | 8.8 |
| Virginia | 10,340 | 9,293 | 8,888 | 9,265 | 9,402 | 156.2 | 139.4 | 132.0 | 136.4 | 138.4 |
| Washington | 2,765 | 2,020 | 1,956 | 1,948 | 2,132 | 50.9 | 36.6 | 34.9 | 34.2 | 37.5 |
| West Virginia | 860 | 736 | 957 | 920 | 584 | 47.0 | 40.4 | 52.7 | 50.8 | 32.2 |
| Wisconsin | 5,524 | 4,481 | 4,316 | 6,365 | 6,662 | 107.8 | 87.1 | 83.5 | 121.9 | 127.5 |
| Wyoming | 51 | 41 | 54 | 36 | 43 | 10.6 | 8.5 | 11.3 | 7.5 | 8.9 |
| U.S. TOTAL[1] | 392,651 | 326,805 | 326,564 | 355,728 | 360,076 | 149.4 | 123.2 | 122.0 | 131.6 | 133.2 |
| Northeast | 52,352 | 46,446 | 45,942 | 44,700 | 47,598 | 101.7 | 90.2 | 89.1 | 86.4 | 92.0 |
| Midwest | 97,653 | 74,843 | 74,502 | 86,955 | 86,849 | 158.0 | 120.4 | 119.3 | 138.3 | 138.1 |
| South | 203,689 | 174,873 | 176,152 | 191,661 | 193,622 | 221.7 | 188.0 | 187.0 | 200.8 | 202.9 |
| West | 38,957 | 30,643 | 29,968 | 32,412 | 32,007 | 67.6 | 52.4 | 50.5 | 53.8 | 53.1 |
| Guam | 90 | 56 | 47 | 72 | 59 | 60.3 | 36.7 | 30.1 | 45.0 | 36.9 |
| Puerto Rico | 618 | 648 | 526 | 400 | 321 | 16.7 | 17.4 | 13.7 | 10.4 | 8.3 |
| Virgin Islands | 31 | 12 | 40 | 39 | 51 | 28.3 | 10.9 | 36.5 | 35.6 | 46.5 |
| OUTLYING AREAS | 739 | 716 | 613 | 511 | 431 | 18.7 | 18.0 | 15.0 | 12.4 | 10.4 |
| TOTAL | 393,390 | 327,521 | 327,177 | 356,239 | 360,507 | 147.5 | 121.7 | 120.4 | 129.8 | 131.4 |

[1]Includes cases reported by Washington, D.C.

*Source*: Centers for Disease Control and Prevention, U.S. Department of Health and Human Services. National Center for HIV, STD, and TB Prevention, Division of STD Prevention. *Sexually Transmitted Disease Surveillance 1999* (Atlanta, GA: CDC, 2000). http://www.cdc.gov/nchstp/dstd/Stats_Trends/1999Surveillance/99PDF/Surv99Master.pdf.

## Table D4.5. Gonorrhea—Reported Cases per 100,000 Population by Sex, United States, 1984–1999

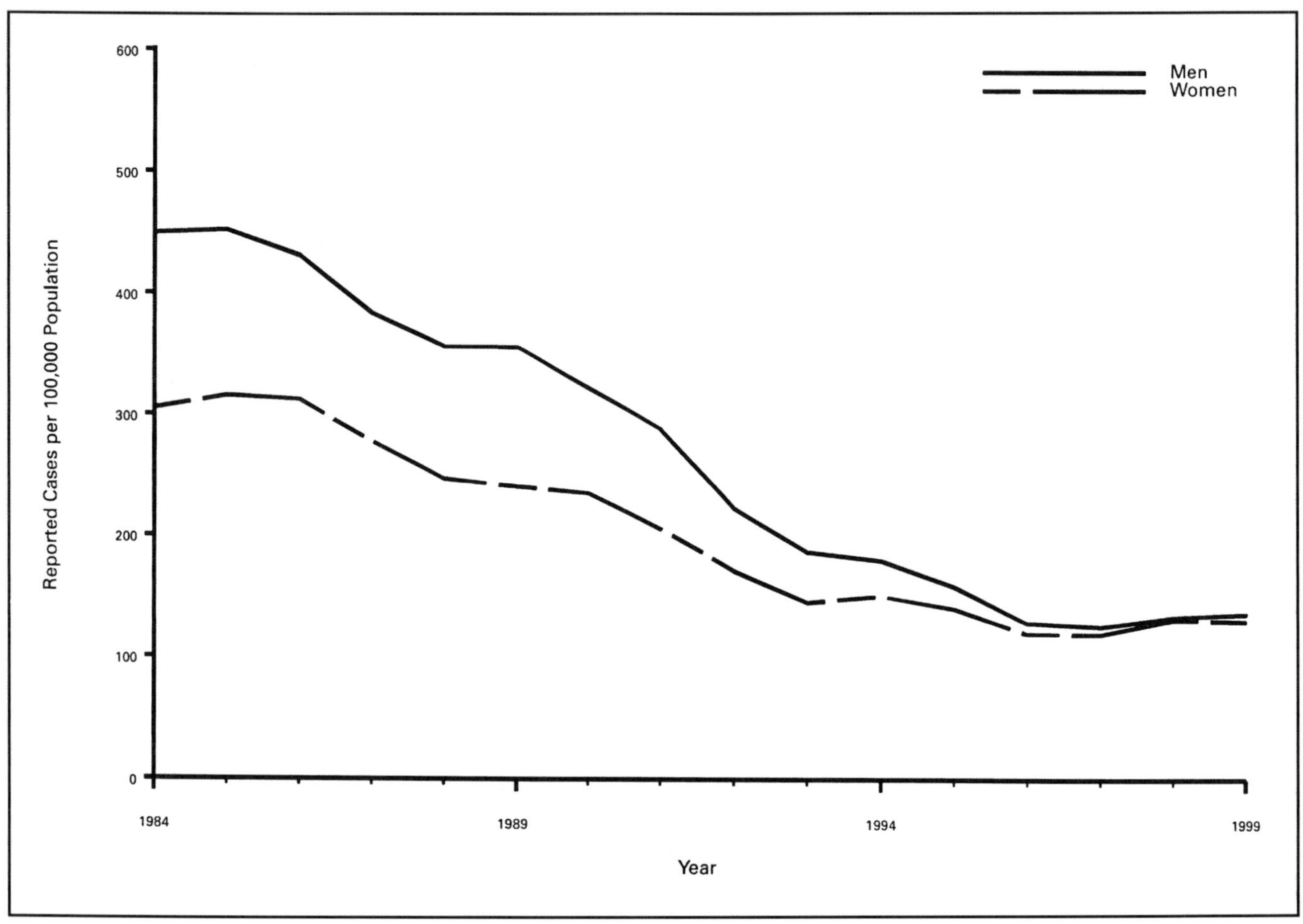


In 1999, the overall U.S. rate of gonorrhea was 133.2 cases/100,000 population, a 1.2% increase from 1998 (131.6). Among men, the rate increased from 132.7 in 1998 to 136.0 in 1999. Among women, the rate decreased only slightly from 130.0 in 1998 to 129.9 in 1999 (Division of Sexually Transmitted Diseases Prevention, National Center for HIV, STD, and TB Prevention).

*Source*: Center for Disease Control and Prevention. U.S. Department of Health and Human Services. *MMWR: Morbidity and Mortality Weekly Review Summary of Notifiable Disease, United States, 1999* 48 no. 53 (2001). http://www.cdc.gov/mmwr/PDF/wk/mm4853.pdf.

## Table D4.6. Gonorrhea—Women—Reported Cases and Rates, by State/Area Listed in Alphabetical Order: United States and Outlying Areas, 1995–1999

| | Cases | | | | | Rates per 100,000 Population | | | | |
|---|---|---|---|---|---|---|---|---|---|---|
| *State/Area* | *1995* | *1996* | *1997* | *1998* | *1999* | *1995* | *1996* | *1997* | *1998* | *1999* |
| Alabama | 6,938 | 6,730 | 5,984 | 6,313 | 5,460 | 313.6 | 302.3 | 266.9 | 278.8 | 241.2 |
| Alaska | 318 | 242 | 230 | 181 | 153 | 111.4 | 84.4 | 79.6 | 62.0 | 52.4 |
| Arizona | 1,700 | 1,690 | 1,625 | 1,730 | 1,760 | 79.7 | 75.5 | 70.8 | 73.3 | 74.6 |
| Arkansas | 2,592 | 2,506 | 2,071 | 1,919 | 1,576 | 201.7 | 193.7 | 159.2 | 146.2 | 120.1 |
| California | 11,349 | 8,847 | 8,462 | 9,345 | 8,903 | 71.9 | 55.6 | 52.5 | 57.2 | 54.5 |
| Colorado | 1,401 | 1,028 | 1,224 | 1,055 | 1,271 | 74.1 | 53.4 | 62.4 | 52.7 | 63.5 |
| Connecticut | 2,075 | 1,815 | 1,642 | 1,714 | 1,796 | 122.9 | 108.1 | 97.7 | 101.7 | 106.6 |
| Delaware | 1,171 | 799 | 705 | 855 | 912 | 318.1 | 215.4 | 188.0 | 223.8 | 238.8 |
| Florida | 9,439 | 9,409 | 9,513 | 8,923 | 11,040 | 129.2 | 126.9 | 126.3 | 116.2 | 143.8 |
| Georgia | 9,995 | 9,806 | 9,532 | 10,056 | 10,092 | 270.2 | 260.7 | 248.5 | 256.3 | 257.2 |
| Hawaii | 290 | 244 | 264 | 278 | 251 | 49.4 | 41.6 | 44.8 | 46.7 | 42.2 |
| Idaho | 68 | 53 | 83 | 74 | 42 | 11.7 | 8.9 | 13.7 | 12.0 | 6.8 |
| Illinois | 11,027 | 9,112 | 6,765 | 11,250 | 11,698 | 181.6 | 150.3 | 111.2 | 182.3 | 189.5 |
| Indiana | 4,143 | 3,305 | 3,141 | 3,308 | 3,254 | 138.9 | 110.6 | 104.5 | 109.2 | 107.4 |
| Iowa | 950 | 666 | 762 | 895 | 759 | 65.1 | 45.6 | 52.2 | 60.9 | 51.7 |
| Kansas | 1,528 | 1,084 | 1,133 | 1,454 | 1,573 | 117.2 | 82.8 | 86.0 | 108.8 | 117.7 |
| Kentucky | 2,259 | 2,013 | 1,882 | 1,866 | 1,626 | 113.6 | 100.9 | 93.7 | 92.1 | 80.2 |
| Louisiana | 4,003 | 3,923 | 5,202 | 6,143 | 6,697 | 177.6 | 174.4 | 230.7 | 270.8 | 295.3 |
| Maine | 56 | 27 | 31 | 31 | 40 | 8.8 | 4.3 | 4.9 | 4.9 | 6.3 |
| Maryland | 6,323 | 5,692 | 5,767 | 5,391 | 4,749 | 243.9 | 219.2 | 220.6 | 204.2 | 179.9 |
| Massachusetts | 1,231 | 1,146 | 1,151 | 1,155 | 1,207 | 39.1 | 36.4 | 36.4 | 36.3 | 37.9 |
| Michigan | 8,117 | 7,780 | 7,969 | 8,265 | 7,771 | 165.5 | 155.9 | 159.1 | 164.0 | 154.2 |
| Minnesota | 1,488 | 1,383 | 1,307 | 1,443 | 1,495 | 63.6 | 58.7 | 55.1 | 60.2 | 62.4 |
| Mississippi | 5,218 | 3,681 | 5,188 | 5,973 | 6,137 | 371.5 | 261.3 | 365.7 | 416.8 | 428.2 |
| Missouri | 5,315 | 4,193 | 4,113 | 4,924 | 4,459 | 193.2 | 151.7 | 147.9 | 175.5 | 159.0 |
| Montana | 27 | 19 | 31 | 33 | 35 | 6.2 | 4.3 | 7.0 | 7.5 | 7.9 |
| Nebraska | 600 | 604 | 670 | 683 | 814 | 71.7 | 71.8 | 79.3 | 80.4 | 95.8 |
| Nevada | 448 | 362 | 317 | 591 | 480 | 59.6 | 46.1 | 38.6 | 68.9 | 56.0 |
| New Hampshire | 70 | 95 | 57 | 47 | 61 | 12.0 | 16.1 | 9.6 | 7.8 | 10.1 |
| New Jersey | 2,706 | 3,743 | 3,564 | 3,763 | 3,824 | 66.0 | 90.8 | 86.0 | 89.9 | 91.4 |
| New Mexico | 583 | 459 | 509 | 530 | 528 | 68.2 | 52.9 | 58.0 | 60.1 | 59.8 |
| New York | 13,999 | 10,952 | 12,833 | 10,586 | 10,639 | 148.7 | 116.5 | 136.6 | 112.2 | 112.8 |
| North Carolina | 11,101 | 8,482 | 7,844 | 9,129 | 9,089 | 299.7 | 225.8 | 205.6 | 234.9 | 233.9 |
| North Dakota | 15 | 18 | 42 | 56 | 46 | 4.7 | 5.6 | 13.1 | 17.5 | 14.3 |
| Ohio | 11,978 | 8,161 | 8,349 | 10,117 | 9,707 | 207.8 | 141.7 | 144.8 | 174.7 | 167.6 |
| Oklahoma | 2,764 | 2,610 | 2,418 | 2,932 | 2,240 | 164.7 | 155.1 | 142.8 | 171.2 | 130.8 |
| Oregon | 387 | 418 | 348 | 430 | 433 | 24.3 | 25.9 | 21.2 | 25.9 | 26.1 |
| Pennsylvania | 6,805 | 5,730 | 5,396 | 6,472 | 7,356 | 108.5 | 91.8 | 86.6 | 103.9 | 118.0 |
| Rhode Island | 274 | 245 | 263 | 258 | 371 | 53.3 | 47.8 | 51.4 | 50.3 | 72.3 |
| South Carolina | 4,597 | 4,807 | 5,128 | 5,730 | 5,874 | 241.9 | 250.2 | 263.9 | 288.3 | 295.6 |
| South Dakota | 117 | 94 | 87 | 124 | 117 | 31.6 | 25.1 | 23.3 | 33.1 | 31.2 |
| Tennessee | 6,197 | 5,106 | 4,940 | 5,263 | 4,965 | 227.7 | 186.3 | 178.2 | 187.3 | 176.7 |
| Texas | 15,008 | 11,933 | 13,797 | 16,704 | 16,819 | 158.2 | 123.6 | 140.4 | 166.8 | 168.0 |
| Utah | 121 | 95 | 84 | 70 | 100 | 12.3 | 9.4 | 8.1 | 6.6 | 9.5 |
| Vermont | 43 | 23 | 32 | 22 | 22 | 14.5 | 7.7 | 10.7 | 7.3 | 7.3 |
| Virginia | 4,886 | 4,495 | 4,290 | 4,543 | 4,566 | 144.6 | 132.2 | 124.9 | 130.7 | 131.4 |
| Washington | 1,301 | 929 | 965 | 863 | 1,009 | 47.6 | 33.5 | 34.3 | 30.2 | 35.3 |
| West Virginia | 459 | 363 | 512 | 549 | 357 | 48.4 | 38.5 | 54.5 | 58.5 | 38.0 |
| Wisconsin | 2,713 | 2,343 | 2,344 | 3,754 | 3,826 | 104.0 | 89.6 | 89.3 | 141.3 | 144.0 |
| Wyoming | 30 | 25 | 30 | 23 | 26 | 12.6 | 10.5 | 12.6 | 9.6 | 10.9 |
| U.S. TOTAL[1] | 188,460 | 161,126 | 162,515 | 179,717 | 179,534 | 140.2 | 119.0 | 119.0 | 130.0 | 129.9 |
| Guam | 49 | 30 | 12 | 25 | 28 | 69.9 | 41.8 | 16.3 | 33.3 | 37.3 |
| Puerto Rico | 205 | 219 | 212 | 163 | 132 | 10.7 | 11.4 | 10.7 | 8.1 | 6.6 |
| Virgin Islands | 14 | 4 | 19 | 16 | 38 | 24.5 | 7.0 | 33.3 | 27.8 | 66.0 |
| OUTLYING AREAS | 268 | 253 | 243 | 204 | 198 | 13.2 | 12.3 | 11.5 | 9.5 | 9.3 |
| TOTAL | 188,728 | 161,379 | 162,758 | 179,921 | 179,732 | 138.3 | 117.4 | 117.3 | 128.2 | 128.0 |

[1]Includes cases reported by Washington, D.C.

Note: Cases and rates underestimated in some areas because of under-reporting or non-reporting by gender.

*Source*: Centers for Disease Control and Prevention, U.S. Department of Health and Human Services. National Center for HIV, STD, and TB Prevention, Division of STD Prevention. *Sexually Transmitted Disease Surveillance 1999* (Atlanta, GA: CDC, 2000). http://www.cdc.gov/nchstp/dstd/Stats_Trends/1999Surveillance/99PDF/Surv99Master.pdf.

## Table D4.7. Gonorrhea—Men—Reported Cases and Rates, by State/Area Listed in Alphabetical Order: United States and Outlying Areas, 1995–1999

| | Cases | | | | | Rates per 100,000 Population | | | | |
|---|---|---|---|---|---|---|---|---|---|---|
| State/Area | 1995 | 1996 | 1997 | 1998 | 1999 | 1995 | 1996 | 1997 | 1998 | 1999 |
| Alabama | 7,698 | 6,409 | 6,022 | 6,411 | 5,399 | 377.2 | 311.0 | 290.0 | 307.1 | 258.6 |
| Alaska | 342 | 224 | 161 | 150 | 149 | 107.5 | 70.4 | 50.3 | 46.6 | 46.2 |
| Arizona | 2,144 | 2,019 | 2,177 | 2,483 | 2,533 | 102.8 | 91.9 | 96.4 | 107.5 | 109.7 |
| Arkansas | 3,031 | 2,536 | 2,295 | 2,029 | 1,650 | 252.9 | 209.1 | 187.9 | 165.5 | 134.6 |
| California | 13,121 | 9,729 | 9,452 | 10,192 | 9,618 | 83.1 | 61.0 | 58.5 | 62.4 | 58.9 |
| Colorado | 1,402 | 992 | 1,091 | 978 | 1,255 | 75.5 | 52.4 | 56.5 | 49.7 | 63.8 |
| Connecticut | 1,980 | 1,573 | 1,512 | 1,463 | 1,525 | 124.8 | 99.1 | 95.1 | 92.1 | 96.0 |
| Delaware | 1,030 | 657 | 568 | 701 | 750 | 295.1 | 186.4 | 159.3 | 193.9 | 207.4 |
| Florida | 11,435 | 9,772 | 9,566 | 10,054 | 11,851 | 166.6 | 139.5 | 134.3 | 138.9 | 163.7 |
| Georgia | 11,030 | 10,000 | 8,916 | 10,525 | 11,039 | 315.0 | 279.8 | 244.2 | 283.1 | 296.9 |
| Hawaii | 273 | 253 | 246 | 228 | 211 | 45.5 | 42.4 | 41.2 | 38.1 | 35.3 |
| Idaho | 81 | 45 | 75 | 108 | 46 | 14.0 | 7.6 | 12.4 | 17.6 | 7.5 |
| Illinois | 10,720 | 8,852 | 11,658 | 10,485 | 11,545 | 186.2 | 153.1 | 200.6 | 178.5 | 196.6 |
| Indiana | 4,737 | 3,331 | 3,006 | 2,991 | 2,836 | 168.0 | 117.3 | 105.1 | 104.2 | 98.8 |
| Iowa | 773 | 479 | 549 | 721 | 606 | 55.9 | 34.5 | 39.4 | 51.7 | 43.5 |
| Kansas | 1,269 | 960 | 942 | 1,168 | 1,092 | 100.6 | 75.6 | 73.7 | 90.4 | 84.5 |
| Kentucky | 2,492 | 2,216 | 2,137 | 1,887 | 1,669 | 133.2 | 117.5 | 112.5 | 98.8 | 87.4 |
| Louisiana | 5,289 | 5,392 | 5,580 | 6,356 | 6,492 | 253.3 | 257.8 | 266.1 | 302.6 | 309.0 |
| Maine | 38 | 28 | 35 | 36 | 43 | 6.3 | 4.6 | 5.8 | 5.9 | 7.1 |
| Maryland | 6,661 | 5,897 | 5,801 | 5,846 | 5,669 | 271.9 | 239.4 | 233.9 | 234.3 | 227.2 |
| Massachusetts | 1,427 | 1,043 | 1,074 | 1,103 | 1,246 | 48.8 | 35.5 | 36.4 | 37.2 | 42.0 |
| Michigan | 10,103 | 7,350 | 7,767 | 8,094 | 8,136 | 217.5 | 155.0 | 163.0 | 169.5 | 170.3 |
| Minnesota | 1,364 | 1,314 | 1,110 | 1,265 | 1,335 | 60.1 | 57.3 | 48.0 | 54.3 | 57.3 |
| Mississippi | 4,284 | 3,266 | 4,049 | 4,653 | 4,184 | 331.4 | 250.9 | 308.6 | 352.8 | 317.2 |
| Missouri | 6,011 | 4,228 | 3,545 | 4,539 | 3,728 | 233.6 | 162.6 | 135.2 | 172.4 | 141.6 |
| Montana | 38 | 19 | 35 | 22 | 18 | 8.8 | 4.3 | 8.0 | 5.0 | 4.1 |
| Nebraska | 532 | 551 | 537 | 520 | 657 | 66.5 | 68.2 | 66.1 | 63.9 | 80.8 |
| Nevada | 789 | 663 | 512 | 854 | 822 | 101.3 | 81.2 | 59.9 | 96.1 | 92.5 |
| New Hampshire | 48 | 58 | 39 | 44 | 54 | 8.5 | 10.2 | 6.7 | 7.5 | 9.3 |
| New Jersey | 3,077 | 4,972 | 3,999 | 4,094 | 4,019 | 80.0 | 128.1 | 102.3 | 104.2 | 102.2 |
| New Mexico | 471 | 431 | 348 | 427 | 445 | 56.7 | 51.1 | 40.8 | 50.0 | 52.1 |
| New York | 11,993 | 9,652 | 9,560 | 8,476 | 9,176 | 137.5 | 110.5 | 109.3 | 96.9 | 105.0 |
| North Carolina | 12,860 | 9,747 | 9,044 | 10,101 | 10,339 | 368.5 | 274.4 | 250.5 | 276.0 | 282.5 |
| North Dakota | 23 | 19 | 26 | 24 | 37 | 7.2 | 5.9 | 8.1 | 7.6 | 11.6 |
| Ohio | 10,940 | 6,672 | 6,506 | 8,023 | 8,245 | 203.1 | 123.5 | 120.1 | 148.1 | 152.2 |
| Oklahoma | 2,313 | 2,287 | 2,342 | 2,311 | 1,781 | 144.6 | 141.9 | 144.3 | 141.4 | 109.0 |
| Oregon | 467 | 469 | 425 | 450 | 470 | 30.2 | 29.7 | 26.5 | 27.8 | 29.0 |
| Pennsylvania | 6,233 | 5,073 | 4,571 | 5,247 | 5,939 | 107.5 | 87.5 | 79.0 | 90.9 | 102.9 |
| Rhode Island | 271 | 241 | 159 | 172 | 230 | 57.0 | 50.7 | 33.4 | 36.2 | 48.4 |
| South Carolina | 7,388 | 6,828 | 6,340 | 5,769 | 9,052 | 416.7 | 380.2 | 349.0 | 312.1 | 489.7 |
| South Dakota | 120 | 82 | 85 | 97 | 75 | 33.4 | 22.6 | 23.4 | 26.7 | 20.7 |
| Tennessee | 7,695 | 6,603 | 6,083 | 6,577 | 6,401 | 303.6 | 257.3 | 234.4 | 251.0 | 244.3 |
| Texas | 15,793 | 11,191 | 12,815 | 15,995 | 15,973 | 171.0 | 118.6 | 133.3 | 164.1 | 163.9 |
| Utah | 185 | 182 | 194 | 166 | 154 | 19.1 | 18.1 | 18.9 | 15.9 | 14.8 |
| Vermont | 26 | 24 | 21 | 16 | 30 | 9.0 | 8.3 | 7.2 | 5.5 | 10.3 |
| Virginia | 5,414 | 4,783 | 4,590 | 4,720 | 4,832 | 167.1 | 146.4 | 139.2 | 142.3 | 145.7 |
| Washington | 1,464 | 1,091 | 991 | 1,085 | 1,123 | 54.3 | 39.7 | 35.4 | 38.4 | 39.7 |
| West Virginia | 401 | 373 | 445 | 369 | 227 | 45.5 | 42.5 | 50.8 | 42.3 | 26.0 |
| Wisconsin | 2,811 | 2,138 | 1,972 | 2,611 | 2,827 | 111.8 | 84.5 | 77.5 | 101.7 | 110.1 |
| Wyoming | 21 | 16 | 24 | 13 | 17 | 8.7 | 6.6 | 9.9 | 5.4 | 7.0 |
| U.S. TOTAL[1] | 203,557 | 165,321 | 163,634 | 175,253 | 179,564 | 158.7 | 127.4 | 124.9 | 132.7 | 136.0 |
| Guam | 41 | 26 | 35 | 47 | 31 | 51.8 | 32.1 | 42.3 | 55.5 | 36.6 |
| Puerto Rico | 413 | 429 | 314 | 237 | 189 | 23.2 | 23.9 | 17.1 | 12.8 | 10.2 |
| Virgin Islands | 17 | 8 | 21 | 23 | 13 | 32.3 | 15.2 | 39.9 | 43.2 | 24.4 |
| OUTLYING AREAS | 471 | 463 | 370 | 307 | 233 | 24.6 | 24.0 | 18.8 | 15.4 | 11.7 |
| TOTAL | 204,028 | 165,784 | 164,004 | 175,560 | 179,797 | 156.7 | 125.9 | 123.3 | 131.0 | 134.1 |

[1]Includes cases reported by Washington, D.C.

Note: Cases and rates underestimated in some areas because of under-reporting or non-reporting by gender.

*Source*: Centers for Disease Control and Prevention, U.S. Department of Health and Human Services. National Center for HIV, STD, and TB Prevention, Division of STD Prevention. *Sexually Transmitted Disease Surveillance 1999* (Atlanta, GA: CDC, 2000). http://www.cdc.gov/nchstp/dstd/Stats_Trends/1999Surveillance/99PDF/Surv99Master.pdf.

**Table D4.8. Gonorrhea—Reported Cases per 100,000 Population, by Race and Ethnicity, United States, 1984–1999**

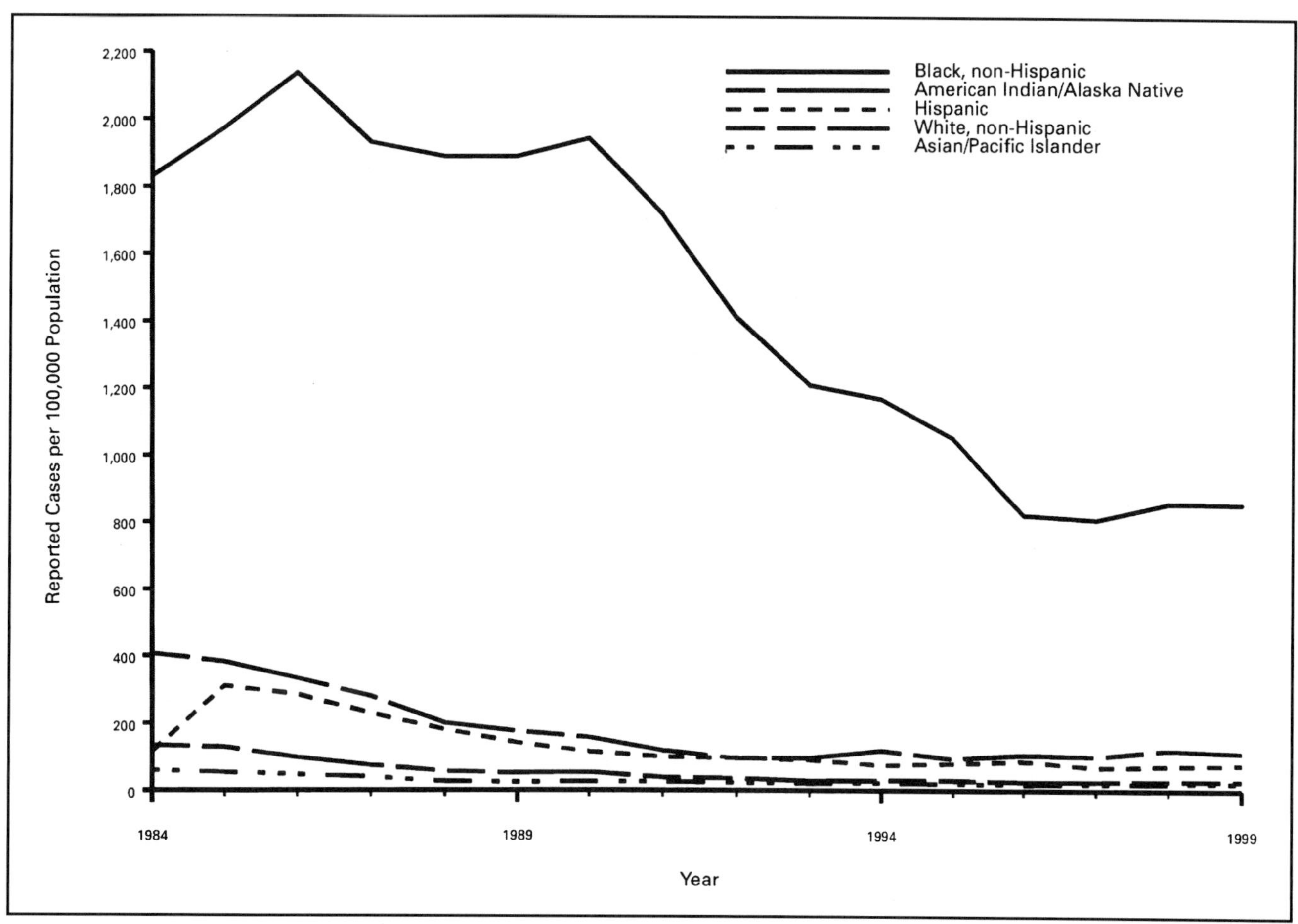


In 1999, gonorrhea rates decreased among non-Hispanic whites, non-Hispanic blacks, and American Indian/Alaska Natives, but increased among Hispanics and Asian/Pacific Islanders.

*Source*: Center for Disease Control and Prevention. U.S. Department of Health and Human Services. *MMWR: Morbidity and Mortality Weekly Review Summary of Notifiable Disease, United States, 1999* 48 no. 53 (2001). http://www.cdc.gov/mmwr/PDF/wk/mm4853.pdf.

## Table D4.9. Gonorrhea—Reported Rates per 100,000 Population, by Age, Gender, and Race/Ethnicity: United States, 1995–1999

| Age | Total | | | White, Non-Hispanic | | | Black, Non-Hispanic | | | Hispanic | | | Asian/Pacific Islander | | | American Indian/ Alaska Native | | | |
|---|---|---|---|---|---|---|---|---|---|---|---|---|---|---|---|---|---|---|---|
| Group | Total | Male | Female | Total | Male | Female | Total | Male | Female | Total | Male | Female | Total | Male | Female | Total | Male | Female | |
| 10-14 | 41.3 | 12.4 | 71.7 | 8.9 | 1.2 | 17.1 | 237.0 | 79.7 | 398.9 | 19.3 | 5.7 | 33.6 | 5.6 | 0.6 | 10.7 | 19.0 | 9.2 | 29.1 | |
| 15-19 | 671.0 | 503.2 | 847.8 | 145.1 | 45.0 | 251.6 | 3,815.3 | 3,234.6 | 4,413.1 | 270.3 | 195.3 | 348.6 | 81.0 | 35.0 | 128.0 | 296.2 | 141.1 | 454.4 | |
| 20-24 | 633.1 | 653.8 | 611.6 | 121.0 | 73.4 | 170.2 | 3,841.8 | 4,376.7 | 3,321.1 | 275.3 | 276.2 | 274.3 | 70.2 | 59.9 | 80.5 | 309.5 | 220.3 | 402.4 | |
| 25-29 | 316.1 | 366.6 | 265.2 | 65.9 | 56.9 | 75.0 | 2,044.9 | 2,623.9 | 1,518.7 | 139.6 | 151.2 | 126.0 | 44.4 | 52.6 | 36.7 | 186.7 | 159.4 | 214.8 | |
| 30-34 | 175.7 | 223.1 | 128.4 | 40.3 | 42.9 | 37.7 | 1,184.0 | 1,665.3 | 761.1 | 86.0 | 103.9 | 66.0 | 23.0 | 28.6 | 17.7 | 138.9 | 117.4 | 159.8 | 1995 |
| 35-39 | 112.9 | 159.0 | 67.0 | 24.7 | 30.0 | 19.3 | 778.5 | 1,205.2 | 402.3 | 58.4 | 75.8 | 39.7 | 10.5 | 14.2 | 7.1 | 97.8 | 104.6 | 91.4 | |
| 40-44 | 66.0 | 105.9 | 26.8 | 12.7 | 17.9 | 7.6 | 491.4 | 866.9 | 165.1 | 34.9 | 47.4 | 22.0 | 7.7 | 10.1 | 5.5 | 46.6 | 59.9 | 34.3 | |
| 45-54 | 28.7 | 50.6 | 7.6 | 6.7 | 10.8 | 2.8 | 236.7 | 462.8 | 47.3 | 18.7 | 29.9 | 8.0 | 4.3 | 6.0 | 2.9 | 20.0 | 26.9 | 13.5 | |
| 55-64 | 10.9 | 20.8 | 1.9 | 2.4 | 4.3 | 0.6 | 91.7 | 194.0 | 12.4 | 9.3 | 16.5 | 2.9 | 1.8 | 4.0 | 0.0 | 3.6 | 7.6 | 0.0 | |
| 65+ | 3.1 | 6.3 | 1.0 | 0.6 | 1.2 | 0.2 | 32.4 | 69.3 | 8.6 | 2.4 | 3.2 | 1.9 | 2.1 | 3.2 | 1.3 | 4.9 | 7.8 | 2.8 | |
| TOTAL | 149.5 | 160.4 | 139.1 | 29.6 | 21.5 | 37.3 | 1,045.9 | 1,230.2 | 879.4 | 79.2 | 80.0 | 78.3 | 20.3 | 18.1 | 22.3 | 92.9 | 70.7 | 114.3 | |
| 10-14 | 33.2 | 9.1 | 58.6 | 7.5 | 1.0 | 14.4 | 179.8 | 55.6 | 307.8 | 15.8 | 3.6 | 28.8 | 3.3 | 1.3 | 5.3 | 21.7 | 5.1 | 38.6 | |
| 15-19 | 543.6 | 373.6 | 724.5 | 125.8 | 44.7 | 211.8 | 2,904.8 | 2,235.0 | 3,594.2 | 222.7 | 152.1 | 302.9 | 64.1 | 21.5 | 107.8 | 329.0 | 147.7 | 513.3 | |
| 20-24 | 537.3 | 532.4 | 542.6 | 109.8 | 67.1 | 154.3 | 3,096.2 | 3,418.2 | 2,783.0 | 218.2 | 200.4 | 239.9 | 64.8 | 53.5 | 76.2 | 364.9 | 238.1 | 494.4 | |
| 25-29 | 260.6 | 297.6 | 223.3 | 57.0 | 51.1 | 62.9 | 1,594.2 | 2,015.2 | 1,212.1 | 121.7 | 124.0 | 118.9 | 36.6 | 39.1 | 34.3 | 215.6 | 174.0 | 258.9 | |
| 30-34 | 147.6 | 186.0 | 109.3 | 36.1 | 39.6 | 32.5 | 916.4 | 1,273.3 | 603.2 | 67.9 | 80.5 | 53.2 | 22.6 | 27.5 | 18.1 | 143.9 | 126.0 | 161.6 | 1996 |
| 35-39 | 91.0 | 125.4 | 56.7 | 21.1 | 25.5 | 16.6 | 591.8 | 902.3 | 319.0 | 45.6 | 53.1 | 37.2 | 13.8 | 16.9 | 10.9 | 101.3 | 111.8 | 91.2 | |
| 40-44 | 54.8 | 85.3 | 24.7 | 11.8 | 16.4 | 7.2 | 380.1 | 652.5 | 142.7 | 28.8 | 36.4 | 20.7 | 8.2 | 10.5 | 6.2 | 57.5 | 74.6 | 41.7 | |
| 45-54 | 24.3 | 42.1 | 7.2 | 6.3 | 9.8 | 2.7 | 183.8 | 354.7 | 41.0 | 14.9 | 22.1 | 7.7 | 4.0 | 5.4 | 2.8 | 20.5 | 22.4 | 18.8 | |
| 55-64 | 9.0 | 17.0 | 1.6 | 2.2 | 3.8 | 0.6 | 72.2 | 153.9 | 9.4 | 6.0 | 10.9 | 1.7 | 2.1 | 2.1 | 2.1 | 3.4 | 3.7 | 3.3 | |
| 65+ | 3.1 | 5.6 | 1.3 | 0.7 | 1.2 | 0.4 | 28.5 | 57.4 | 9.9 | 4.4 | 5.5 | 3.5 | 1.0 | 1.6 | 0.6 | 1.6 | 0.0 | 2.7 | |
| TOTAL | 124.0 | 127.9 | 120.2 | 26.1 | 19.6 | 32.4 | 816.8 | 923.4 | 720.7 | 66.0 | 62.6 | 69.6 | 18.0 | 15.3 | 20.5 | 104.8 | 75.1 | 133.7 | |
| 10-14 | 30.7 | 8.5 | 54.1 | 7.2 | 1.0 | 13.8 | 162.2 | 49.6 | 278.3 | 15.0 | 4.4 | 26.1 | 3.5 | 0.9 | 6.2 | 23.7 | 4.1 | 43.8 | |
| 15-19 | 521.6 | 348.1 | 706.2 | 117.4 | 39.7 | 199.7 | 2,780.0 | 2,077.3 | 3,504.3 | 223.5 | 142.3 | 315.6 | 68.6 | 31.5 | 106.5 | 342.9 | 150.3 | 537.2 | |
| 20-24 | 548.4 | 537.1 | 560.4 | 114.0 | 69.6 | 160.5 | 3,124.8 | 3,404.5 | 2,852.4 | 220.2 | 201.6 | 242.7 | 74.5 | 69.7 | 79.4 | 342.6 | 225.5 | 461.4 | |
| 25-29 | 268.8 | 310.5 | 226.8 | 60.2 | 52.3 | 68.0 | 1,606.8 | 2,059.4 | 1,195.3 | 130.4 | 141.0 | 117.5 | 38.1 | 37.4 | 38.8 | 189.8 | 150.0 | 231.5 | |
| 30-34 | 148.7 | 188.5 | 109.0 | 37.3 | 40.9 | 33.7 | 897.0 | 1,255.2 | 582.7 | 74.4 | 88.6 | 57.9 | 27.9 | 37.6 | 19.0 | 141.7 | 129.1 | 154.2 | 1997 |
| 35-39 | 92.1 | 126.5 | 57.7 | 23.8 | 28.3 | 19.2 | 577.4 | 880.4 | 311.1 | 50.1 | 63.2 | 35.5 | 12.6 | 15.3 | 10.2 | 72.3 | 63.4 | 81.0 | |
| 40-44 | 55.0 | 86.2 | 24.1 | 12.6 | 17.7 | 7.6 | 368.9 | 636.7 | 134.4 | 29.6 | 40.0 | 18.4 | 9.5 | 12.6 | 6.8 | 48.6 | 47.3 | 49.7 | |
| 45-54 | 24.7 | 42.9 | 7.2 | 6.0 | 9.7 | 2.5 | 186.3 | 359.7 | 41.4 | 14.6 | 20.7 | 8.5 | 5.2 | 8.0 | 2.9 | 18.5 | 18.6 | 18.3 | |
| 55-64 | 9.3 | 17.4 | 2.0 | 2.4 | 3.8 | 1.0 | 73.4 | 156.1 | 9.8 | 6.5 | 11.6 | 1.9 | 1.6 | 2.7 | 0.7 | 7.6 | 12.6 | 3.2 | |
| 65+ | 4.1 | 6.9 | 2.2 | 0.9 | 1.4 | 0.5 | 39.2 | 70.1 | 19.3 | 5.5 | 9.0 | 2.9 | 0.5 | 0.4 | 0.6 | 1.5 | 3.6 | 0.0 | |
| TOTAL | 123.3 | 127.0 | 119.8 | 26.2 | 19.7 | 32.4 | 802.4 | 904.5 | 710.2 | 67.4 | 64.9 | 70.0 | 19.5 | 18.1 | 20.8 | 99.4 | 66.4 | 131.3 | |
| 10-14 | 32.4 | 8.4 | 57.5 | 6.8 | 0.9 | 13.0 | 173.2 | 49.0 | 301.1 | 13.4 | 4.2 | 23.1 | 3.4 | 0.8 | 6.1 | 24.9 | 3.9 | 46.5 | |
| 15-19 | 547.0 | 347.0 | 758.7 | 125.1 | 40.9 | 214.4 | 2,892.2 | 2,034.2 | 3,777.2 | 222.6 | 151.1 | 300.3 | 66.0 | 22.9 | 110.0 | 390.7 | 152.3 | 630.5 | |
| 20-24 | 605.2 | 576.4 | 635.1 | 125.8 | 75.7 | 178.1 | 3,371.6 | 3,529.5 | 3,218.0 | 257.3 | 250.9 | 264.2 | 86.6 | 61.2 | 111.4 | 414.5 | 266.5 | 563.8 | |
| 25-29 | 302.9 | 350.2 | 256.1 | 65.3 | 57.9 | 72.7 | 1,754.4 | 2,217.8 | 1,332.7 | 149.3 | 168.7 | 128.3 | 45.6 | 45.8 | 45.4 | 241.0 | 153.3 | 332.8 | |
| 30-34 | 162.1 | 205.1 | 119.9 | 41.3 | 46.0 | 36.6 | 946.0 | 1,306.1 | 630.9 | 83.2 | 104.6 | 60.2 | 25.3 | 27.4 | 23.4 | 138.0 | 123.7 | 152.2 | 1998 |
| 35-39 | 102.8 | 140.6 | 65.4 | 26.1 | 32.4 | 19.7 | 632.2 | 945.8 | 357.3 | 54.4 | 70.3 | 37.5 | 18.5 | 23.1 | 14.2 | 105.6 | 92.4 | 118.6 | |
| 40-44 | 60.7 | 92.3 | 29.6 | 14.1 | 18.8 | 9.4 | 396.0 | 663.0 | 163.1 | 32.9 | 44.9 | 20.7 | 11.1 | 15.4 | 7.2 | 58.0 | 70.8 | 46.0 | |
| 45-54 | 27.2 | 46.6 | 8.7 | 6.3 | 9.8 | 2.9 | 199.2 | 380.3 | 49.6 | 17.5 | 25.6 | 9.8 | 4.1 | 4.6 | 3.7 | 27.7 | 40.0 | 16.2 | |
| 55-64 | 9.7 | 18.2 | 2.0 | 2.4 | 4.2 | 0.6 | 75.2 | 157.8 | 12.2 | 7.3 | 12.3 | 3.1 | 1.5 | 1.9 | 1.1 | 10.3 | 13.5 | 7.4 | |
| 65+ | 3.6 | 6.3 | 1.7 | 0.9 | 1.5 | 0.4 | 31.5 | 59.5 | 13.6 | 4.9 | 8.8 | 2.0 | 1.3 | 1.0 | 1.5 | 12.1 | 1.7 | 19.6 | |
| TOTAL | 133.3 | 134.5 | 132.1 | 28.2 | 21.2 | 34.8 | 851.2 | 933.2 | 777.5 | 72.3 | 72.9 | 71.6 | 20.9 | 16.7 | 24.8 | 119.4 | 77.0 | 160.3 | |
| 10-14 | 30.9 | 8.4 | 54.6 | 6.6 | 0.9 | 12.7 | 163.7 | 48.6 | 282.4 | 14.4 | 4.6 | 24.6 | 4.7 | 0.5 | 9.1 | 19.2 | 2.9 | 36.0 | |
| 15-19 | 534.0 | 341.1 | 738.1 | 116.1 | 38.6 | 198.3 | 2,830.6 | 1,996.5 | 3,691.0 | 242.8 | 160.9 | 331.8 | 76.6 | 37.2 | 117.0 | 365.0 | 128.5 | 602.6 | |
| 20-24 | 614.7 | 585.6 | 644.9 | 126.3 | 76.6 | 178.4 | 3,425.8 | 3,582.4 | 3,273.1 | 266.9 | 255.0 | 279.6 | 96.6 | 86.1 | 106.8 | 420.8 | 252.7 | 590.3 | |
| 25-29 | 301.7 | 352.3 | 251.7 | 65.3 | 58.6 | 72.1 | 1,743.8 | 2,225.7 | 1,304.6 | 154.5 | 170.3 | 137.6 | 38.0 | 46.1 | 31.1 | 187.8 | 130.2 | 248.1 | |
| 30-34 | 160.2 | 206.7 | 114.5 | 40.7 | 44.9 | 36.4 | 930.1 | 1,323.8 | 585.5 | 85.7 | 103.5 | 66.6 | 29.1 | 35.9 | 23.3 | 141.2 | 129.7 | 152.6 | 1999 |
| 35-39 | 103.6 | 144.0 | 63.5 | 27.8 | 33.9 | 21.8 | 630.2 | 970.0 | 332.2 | 53.9 | 68.6 | 38.4 | 18.0 | 23.4 | 13.1 | 88.0 | 75.4 | 100.3 | |
| 40-44 | 64.0 | 98.2 | 30.4 | 15.5 | 21.9 | 9.1 | 417.5 | 701.8 | 169.6 | 33.1 | 42.6 | 23.4 | 8.8 | 9.7 | 8.0 | 50.9 | 64.1 | 38.7 | |
| 45-54 | 29.9 | 51.2 | 9.5 | 7.3 | 11.3 | 3.3 | 217.9 | 416.6 | 54.1 | 16.5 | 24.6 | 8.8 | 5.3 | 7.7 | 3.2 | 33.7 | 39.4 | 28.4 | |
| 55-64 | 10.4 | 19.6 | 2.0 | 3.0 | 5.3 | 0.8 | 76.7 | 163.8 | 10.3 | 7.3 | 12.1 | 3.0 | 2.3 | 3.7 | 1.1 | 8.6 | 13.3 | 4.4 | |
| 65+ | 2.6 | 5.1 | 0.9 | 0.7 | 1.3 | 0.2 | 22.5 | 46.7 | 6.9 | 4.1 | 7.7 | 1.5 | 0.9 | 0.6 | 1.2 | 7.0 | 5.0 | 8.4 | |
| TOTAL | 133.0 | 136.1 | 130.0 | 27.9 | 21.7 | 33.9 | 848.8 | 943.7 | 763.5 | 75.3 | 73.7 | 77.0 | 22.1 | 20.4 | 23.7 | 110.7 | 69.7 | 150.4 | |

Note: These tables should be used only for race/ethnicity and age comparisons, not for overall totals or gender totals. This is because, if age or race/ethnicity was not specified, cases were prorated according to the distribution of cases for which these variables were specified. For the following years the states listed did not report race/ethnicity for most cases and were excluded: 1995 (Georgia, New Jersey, and New York); 1996 (New Jersey and New York); 1997 (Idaho, New Jersey, and New York); 1998 (Idaho and New Jersey). Cases and population denominators have been excluded for these states/areas. Differences between total cases from this table and others in the report are due to different reporting forms and above listed exclusions. The 0 to 9 year age group is not shown because some of these may not be due to sexual transmission; however, they are included in the totals.

*Source*: Centers for Disease Control and Prevention, U.S. Department of Health and Human Services. National Center for HIV, STD, and TB Prevention, Division of STD Prevention. *Sexually Transmitted Disease Surveillance 1999* (Atlanta, GA: CDC, 2000). http://www.cdc.gov/nchstp/dstd/Stats_Trends/1999Surveillance/99PDF/Surv99Master.pdf.

## Table D4.10. Gonorrhea—Reported Cases, by Age, Gender, and Race/Ethnicity: United States, 1995–1999

| Year | Age Group | Total: Total | Total: Male | Total: Female | White, Non-Hispanic: Total | White, Non-Hispanic: Male | White, Non-Hispanic: Female | Black, Non-Hispanic: Total | Black, Non-Hispanic: Male | Black, Non-Hispanic: Female | Hispanic: Total | Hispanic: Male | Hispanic: Female | Asian/Pacific Islander: Total | Asian/Pacific Islander: Male | Asian/Pacific Islander: Female | American Indian/ Alaska Native: Total | American Indian/ Alaska Native: Male | American Indian/ Alaska Native: Female |
|---|---|---|---|---|---|---|---|---|---|---|---|---|---|---|---|---|---|---|---|
| 1995 | 10-14 | 6,965 | 1,072 | 5,893 | 1,033 | 71 | 962 | 5,445 | 928 | 4,517 | 415 | 62 | 353 | 35 | 2 | 33 | 37 | 9 | 28 |
| | 15-19 | 104,753 | 40,311 | 64,442 | 15,661 | 2,500 | 13,161 | 82,894 | 35,649 | 47,245 | 5,290 | 1,953 | 3,337 | 430 | 94 | 336 | 478 | 115 | 363 |
| | 20-24 | 100,107 | 52,577 | 47,530 | 13,213 | 4,071 | 9,142 | 80,385 | 45,171 | 35,214 | 5,600 | 2,978 | 2,622 | 430 | 183 | 247 | 479 | 174 | 305 |
| | 25-29 | 51,167 | 29,789 | 21,378 | 7,440 | 3,212 | 4,228 | 40,158 | 24,532 | 15,626 | 3,027 | 1,771 | 1,256 | 281 | 161 | 120 | 261 | 113 | 148 |
| | 30-34 | 33,761 | 21,411 | 12,350 | 5,638 | 3,008 | 2,630 | 25,865 | 17,015 | 8,850 | 1,887 | 1,204 | 683 | 160 | 96 | 64 | 211 | 88 | 123 |
| | 35-39 | 22,045 | 15,479 | 6,566 | 3,616 | 2,204 | 1,412 | 17,135 | 12,429 | 4,706 | 1,082 | 727 | 355 | 70 | 45 | 25 | 142 | 74 | 68 |
| | 40-44 | 11,528 | 9,164 | 2,364 | 1,707 | 1,197 | 510 | 9,205 | 7,551 | 1,654 | 510 | 351 | 159 | 46 | 28 | 18 | 60 | 37 | 23 |
| | 45-54 | 7,778 | 6,726 | 1,052 | 1,465 | 1,156 | 309 | 5,884 | 5,244 | 640 | 356 | 279 | 77 | 36 | 23 | 13 | 37 | 24 | 13 |
| | 55-64 | 1,990 | 1,810 | 180 | 358 | 311 | 47 | 1,511 | 1,396 | 115 | 108 | 90 | 18 | 9 | 9 | 0 | 4 | 4 | 0 |
| | 65+ | 920 | 754 | 166 | 160 | 129 | 31 | 712 | 597 | 115 | 31 | 17 | 14 | 11 | 7 | 4 | 6 | 4 | 2 |
| | TOTAL | 343,127 | 179,985 | 163,142 | 50,565 | 17,956 | 32,609 | 270,898 | 151,263 | 119,635 | 18,430 | 9,472 | 8,958 | 1,514 | 650 | 864 | 1,720 | 644 | 1,076 |
| 1996 | 10-14 | 5,725 | 807 | 4,918 | 884 | 62 | 822 | 4,433 | 696 | 3,737 | 346 | 40 | 306 | 20 | 4 | 16 | 42 | 5 | 37 |
| | 15-19 | 92,253 | 32,683 | 59,570 | 14,517 | 2,655 | 11,862 | 71,870 | 28,047 | 43,823 | 4,932 | 1,790 | 3,142 | 364 | 62 | 302 | 570 | 129 | 441 |
| | 20-24 | 85,731 | 43,556 | 42,175 | 11,801 | 3,677 | 8,124 | 68,108 | 37,077 | 31,031 | 4,866 | 2,452 | 2,414 | 407 | 169 | 238 | 549 | 181 | 368 |
| | 25-29 | 44,639 | 25,609 | 19,030 | 6,764 | 3,029 | 3,735 | 34,569 | 20,789 | 13,780 | 2,728 | 1,527 | 1,201 | 258 | 132 | 126 | 320 | 132 | 188 |
| | 30-34 | 28,257 | 17,777 | 10,480 | 4,930 | 2,704 | 2,226 | 21,402 | 13,900 | 7,502 | 1,553 | 988 | 565 | 158 | 92 | 66 | 214 | 93 | 121 |
| | 35-39 | 18,464 | 12,702 | 5,762 | 3,174 | 1,927 | 1,247 | 14,125 | 10,073 | 4,052 | 921 | 566 | 355 | 94 | 55 | 39 | 150 | 81 | 69 |
| | 40-44 | 10,289 | 7,953 | 2,336 | 1,689 | 1,172 | 517 | 8,003 | 6,397 | 1,606 | 468 | 305 | 163 | 52 | 31 | 21 | 77 | 48 | 29 |
| | 45-54 | 7,069 | 5,999 | 1,070 | 1,441 | 1,122 | 319 | 5,238 | 4,601 | 637 | 313 | 232 | 81 | 37 | 23 | 14 | 40 | 21 | 19 |
| | 55-64 | 1,717 | 1,552 | 165 | 333 | 282 | 51 | 1,295 | 1,200 | 95 | 74 | 63 | 11 | 11 | 5 | 6 | 4 | 2 | 2 |
| | 65+ | 930 | 701 | 229 | 187 | 133 | 54 | 675 | 532 | 143 | 60 | 32 | 28 | 6 | 4 | 2 | 2 | 0 | 2 |
| | TOTAL | 296,393 | 149,814 | 146,579 | 45,991 | 16,852 | 29,139 | 230,616 | 123,656 | 106,960 | 16,394 | 8,031 | 8,363 | 1,416 | 579 | 837 | 1,976 | 696 | 1,280 |
| 1997 | 10-14 | 5,283 | 746 | 4,537 | 842 | 61 | 781 | 4,038 | 627 | 3,411 | 335 | 51 | 284 | 22 | 3 | 19 | 46 | 4 | 42 |
| | 15-19 | 90,096 | 30,995 | 59,101 | 13,710 | 2,389 | 11,321 | 70,242 | 26,642 | 43,600 | 5,127 | 1,735 | 3,392 | 408 | 95 | 313 | 609 | 134 | 475 |
| | 20-24 | 86,853 | 43,644 | 43,209 | 12,068 | 3,760 | 8,308 | 68,778 | 36,978 | 31,800 | 5,038 | 2,522 | 2,516 | 459 | 215 | 244 | 510 | 169 | 341 |
| | 25-29 | 45,645 | 26,478 | 19,167 | 7,012 | 3,047 | 3,965 | 35,121 | 21,434 | 13,687 | 2,950 | 1,752 | 1,198 | 278 | 130 | 148 | 284 | 115 | 169 |
| | 30-34 | 27,570 | 17,441 | 10,129 | 4,871 | 2,664 | 2,207 | 20,561 | 13,446 | 7,115 | 1,735 | 1,111 | 624 | 198 | 127 | 71 | 205 | 93 | 112 |
| | 35-39 | 18,666 | 12,810 | 5,856 | 3,547 | 2,118 | 1,429 | 13,868 | 9,892 | 3,976 | 1,056 | 703 | 353 | 88 | 51 | 37 | 107 | 46 | 61 |
| | 40-44 | 10,556 | 8,225 | 2,331 | 1,830 | 1,282 | 548 | 8,088 | 6,517 | 1,571 | 509 | 356 | 153 | 63 | 39 | 24 | 66 | 31 | 35 |
| | 45-54 | 7,433 | 6,331 | 1,102 | 1,433 | 1,136 | 297 | 5,586 | 4,910 | 676 | 326 | 231 | 95 | 51 | 36 | 15 | 37 | 18 | 19 |
| | 55-64 | 1,820 | 1,617 | 203 | 370 | 286 | 84 | 1,349 | 1,247 | 102 | 83 | 70 | 13 | 9 | 7 | 2 | 9 | 7 | 2 |
| | 65+ | 1,251 | 866 | 385 | 228 | 150 | 78 | 939 | 658 | 281 | 79 | 55 | 24 | 3 | 1 | 2 | 2 | 2 | 0 |
| | TOTAL | 296,222 | 149,547 | 146,675 | 46,068 | 16,933 | 29,135 | 229,358 | 122,665 | 106,693 | 17,331 | 8,624 | 8,707 | 1,583 | 706 | 877 | 1,882 | 619 | 1,263 |
| 1998 | 10-14 | 6,019 | 803 | 5,216 | 838 | 57 | 781 | 4,765 | 684 | 4,081 | 342 | 55 | 287 | 24 | 3 | 21 | 50 | 4 | 46 |
| | 15-19 | 103,442 | 33,741 | 69,701 | 15,777 | 2,659 | 13,118 | 80,643 | 28,799 | 51,844 | 5,819 | 2,057 | 3,762 | 466 | 82 | 384 | 737 | 144 | 593 |
| | 20-24 | 103,566 | 50,207 | 53,359 | 14,271 | 4,394 | 9,877 | 81,613 | 42,139 | 39,474 | 6,452 | 3,261 | 3,191 | 589 | 206 | 383 | 641 | 207 | 434 |
| | 25-29 | 54,544 | 31,369 | 23,175 | 7,953 | 3,523 | 4,430 | 42,184 | 25,406 | 16,778 | 3,657 | 2,144 | 1,513 | 372 | 173 | 199 | 378 | 123 | 255 |
| | 30-34 | 31,574 | 19,800 | 11,774 | 5,563 | 3,093 | 2,470 | 23,487 | 15,133 | 8,354 | 2,111 | 1,377 | 734 | 210 | 106 | 104 | 203 | 91 | 112 |
| | 35-39 | 22,413 | 15,252 | 7,161 | 4,115 | 2,566 | 1,549 | 16,685 | 11,661 | 5,024 | 1,297 | 863 | 434 | 154 | 92 | 62 | 162 | 70 | 92 |
| | 40-44 | 12,807 | 9,652 | 3,155 | 2,217 | 1,478 | 739 | 9,768 | 7,619 | 2,149 | 652 | 449 | 203 | 87 | 57 | 30 | 83 | 49 | 34 |
| | 45-54 | 9,087 | 7,596 | 1,491 | 1,635 | 1,256 | 379 | 6,884 | 5,945 | 939 | 461 | 329 | 132 | 48 | 25 | 23 | 59 | 41 | 18 |
| | 55-64 | 2,128 | 1,894 | 234 | 412 | 358 | 54 | 1,581 | 1,435 | 146 | 112 | 87 | 25 | 10 | 6 | 4 | 13 | 8 | 5 |
| | 65+ | 1,193 | 857 | 336 | 241 | 168 | 73 | 843 | 622 | 221 | 83 | 63 | 20 | 9 | 3 | 6 | 17 | 1 | 16 |
| | TOTAL | 347,882 | 171,553 | 176,329 | 53,195 | 19,602 | 33,593 | 269,287 | 139,738 | 129,549 | 21,068 | 10,709 | 10,359 | 1,978 | 757 | 1,221 | 2,354 | 747 | 1,607 |
| 1999 | 10-14 | 5,952 | 824 | 5,128 | 850 | 56 | 794 | 4,649 | 701 | 3,948 | 379 | 62 | 317 | 35 | 2 | 33 | 39 | 3 | 36 |
| | 15-19 | 104,336 | 34,266 | 70,070 | 15,132 | 2,593 | 12,539 | 81,376 | 29,147 | 52,229 | 6,565 | 2,264 | 4,301 | 566 | 139 | 427 | 697 | 123 | 574 |
| | 20-24 | 108,639 | 52,677 | 55,962 | 14,800 | 4,587 | 10,213 | 85,570 | 44,163 | 41,407 | 6,924 | 3,426 | 3,498 | 685 | 302 | 383 | 660 | 199 | 461 |
| | 25-29 | 56,082 | 32,574 | 23,508 | 8,202 | 3,673 | 4,529 | 43,337 | 26,376 | 16,961 | 3,921 | 2,238 | 1,683 | 323 | 181 | 142 | 299 | 106 | 193 |
| | 30-34 | 32,340 | 20,685 | 11,655 | 5,673 | 3,124 | 2,549 | 23,940 | 15,903 | 8,037 | 2,261 | 1,415 | 846 | 255 | 146 | 109 | 211 | 97 | 114 |
| | 35-39 | 23,432 | 16,210 | 7,222 | 4,558 | 2,779 | 1,779 | 17,238 | 12,398 | 4,840 | 1,341 | 877 | 464 | 158 | 98 | 60 | 137 | 58 | 79 |
| | 40-44 | 14,004 | 10,648 | 3,356 | 2,527 | 1,786 | 741 | 10,648 | 8,336 | 2,312 | 682 | 443 | 239 | 73 | 38 | 35 | 74 | 45 | 29 |
| | 45-54 | 10,341 | 8,657 | 1,684 | 1,946 | 1,502 | 444 | 7,803 | 6,740 | 1,063 | 454 | 330 | 124 | 65 | 44 | 21 | 73 | 41 | 32 |
| | 55-64 | 2,355 | 2,122 | 233 | 536 | 464 | 72 | 1,676 | 1,548 | 128 | 116 | 90 | 26 | 16 | 12 | 4 | 11 | 8 | 3 |
| | 65+ | 907 | 725 | 182 | 197 | 158 | 39 | 621 | 505 | 116 | 72 | 57 | 15 | 7 | 2 | 5 | 10 | 3 | 7 |
| | TOTAL | 359,463 | 179,780 | 179,683 | 54,574 | 20,773 | 33,801 | 277,695 | 146,123 | 131,572 | 22,790 | 11,230 | 11,560 | 2,189 | 969 | 1,220 | 2,215 | 685 | 1,530 |

Note: These tables should be used only for race/ethnicity and age comparisons, not for overall totals or gender totals. This is because, if age or race/ethnicity was not specified, cases were prorated according to the distribution of cases for which these variables were specified. For the following years the states listed did not report race/ethnicity for most cases and were excluded: 1995 (Georgia, New Jersey, and New York); 1996 (New Jersey and New York); 1997 (Idaho, New Jersey, and New York); 1998 (Idaho and New Jersey). Cases and population denominators have been excluded for these states/areas. Differences between total cases from this table and others in the report are due to different reporting forms and above listed exclusions. The 0 to 9 year age group is not shown because some of these may not be due to sexual transmission; however, they are included in the totals.

*Source*: Centers for Disease Control and Prevention, U.S. Department of Health and Human Services. National Center for HIV, STD, and TB Prevention, Division of STD Prevention. *Sexually Transmitted Disease Surveillance 1999* (Atlanta, GA: CDC, 2000). http://www.cdc.gov/nchstp/dstd/Stats_Trends/1999Surveillance/99PDF/Surv99Master.pdf.

## Table D5.1. Primary and Secondary Syphilis—Reported Rates: United States, 1970–1999, and the Healthy People Year 2000 Objective

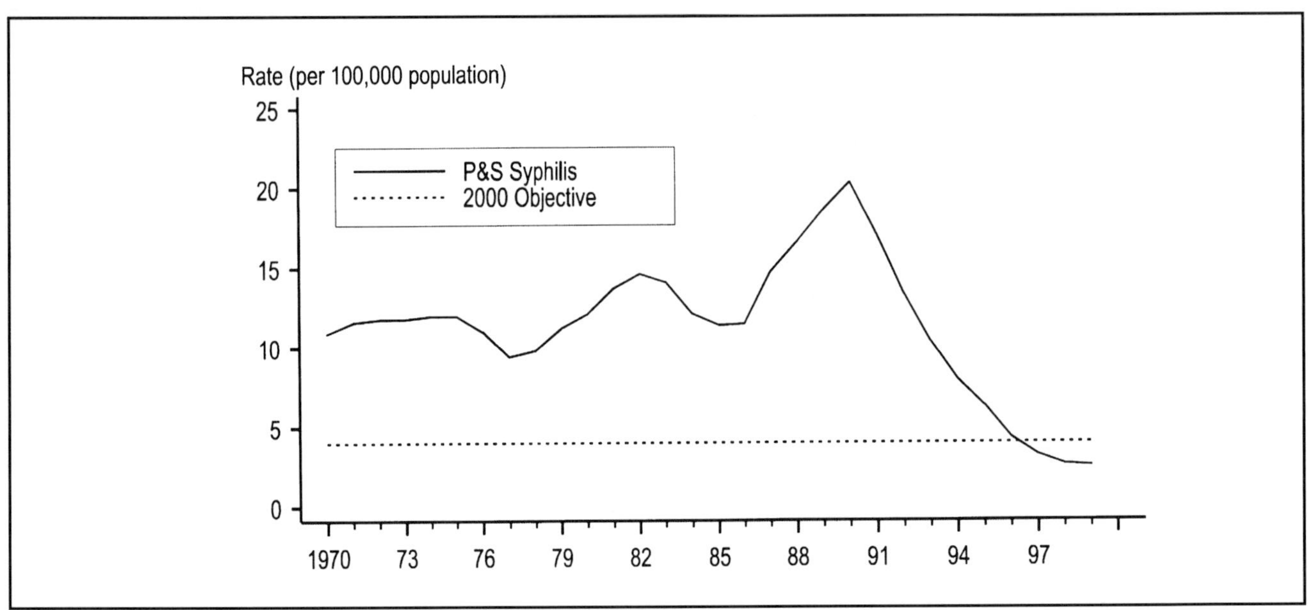


*Source*: Centers for Disease Control and Prevention, U.S. Department of Health and Human Services. National Center for HIV, STD, and TB Prevention, Division of STD Prevention. *Sexually Transmitted Disease Surveillance 1999* (Atlanta, GA: CDC, 2000). http://www.cdc.gov//nchstp/dstd/Stats_Trends/1999Surveillance/99PDF/Surv99Master.pdf.

## Table D5.2. Syphilis, Primary and Secondary—Reported Cases per 100,000 Population, United States, 1999

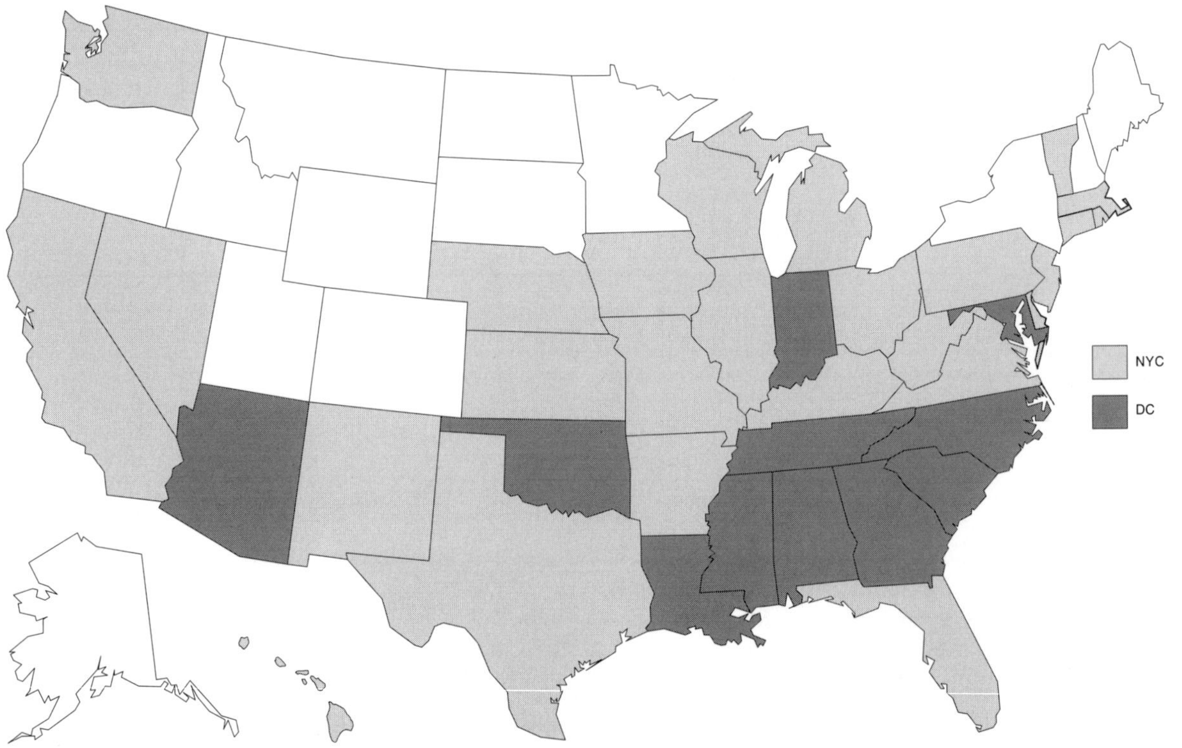

NYC

DC

≤ 0.2 0.3-4 >4

In 1999, the U.S. rate of primary and secondary syphilis was 2.5 cases/100,000 population, which is below the revised *Healthy People 2000* national objective of 4.0 cases/100,000 population. Thirty-nine states reported rates below the national objective, and 14 states reported <5 cases.

*Source*: Center for Disease Control and Prevention. U.S. Department of Health and Human Services. *MMWR: Morbidity and Mortality Weekly Review Summary of Notifiable Disease, United States, 1999* 48 no. 53 (2001). http://www.cdc.gov/mmwr/PDF/wk/mm4853.pdf.

## Table D5.3. Primary and Secondary Syphilis—Reported Cases and Rates, by State/Area Ranked According to Rates: United State and Outlying Areas, 1999

| *Rank* | *State/Area* | *Cases* | *Rate per 100,000 Population* |
|---|---|---|---|
| 1 | Tennessee | 641 | 11.8 |
| 2 | Indiana | 450 | 7.6 |
| 3 | Louisiana | 306 | 7.0 |
| 4 | Mississippi | 194 | 7.0 |
| 5 | South Carolina | 269 | 7.0 |
| 6 | Maryland | 343 | 6.7 |
| 7 | North Carolina | 464 | 6.1 |
| 8 | Georgia | 430 | 5.6 |
| 9 | Oklahoma | 187 | 5.6 |
| 10 | Alabama | 202 | 4.6 |
| 11 | Arizona | 212 | 4.5 |
| | **YEAR 2000 OBJECTIVE** | | **4.0** |
| 12 | Puerto Rico | 146 | 3.8 |
| 13 | Illinois | 422 | 3.5 |
| 14 | Arkansas | 87 | 3.4 |
| 15 | Florida | 383 | 2.6 |
| 16 | Kentucky | 101 | 2.6 |
| 17 | Michigan | 249 | 2.5 |
| | **U.S. TOTAL[1]** | **6,657** | **2.5** |
| 18 | Texas | 473 | 2.4 |
| 19 | Virginia | 153 | 2.3 |
| 20 | Missouri | 96 | 1.8 |
| 21 | Washington | 77 | 1.4 |
| 22 | Delaware | 10 | 1.3 |
| 23 | Guam | 2 | 1.3 |
| 24 | California | 283 | 0.9 |
| 25 | Virgin Islands | 1 | 0.9 |
| 26 | New Jersey | 68 | 0.8 |
| 27 | New York | 150 | 0.8 |
| 28 | Ohio | 92 | 0.8 |
| 29 | Wisconsin | 41 | 0.8 |
| 30 | New Mexico | 12 | 0.7 |
| 31 | Pennsylvania | 84 | 0.7 |
| 32 | Massachusetts | 37 | 0.6 |
| 33 | Connecticut | 16 | 0.5 |
| 34 | Kansas | 14 | 0.5 |
| 35 | Vermont | 3 | 0.5 |
| 36 | Nebraska | 6 | 0.4 |
| 37 | Hawaii | 3 | 0.3 |
| 38 | Iowa | 9 | 0.3 |
| 39 | Nevada | 5 | 0.3 |
| 40 | Rhode Island | 3 | 0.3 |
| 41 | West Virginia | 5 | 0.3 |
| 42 | Alaska | 1 | 0.2 |
| 43 | Colorado | 8 | 0.2 |
| 44 | Minnesota | 10 | 0.2 |
| 45 | Oregon | 8 | 0.2 |
| 46 | Idaho | 1 | 0.1 |
| 47 | Montana | 1 | 0.1 |
| 48 | New Hampshire | 1 | 0.1 |
| 49 | Utah | 2 | 0.1 |
| 50 | Maine | 0 | 0.0 |
| 51 | North Dakota | 0 | 0.0 |
| 52 | South Dakota | 0 | 0.0 |
| 53 | Wyoming | 0 | 0.0 |

[1]Includes cases reported by Washington, D.C., but excludes outlying areas (Guam, Puerto Rico and Virgin Islands).

*Source*: Centers for Disease Control and Prevention, U.S. Department of Health and Human Services. National Center for HIV, STD, and TB Prevention, Division of STD Prevention. *Sexually Transmitted Disease Surveillance 1999* (Atlanta, GA: CDC, 2000). http://www.cdc.gov/nchstp/dstd/Stats_Trends/1999Surveillance/99PDF/Surv99Master.pdf.

## Table D5.4. Syphilis, Primary and Secondary—Reported Cases per 100,000 Population by Sex, United States, 1984–1999

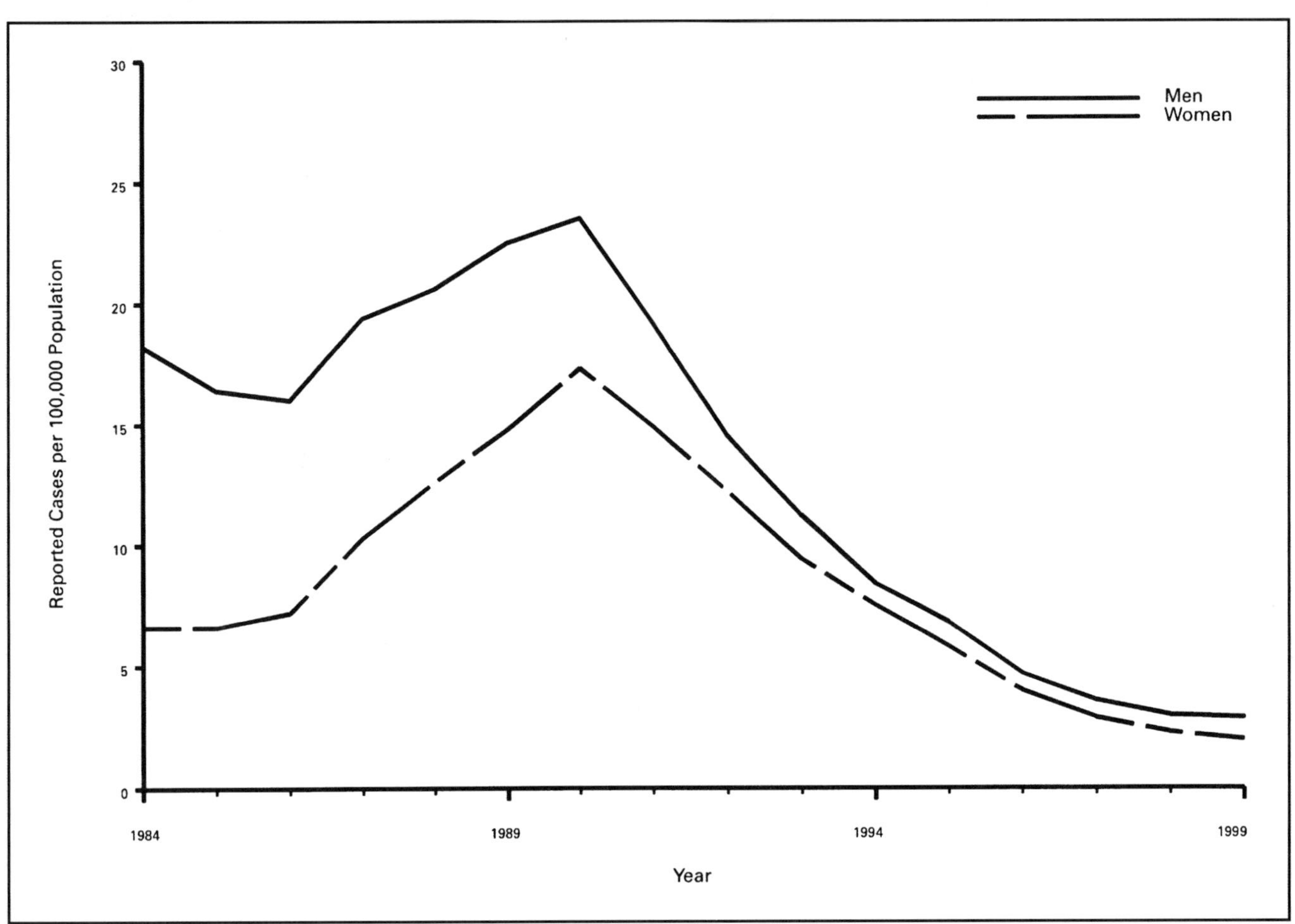


The reported U.S. rate of primary and secondary syphilis continues to decline, with 1999 rates among both males and females below the *Healthy People 2000* national objective of 4.0 cases/100,000 population. Rates decreased from 3.0 cases/100,000 in 1998 to 2.9 in 1999 among men and from 2.2 cases/100,000 in 1998 to 2.0 cases in 1999 among women.

*Source*: Center for Disease Control and Prevention. U.S. Department of Health and Human Services. *MMWR: Morbidity and Mortality Weekly Review Summary of Notifiable Disease, United States, 1999* 48 no. 53 (2001). http://www.cdc.gov/mmwr/PDF/wk/mm4853.pdf.

# Table D5.5. Primary and Secondary Syphilis—Women—Reported Cases and Rates, by State/Area Listed in Alphabetical Order: United States and Outlying Areas, 1995–1999

| | Cases | | | | | Rates per 100,000 Population | | | | |
|---|---|---|---|---|---|---|---|---|---|---|
| *State/Area* | *1995* | *1996* | *1997* | *1998* | *1999* | *1995* | *1996* | *1997* | *1998* | *1999* |
| Alabama | 257 | 244 | 183 | 133 | 102 | 11.6 | 11.0 | 8.2 | 5.9 | 4.5 |
| Alaska | 1 | 0 | 0 | 0 | 0 | 0.4 | 0.0 | 0.0 | 0.0 | 0.0 |
| Arizona | 14 | 43 | 37 | 67 | 65 | 0.7 | 1.9 | 1.6 | 2.8 | 2.8 |
| Arkansas | 267 | 144 | 103 | 59 | 44 | 20.8 | 11.1 | 7.9 | 4.5 | 3.4 |
| California | 219 | 187 | 116 | 132 | 76 | 1.4 | 1.2 | 0.7 | 0.8 | 0.5 |
| Colorado | 42 | 10 | 5 | 3 | 6 | 2.2 | 0.5 | 0.3 | 0.1 | 0.3 |
| Connecticut | 34 | 58 | 25 | 16 | 6 | 2.0 | 3.5 | 1.5 | 0.9 | 0.4 |
| Delaware | 7 | 14 | 10 | 11 | 1 | 1.9 | 3.8 | 2.7 | 2.9 | 0.3 |
| Florida | 189 | 172 | 131 | 116 | 162 | 2.6 | 2.3 | 1.7 | 1.5 | 2.1 |
| Georgia | 360 | 284 | 194 | 130 | 160 | 9.7 | 7.6 | 5.1 | 3.3 | 4.1 |
| Hawaii | 0 | 1 | 0 | 0 | 2 | 0.0 | 0.2 | 0.0 | 0.0 | 0.3 |
| Idaho | 0 | 3 | 0 | 0 | 0 | 0.0 | 0.5 | 0.0 | 0.0 | 0.0 |
| Illinois | 500 | 246 | 194 | 171 | 180 | 8.2 | 4.1 | 3.2 | 2.8 | 2.9 |
| Indiana | 151 | 115 | 82 | 113 | 225 | 5.1 | 3.8 | 2.7 | 3.7 | 7.4 |
| Iowa | 31 | 16 | 4 | 0 | 6 | 2.1 | 1.1 | 0.3 | 0.0 | 0.4 |
| Kansas | 22 | 10 | 12 | 6 | 8 | 1.7 | 0.8 | 0.9 | 0.4 | 0.6 |
| Kentucky | 83 | 81 | 66 | 49 | 45 | 4.2 | 4.1 | 3.3 | 2.4 | 2.2 |
| Louisiana | 505 | 271 | 187 | 196 | 153 | 22.4 | 12.0 | 8.3 | 8.6 | 6.7 |
| Maine | 0 | 0 | 1 | 0 | 0 | 0.0 | 0.0 | 0.2 | 0.0 | 0.0 |
| Maryland | 233 | 329 | 400 | 302 | 164 | 9.0 | 12.7 | 15.3 | 11.4 | 6.2 |
| Massachusetts | 27 | 30 | 33 | 15 | 15 | 0.9 | 1.0 | 1.0 | 0.5 | 0.5 |
| Michigan | 132 | 82 | 68 | 86 | 95 | 2.7 | 1.6 | 1.4 | 1.7 | 1.9 |
| Minnesota | 25 | 8 | 4 | 4 | 5 | 1.1 | 0.3 | 0.2 | 0.2 | 0.2 |
| Mississippi | 1,000 | 427 | 201 | 128 | 93 | 71.2 | 30.3 | 14.2 | 8.9 | 6.5 |
| Missouri | 283 | 103 | 63 | 50 | 49 | 10.3 | 3.7 | 2.3 | 1.8 | 1.7 |
| Montana | 2 | 0 | 0 | 0 | 0 | 0.5 | 0.0 | 0.0 | 0.0 | 0.0 |
| Nebraska | 4 | 4 | 0 | 3 | 3 | 0.5 | 0.5 | 0.0 | 0.4 | 0.4 |
| Nevada | 12 | 10 | 6 | 3 | 3 | 1.6 | 1.3 | 0.7 | 0.3 | 0.3 |
| New Hampshire | 0 | 0 | 0 | 1 | 1 | 0.0 | 0.0 | 0.0 | 0.2 | 0.2 |
| New Jersey | 72 | 81 | 59 | 37 | 32 | 1.8 | 2.0 | 1.4 | 0.9 | 0.8 |
| New Mexico | 3 | 1 | 5 | 8 | 3 | 0.4 | 0.1 | 0.6 | 0.9 | 0.3 |
| New York | 218 | 92 | 56 | 28 | 34 | 2.3 | 1.0 | 0.6 | 0.3 | 0.4 |
| North Carolina | 536 | 484 | 353 | 347 | 202 | 14.5 | 12.9 | 9.3 | 8.9 | 5.2 |
| North Dakota | 0 | 0 | 0 | 0 | 0 | 0.0 | 0.0 | 0.0 | 0.0 | 0.0 |
| Ohio | 417 | 287 | 101 | 72 | 43 | 7.2 | 5.0 | 1.8 | 1.2 | 0.7 |
| Oklahoma | 90 | 80 | 53 | 45 | 77 | 5.4 | 4.8 | 3.1 | 2.6 | 4.5 |
| Oregon | 2 | 3 | 2 | 2 | 5 | 0.1 | 0.2 | 0.1 | 0.1 | 0.3 |
| Pennsylvania | 92 | 62 | 52 | 31 | 27 | 1.5 | 1.0 | 0.8 | 0.5 | 0.4 |
| Rhode Island | 2 | 1 | 1 | 1 | 1 | 0.4 | 0.2 | 0.2 | 0.2 | 0.2 |
| South Carolina | 285 | 182 | 173 | 131 | 117 | 15.0 | 9.5 | 8.9 | 6.6 | 5.9 |
| South Dakota | 0 | 0 | 0 | 1 | 0 | 0.0 | 0.0 | 0.0 | 0.3 | 0.0 |
| Tennessee | 432 | 422 | 370 | 284 | 283 | 15.9 | 15.4 | 13.3 | 10.1 | 10.1 |
| Texas | 770 | 437 | 315 | 183 | 182 | 8.1 | 4.5 | 3.2 | 1.8 | 1.8 |
| Utah | 0 | 0 | 2 | 0 | 0 | 0.0 | 0.0 | 0.2 | 0.0 | 0.0 |
| Vermont | 0 | 0 | 0 | 1 | 2 | 0.0 | 0.0 | 0.0 | 0.3 | 0.7 |
| Virginia | 299 | 204 | 112 | 61 | 71 | 8.8 | 6.0 | 3.3 | 1.8 | 2.0 |
| Washington | 6 | 2 | 8 | 7 | 3 | 0.2 | 0.1 | 0.3 | 0.2 | 0.1 |
| West Virginia | 11 | 6 | 1 | 2 | 3 | 1.2 | 0.6 | 0.1 | 0.2 | 0.3 |
| Wisconsin | 93 | 85 | 49 | 40 | 18 | 3.6 | 3.3 | 1.9 | 1.5 | 0.7 |
| Wyoming | 0 | 1 | 0 | 0 | 0 | 0.0 | 0.4 | 0.0 | 0.0 | 0.0 |
| U.S. TOTAL[1] | 7,776 | 5,379 | 3,895 | 3,109 | 2,796 | 5.8 | 4.0 | 2.9 | 2.2 | 2.0 |
| Guam | 0 | 0 | 0 | 0 | 0 | 0.0 | 0.0 | 0.0 | 0.0 | 0.0 |
| Puerto Rico | 141 | 100 | 116 | 81 | 73 | 7.4 | 5.2 | 5.8 | 4.0 | 3.6 |
| Virgin Islands | 0 | 5 | 0 | 1 | 1 | 0.0 | 8.8 | 0.0 | 1.7 | 1.7 |
| OUTLYING AREAS | 141 | 105 | 116 | 82 | 74 | 6.9 | 5.1 | 5.5 | 3.8 | 3.5 |
| TOTAL | 7,917 | 5,484 | 4,011 | 3,191 | 2,870 | 5.8 | 4.0 | 2.9 | 2.3 | 2.0 |

[1]Includes cases reported by Washington, D.C.

Note: Cases and rates underestimated in some areas because of under-reporting or non-reporting by gender.

*Source*: Centers for Disease Control and Prevention, U.S. Department of Health and Human Services. National Center for HIV, STD, and TB Prevention, Division of STD Prevention. *Sexually Transmitted Disease Surveillance 1999* (Atlanta, GA: CDC, 2000). http://www.cdc.gov/nchstp/dstd/Stats_Trends/1999Surveillance/99PDF/Surv99Master.pdf.

## Table D5.6. Primary and Secondary Syphilis—Men—Reported Cases and Rates, by State/Area Listed in Alphabetical Order: United States and Outlying Areas, 1995–1999

| | Cases | | | | | Rates per 100,000 Population | | | | |
|---|---|---|---|---|---|---|---|---|---|---|
| State/Area | 1995 | 1996 | 1997 | 1998 | 1999 | 1995 | 1996 | 1997 | 1998 | 1999 |
| Alabama | 355 | 284 | 227 | 141 | 100 | 17.4 | 13.8 | 10.9 | 6.8 | 4.8 |
| Alaska | 1 | 0 | 1 | 1 | 1 | 0.3 | 0.0 | 0.3 | 0.3 | 0.3 |
| Arizona | 32 | 59 | 95 | 118 | 147 | 1.5 | 2.7 | 4.2 | 5.1 | 6.4 |
| Arkansas | 228 | 118 | 70 | 49 | 43 | 19.0 | 9.7 | 5.7 | 4.0 | 3.5 |
| California | 363 | 322 | 270 | 195 | 206 | 2.3 | 2.0 | 1.7 | 1.2 | 1.3 |
| Colorado | 58 | 16 | 10 | 7 | 2 | 3.1 | 0.8 | 0.5 | 0.4 | 0.1 |
| Connecticut | 52 | 45 | 37 | 10 | 10 | 3.3 | 2.8 | 2.3 | 0.6 | 0.6 |
| Delaware | 12 | 21 | 12 | 10 | 9 | 3.4 | 6.0 | 3.4 | 2.8 | 2.5 |
| Florida | 194 | 196 | 165 | 178 | 220 | 2.8 | 2.8 | 2.3 | 2.5 | 3.0 |
| Georgia | 541 | 405 | 321 | 203 | 269 | 15.5 | 11.3 | 8.8 | 5.5 | 7.2 |
| Hawaii | 0 | 2 | 1 | 4 | 1 | 0.0 | 0.3 | 0.2 | 0.7 | 0.2 |
| Idaho | 0 | 1 | 1 | 2 | 1 | 0.0 | 0.2 | 0.2 | 0.3 | 0.2 |
| Illinois | 526 | 255 | 241 | 253 | 242 | 9.1 | 4.4 | 4.1 | 4.3 | 4.1 |
| Indiana | 169 | 92 | 69 | 102 | 225 | 6.0 | 3.2 | 2.4 | 3.6 | 7.8 |
| Iowa | 17 | 7 | 3 | 5 | 3 | 1.2 | 0.5 | 0.2 | 0.4 | 0.2 |
| Kansas | 25 | 18 | 20 | 8 | 6 | 2.0 | 1.4 | 1.6 | 0.6 | 0.5 |
| Kentucky | 102 | 73 | 69 | 57 | 56 | 5.5 | 3.9 | 3.6 | 3.0 | 2.9 |
| Louisiana | 519 | 262 | 177 | 234 | 153 | 24.9 | 12.5 | 8.4 | 11.1 | 7.3 |
| Maine | 2 | 1 | 1 | 1 | 0 | 0.3 | 0.2 | 0.2 | 0.2 | 0.0 |
| Maryland | 321 | 400 | 490 | 346 | 179 | 13.1 | 16.2 | 19.8 | 13.9 | 7.2 |
| Massachusetts | 42 | 55 | 45 | 31 | 22 | 1.4 | 1.9 | 1.5 | 1.0 | 0.7 |
| Michigan | 172 | 101 | 85 | 125 | 154 | 3.7 | 2.1 | 1.8 | 2.6 | 3.2 |
| Minnesota | 20 | 8 | 12 | 5 | 5 | 0.9 | 0.3 | 0.5 | 0.2 | 0.2 |
| Mississippi | 952 | 390 | 189 | 131 | 101 | 73.6 | 30.0 | 14.4 | 9.9 | 7.7 |
| Missouri | 301 | 118 | 55 | 59 | 47 | 11.7 | 4.5 | 2.1 | 2.2 | 1.8 |
| Montana | 2 | 0 | 0 | 0 | 1 | 0.5 | 0.0 | 0.0 | 0.0 | 0.2 |
| Nebraska | 10 | 2 | 3 | 5 | 3 | 1.3 | 0.2 | 0.4 | 0.6 | 0.4 |
| Nevada | 24 | 10 | 5 | 12 | 2 | 3.1 | 1.2 | 0.6 | 1.3 | 0.2 |
| New Hampshire | 0 | 1 | 0 | 1 | 0 | 0.0 | 0.2 | 0.0 | 0.2 | 0.0 |
| New Jersey | 116 | 96 | 91 | 70 | 36 | 3.0 | 2.5 | 2.3 | 1.8 | 0.9 |
| New Mexico | 10 | 2 | 4 | 6 | 9 | 1.2 | 0.2 | 0.5 | 0.7 | 1.1 |
| New York | 231 | 122 | 82 | 91 | 116 | 2.6 | 1.4 | 0.9 | 1.0 | 1.3 |
| North Carolina | 596 | 568 | 368 | 376 | 262 | 17.1 | 16.0 | 10.2 | 10.3 | 7.2 |
| North Dakota | 0 | 0 | 0 | 0 | 0 | 0.0 | 0.0 | 0.0 | 0.0 | 0.0 |
| Ohio | 479 | 297 | 117 | 62 | 49 | 8.9 | 5.5 | 2.2 | 1.1 | 0.9 |
| Oklahoma | 107 | 99 | 64 | 53 | 110 | 6.7 | 6.1 | 3.9 | 3.2 | 6.7 |
| Oregon | 3 | 6 | 8 | 4 | 3 | 0.2 | 0.4 | 0.5 | 0.2 | 0.2 |
| Pennsylvania | 156 | 102 | 71 | 67 | 57 | 2.7 | 1.8 | 1.2 | 1.2 | 1.0 |
| Rhode Island | 2 | 3 | 1 | 0 | 2 | 0.4 | 0.6 | 0.2 | 0.0 | 0.4 |
| South Carolina | 285 | 220 | 205 | 140 | 152 | 16.1 | 12.3 | 11.3 | 7.6 | 8.2 |
| South Dakota | 0 | 0 | 1 | 0 | 0 | 0.0 | 0.0 | 0.3 | 0.0 | 0.0 |
| Tennessee | 474 | 428 | 377 | 283 | 358 | 18.7 | 16.7 | 14.5 | 10.8 | 13.7 |
| Texas | 787 | 453 | 361 | 260 | 289 | 8.5 | 4.8 | 3.8 | 2.7 | 3.0 |
| Utah | 4 | 3 | 3 | 4 | 2 | 0.4 | 0.3 | 0.3 | 0.4 | 0.2 |
| Vermont | 0 | 0 | 0 | 3 | 1 | 0.0 | 0.0 | 0.0 | 1.0 | 0.3 |
| Virginia | 301 | 189 | 125 | 88 | 82 | 9.3 | 5.8 | 3.8 | 2.7 | 2.5 |
| Washington | 11 | 7 | 9 | 37 | 74 | 0.4 | 0.3 | 0.3 | 1.3 | 2.6 |
| West Virginia | 5 | 1 | 0 | 1 | 2 | 0.6 | 0.1 | 0.0 | 0.1 | 0.2 |
| Wisconsin | 92 | 91 | 40 | 38 | 23 | 3.7 | 3.6 | 1.6 | 1.5 | 0.9 |
| Wyoming | 1 | 1 | 0 | 1 | 0 | 0.4 | 0.4 | 0.0 | 0.4 | 0.0 |
| U.S. TOTAL[1] | 8,764 | 6,009 | 4,660 | 3,924 | 3,856 | 6.8 | 4.6 | 3.6 | 3.0 | 2.9 |
| Guam | 0 | 0 | 0 | 0 | 2 | 0.0 | 0.0 | 0.0 | 0.0 | 2.4 |
| Puerto Rico | 144 | 108 | 133 | 96 | 73 | 8.1 | 6.0 | 7.2 | 5.2 | 3.9 |
| Virgin Islands | 2 | 6 | 2 | 6 | 0 | 3.8 | 11.4 | 3.8 | 11.3 | 0.0 |
| OUTLYING AREAS | 146 | 114 | 135 | 102 | 75 | 7.6 | 5.9 | 6.8 | 5.1 | 3.8 |
| TOTAL | 8,910 | 6,123 | 4,795 | 4,026 | 3,931 | 6.8 | 4.7 | 3.6 | 3.0 | 2.9 |

[1]Includes cases reported by Washington, D.C.

Note: Cases and rates underestimated in some areas because of under-reporting or non-reporting by gender.

*Source*: Centers for Disease Control and Prevention, U.S. Department of Health and Human Services. National Center for HIV, STD, and TB Prevention, Division of STD Prevention. *Sexually Transmitted Disease Surveillance 1999* (Atlanta, GA: CDC, 2000). http://www.cdc.gov/nchstp/dstd/Stats_Trends/1999Surveillance/99PDF/Surv99Master.pdf.

# Table D5.7. All Stages of Syphilis—Reported Cases and Rates, by State/Area Listed in Alphabetical Order: United States and Outlying Areas, 1995–1999

| State/Area | Cases | | | | | Rates per 100,000 Population | | | | |
|---|---|---|---|---|---|---|---|---|---|---|
| | 1995 | 1996 | 1997 | 1998 | 1999 | 1995 | 1996 | 1997 | 1998 | 1999 |
| Alabama | 1,640 | 1,889 | 1,486 | 1,139 | 1,018 | 38.6 | 44.1 | 34.4 | 26.2 | 23.4 |
| Alaska | 20 | 15 | 12 | 13 | 13 | 3.3 | 2.5 | 2.0 | 2.1 | 2.1 |
| Arizona | 417 | 468 | 600 | 697 | 833 | 9.9 | 10.6 | 13.2 | 14.9 | 17.8 |
| Arkansas | 1,270 | 843 | 572 | 506 | 364 | 51.1 | 33.6 | 22.7 | 19.9 | 14.3 |
| California | 5,771 | 4,420 | 3,827 | 2,869 | 2,859 | 18.3 | 13.9 | 11.9 | 8.8 | 8.8 |
| Colorado | 304 | 165 | 153 | 122 | 91 | 8.1 | 4.3 | 3.9 | 3.1 | 2.3 |
| Connecticut | 270 | 334 | 325 | 177 | 126 | 8.2 | 10.2 | 9.9 | 5.4 | 3.8 |
| Delaware | 129 | 124 | 113 | 114 | 72 | 18.0 | 17.1 | 15.4 | 15.3 | 9.7 |
| Florida | 3,468 | 2,912 | 2,746 | 2,539 | 2,957 | 24.5 | 20.2 | 18.7 | 17.0 | 19.8 |
| Georgia | 3,666 | 2,953 | 2,835 | 1,836 | 1,973 | 50.9 | 40.3 | 37.9 | 24.0 | 25.8 |
| Hawaii | 25 | 30 | 47 | 18 | 11 | 2.1 | 2.5 | 4.0 | 1.5 | 0.9 |
| Idaho | 12 | 24 | 24 | 15 | 13 | 1.0 | 2.0 | 2.0 | 1.2 | 1.1 |
| Illinois | 3,712 | 2,071 | 1,954 | 2,028 | 1,967 | 31.4 | 17.5 | 16.4 | 16.8 | 16.3 |
| Indiana | 870 | 675 | 522 | 509 | 802 | 15.0 | 11.6 | 8.9 | 8.6 | 13.6 |
| Iowa | 170 | 86 | 72 | 48 | 37 | 6.0 | 3.0 | 2.5 | 1.7 | 1.3 |
| Kansas | 150 | 136 | 169 | 116 | 95 | 5.8 | 5.3 | 6.5 | 4.4 | 3.6 |
| Kentucky | 501 | 398 | 403 | 339 | 302 | 13.0 | 10.3 | 10.3 | 8.6 | 7.7 |
| Louisiana | 3,692 | 2,409 | 1,808 | 1,651 | 1,423 | 85.0 | 55.5 | 41.5 | 37.8 | 32.6 |
| Maine | 4 | 4 | 13 | 4 | 1 | 0.3 | 0.3 | 1.0 | 0.3 | 0.1 |
| Maryland | 1,679 | 2,234 | 2,455 | 2,156 | 1,385 | 33.3 | 44.1 | 48.2 | 42.0 | 27.0 |
| Massachusetts | 506 | 633 | 730 | 568 | 385 | 8.3 | 10.4 | 11.9 | 9.2 | 6.3 |
| Michigan | 1,203 | 851 | 794 | 692 | 778 | 12.6 | 8.7 | 8.1 | 7.0 | 7.9 |
| Minnesota | 187 | 116 | 124 | 75 | 71 | 4.1 | 2.5 | 2.6 | 1.6 | 1.5 |
| Mississippi | 4,532 | 2,365 | 1,441 | 1,161 | 906 | 168.0 | 87.2 | 52.8 | 42.2 | 32.9 |
| Missouri | 1,265 | 618 | 503 | 379 | 395 | 23.8 | 11.5 | 9.3 | 7.0 | 7.3 |
| Montana | 13 | 4 | 5 | 0 | 3 | 1.5 | 0.5 | 0.6 | 0.0 | 0.3 |
| Nebraska | 35 | 27 | 34 | 35 | 24 | 2.1 | 1.6 | 2.1 | 2.1 | 1.4 |
| Nevada | 193 | 142 | 120 | 139 | 92 | 12.6 | 8.9 | 7.2 | 8.0 | 5.3 |
| New Hampshire | 32 | 29 | 26 | 14 | 17 | 2.8 | 2.5 | 2.2 | 1.2 | 1.4 |
| New Jersey | 1,470 | 1,448 | 1,166 | 836 | 800 | 18.5 | 18.1 | 14.5 | 10.3 | 9.9 |
| New Mexico | 138 | 78 | 103 | 76 | 80 | 8.2 | 4.6 | 6.0 | 4.4 | 4.6 |
| New York | 8,880 | 6,529 | 5,645 | 5,147 | 4,094 | 49.0 | 36.0 | 31.1 | 28.3 | 22.5 |
| North Carolina | 3,066 | 2,670 | 2,202 | 2,133 | 1,713 | 42.6 | 36.5 | 29.7 | 28.3 | 22.7 |
| North Dakota | 0 | 0 | 0 | 0 | 0 | 0.0 | 0.0 | 0.0 | 0.0 | 0.0 |
| Ohio | 1,938 | 1,324 | 761 | 474 | 364 | 17.4 | 11.9 | 6.8 | 4.2 | 3.2 |
| Oklahoma | 589 | 467 | 410 | 369 | 538 | 18.0 | 14.2 | 12.4 | 11.0 | 16.1 |
| Oregon | 67 | 70 | 48 | 32 | 37 | 2.1 | 2.2 | 1.5 | 1.0 | 1.1 |
| Pennsylvania | 1,948 | 1,440 | 1,182 | 910 | 932 | 16.1 | 12.0 | 9.8 | 7.6 | 7.8 |
| Rhode Island | 90 | 72 | 84 | 55 | 55 | 9.1 | 7.3 | 8.5 | 5.6 | 5.6 |
| South Carolina | 1,669 | 1,286 | 1,139 | 876 | 925 | 45.4 | 34.6 | 30.3 | 22.8 | 24.1 |
| South Dakota | 7 | 2 | 8 | 3 | 3 | 1.0 | 0.3 | 1.1 | 0.4 | 0.4 |
| Tennessee | 2,604 | 2,322 | 2,368 | 1,754 | 1,734 | 49.5 | 43.8 | 44.1 | 32.3 | 31.9 |
| Texas | 7,926 | 5,897 | 5,382 | 3,967 | 3,699 | 42.3 | 30.9 | 27.7 | 20.1 | 18.7 |
| Utah | 50 | 49 | 56 | 58 | 49 | 2.6 | 2.4 | 2.7 | 2.8 | 2.3 |
| Vermont | 0 | 1 | 1 | 6 | 3 | 0.0 | 0.2 | 0.2 | 1.0 | 0.5 |
| Virginia | 1,590 | 1,265 | 1,118 | 719 | 722 | 24.0 | 19.0 | 16.6 | 10.6 | 10.6 |
| Washington | 211 | 134 | 137 | 143 | 204 | 3.9 | 2.4 | 2.4 | 2.5 | 3.6 |
| West Virginia | 65 | 59 | 20 | 11 | 15 | 3.6 | 3.2 | 1.1 | 0.6 | 0.8 |
| Wisconsin | 585 | 496 | 317 | 257 | 190 | 11.4 | 9.6 | 6.1 | 4.9 | 3.6 |
| Wyoming | 2 | 8 | 4 | 2 | 0 | 0.4 | 1.7 | 0.8 | 0.4 | 0.0 |
| U.S. TOTAL[1] | 69,353 | 53,218 | 46,708 | 38,366 | 35,628 | 26.4 | 20.1 | 17.5 | 14.2 | 13.2 |
| Guam | 6 | 3 | 1 | 3 | 12 | 4.0 | 2.0 | 0.6 | 1.9 | 7.5 |
| Puerto Rico | 1,619 | 1,469 | 1,577 | 1,461 | 1,457 | 43.9 | 39.5 | 41.2 | 37.8 | 37.7 |
| Virgin Islands | 19 | 17 | 10 | 35 | 13 | 17.3 | 15.5 | 9.1 | 31.9 | 11.9 |
| OUTLYING AREAS | 1,644 | 1,489 | 1,588 | 1,499 | 1,482 | 41.6 | 37.4 | 38.8 | 36.3 | 35.9 |
| TOTAL | 70,997 | 54,707 | 48,296 | 39,865 | 37,110 | 26.6 | 20.3 | 17.8 | 14.5 | 13.5 |

[1]Includes cases reported by Washington, D.C.

*Source*: Centers for Disease Control and Prevention, U.S. Department of Health and Human Services. National Center for HIV, STD, and TB Prevention, Division of STD Prevention. *Sexually Transmitted Disease Surveillance 1999* (Atlanta, GA: CDC, 2000). http://www.cdc.gov/nchstp/dstd/Stats_Trends/1999Surveillance/99PDF/Surv99Master.pdf.

## Table D5.8. All Stages of Syphilis—Reported Cases and Rates in Selected Cities of >200,000 Population Listed in Alphabetical Order: United States and Outlying Areas, 1995–1999

| | Cases | | | | | Rates per 100,000 Population | | | | |
|---|---|---|---|---|---|---|---|---|---|---|
| *City* | *1995* | *1996* | *1997* | *1998* | *1999* | *1995* | *1996* | *1997* | *1998* | *1999* |
| Akron, OH | 8 | 8 | 4 | 7 | 6 | 1.5 | 1.5 | 0.8 | 1.3 | 1.1 |
| Albuquerque, NM | 41 | 33 | 56 | 45 | 50 | 7.8 | 6.3 | 10.6 | 8.6 | 9.5 |
| Atlanta, GA | 1,074 | 835 | 872 | 591 | 580 | 153.3 | 116.9 | 120.7 | 79.9 | 78.4 |
| Austin, TX | 183 | 88 | 98 | 56 | 62 | 27.5 | 12.9 | 14.1 | 7.9 | 8.7 |
| Baltimore, MD | 1,089 | 1,552 | 1,781 | 1,472 | 941 | 157.6 | 231.0 | 271.0 | 228.0 | 145.8 |
| Birmingham, AL | 640 | 703 | 474 | 246 | 278 | 97.3 | 106.4 | 72.0 | 37.3 | 42.2 |
| Boston, MA | 193 | 257 | 305 | 240 | 164 | 34.7 | 46.1 | 54.7 | 43.1 | 29.5 |
| Buffalo, NY | 32 | 22 | 23 | 12 | 6 | 9.8 | 6.8 | 7.2 | 3.8 | 1.9 |
| Charlotte, NC | 347 | 312 | 153 | 211 | 194 | 59.9 | 52.3 | 24.9 | 33.4 | 30.8 |
| Chicago, IL | 2,244 | 1,254 | 1,314 | 1,457 | 1,324 | 76.1 | 43.0 | 45.1 | 48.9 | 44.4 |
| Cincinnati, OH | 399 | 166 | 93 | 32 | 12 | 46.2 | 19.4 | 10.9 | 3.8 | 1.4 |
| Cleveland, OH | 750 | 377 | 250 | 151 | 88 | 53.6 | 27.0 | 18.0 | 10.9 | 6.4 |
| Columbus, OH | 31 | 89 | 117 | 115 | 109 | 3.1 | 8.8 | 11.5 | 11.3 | 10.7 |
| Corpus Christi, TX | 62 | 29 | 22 | 27 | 20 | 19.8 | 9.2 | 6.9 | 8.5 | 6.3 |
| Dallas, TX | 1,022 | 790 | 717 | 736 | 695 | 52.2 | 39.6 | 35.4 | 35.9 | 33.9 |
| Dayton, OH | 399 | 367 | 126 | 39 | 16 | 69.9 | 64.9 | 22.4 | 7.0 | 2.9 |
| Denver, CO | 179 | 67 | 72 | 35 | 46 | 36.2 | 13.5 | 14.4 | 7.0 | 9.2 |
| Des Moines, IA | 92 | 34 | 26 | 20 | 7 | 26.3 | 9.6 | 7.3 | 5.6 | 1.9 |
| Detroit, MI | 707 | 522 | 548 | 477 | 567 | 67.2 | 47.7 | 50.3 | 37.8 | 45.0 |
| El Paso, TX | 142 | 118 | 112 | 81 | 79 | 20.9 | 17.2 | 16.0 | 11.5 | 11.2 |
| Fort Worth, TX | 489 | 379 | 299 | 175 | 177 | 38.2 | 29.2 | 22.5 | 12.9 | 13.1 |
| Honolulu, HI | 22 | 26 | 42 | 18 | 8 | 2.5 | 3.0 | 4.8 | 2.1 | 0.9 |
| Houston, TX | 2,691 | 2,047 | 1,937 | 1,401 | 1,111 | 87.5 | 65.7 | 61.3 | 43.7 | 34.7 |
| Indianapolis, IN | 168 | 186 | 125 | 239 | 553 | 20.5 | 22.8 | 15.4 | 29.4 | 68.0 |
| Jacksonville, FL | 192 | 228 | 206 | 154 | 79 | 27.4 | 31.4 | 28.1 | 20.9 | 10.7 |
| Jersey City, NJ | 136 | 96 | 85 | 34 | 42 | 62.6 | 44.2 | 39.0 | 15.4 | 19.1 |
| Kansas City, MO | 68 | 38 | 13 | 14 | 66 | 15.5 | 8.5 | 2.9 | 3.1 | 14.6 |
| Los Angeles, CA | 3,009 | 2,193 | 1,630 | 1,264 | 1,189 | 35.2 | 25.8 | 19.0 | 14.7 | 13.8 |
| Louisville, KY | 272 | 227 | 232 | 213 | 174 | 40.4 | 33.8 | 34.6 | 31.7 | 25.9 |
| Memphis, TN | 1,596 | 1,371 | 1,435 | 1,036 | 924 | 184.5 | 158.5 | 165.7 | 119.2 | 106.4 |
| Miami, FL | 1,008 | 876 | 874 | 773 | 888 | 49.6 | 43.0 | 42.7 | 35.9 | 41.3 |
| Milwaukee, WI | 464 | 397 | 275 | 233 | 166 | 49.8 | 43.2 | 30.3 | 25.6 | 18.2 |
| Minneapolis, MN | 86 | 52 | 53 | 34 | 28 | 22.4 | 13.6 | 13.8 | 9.3 | 7.7 |
| Nashville, TN | 202 | 293 | 412 | 416 | 505 | 38.1 | 55.0 | 77.2 | 77.9 | 94.6 |
| New Orleans, LA | 649 | 520 | 463 | 348 | 228 | 134.7 | 109.7 | 98.7 | 74.8 | 49.0 |
| New York City, NY | 7,881 | 5,801 | 4,961 | 4,652 | 3,737 | 107.8 | 79.1 | 67.6 | 62.7 | 50.4 |
| Newark, NJ | 392 | 363 | 241 | 191 | 171 | 136.3 | 127.1 | 84.7 | 67.2 | 60.1 |
| Norfolk, VA | 278 | 222 | 158 | 108 | 84 | 117.0 | 95.4 | 68.9 | 50.2 | 39.0 |
| Oakland, CA | 185 | 139 | 128 | 129 | 127 | 15.3 | 11.2 | 10.2 | 10.1 | 9.9 |
| Oklahoma City, OK | 291 | 227 | 110 | 181 | 300 | 66.6 | 51.7 | 25.0 | 44.4 | 73.6 |
| Omaha, NE | 21 | 1 | 17 | 26 | 10 | 4.8 | 0.2 | 3.9 | 5.9 | 2.3 |
| Philadelphia, PA | 1,696 | 1,293 | 1,093 | 804 | 825 | 113.1 | 87.8 | 75.3 | 56.0 | 57.4 |
| Phoenix, AZ | 270 | 342 | 473 | 572 | 722 | 11.1 | 13.1 | 17.5 | 20.5 | 25.9 |
| Pittsburgh, PA | 27 | 16 | 21 | 12 | 7 | 2.1 | 1.2 | 1.6 | 0.9 | 0.6 |
| Portland, OR | 42 | 45 | 23 | 17 | 19 | 8.7 | 9.2 | 4.7 | 3.4 | 3.8 |
| Richmond, VA | 122 | 171 | 137 | 81 | 64 | 61.5 | 89.5 | 71.2 | 41.7 | 33.0 |
| Rochester, NY | 104 | 68 | 32 | 39 | 16 | 42.8 | 28.1 | 13.3 | 16.2 | 6.7 |
| Sacramento, CA | 86 | 58 | 55 | 31 | 20 | 7.8 | 5.2 | 4.9 | 2.7 | 1.7 |
| San Antonio, TX | 394 | 378 | 309 | 237 | 228 | 30.4 | 28.8 | 23.2 | 17.5 | 16.9 |
| San Diego, CA | 371 | 227 | 259 | 187 | 251 | 14.0 | 8.5 | 9.5 | 6.7 | 9.0 |
| San Francisco, CA | 84 | 151 | 171 | 129 | 128 | 11.5 | 20.7 | 23.4 | 17.3 | 17.2 |
| San Jose, CA | 78 | 70 | 93 | 62 | 56 | 5.0 | 4.4 | 5.8 | 3.8 | 3.4 |
| Seattle, WA | 93 | 61 | 62 | 69 | 122 | 5.8 | 3.8 | 3.8 | 4.2 | 7.4 |
| St Louis, MO | 734 | 329 | 261 | 170 | 165 | 204.6 | 94.2 | 76.3 | 50.1 | 48.6 |
| St Paul, MN | 28 | 17 | 8 | 10 | 6 | 10.2 | 6.2 | 2.9 | 3.7 | 2.2 |
| St Petersburg, FL | 168 | 86 | 79 | 56 | 39 | 19.3 | 9.9 | 9.1 | 6.4 | 4.4 |
| Tampa, FL | 277 | 314 | 207 | 177 | 117 | 31.3 | 35.1 | 22.8 | 19.1 | 12.6 |
| Toledo, OH | 52 | 63 | 25 | 23 | 21 | 11.4 | 13.9 | 5.5 | 5.1 | 4.7 |
| Tucson, AZ | 78 | 61 | 52 | 36 | 42 | 10.4 | 7.9 | 6.7 | 4.6 | 5.3 |
| Tulsa, OK | 105 | 109 | 36 | 75 | 109 | 27.8 | 28.6 | 9.3 | 19.7 | 28.6 |
| Washington, DC | 722 | 626 | 644 | 579 | 458 | 130.3 | 116.1 | 121.7 | 110.7 | 87.6 |
| Wichita, KS | 42 | 58 | 85 | 21 | 34 | 10.0 | 13.4 | 19.4 | 4.7 | 7.6 |
| Yonkers, NY | 64 | 33 | 34 | 22 | 12 | 33.4 | 17.2 | 17.6 | 11.4 | 6.2 |
| U.S. CITY TOTAL | 35,371 | 27,881 | 25,018 | 21,098 | 19,272 | 51.3 | 40.2 | 35.9 | 29.9 | 27.3 |
| San Juan, PR | 692 | 722 | 719 | 673 | 681 | 79.3 | 82.8 | 82.4 | 64.3 | 65.1 |
| TOTAL | 36,063 | 28,603 | 25,737 | 21,771 | 19,953 | 51.7 | 40.8 | 36.5 | 30.4 | 27.9 |

*Source*: Centers for Disease Control and Prevention, U.S. Department of Health and Human Services. National Center for HIV, STD, and TB Prevention, Division of STD Prevention. *Sexually Transmitted Disease Surveillance 1999* (Atlanta, GA: CDC, 2000). http://www.cdc.gov/nchstp/dstd/Stats_Trends/1999Surveillance/99PDF/Surv99Master.pdf.

# Table D5.9. Primary and Secondary Syphilis—Reported Cases and Rates, by State/Area and Region Listed in Alphabetical Order: United States and Outlying Areas, 1995–1999

| | *Cases* | | | | | *Rates per 100,000 Population* | | | | |
|---|---|---|---|---|---|---|---|---|---|---|
| *State/Area* | *1995* | *1996* | *1997* | *1998* | *1999* | *1995* | *1996* | *1997* | *1998* | *1999* |
| Alabama | 612 | 528 | 410 | 274 | 202 | 14.4 | 12.3 | 9.5 | 6.3 | 4.6 |
| Alaska | 2 | 0 | 1 | 1 | 1 | 0.3 | 0.0 | 0.2 | 0.2 | 0.2 |
| Arizona | 46 | 102 | 132 | 185 | 212 | 1.1 | 2.3 | 2.9 | 4.0 | 4.5 |
| Arkansas | 495 | 262 | 173 | 108 | 87 | 19.9 | 10.5 | 6.9 | 4.3 | 3.4 |
| California | 584 | 509 | 386 | 327 | 283 | 1.8 | 1.6 | 1.2 | 1.0 | 0.9 |
| Colorado | 100 | 26 | 15 | 10 | 8 | 2.7 | 0.7 | 0.4 | 0.3 | 0.2 |
| Connecticut | 86 | 103 | 62 | 26 | 16 | 2.6 | 3.2 | 1.9 | 0.8 | 0.5 |
| Delaware | 19 | 35 | 22 | 21 | 10 | 2.6 | 4.8 | 3.0 | 2.8 | 1.3 |
| Florida | 383 | 368 | 296 | 294 | 383 | 2.7 | 2.6 | 2.0 | 2.0 | 2.6 |
| Georgia | 901 | 689 | 515 | 333 | 430 | 12.5 | 9.4 | 6.9 | 4.4 | 5.6 |
| Hawaii | 0 | 3 | 1 | 4 | 3 | 0.0 | 0.3 | 0.1 | 0.3 | 0.3 |
| Idaho | 0 | 4 | 1 | 2 | 1 | 0.0 | 0.3 | 0.1 | 0.2 | 0.1 |
| Illinois | 1,026 | 501 | 435 | 424 | 422 | 8.7 | 4.2 | 3.7 | 3.5 | 3.5 |
| Indiana | 321 | 207 | 151 | 215 | 450 | 5.5 | 3.6 | 2.6 | 3.6 | 7.6 |
| Iowa | 48 | 23 | 7 | 5 | 9 | 1.7 | 0.8 | 0.2 | 0.2 | 0.3 |
| Kansas | 47 | 28 | 32 | 14 | 14 | 1.8 | 1.1 | 1.2 | 0.5 | 0.5 |
| Kentucky | 185 | 154 | 135 | 106 | 101 | 4.8 | 4.0 | 3.5 | 2.7 | 2.6 |
| Louisiana | 1,024 | 533 | 364 | 430 | 306 | 23.6 | 12.3 | 8.4 | 9.8 | 7.0 |
| Maine | 2 | 1 | 2 | 1 | 0 | 0.2 | 0.1 | 0.2 | 0.1 | 0.0 |
| Maryland | 554 | 729 | 891 | 648 | 343 | 11.0 | 14.4 | 17.5 | 12.6 | 6.7 |
| Massachusetts | 69 | 85 | 78 | 46 | 37 | 1.1 | 1.4 | 1.3 | 0.7 | 0.6 |
| Michigan | 304 | 183 | 153 | 211 | 249 | 3.2 | 1.9 | 1.6 | 2.1 | 2.5 |
| Minnesota | 45 | 16 | 16 | 9 | 10 | 1.0 | 0.3 | 0.3 | 0.2 | 0.2 |
| Mississippi | 1,952 | 817 | 390 | 261 | 194 | 72.4 | 30.1 | 14.3 | 9.5 | 7.0 |
| Missouri | 584 | 221 | 118 | 109 | 96 | 11.0 | 4.1 | 2.2 | 2.0 | 1.8 |
| Montana | 4 | 0 | 0 | 0 | 1 | 0.5 | 0.0 | 0.0 | 0.0 | 0.1 |
| Nebraska | 14 | 6 | 3 | 8 | 6 | 0.9 | 0.4 | 0.2 | 0.5 | 0.4 |
| Nevada | 36 | 20 | 11 | 15 | 5 | 2.4 | 1.2 | 0.7 | 0.9 | 0.3 |
| New Hampshire | 0 | 1 | 0 | 2 | 1 | 0.0 | 0.1 | 0.0 | 0.2 | 0.1 |
| New Jersey | 188 | 177 | 150 | 107 | 68 | 2.4 | 2.2 | 1.9 | 1.3 | 0.8 |
| New Mexico | 13 | 3 | 9 | 14 | 12 | 0.8 | 0.2 | 0.5 | 0.8 | 0.7 |
| New York | 449 | 214 | 138 | 119 | 150 | 2.5 | 1.2 | 0.8 | 0.7 | 0.8 |
| North Carolina | 1,132 | 1,052 | 721 | 723 | 464 | 15.7 | 14.4 | 9.7 | 9.6 | 6.1 |
| North Dakota | 0 | 0 | 0 | 0 | 0 | 0.0 | 0.0 | 0.0 | 0.0 | 0.0 |
| Ohio | 896 | 584 | 218 | 134 | 92 | 8.0 | 5.2 | 1.9 | 1.2 | 0.8 |
| Oklahoma | 197 | 179 | 117 | 98 | 187 | 6.0 | 5.4 | 3.5 | 2.9 | 5.6 |
| Oregon | 5 | 9 | 10 | 6 | 8 | 0.2 | 0.3 | 0.3 | 0.2 | 0.2 |
| Pennsylvania | 248 | 164 | 123 | 98 | 84 | 2.1 | 1.4 | 1.0 | 0.8 | 0.7 |
| Rhode Island | 4 | 4 | 2 | 1 | 3 | 0.4 | 0.4 | 0.2 | 0.1 | 0.3 |
| South Carolina | 570 | 402 | 378 | 271 | 269 | 15.5 | 10.8 | 10.1 | 7.1 | 7.0 |
| South Dakota | 0 | 0 | 1 | 1 | 0 | 0.0 | 0.0 | 0.1 | 0.1 | 0.0 |
| Tennessee | 906 | 850 | 747 | 567 | 641 | 17.2 | 16.0 | 13.9 | 10.4 | 11.8 |
| Texas | 1,557 | 890 | 676 | 443 | 473 | 8.3 | 4.7 | 3.5 | 2.2 | 2.4 |
| Utah | 4 | 3 | 5 | 4 | 2 | 0.2 | 0.1 | 0.2 | 0.2 | 0.1 |
| Vermont | 0 | 0 | 0 | 4 | 3 | 0.0 | 0.0 | 0.0 | 0.7 | 0.5 |
| Virginia | 600 | 393 | 237 | 149 | 153 | 9.1 | 5.9 | 3.5 | 2.2 | 2.3 |
| Washington | 17 | 9 | 17 | 44 | 77 | 0.3 | 0.2 | 0.3 | 0.8 | 1.4 |
| West Virginia | 16 | 7 | 1 | 3 | 5 | 0.9 | 0.4 | 0.1 | 0.2 | 0.3 |
| Wisconsin | 185 | 176 | 89 | 78 | 41 | 3.6 | 3.4 | 1.7 | 1.5 | 0.8 |
| Wyoming | 1 | 2 | 0 | 1 | 0 | 0.2 | 0.4 | 0.0 | 0.2 | 0.0 |
| U.S. TOTAL[1] | 16,543 | 11,388 | 8,556 | 7,035 | 6,657 | 6.3 | 4.3 | 3.2 | 2.6 | 2.5 |
| Northeast | 1,046 | 749 | 555 | 404 | 362 | 2.0 | 1.5 | 1.1 | 0.8 | 0.7 |
| Midwest | 3,470 | 1,945 | 1,223 | 1,208 | 1,389 | 5.6 | 3.1 | 2.0 | 1.9 | 2.2 |
| South | 11,215 | 8,004 | 6,190 | 4,810 | 4,293 | 12.2 | 8.6 | 6.6 | 5.0 | 4.5 |
| West | 812 | 690 | 588 | 613 | 613 | 1.4 | 1.2 | 1.0 | 1.0 | 1.0 |
| Guam | 0 | 0 | 0 | 0 | 2 | 0.0 | 0.0 | 0.0 | 0.0 | 1.3 |
| Puerto Rico | 285 | 208 | 249 | 177 | 146 | 7.7 | 5.6 | 6.5 | 4.6 | 3.8 |
| Virgin Islands | 2 | 11 | 2 | 7 | 1 | 1.8 | 10.0 | 1.8 | 6.4 | 0.9 |
| OUTLYING AREAS | 287 | 219 | 251 | 184 | 149 | 7.3 | 5.5 | 6.1 | 4.5 | 3.6 |
| TOTAL | 16,830 | 11,607 | 8,807 | 7,219 | 6,806 | 6.3 | 4.3 | 3.2 | 2.6 | 2.5 |

[1]Includes cases reported by Washington, D.C.

*Source*: Centers for Disease Control and Prevention, U.S. Department of Health and Human Services. National Center for HIV, STD, and TB Prevention, Division of STD Prevention. *Sexually Transmitted Disease Surveillance 1999* (Atlanta, GA: CDC, 2000). http://www.cdc.gov/nchstp/dstd/Stats_Trends/1999Surveillance/99PDF/Surv99Master.pdf.

**Table D5.10. Early Latent Syphilis—Reported Cases and Rates in Selected Cities of >200,000 Population Listed in Alphabetical Order: United States and Outlying Areas, 1995–1999**

| | Cases | | | | | Rates per 100,000 Population | | | | |
|---|---|---|---|---|---|---|---|---|---|---|
| City | 1995 | 1996 | 1997 | 1998 | 1999 | 1995 | 1996 | 1997 | 1998 | 1999 |
| Akron, OH | 6 | 4 | 0 | 4 | 6 | 1.1 | 0.8 | 0.0 | 0.7 | 1.1 |
| Albuquerque, NM | 9 | 0 | 6 | 5 | 2 | 1.7 | 0.0 | 1.1 | 1.0 | 0.4 |
| Atlanta, GA | 531 | 383 | 367 | 303 | 241 | 75.8 | 53.6 | 50.8 | 41.0 | 32.6 |
| Austin, TX | 79 | 49 | 33 | 19 | 23 | 11.9 | 7.2 | 4.8 | 2.7 | 3.2 |
| Baltimore, MD | 466 | 896 | 975 | 646 | 472 | 67.4 | 133.4 | 148.3 | 100.1 | 73.1 |
| Birmingham, AL | 289 | 341 | 225 | 95 | 103 | 43.9 | 51.6 | 34.2 | 14.4 | 15.6 |
| Boston, MA | 65 | 83 | 62 | 60 | 41 | 11.7 | 14.9 | 11.1 | 10.8 | 7.4 |
| Buffalo, NY | 6 | 6 | 5 | 2 | 1 | 1.8 | 1.9 | 1.6 | 0.6 | 0.3 |
| Charlotte, NC | 180 | 144 | 86 | 97 | 99 | 31.1 | 24.2 | 14.0 | 15.4 | 15.7 |
| Chicago, IL | 1,400 | 745 | 918 | 563 | 522 | 47.5 | 25.5 | 31.5 | 18.9 | 17.5 |
| Cincinnati, OH | 115 | 43 | 26 | 11 | 5 | 13.3 | 5.0 | 3.1 | 1.3 | 0.6 |
| Cleveland, OH | 361 | 202 | 164 | 98 | 63 | 25.8 | 14.5 | 11.8 | 7.1 | 4.6 |
| Columbus, OH | 11 | 32 | 34 | 42 | 34 | 1.1 | 3.2 | 3.3 | 4.1 | 3.3 |
| Corpus Christi, TX | 29 | 10 | 6 | 13 | 9 | 9.3 | 3.2 | 1.9 | 4.1 | 2.8 |
| Dallas, TX | 410 | 335 | 306 | 405 | 384 | 20.9 | 16.8 | 15.1 | 19.7 | 18.7 |
| Dayton, OH | 98 | 93 | 28 | 5 | 5 | 17.2 | 16.4 | 5.0 | 0.9 | 0.9 |
| Denver, CO | 46 | 7 | 7 | 7 | 4 | 9.3 | 1.4 | 1.4 | 1.4 | 0.8 |
| Des Moines, IA | 54 | 23 | 19 | 11 | 2 | 15.4 | 6.5 | 5.4 | 3.1 | 0.6 |
| Detroit, MI | 364 | 271 | 254 | 180 | 223 | 34.6 | 24.8 | 23.3 | 14.3 | 17.7 |
| El Paso, TX | 21 | 44 | 34 | 14 | 9 | 3.1 | 6.4 | 4.8 | 2.0 | 1.3 |
| Fort Worth, TX | 280 | 216 | 192 | 121 | 66 | 21.9 | 16.6 | 14.5 | 8.9 | 4.9 |
| Honolulu, HI | 0 | 0 | 0 | 0 | 1 | 0.0 | 0.0 | 0.0 | 0.0 | 0.1 |
| Houston, TX | 892 | 703 | 528 | 367 | 248 | 29.0 | 22.6 | 16.7 | 11.4 | 7.7 |
| Indianapolis, IN | 55 | 56 | 33 | 44 | 102 | 6.7 | 6.9 | 4.1 | 5.4 | 12.5 |
| Jacksonville, FL | 111 | 104 | 81 | 69 | 42 | 15.8 | 14.3 | 11.1 | 9.4 | 5.7 |
| Jersey City, NJ | 30 | 17 | 10 | 2 | 1 | 13.8 | 7.8 | 4.6 | 0.9 | 0.5 |
| Kansas City, MO | 29 | 13 | 6 | 6 | 16 | 6.6 | 2.9 | 1.3 | 1.3 | 3.5 |
| Los Angeles, CA | 952 | 718 | 649 | 525 | 330 | 11.1 | 8.4 | 7.6 | 6.1 | 3.8 |
| Louisville, KY | 81 | 71 | 66 | 64 | 38 | 12.0 | 10.6 | 9.8 | 9.5 | 5.7 |
| Memphis, TN | 652 | 548 | 591 | 382 | 338 | 75.4 | 63.4 | 68.2 | 44.0 | 38.9 |
| Miami, FL | 499 | 437 | 427 | 242 | 331 | 24.6 | 21.4 | 20.9 | 11.2 | 15.4 |
| Milwaukee, WI | 229 | 183 | 140 | 94 | 84 | 24.6 | 19.9 | 15.4 | 10.3 | 9.2 |
| Minneapolis, MN | 24 | 16 | 14 | 5 | 7 | 6.3 | 4.2 | 3.7 | 1.4 | 1.9 |
| Nashville, TN | 97 | 99 | 173 | 148 | 201 | 18.3 | 18.6 | 32.4 | 27.7 | 37.6 |
| New Orleans, LA | 215 | 153 | 119 | 84 | 65 | 44.6 | 32.3 | 25.4 | 18.0 | 14.0 |
| New York City, NY | 1,945 | 1,077 | 670 | 645 | 659 | 26.6 | 14.7 | 9.1 | 8.7 | 8.9 |
| Newark, NJ | 77 | 55 | 30 | 56 | 23 | 26.8 | 19.3 | 10.5 | 19.7 | 8.1 |
| Norfolk, VA | 110 | 101 | 87 | 50 | 34 | 46.3 | 43.4 | 37.9 | 23.2 | 15.8 |
| Oakland, CA | 55 | 25 | 33 | 25 | 22 | 4.5 | 2.0 | 2.6 | 2.0 | 1.7 |
| Oklahoma City, OK | 140 | 89 | 50 | 70 | 147 | 32.0 | 20.3 | 11.3 | 17.2 | 36.1 |
| Omaha, NE | 3 | 0 | 2 | 3 | 2 | 0.7 | 0.0 | 0.5 | 0.7 | 0.5 |
| Philadelphia, PA | 1,100 | 839 | 648 | 407 | 394 | 73.4 | 56.9 | 44.6 | 28.3 | 27.4 |
| Phoenix, AZ | 79 | 108 | 189 | 193 | 266 | 3.2 | 4.1 | 7.0 | 6.9 | 9.6 |
| Pittsburgh, PA | 13 | 3 | 2 | 1 | 1 | 1.0 | 0.2 | 0.2 | 0.1 | 0.1 |
| Portland, OR | 11 | 6 | 8 | 5 | 5 | 2.3 | 1.2 | 1.6 | 1.0 | 1.0 |
| Richmond, VA | 70 | 78 | 58 | 36 | 34 | 35.3 | 40.8 | 30.1 | 18.5 | 17.5 |
| Rochester, NY | 23 | 23 | 9 | 9 | 2 | 9.5 | 9.5 | 3.7 | 3.7 | 0.8 |
| Sacramento, CA | 21 | 15 | 10 | 12 | 3 | 1.9 | 1.3 | 0.9 | 1.0 | 0.3 |
| San Antonio, TX | 161 | 115 | 96 | 63 | 72 | 12.4 | 8.8 | 7.2 | 4.7 | 5.3 |
| San Diego, CA | 60 | 43 | 17 | 21 | 23 | 2.3 | 1.6 | 0.6 | 0.8 | 0.8 |
| San Francisco, CA | 14 | 11 | 16 | 15 | 14 | 1.9 | 1.5 | 2.2 | 2.0 | 1.9 |
| San Jose, CA | 4 | 6 | 4 | 5 | 11 | 0.3 | 0.4 | 0.2 | 0.3 | 0.7 |
| Seattle, WA | 1 | 0 | 5 | 8 | 6 | 0.1 | 0.0 | 0.3 | 0.5 | 0.4 |
| St Louis, MO | 289 | 136 | 83 | 63 | 40 | 80.6 | 38.9 | 24.3 | 18.6 | 11.8 |
| St Paul, MN | 9 | 2 | 1 | 1 | 1 | 3.3 | 0.7 | 0.4 | 0.4 | 0.4 |
| St Petersburg, FL | 83 | 35 | 28 | 19 | 16 | 9.5 | 4.0 | 3.2 | 2.2 | 1.8 |
| Tampa, FL | 79 | 139 | 83 | 76 | 57 | 8.9 | 15.5 | 9.1 | 8.2 | 6.2 |
| Toledo, OH | 27 | 23 | 6 | 5 | 5 | 5.9 | 5.1 | 1.3 | 1.1 | 1.1 |
| Tucson, AZ | 29 | 14 | 6 | 6 | 14 | 3.9 | 1.8 | 0.8 | 0.8 | 1.8 |
| Tulsa, OK | 44 | 48 | 16 | 44 | 40 | 11.6 | 12.6 | 4.1 | 11.6 | 10.5 |
| Washington, DC | 396 | 371 | 348 | 288 | 284 | 71.4 | 68.8 | 65.8 | 55.1 | 54.3 |
| Wichita, KS | 12 | 30 | 45 | 13 | 11 | 2.9 | 6.9 | 10.3 | 2.9 | 2.5 |
| Yonkers, NY | 16 | 12 | 5 | 2 | 2 | 8.4 | 6.3 | 2.6 | 1.0 | 1.0 |
| U.S. CITY TOTAL | 13,557 | 10,449 | 9,139 | 6,874 | 6,306 | 19.7 | 15.1 | 13.1 | 9.7 | 8.9 |
| San Juan, PR | 313 | 308 | 305 | 300 | 296 | 35.9 | 35.3 | 35.0 | 28.7 | 28.3 |
| TOTAL | 13,870 | 10,757 | 9,444 | 7,174 | 6,602 | 19.9 | 15.3 | 13.4 | 10.0 | 9.2 |

*Source*: Centers for Disease Control and Prevention, U.S. Department of Health and Human Services. National Center for HIV, STD, and TB Prevention, Division of STD Prevention. *Sexually Transmitted Disease Surveillance 1999* (Atlanta, GA: CDC, 2000). http://www.cdc.gov/nchstp/dstd/Stats_Trends/1999Surveillance/99PDF/Surv99Master.pdf.

# Table D5.11. Late and Late Latent Syphilis—Reported Cases and Rates, by State/Area Listed in Alphabetical Order: United States and Outlying Areas, 1995–1999

| | Cases | | | | | Rates per 100,000 Population | | | | |
|---|---|---|---|---|---|---|---|---|---|---|
| State/Area | 1995 | 1996 | 1997 | 1998 | 1999 | 1995 | 1996 | 1997 | 1998 | 1999 |
| Alabama | 334 | 538 | 422 | 413 | 443 | 7.9 | 12.5 | 9.8 | 9.5 | 10.2 |
| Alaska | 15 | 15 | 11 | 12 | 11 | 2.5 | 2.5 | 1.8 | 2.0 | 1.8 |
| Arizona | 248 | 231 | 255 | 281 | 307 | 5.9 | 5.2 | 5.6 | 6.0 | 6.6 |
| Arkansas | 217 | 103 | 121 | 183 | 140 | 8.7 | 4.1 | 4.8 | 7.2 | 5.5 |
| California | 3,417 | 2,567 | 2,319 | 1,637 | 1,897 | 10.8 | 8.1 | 7.2 | 5.0 | 5.8 |
| Colorado | 135 | 115 | 125 | 100 | 76 | 3.6 | 3.0 | 3.2 | 2.5 | 1.9 |
| Connecticut | 86 | 125 | 175 | 114 | 97 | 2.6 | 3.8 | 5.4 | 3.5 | 3.0 |
| Delaware | 52 | 49 | 52 | 49 | 46 | 7.3 | 6.8 | 7.1 | 6.6 | 6.2 |
| Florida | 1,489 | 1,128 | 1,198 | 1,082 | 1,315 | 10.5 | 7.8 | 8.2 | 7.3 | 8.8 |
| Georgia | 1,104 | 931 | 1,218 | 749 | 799 | 15.3 | 12.7 | 16.3 | 9.8 | 10.5 |
| Hawaii | 25 | 25 | 46 | 14 | 7 | 2.1 | 2.1 | 3.9 | 1.2 | 0.6 |
| Idaho | 11 | 14 | 18 | 13 | 11 | 0.9 | 1.2 | 1.5 | 1.1 | 0.9 |
| Illinois | 728 | 549 | 414 | 892 | 852 | 6.2 | 4.6 | 3.5 | 7.4 | 7.1 |
| Indiana | 172 | 197 | 199 | 173 | 173 | 3.0 | 3.4 | 3.4 | 2.9 | 2.9 |
| Iowa | 45 | 25 | 38 | 23 | 24 | 1.6 | 0.9 | 1.3 | 0.8 | 0.8 |
| Kansas | 62 | 62 | 77 | 63 | 62 | 2.4 | 2.4 | 3.0 | 2.4 | 2.4 |
| Kentucky | 143 | 113 | 141 | 127 | 120 | 3.7 | 2.9 | 3.6 | 3.2 | 3.0 |
| Louisiana | 1,034 | 902 | 872 | 767 | 701 | 23.8 | 20.8 | 20.0 | 17.6 | 16.0 |
| Maine | 2 | 1 | 9 | 3 | 1 | 0.2 | 0.1 | 0.7 | 0.2 | 0.1 |
| Maryland | 394 | 317 | 288 | 616 | 405 | 7.8 | 6.3 | 5.7 | 12.0 | 7.9 |
| Massachusetts | 283 | 364 | 524 | 416 | 283 | 4.7 | 6.0 | 8.6 | 6.8 | 4.6 |
| Michigan | 304 | 233 | 258 | 202 | 207 | 3.2 | 2.4 | 2.6 | 2.1 | 2.1 |
| Minnesota | 85 | 69 | 87 | 58 | 52 | 1.8 | 1.5 | 1.9 | 1.2 | 1.1 |
| Mississippi | 126 | 10 | 48 | 235 | 147 | 4.7 | 0.4 | 1.8 | 8.5 | 5.3 |
| Missouri | 135 | 123 | 173 | 90 | 191 | 2.5 | 2.3 | 3.2 | 1.7 | 3.5 |
| Montana | 0 | 0 | 1 | 0 | 0 | 0.0 | 0.0 | 0.1 | 0.0 | 0.0 |
| Nebraska | 18 | 16 | 26 | 24 | 12 | 1.1 | 1.0 | 1.6 | 1.4 | 0.7 |
| Nevada | 89 | 89 | 85 | 86 | 59 | 5.8 | 5.6 | 5.1 | 4.9 | 3.4 |
| New Hampshire | 29 | 25 | 26 | 11 | 14 | 2.5 | 2.2 | 2.2 | 0.9 | 1.2 |
| New Jersey | 893 | 888 | 696 | 411 | 587 | 11.2 | 11.1 | 8.6 | 5.1 | 7.2 |
| New Mexico | 100 | 70 | 86 | 54 | 66 | 5.9 | 4.1 | 5.0 | 3.1 | 3.8 |
| New York | 6,005 | 4,957 | 4,639 | 4,291 | 3,201 | 33.1 | 27.3 | 25.6 | 23.6 | 17.6 |
| North Carolina | 670 | 516 | 584 | 540 | 490 | 9.3 | 7.1 | 7.9 | 7.2 | 6.5 |
| North Dakota | 0 | 0 | 0 | 0 | 0 | 0.0 | 0.0 | 0.0 | 0.0 | 0.0 |
| Ohio | 281 | 217 | 202 | 109 | 98 | 2.5 | 1.9 | 1.8 | 1.0 | 0.9 |
| Oklahoma | 95 | 62 | 105 | 97 | 94 | 2.9 | 1.9 | 3.2 | 2.9 | 2.8 |
| Oregon | 45 | 52 | 23 | 19 | 23 | 1.4 | 1.6 | 0.7 | 0.6 | 0.7 |
| Pennsylvania | 420 | 335 | 354 | 367 | 427 | 3.5 | 2.8 | 2.9 | 3.1 | 3.6 |
| Rhode Island | 72 | 60 | 75 | 54 | 51 | 7.3 | 6.1 | 7.6 | 5.5 | 5.2 |
| South Carolina | 266 | 259 | 261 | 198 | 230 | 7.2 | 7.0 | 6.9 | 5.2 | 6.0 |
| South Dakota | 6 | 2 | 5 | 1 | 1 | 0.8 | 0.3 | 0.7 | 0.1 | 0.1 |
| Tennessee | 540 | 480 | 605 | 515 | 439 | 10.3 | 9.0 | 11.3 | 9.5 | 8.1 |
| Texas | 3,152 | 2,674 | 2,694 | 1,930 | 1,885 | 16.8 | 14.0 | 13.9 | 9.8 | 9.5 |
| Utah | 39 | 38 | 49 | 50 | 42 | 2.0 | 1.9 | 2.4 | 2.4 | 2.0 |
| Vermont | 0 | 0 | 1 | 0 | 0 | 0.0 | 0.0 | 0.2 | 0.0 | 0.0 |
| Virginia | 419 | 450 | 495 | 334 | 354 | 6.3 | 6.8 | 7.4 | 4.9 | 5.2 |
| Washington | 181 | 119 | 107 | 82 | 110 | 3.3 | 2.2 | 1.9 | 1.4 | 1.9 |
| West Virginia | 38 | 44 | 17 | 6 | 7 | 2.1 | 2.4 | 0.9 | 0.3 | 0.4 |
| Wisconsin | 90 | 74 | 50 | 58 | 52 | 1.8 | 1.4 | 1.0 | 1.1 | 1.0 |
| Wyoming | 1 | 6 | 4 | 1 | 0 | 0.2 | 1.2 | 0.8 | 0.2 | 0.0 |
| U.S. TOTAL[1] | 24,296 | 20,364 | 20,446 | 17,752 | 16,738 | 9.2 | 7.7 | 7.6 | 6.6 | 6.2 |
| Guam | 6 | 3 | 1 | 3 | 10 | 4.0 | 2.0 | 0.6 | 1.9 | 6.3 |
| Puerto Rico | 582 | 620 | 640 | 597 | 614 | 15.8 | 16.7 | 16.7 | 15.5 | 15.9 |
| Virgin Islands | 0 | 0 | 0 | 0 | 0 | 0.0 | 0.0 | 0.0 | 0.0 | 0.0 |
| OUTLYING AREAS | 588 | 623 | 641 | 600 | 624 | 14.9 | 15.6 | 15.7 | 14.5 | 15.1 |
| TOTAL | 24,884 | 20,987 | 21,087 | 18,352 | 17,362 | 9.3 | 7.8 | 7.8 | 6.7 | 6.3 |

[1]Includes cases reported by Washington, D.C.

*Source*: Centers for Disease Control and Prevention, U.S. Department of Health and Human Services. National Center for HIV, STD, and TB Prevention, Division of STD Prevention. *Sexually Transmitted Disease Surveillance 1999* (Atlanta, GA: CDC, 2000). http://www.cdc.gov/nchstp/dstd/Stats_Trends/1999Surveillance/99PDF/Surv99Master.pdf.

## Table D5.12. Late and Late Latent Syphilis—Reported Cases and Rates in Selected Cities of >200,000 Population Listed in Alphabetical Order: United States and Outlying Areas, 1995–1999

| | Cases | | | | | Rates per 100,000 Population | | | | |
|---|---|---|---|---|---|---|---|---|---|---|
| City | 1995 | 1996 | 1997 | 1998 | 1999 | 1995 | 1996 | 1997 | 1998 | 1999 |
| Akron, OH | 1 | 4 | 0 | 0 | 0 | 0.2 | 0.8 | 0.0 | 0.0 | 0.0 |
| Albuquerque, NM | 26 | 31 | 41 | 29 | 37 | 5.0 | 5.9 | 7.8 | 5.5 | 7.0 |
| Atlanta, GA | 207 | 190 | 289 | 120 | 119 | 29.5 | 26.6 | 40.0 | 16.2 | 16.1 |
| Austin, TX | 87 | 30 | 57 | 22 | 20 | 13.1 | 4.4 | 8.2 | 3.1 | 2.8 |
| Baltimore, MD | 191 | 73 | 81 | 331 | 202 | 27.6 | 10.9 | 12.3 | 51.3 | 31.3 |
| Birmingham, AL | 78 | 149 | 136 | 110 | 149 | 11.9 | 22.5 | 20.6 | 16.7 | 22.6 |
| Boston, MA | 88 | 130 | 191 | 155 | 107 | 15.8 | 23.3 | 34.3 | 27.9 | 19.2 |
| Buffalo, NY | 23 | 8 | 13 | 6 | 4 | 7.1 | 2.5 | 4.1 | 1.9 | 1.3 |
| Charlotte, NC | 41 | 31 | 19 | 44 | 39 | 7.1 | 5.2 | 3.1 | 7.0 | 6.2 |
| Chicago, IL | 141 | 100 | 0 | 507 | 476 | 4.8 | 3.4 | 0.0 | 17.0 | 16.0 |
| Cincinnati, OH | 26 | 46 | 33 | 9 | 6 | 3.0 | 5.4 | 3.9 | 1.1 | 0.7 |
| Cleveland, OH | 108 | 40 | 19 | 20 | 11 | 7.7 | 2.9 | 1.4 | 1.4 | 0.8 |
| Columbus, OH | 13 | 3 | 28 | 17 | 30 | 1.3 | 0.3 | 2.8 | 1.7 | 2.9 |
| Corpus Christi, TX | 24 | 19 | 14 | 13 | 10 | 7.7 | 6.0 | 4.4 | 4.1 | 3.2 |
| Dallas, TX | 334 | 217 | 260 | 187 | 156 | 17.0 | 10.9 | 12.9 | 9.1 | 7.6 |
| Dayton, OH | 50 | 66 | 70 | 28 | 9 | 8.8 | 11.7 | 12.5 | 5.0 | 1.6 |
| Denver, CO | 65 | 48 | 57 | 24 | 37 | 13.1 | 9.7 | 11.4 | 4.8 | 7.4 |
| Des Moines, IA | 11 | 5 | 7 | 6 | 5 | 3.1 | 1.4 | 2.0 | 1.7 | 1.4 |
| Detroit, MI | 192 | 144 | 175 | 131 | 136 | 18.2 | 13.2 | 16.1 | 10.4 | 10.8 |
| El Paso, TX | 115 | 60 | 73 | 65 | 60 | 17.0 | 8.8 | 10.4 | 9.2 | 8.5 |
| Fort Worth, TX | 60 | 63 | 62 | 27 | 87 | 4.7 | 4.8 | 4.7 | 2.0 | 6.4 |
| Honolulu, HI | 22 | 23 | 41 | 14 | 4 | 2.5 | 2.6 | 4.7 | 1.6 | 0.5 |
| Houston, TX | 1,283 | 1,095 | 1,128 | 879 | 755 | 41.7 | 35.2 | 35.7 | 27.4 | 23.5 |
| Indianapolis, IN | 39 | 45 | 21 | 30 | 38 | 4.8 | 5.5 | 2.6 | 3.7 | 4.7 |
| Jacksonville, FL | 30 | 48 | 89 | 69 | 30 | 4.3 | 6.6 | 12.1 | 9.4 | 4.1 |
| Jersey City, NJ | 70 | 68 | 62 | 28 | 38 | 32.2 | 31.3 | 28.5 | 12.7 | 17.3 |
| Kansas City, MO | 13 | 18 | 4 | 2 | 41 | 3.0 | 4.0 | 0.9 | 0.4 | 9.1 |
| Los Angeles, CA | 1,605 | 1,165 | 806 | 557 | 740 | 18.8 | 13.7 | 9.4 | 6.5 | 8.6 |
| Louisville, KY | 59 | 49 | 56 | 54 | 69 | 8.8 | 7.3 | 8.4 | 8.0 | 10.3 |
| Memphis, TN | 442 | 399 | 473 | 383 | 321 | 51.1 | 46.1 | 54.6 | 44.1 | 36.9 |
| Miami, FL | 409 | 364 | 367 | 463 | 456 | 20.1 | 17.9 | 17.9 | 21.5 | 21.2 |
| Milwaukee, WI | 74 | 53 | 42 | 62 | 36 | 7.9 | 5.8 | 4.6 | 6.8 | 3.9 |
| Minneapolis, MN | 36 | 31 | 27 | 25 | 15 | 9.4 | 8.1 | 7.0 | 6.9 | 4.1 |
| Nashville, TN | 7 | 0 | 36 | 58 | 54 | 1.3 | 0.0 | 6.7 | 10.9 | 10.1 |
| New Orleans, LA | 213 | 198 | 208 | 157 | 108 | 44.2 | 41.8 | 44.3 | 33.7 | 23.2 |
| New York City, NY | 5,291 | 4,455 | 4,110 | 3,881 | 2,907 | 72.4 | 60.7 | 56.0 | 52.3 | 39.2 |
| Newark, NJ | 232 | 256 | 159 | 82 | 115 | 80.7 | 89.6 | 55.9 | 28.8 | 40.4 |
| Norfolk, VA | 31 | 24 | 26 | 25 | 30 | 13.0 | 10.3 | 11.3 | 11.6 | 13.9 |
| Oakland, CA | 91 | 96 | 86 | 91 | 92 | 7.5 | 7.8 | 6.9 | 7.1 | 7.2 |
| Oklahoma City, OK | 32 | 20 | 16 | 39 | 34 | 7.3 | 4.6 | 3.6 | 9.6 | 8.3 |
| Omaha, NE | 11 | 1 | 14 | 19 | 3 | 2.5 | 0.2 | 3.2 | 4.3 | 0.7 |
| Philadelphia, PA | 329 | 255 | 300 | 287 | 355 | 21.9 | 17.3 | 20.7 | 20.0 | 24.7 |
| Phoenix, AZ | 142 | 143 | 156 | 187 | 245 | 5.8 | 5.5 | 5.8 | 6.7 | 8.8 |
| Pittsburgh, PA | 10 | 11 | 14 | 11 | 4 | 0.8 | 0.9 | 1.1 | 0.9 | 0.3 |
| Portland, OR | 27 | 32 | 11 | 8 | 9 | 5.6 | 6.5 | 2.2 | 1.6 | 1.8 |
| Richmond, VA | 14 | 27 | 29 | 20 | 17 | 7.1 | 14.1 | 15.1 | 10.3 | 8.8 |
| Rochester, NY | 59 | 31 | 21 | 21 | 13 | 24.3 | 12.8 | 8.7 | 8.7 | 5.4 |
| Sacramento, CA | 54 | 34 | 36 | 16 | 13 | 4.9 | 3.0 | 3.2 | 1.4 | 1.1 |
| San Antonio, TX | 174 | 231 | 182 | 143 | 121 | 13.4 | 17.6 | 13.7 | 10.6 | 8.9 |
| San Diego, CA | 252 | 143 | 206 | 135 | 196 | 9.5 | 5.3 | 7.6 | 4.9 | 7.0 |
| San Francisco, CA | 37 | 105 | 101 | 88 | 84 | 5.1 | 14.4 | 13.8 | 11.8 | 11.3 |
| San Jose, CA | 68 | 59 | 83 | 54 | 40 | 4.3 | 3.7 | 5.2 | 3.3 | 2.4 |
| Seattle, WA | 87 | 60 | 46 | 28 | 51 | 5.5 | 3.7 | 2.8 | 1.7 | 3.1 |
| St Louis, MO | 60 | 43 | 109 | 46 | 69 | 16.7 | 12.3 | 31.9 | 13.6 | 20.3 |
| St Paul, MN | 12 | 12 | 7 | 6 | 3 | 4.4 | 4.4 | 2.5 | 2.2 | 1.1 |
| St Petersburg, FL | 63 | 42 | 40 | 29 | 18 | 7.2 | 4.8 | 4.6 | 3.3 | 2.0 |
| Tampa, FL | 156 | 115 | 83 | 65 | 41 | 17.6 | 12.9 | 9.1 | 7.0 | 4.4 |
| Toledo, OH | 3 | 10 | 13 | 10 | 10 | 0.7 | 2.2 | 2.9 | 2.2 | 2.2 |
| Tucson, AZ | 47 | 35 | 34 | 23 | 20 | 6.2 | 4.6 | 4.4 | 2.9 | 2.5 |
| Tulsa, OK | 13 | 18 | 11 | 14 | 23 | 3.4 | 4.7 | 2.9 | 3.7 | 6.0 |
| Washington, DC | 201 | 125 | 168 | 202 | 129 | 36.3 | 23.2 | 31.8 | 38.6 | 24.7 |
| Wichita, KS | 14 | 13 | 22 | 5 | 16 | 3.3 | 3.0 | 5.0 | 1.1 | 3.6 |
| Yonkers, NY | 43 | 21 | 27 | 17 | 9 | 22.4 | 10.9 | 14.0 | 8.8 | 4.7 |
| U.S. CITY TOTAL | 13,736 | 11,430 | 11,095 | 10,184 | 9,072 | 19.9 | 16.5 | 15.9 | 14.4 | 12.9 |
| San Juan, PR | 309 | 339 | 312 | 293 | 322 | 35.4 | 38.9 | 35.8 | 28.0 | 30.8 |
| TOTAL | 14,045 | 11,769 | 11,407 | 10,477 | 9,394 | 20.1 | 16.8 | 16.2 | 14.6 | 13.1 |

*Source*: Centers for Disease Control and Prevention, U.S. Department of Health and Human Services. National Center for HIV, STD, and TB Prevention, Division of STD Prevention. *Sexually Transmitted Disease Surveillance 1999* (Atlanta, GA: CDC, 2000). http://www.cdc.gov/nchstp/dstd/Stats_Trends/1999Surveillance/99PDF/Surv99Master.pdf.

## Table D5.13. Primary and Secondary Syphilis—Rates, by Race and Ethnicity: United States, 1981–1999, and the Healthy People Year 2000 Objective

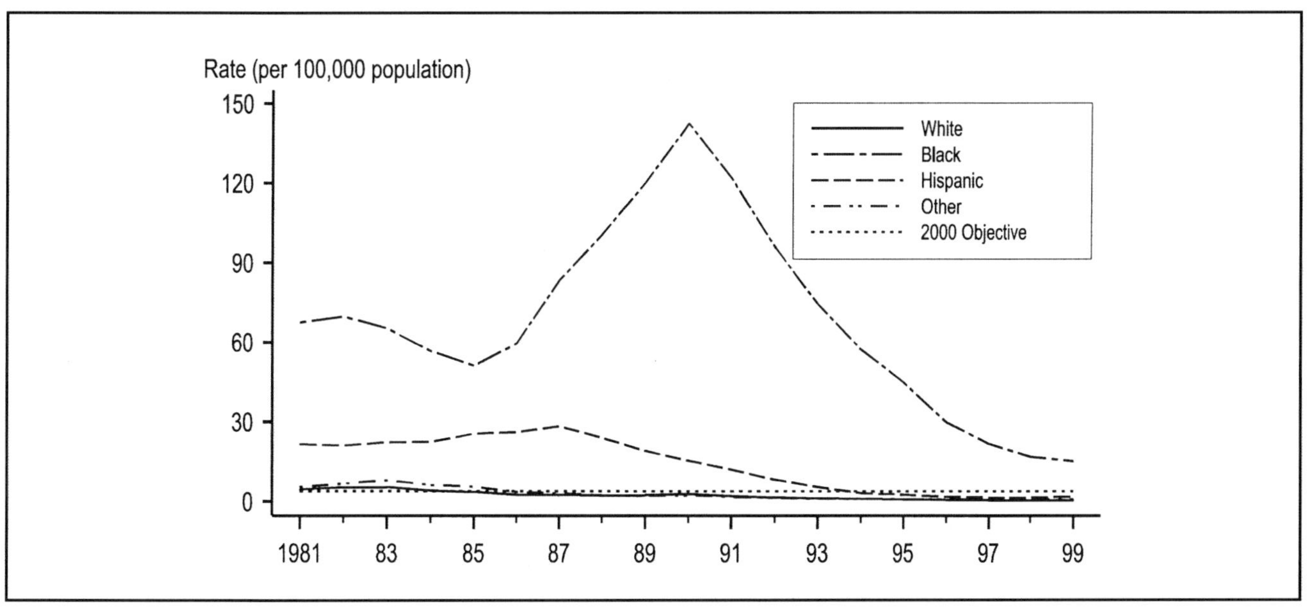


Note: "Other" includes Asian/Pacific Islander and American Indian/Alaska Native populations. Black, White, and Other are non-Hispanic.
*Source*: Centers for Disease Control and Prevention, U.S. Department of Health and Human Services. National Center for HIV, STD, and TB Prevention, Division of STD Prevention. *Sexually Transmitted Disease Surveillance 1999* (Atlanta, GA: CDC, 2000). http://www.cdc.gov/nchstp/dstd/Stats_Trends/1999Surveillance/99PDF/Surv99Master.pdf.

## Table D5.14. Syphilis, Primary and Secondary—Reported Cases per 100,000 Population, by Race and Ethnicity, United States, 1984–1999

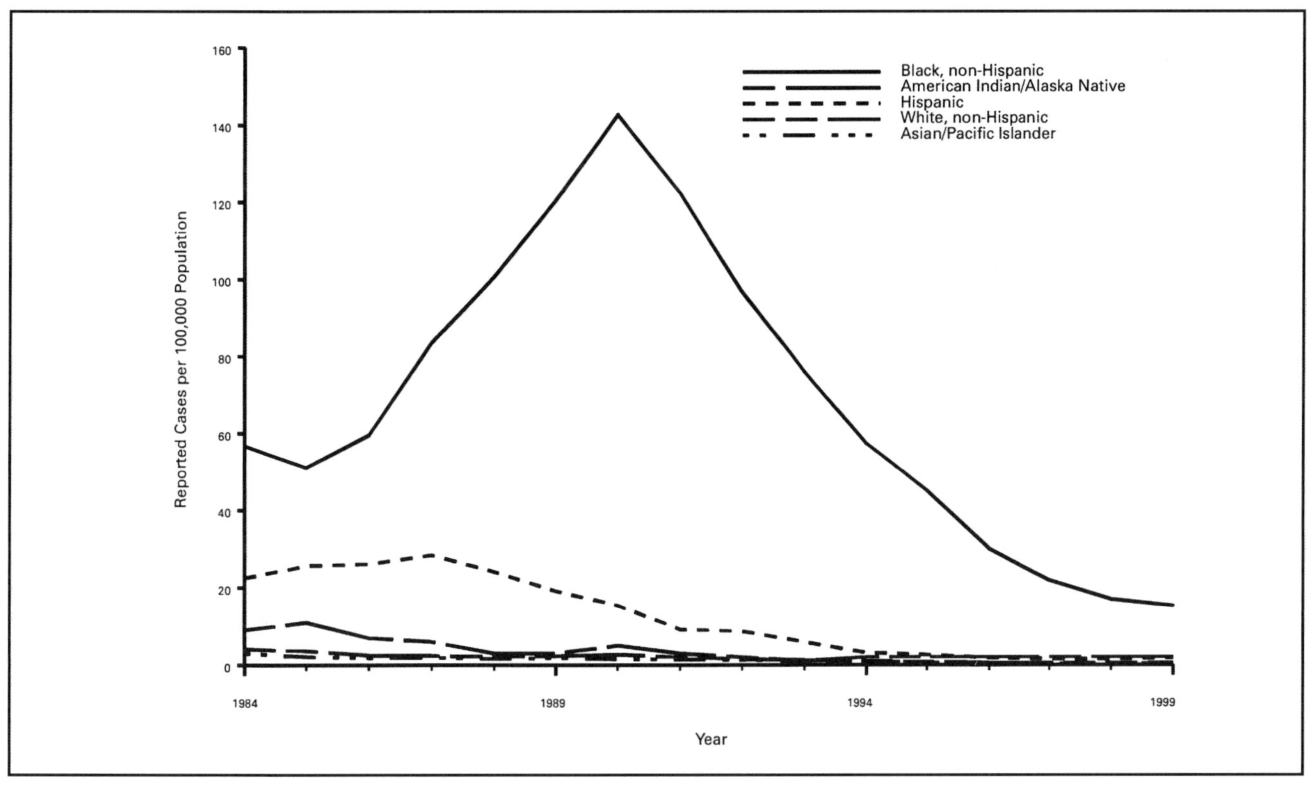


In 1999, primary and secondary syphilis rates declined or remained the same except among Hispanics. The reported rate among Hispanic blacks (15.2 cases/100,000 persons) decreased 10% during 1998–1999 but was 30 times greater than the rate among non-Hispanic whites.
*Source*: Center for Disease Control and Prevention. U.S. Department of Health and Human Services. *MMWR: Morbidity and Mortality Weekly Review Summary of Notifiable Disease, United States, 1999* 48 no. 53 (2001). http://www.cdc.gov/mmwr/PDF/wk/mm4853.pdf.

## Table D5.15. Primary and Secondary Syphilis—Reported Cases, by Age, Gender, and Race/Ethnicity: United States, 1995–1999

| | Age | Total | | | White, Non-Hispanic | | | Black, Non-Hispanic | | | Hispanic | | | Asian/Pacific Islander | | | American Indian/ Alaska Native | | |
|---|---|---|---|---|---|---|---|---|---|---|---|---|---|---|---|---|---|---|---|
| | Group | Total | Male | Female | Total | Male | Female | Total | Male | Female | Total | Male | Female | Total | Male | Female | Total | Male | Female |
| 1995 | 10-14 | 106 | 11 | 95 | 5 | 0 | 5 | 98 | 11 | 87 | 3 | 0 | 3 | 0 | 0 | 0 | 0 | 0 | 0 |
| | 15-19 | 1,796 | 604 | 1,192 | 132 | 28 | 104 | 1,601 | 555 | 1,046 | 53 | 20 | 33 | 3 | 0 | 3 | 7 | 1 | 6 |
| | 20-24 | 3,067 | 1,476 | 1,591 | 242 | 99 | 143 | 2,683 | 1,303 | 1,380 | 126 | 70 | 56 | 12 | 1 | 11 | 4 | 3 | 1 |
| | 25-29 | 2,853 | 1,390 | 1,463 | 258 | 121 | 137 | 2,433 | 1,174 | 1,259 | 141 | 86 | 55 | 9 | 3 | 6 | 12 | 6 | 6 |
| | 30-34 | 2,919 | 1,482 | 1,437 | 255 | 130 | 125 | 2,506 | 1,260 | 1,246 | 134 | 81 | 53 | 15 | 6 | 9 | 9 | 5 | 4 |
| | 35-39 | 2,412 | 1,369 | 1,043 | 253 | 146 | 107 | 2,043 | 1,148 | 895 | 108 | 72 | 36 | 5 | 1 | 4 | 3 | 2 | 1 |
| | 40-44 | 1,472 | 980 | 492 | 153 | 100 | 53 | 1,265 | 840 | 425 | 46 | 36 | 10 | 4 | 2 | 2 | 4 | 2 | 2 |
| | 45-54 | 1,272 | 939 | 333 | 140 | 108 | 32 | 1,067 | 784 | 283 | 57 | 43 | 14 | 3 | 1 | 2 | 5 | 3 | 2 |
| | 55-64 | 385 | 311 | 74 | 51 | 45 | 6 | 317 | 254 | 63 | 16 | 11 | 5 | 1 | 1 | 0 | 0 | 0 | 0 |
| | 65+ | 186 | 149 | 37 | 29 | 23 | 6 | 139 | 111 | 28 | 14 | 11 | 3 | 2 | 2 | 0 | 2 | 2 | 0 |
| | TOTAL | 16,503 | 8,729 | 7,774 | 1,519 | 801 | 718 | 14,186 | 7,457 | 6,729 | 698 | 430 | 268 | 54 | 17 | 37 | 46 | 24 | 22 |
| 1996 | 10-14 | 49 | 6 | 43 | 3 | 0 | 3 | 43 | 6 | 37 | 3 | 0 | 3 | 0 | 0 | 0 | 0 | 0 | 0 |
| | 15-19 | 1,125 | 388 | 737 | 107 | 28 | 79 | 968 | 340 | 628 | 43 | 18 | 25 | 5 | 1 | 4 | 2 | 1 | 1 |
| | 20-24 | 1,933 | 875 | 1,058 | 162 | 41 | 121 | 1,645 | 762 | 883 | 106 | 65 | 41 | 13 | 5 | 8 | 7 | 2 | 5 |
| | 25-29 | 1,889 | 919 | 970 | 211 | 99 | 112 | 1,562 | 738 | 824 | 100 | 72 | 28 | 10 | 6 | 4 | 6 | 4 | 2 |
| | 30-34 | 2,001 | 1,026 | 975 | 197 | 103 | 94 | 1,704 | 853 | 851 | 85 | 63 | 22 | 6 | 3 | 3 | 9 | 4 | 5 |
| | 35-39 | 1,854 | 1,022 | 832 | 203 | 107 | 96 | 1,563 | 854 | 709 | 78 | 55 | 23 | 6 | 4 | 2 | 4 | 2 | 2 |
| | 40-44 | 1,122 | 703 | 419 | 110 | 65 | 45 | 962 | 605 | 357 | 40 | 30 | 10 | 5 | 3 | 2 | 5 | 0 | 5 |
| | 45-54 | 967 | 714 | 253 | 130 | 97 | 33 | 795 | 585 | 210 | 32 | 22 | 10 | 3 | 3 | 0 | 7 | 7 | 0 |
| | 55-64 | 281 | 234 | 47 | 55 | 48 | 7 | 210 | 172 | 38 | 16 | 14 | 2 | 0 | 0 | 0 | 0 | 0 | 0 |
| | 65+ | 107 | 93 | 14 | 18 | 18 | 0 | 78 | 66 | 12 | 9 | 7 | 2 | 2 | 2 | 0 | 0 | 0 | 0 |
| | TOTAL | 11,339 | 5,982 | 5,357 | 1,197 | 606 | 591 | 9,540 | 4,983 | 4,557 | 512 | 346 | 166 | 50 | 27 | 23 | 40 | 20 | 20 |
| 1997 | 10-14 | 43 | 4 | 39 | 4 | 0 | 4 | 36 | 3 | 33 | 3 | 1 | 2 | 0 | 0 | 0 | 0 | 0 | 0 |
| | 15-19 | 775 | 253 | 522 | 69 | 16 | 53 | 648 | 213 | 435 | 54 | 23 | 31 | 3 | 1 | 2 | 1 | 0 | 1 |
| | 20-24 | 1,318 | 619 | 699 | 110 | 44 | 66 | 1,116 | 518 | 598 | 79 | 53 | 26 | 6 | 1 | 5 | 7 | 3 | 4 |
| | 25-29 | 1,434 | 720 | 714 | 143 | 67 | 76 | 1,179 | 568 | 611 | 101 | 76 | 25 | 4 | 4 | 0 | 7 | 5 | 2 |
| | 30-34 | 1,475 | 759 | 716 | 162 | 73 | 89 | 1,227 | 630 | 597 | 73 | 51 | 22 | 7 | 3 | 4 | 6 | 2 | 4 |
| | 35-39 | 1,405 | 779 | 626 | 197 | 101 | 96 | 1,151 | 637 | 514 | 49 | 37 | 12 | 3 | 2 | 1 | 5 | 2 | 3 |
| | 40-44 | 942 | 626 | 316 | 106 | 74 | 32 | 786 | 521 | 265 | 38 | 24 | 14 | 5 | 2 | 3 | 7 | 5 | 2 |
| | 45-54 | 770 | 565 | 205 | 108 | 82 | 26 | 621 | 456 | 165 | 30 | 20 | 10 | 4 | 2 | 2 | 7 | 5 | 2 |
| | 55-64 | 255 | 223 | 32 | 52 | 44 | 8 | 186 | 162 | 24 | 17 | 17 | 0 | 0 | 0 | 0 | 0 | 0 | 0 |
| | 65+ | 107 | 99 | 8 | 25 | 24 | 1 | 74 | 67 | 7 | 8 | 8 | 0 | 0 | 0 | 0 | 0 | 0 | 0 |
| | TOTAL | 8,536 | 4,652 | 3,884 | 977 | 525 | 452 | 7,035 | 3,780 | 3,255 | 452 | 310 | 142 | 32 | 15 | 17 | 40 | 22 | 18 |
| 1998 | 10-14 | 39 | 5 | 34 | 4 | 0 | 4 | 34 | 5 | 29 | 1 | 0 | 1 | 0 | 0 | 0 | 0 | 0 | 0 |
| | 15-19 | 610 | 193 | 417 | 53 | 11 | 42 | 505 | 163 | 342 | 42 | 16 | 26 | 3 | 0 | 3 | 7 | 3 | 4 |
| | 20-24 | 1,027 | 508 | 519 | 104 | 30 | 74 | 835 | 418 | 417 | 72 | 51 | 21 | 5 | 3 | 2 | 11 | 6 | 5 |
| | 25-29 | 1,026 | 507 | 519 | 129 | 50 | 79 | 781 | 383 | 398 | 99 | 65 | 34 | 5 | 4 | 1 | 12 | 5 | 7 |
| | 30-34 | 1,177 | 625 | 552 | 146 | 77 | 69 | 949 | 484 | 465 | 64 | 53 | 11 | 9 | 7 | 2 | 9 | 4 | 5 |
| | 35-39 | 1,177 | 683 | 494 | 173 | 105 | 68 | 926 | 522 | 404 | 64 | 46 | 18 | 7 | 6 | 1 | 7 | 4 | 3 |
| | 40-44 | 830 | 533 | 297 | 129 | 95 | 34 | 653 | 403 | 250 | 40 | 30 | 10 | 3 | 2 | 1 | 5 | 3 | 2 |
| | 45-54 | 777 | 576 | 201 | 122 | 102 | 20 | 609 | 439 | 170 | 44 | 34 | 10 | 1 | 1 | 0 | 1 | 0 | 1 |
| | 55-64 | 231 | 194 | 37 | 50 | 47 | 3 | 161 | 129 | 32 | 16 | 14 | 2 | 2 | 2 | 0 | 2 | 2 | 0 |
| | 65+ | 102 | 86 | 16 | 21 | 18 | 3 | 71 | 60 | 11 | 9 | 7 | 2 | 0 | 0 | 0 | 1 | 1 | 0 |
| | TOTAL | 7,004 | 3,912 | 3,092 | 932 | 535 | 397 | 5,531 | 3,008 | 2,523 | 451 | 316 | 135 | 35 | 25 | 10 | 55 | 28 | 27 |
| 1999 | 10-14 | 25 | 2 | 23 | 3 | 1 | 2 | 21 | 1 | 20 | 1 | 0 | 1 | 0 | 0 | 0 | 0 | 0 | 0 |
| | 15-19 | 524 | 182 | 342 | 48 | 16 | 32 | 424 | 139 | 285 | 43 | 24 | 19 | 1 | 1 | 0 | 8 | 2 | 6 |
| | 20-24 | 963 | 512 | 451 | 120 | 46 | 74 | 719 | 383 | 336 | 109 | 75 | 34 | 5 | 3 | 2 | 10 | 5 | 5 |
| | 25-29 | 994 | 509 | 485 | 139 | 69 | 70 | 744 | 364 | 380 | 93 | 67 | 26 | 7 | 7 | 0 | 11 | 2 | 9 |
| | 30-34 | 1,091 | 593 | 498 | 169 | 99 | 70 | 808 | 415 | 393 | 96 | 72 | 24 | 12 | 6 | 6 | 6 | 1 | 5 |
| | 35-39 | 1,158 | 679 | 479 | 192 | 115 | 77 | 885 | 501 | 384 | 70 | 57 | 13 | 3 | 3 | 0 | 8 | 3 | 5 |
| | 40-44 | 809 | 539 | 270 | 142 | 99 | 43 | 603 | 391 | 212 | 55 | 46 | 9 | 7 | 3 | 4 | 2 | 0 | 2 |
| | 45-54 | 756 | 573 | 183 | 140 | 97 | 43 | 562 | 431 | 131 | 42 | 36 | 6 | 5 | 5 | 0 | 7 | 4 | 3 |
| | 55-64 | 228 | 187 | 41 | 54 | 41 | 13 | 151 | 129 | 22 | 21 | 16 | 5 | 1 | 0 | 1 | 1 | 1 | 0 |
| | 65+ | 74 | 65 | 9 | 24 | 22 | 2 | 46 | 39 | 7 | 4 | 4 | 0 | 0 | 0 | 0 | 0 | 0 | 0 |
| | TOTAL | 6,634 | 3,844 | 2,790 | 1,033 | 605 | 428 | 4,972 | 2,795 | 2,177 | 535 | 398 | 137 | 41 | 28 | 13 | 53 | 18 | 35 |

Note: These tables should be used only for race/ethnicity and age comparisons, not for overall totals or gender totals. This is because, if age or race/ethnicity was not specified, cases were prorated according to the distribution of cases for which these variables were specified. For the following years the states listed did not report race/ethnicity for most cases and were excluded: 1996 (Rhode Island); 1999 (New Hampshire). Differences between total cases from this table and others in the report are due to different reporting forms and above listed exclusions. The 0 to 9 year age group is not shown because some of these may not be due to sexual transmission; however, they are included in the totals.

*Source*: Centers for Disease Control and Prevention, U.S. Department of Health and Human Services. National Center for HIV, STD, and TB Prevention, Division of STD Prevention. *Sexually Transmitted Disease Surveillance 1999* (Atlanta, GA: CDC, 2000). http://www.cdc.gov/nchstp/dstd/Stats_Trends/1999Surveillance/99PDF/Surv99Master.pdf.

**Table D5.16. Congenital Syphilis—Rates for Infants <1 Year of Age: United States, 1981–1999, and the Healthy People Year 2000 Objective**

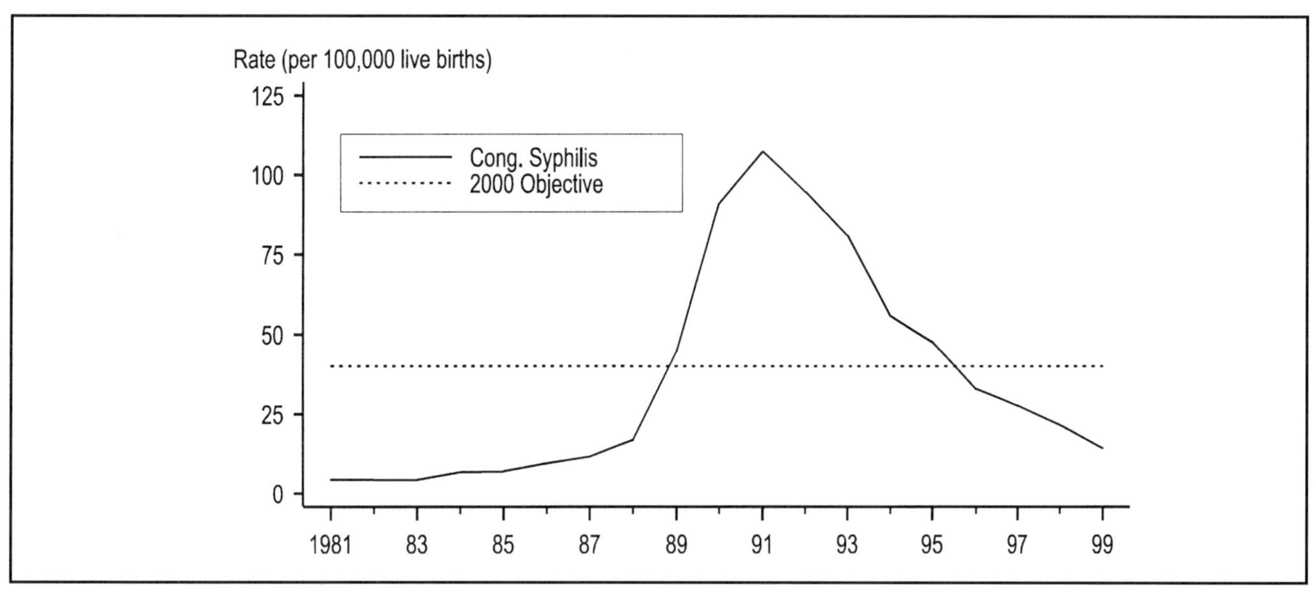


Note: The surveillance case definition for congenital syphilis changed in 1988 (see Appendix).
*Source*: Centers for Disease Control and Prevention, U.S. Department of Health and Human Services. National Center for HIV, STD, and TB Prevention, Division of STD Prevention. *Sexually Transmitted Disease Surveillance 1999* (Atlanta, GA: CDC, 2000). http://www.cdc.gov/nchstp/dstd/Stats_Trends/1999Surveillance/99PDF/Surv99Master.pdf.

**Table D5.17. Congenital Syphilis—Reported Cases per 100,000 Live Births among Infants Aged <1 Year, United States, 1969–1999**

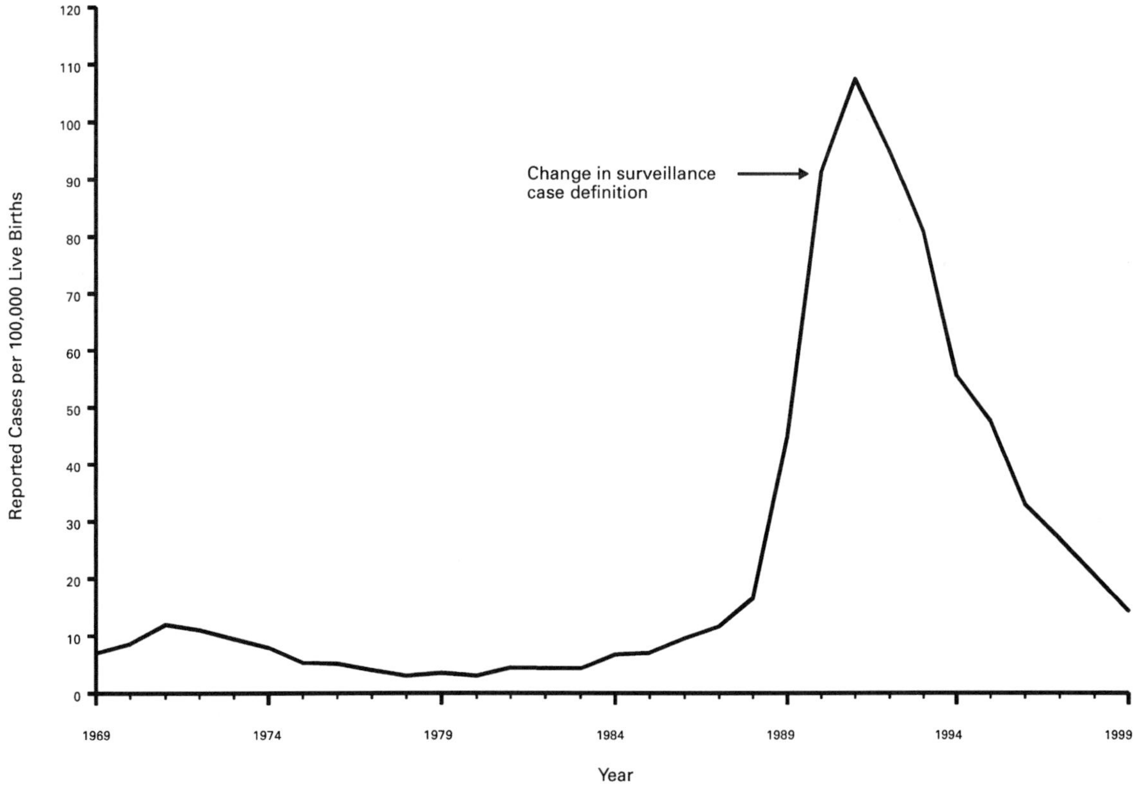

The rate of congenital syphilis decreased from 21.6 cases/100,000 live births in 1998 to 14.3/100,000 in 1999 (Division of Sexually Transmitted Diseases Prevention, National Center for HIV, STD, and TB Prevention).
*Source*: Center for Disease Control and Prevention. U.S. Department of Health and Human Services. *MMWR: Morbidity and Mortality Weekly Review Summary of Notifiable Disease, United States, 1999* 48 no. 53 (2001). http://www.cdc.gov/mmwr/PDF/wk/mm4853.pdf.

## Table D5.18. Congenital Syphilis—Reported Cases and Rates in Infants <1 Year of Age: United States (Excluding Outlying Areas). 1963–1999

| *Year* | *Cases* | *Rate per 100,000 Live Births* |
|---|---|---|
| 1963 | 367 | 9.2 |
| 1964 | 336 | 8.7 |
| 1965 | 335 | 8.9 |
| 1966 | 333 | 8.8 |
| 1967 | 156 | 4.1 |
| 1968 | 274 | 7.3 |
| 1969 | 264 | 7.0 |
| 1970 | 323 | 8.6 |
| 1971 | 422 | 11.9 |
| 1972 | 360 | 11.0 |
| 1973 | 295 | 9.4 |
| 1974 | 250 | 7.9 |
| 1975 | 169 | 5.3 |
| 1976 | 160 | 5.1 |
| 1977 | 134 | 4.0 |
| 1978 | 104 | 3.0 |
| 1979 | 123 | 3.5 |
| 1980 | 107 | 3.0 |
| 1981 | 160 | 4.4 |
| 1982 | 159 | 4.3 |
| 1983 | 158 | 4.3 |
| 1984 | 247 | 6.7 |
| 1985 | 266 | 7.0 |
| 1986 | 357 | 9.5 |
| 1987 | 444 | 11.6 |
| 1988 | 658 | 16.8 |
| 1989 | 1,807 | 44.7 |
| 1990 | 3,816 | 91.0 |
| 1991 | 4,410 | 107.3 |
| 1992 | 3,851 | 94.7 |
| 1993 | 3,237 | 80.9 |
| 1994 | 2,204 | 55.8 |
| 1995 | 1,857 | 47.6 |
| 1996 | 1,279 | 32.9 |
| 1997 | 1,075 | 27.7 |
| 1998 | 838 | 21.6 |
| 1999 | 556 | 14.3 |

Years 1963-1966 are fiscal years.

Note: The surveillance case definition for congenital syphilis changed in 1988 (see Appendix). As of 1995, cases of congenital syphilis <1 year of age are obtained using case reporting from CDC 73.126. Yearly case counts in this table correspond to confirmed diagnoses of congenital syphilis among those known to be less than one year of age. As a result, the case counts in this table are a subset of those listed in Table 1 for the years prior to 1995.

*Source*: Centers for Disease Control and Prevention, U.S. Department of Health and Human Services. National Center for HIV, STD, and TB Prevention, Division of STD Prevention. *Sexually Transmitted Disease Surveillance 1999* (Atlanta, GA: CDC, 2000). http://www.cdc.gov/nchstp/dstd/Stats_Trends/1999Surveillance/99PDF/Surv99Master.pdf.

## Table D5.19. Congenital Syphilis—Reported Cases and Rates in Infants <1 Year of Age, by State/Area Listed in Alphabetical Order: United States and Outlying Areas, 1995–1999

| | Cases | | | | | Rates per 100,000 Live Births | | | | |
|---|---|---|---|---|---|---|---|---|---|---|
| *State/Area** | *1995* | *1996* | *1997* | *1998* | *1999* | *1995* | *1996* | *1997* | *1998* | *1999* |
| Alabama | 18 | 22 | 31 | 12 | 6 | 29.8 | 36.4 | 50.9 | 19.7 | 9.8 |
| Alaska | 0 | 0 | 0 | 0 | 0 | 0.0 | 0.0 | 0.0 | 0.0 | 0.0 |
| Arizona | 10 | 6 | 12 | 25 | 24 | 13.8 | 8.0 | 15.9 | 33.0 | 31.7 |
| Arkansas | 29 | 32 | 41 | 30 | 14 | 82.4 | 88.0 | 112.4 | 82.2 | 38.4 |
| California | 344 | 196 | 161 | 122 | 88 | 62.3 | 36.3 | 30.7 | 23.2 | 16.8 |
| Colorado | 1 | 3 | 0 | 2 | 1 | 1.8 | 5.4 | 0.0 | 3.5 | 1.8 |
| Connecticut | 6 | 2 | 2 | 0 | 1 | 13.5 | 4.5 | 4.6 | 0.0 | 2.3 |
| Delaware | 1 | 0 | 2 | 0 | 0 | 9.7 | 0.0 | 19.5 | 0.0 | 0.0 |
| Florida | 112 | 93 | 73 | 71 | 32 | 59.3 | 49.1 | 37.9 | 36.9 | 16.6 |
| Georgia | 45 | 29 | 17 | 14 | 15 | 40.1 | 25.4 | 14.4 | 11.8 | 12.7 |
| Hawaii | 0 | 0 | 0 | 0 | 0 | 0.0 | 0.0 | 0.0 | 0.0 | 0.0 |
| Idaho | 0 | 1 | 0 | 0 | 0 | 0.0 | 5.4 | 0.0 | 0.0 | 0.0 |
| Illinois | 184 | 104 | 73 | 71 | 53 | 99.0 | 56.8 | 40.4 | 39.3 | 29.3 |
| Indiana | 0 | 6 | 3 | 0 | 7 | 0.0 | 7.2 | 3.6 | 0.0 | 8.4 |
| Iowa | 0 | 0 | 0 | 0 | 0 | 0.0 | 0.0 | 0.0 | 0.0 | 0.0 |
| Kansas | 1 | 0 | 2 | 0 | 0 | 2.7 | 0.0 | 5.4 | 0.0 | 0.0 |
| Kentucky | 7 | 5 | 5 | 5 | 0 | 13.4 | 9.5 | 9.4 | 9.4 | 0.0 |
| Louisiana | 36 | 15 | 22 | 8 | 12 | 54.8 | 23.0 | 33.3 | 12.1 | 18.2 |
| Maine | 0 | 0 | 0 | 0 | 0 | 0.0 | 0.0 | 0.0 | 0.0 | 0.0 |
| Maryland | 28 | 36 | 58 | 44 | 27 | 38.7 | 50.3 | 82.6 | 62.7 | 38.5 |
| Massachusetts | 0 | 6 | 1 | 2 | 0 | 0.0 | 7.5 | 1.2 | 2.5 | 0.0 |
| Michigan | 28 | 22 | 29 | 18 | 20 | 20.8 | 16.5 | 21.7 | 13.5 | 15.0 |
| Minnesota | 2 | 2 | 0 | 0 | 0 | 3.2 | 3.1 | 0.0 | 0.0 | 0.0 |
| Mississippi | 65 | 54 | 41 | 15 | 12 | 157.2 | 131.7 | 98.7 | 36.1 | 28.9 |
| Missouri | 40 | 15 | 10 | 15 | 9 | 54.8 | 20.3 | 13.5 | 20.3 | 12.2 |
| Montana | 0 | 0 | 0 | 0 | 0 | 0.0 | 0.0 | 0.0 | 0.0 | 0.0 |
| Nebraska | 0 | 0 | 0 | 0 | 0 | 0.0 | 0.0 | 0.0 | 0.0 | 0.0 |
| Nevada | 0 | 1 | 0 | 0 | 0 | 0.0 | 3.8 | 0.0 | 0.0 | 0.0 |
| New Hampshire | 0 | 0 | 0 | 0 | 1 | 0.0 | 0.0 | 0.0 | 0.0 | 7.0 |
| New Jersey | 95 | 80 | 84 | 87 | 46 | 82.7 | 70.0 | 74.2 | 76.8 | 40.6 |
| New Mexico | 0 | 0 | 0 | 0 | 0 | 0.0 | 0.0 | 0.0 | 0.0 | 0.0 |
| New York | 326 | 155 | 105 | 58 | 43 | 120.1 | 58.7 | 40.8 | 22.5 | 16.7 |
| North Carolina | 33 | 31 | 18 | 24 | 19 | 32.5 | 29.7 | 16.8 | 22.4 | 17.8 |
| North Dakota | 0 | 0 | 0 | 0 | 0 | 0.0 | 0.0 | 0.0 | 0.0 | 0.0 |
| Ohio | 38 | 15 | 10 | 4 | 6 | 24.7 | 9.9 | 6.6 | 2.6 | 3.9 |
| Oklahoma | 17 | 10 | 9 | 16 | 8 | 37.2 | 21.6 | 18.6 | 33.1 | 16.6 |
| Oregon | 0 | 0 | 1 | 0 | 0 | 0.0 | 0.0 | 2.3 | 0.0 | 0.0 |
| Pennsylvania | 68 | 58 | 37 | 21 | 7 | 44.8 | 39.1 | 25.7 | 14.6 | 4.9 |
| Rhode Island | 0 | 0 | 0 | 0 | 0 | 0.0 | 0.0 | 0.0 | 0.0 | 0.0 |
| South Carolina | 42 | 44 | 19 | 24 | 19 | 82.5 | 86.1 | 36.4 | 46.0 | 36.4 |
| South Dakota | 0 | 0 | 0 | 1 | 1 | 0.0 | 0.0 | 0.0 | 9.8 | 9.8 |
| Tennessee | 29 | 35 | 32 | 13 | 7 | 39.6 | 47.5 | 43.0 | 17.5 | 9.4 |
| Texas | 202 | 166 | 149 | 114 | 68 | 62.6 | 50.2 | 44.6 | 34.1 | 20.4 |
| Utah | 0 | 0 | 0 | 1 | 0 | 0.0 | 0.0 | 0.0 | 2.3 | 0.0 |
| Vermont | 0 | 1 | 0 | 0 | 0 | 0.0 | 14.8 | 0.0 | 0.0 | 0.0 |
| Virginia | 25 | 16 | 7 | 6 | 3 | 27.0 | 17.3 | 7.6 | 6.5 | 3.3 |
| Washington | 1 | 1 | 0 | 1 | 0 | 1.3 | 1.3 | 0.0 | 1.3 | 0.0 |
| West Virginia | 0 | 0 | 1 | 0 | 0 | 0.0 | 0.0 | 4.8 | 0.0 | 0.0 |
| Wisconsin | 11 | 3 | 9 | 6 | 7 | 16.3 | 4.5 | 13.5 | 9.0 | 10.5 |
| Wyoming | 0 | 0 | 0 | 0 | 0 | 0.0 | 0.0 | 0.0 | 0.0 | 0.0 |
| U.S. TOTAL[†] | 1,857 | 1,279 | 1,075 | 838 | 556 | 47.6 | 32.9 | 27.7 | 21.6 | 14.3 |
| Guam | 0 | 0 | 0 | 0 | 0 | 0.0 | 0.0 | 0.0 | 0.0 | 0.0 |
| Puerto Rico | 14 | 10 | 9 | 28 | 17 | 22.1 | 15.8 | 14.0 | 43.7 | 26.5 |
| Virgin Islands | 0 | 0 | 0 | 0 | 0 | 0.0 | 0.0 | 0.0 | 0.0 | 0.0 |
| OUTLYING AREAS | 14 | 10 | 9 | 28 | 17 | 20.1 | 14.4 | 12.8 | 39.8 | 24.1 |
| TOTAL | 1,871 | 1,289 | 1,084 | 866 | 573 | 47.1 | 32.5 | 27.4 | 21.9 | 14.5 |

*Mother's state of residence used to assign case.

†Includes cases reported by Washington, D.C.

Note: As of 1995, cases of congenital syphilis <1 year of age are obtained using case reporting form CDC 73.126.

*Source*: Centers for Disease Control and Prevention, U.S. Department of Health and Human Services. National Center for HIV, STD, and TB Prevention, Division of STD Prevention. *Sexually Transmitted Disease Surveillance 1999* (Atlanta, GA: CDC, 2000). http://www.cdc.gov/nchstp/dstd/Stats_Trends/1999Surveillance/99PDF/Surv99Master.pdf.

## Table D5.20. Congenital Syphilis—Reported Cases and Rates in Infants <1 Year of Age by State/Area, Ranked according to Rates: United States and Outlying Areas, 1999

| Rank | State/Area* | Cases | Rate per 100,000 Live Births |
|---|---|---|---|
| 1 | New Jersey | 46 | 40.6 |
| | **YEAR 2000 OBJECTIVE** | | **40.0** |
| 2 | Maryland | 27 | 38.5 |
| 3 | Arkansas | 14 | 38.4 |
| 4 | South Carolina | 19 | 36.4 |
| 5 | Arizona | 24 | 31.7 |
| 6 | Illinois | 53 | 29.3 |
| 7 | Mississippi | 12 | 28.9 |
| 8 | Puerto Rico | 17 | 26.5 |
| 9 | Texas | 68 | 20.4 |
| 10 | Louisiana | 12 | 18.2 |
| 11 | North Carolina | 19 | 17.8 |
| 12 | California | 88 | 16.8 |
| 13 | New York | 43 | 16.7 |
| 14 | Florida | 32 | 16.6 |
| 15 | Oklahoma | 8 | 16.6 |
| 16 | Michigan | 20 | 15.0 |
| | **U.S. TOTAL**[1] | **556** | **14.3** |
| 17 | Georgia | 15 | 12.7 |
| 18 | Missouri | 9 | 12.2 |
| 19 | Wisconsin | 7 | 10.5 |
| 20 | Alabama | 6 | 9.8 |
| 21 | South Dakota | 1 | 9.8 |
| 22 | Tennessee | 7 | 9.4 |
| 23 | Indiana | 7 | 8.4 |
| 24 | New Hampshire | 1 | 7.0 |
| 25 | Pennsylvania | 7 | 4.9 |
| 26 | Ohio | 6 | 3.9 |
| 27 | Virginia | 3 | 3.3 |
| 28 | Connecticut | 1 | 2.3 |
| 29 | Colorado | 1 | 1.8 |
| 30 | Alaska | 0 | 0.0 |
| 31 | Delaware | 0 | 0.0 |
| 32 | Hawaii | 0 | 0.0 |
| 33 | Idaho | 0 | 0.0 |
| 34 | Iowa | 0 | 0.0 |
| 35 | Kansas | 0 | 0.0 |
| 36 | Kentucky | 0 | 0.0 |
| 37 | Maine | 0 | 0.0 |
| 38 | Massachusetts | 0 | 0.0 |
| 39 | Minnesota | 0 | 0.0 |
| 40 | Montana | 0 | 0.0 |
| 41 | Nebraska | 0 | 0.0 |
| 42 | Nevada | 0 | 0.0 |
| 43 | New Mexico | 0 | 0.0 |
| 44 | North Dakota | 0 | 0.0 |
| 45 | Oregon | 0 | 0.0 |
| 46 | Rhode Island | 0 | 0.0 |
| 47 | Utah | 0 | 0.0 |
| 48 | Vermont | 0 | 0.0 |
| 49 | Washington | 0 | 0.0 |
| 50 | West Virginia | 0 | 0.0 |
| 51 | Wyoming | 0 | 0.0 |
| 52 | Guam | 0 | 0.0 |
| 53 | Virgin Islands | 0 | 0.0 |

*Mother's state of residence used to assign case.

†Includes cases reported by Washington, D.C. but excludes outlying areas (Guam, Puerto Rico and Virgin Islands).

*Source*: Centers for Disease Control and Prevention, U.S. Department of Health and Human Services. National Center for HIV, STD, and TB Prevention, Division of STD Prevention. *Sexually Transmitted Disease Surveillance 1999* (Atlanta, GA: CDC, 2000). http://www.cdc.gov/nchstp/dstd/Stats_Trends/1999Surveillance/99PDF/Surv99Master.pdf.

## Table D6.1. Chancroid—Reported Cases and Rates, by State/Area Listed in Alphabetical Order: United States and Outlying Areas, 1995–1999

| | Cases | | | | | Rates per 100,000 Population | | | | |
|---|---|---|---|---|---|---|---|---|---|---|
| State/Area | 1995 | 1996 | 1997 | 1998 | 1999 | 1995 | 1996 | 1997 | 1998 | 1999 |
| Alabama | 7 | 0 | 1 | 1 | 1 | 0.2 | 0.0 | 0.0 | 0.0 | 0.0 |
| Alaska | 0 | 0 | 0 | 0 | 0 | 0.0 | 0.0 | 0.0 | 0.0 | 0.0 |
| Arizona | 2 | 2 | 0 | 2 | 0 | 0.0 | 0.0 | 0.0 | 0.0 | 0.0 |
| Arkansas | 1 | 1 | 1 | 7 | 0 | 0.0 | 0.0 | 0.0 | 0.3 | 0.0 |
| California | 8 | 8 | 19 | 7 | 7 | 0.0 | 0.0 | 0.1 | 0.0 | 0.0 |
| Colorado | 0 | 0 | 0 | 0 | 0 | 0.0 | 0.0 | 0.0 | 0.0 | 0.0 |
| Connecticut | 0 | 0 | 0 | 2 | 0 | 0.0 | 0.0 | 0.0 | 0.1 | 0.0 |
| Delaware | 0 | 0 | 0 | 0 | 0 | 0.0 | 0.0 | 0.0 | 0.0 | 0.0 |
| Florida | 24 | 3 | 3 | 3 | 3 | 0.2 | 0.0 | 0.0 | 0.0 | 0.0 |
| Georgia | 2 | 0 | 1 | 2 | 1 | 0.0 | 0.0 | 0.0 | 0.0 | 0.0 |
| Hawaii | 0 | 0 | 0 | 0 | 0 | 0.0 | 0.0 | 0.0 | 0.0 | 0.0 |
| Idaho | 0 | 0 | 0 | 0 | 0 | 0.0 | 0.0 | 0.0 | 0.0 | 0.0 |
| Illinois | 21 | 20 | 5 | 0 | 0 | 0.2 | 0.2 | 0.0 | 0.0 | 0.0 |
| Indiana | 0 | 1 | 0 | 1 | 0 | 0.0 | 0.0 | 0.0 | 0.0 | 0.0 |
| Iowa | 0 | 0 | 0 | 0 | 0 | 0.0 | 0.0 | 0.0 | 0.0 | 0.0 |
| Kansas | 2 | 2 | 0 | 1 | 0 | 0.1 | 0.1 | 0.0 | 0.0 | 0.0 |
| Kentucky | 0 | 0 | 0 | 0 | 0 | 0.0 | 0.0 | 0.0 | 0.0 | 0.0 |
| Louisiana | 129 | 58 | 3 | 1 | 9 | 3.0 | 1.3 | 0.1 | 0.0 | 0.2 |
| Maine | 0 | 0 | 0 | 0 | 0 | 0.0 | 0.0 | 0.0 | 0.0 | 0.0 |
| Maryland | 0 | 2 | 1 | 0 | 0 | 0.0 | 0.0 | 0.0 | 0.0 | 0.0 |
| Massachusetts | 7 | 2 | 4 | 0 | 1 | 0.1 | 0.0 | 0.1 | 0.0 | 0.0 |
| Michigan | 0 | 0 | 0 | 0 | 0 | 0.0 | 0.0 | 0.0 | 0.0 | 0.0 |
| Minnesota | 0 | 0 | 0 | 0 | 1 | 0.0 | 0.0 | 0.0 | 0.0 | 0.0 |
| Mississippi | 0 | 1 | 1 | 3 | 0 | 0.0 | 0.0 | 0.0 | 0.1 | 0.0 |
| Missouri | 0 | 0 | 0 | 0 | 0 | 0.0 | 0.0 | 0.0 | 0.0 | 0.0 |
| Montana | 0 | 0 | 0 | 0 | 0 | 0.0 | 0.0 | 0.0 | 0.0 | 0.0 |
| Nebraska | 0 | 0 | 0 | 0 | 0 | 0.0 | 0.0 | 0.0 | 0.0 | 0.0 |
| Nevada | 2 | 0 | 2 | 0 | 0 | 0.1 | 0.0 | 0.1 | 0.0 | 0.0 |
| New Hampshire | 0 | 1 | 0 | 0 | 0 | 0.0 | 0.1 | 0.0 | 0.0 | 0.0 |
| New Jersey | 4 | 4 | 0 | 0 | 0 | 0.1 | 0.0 | 0.0 | 0.0 | 0.0 |
| New Mexico | 0 | 0 | 0 | 0 | 0 | 0.0 | 0.0 | 0.0 | 0.0 | 0.0 |
| New York | 336 | 182 | 119 | 82 | 39 | 1.9 | 1.0 | 0.7 | 0.5 | 0.2 |
| North Carolina | 18 | 14 | 9 | 9 | 7 | 0.3 | 0.2 | 0.1 | 0.1 | 0.1 |
| North Dakota | 0 | 0 | 0 | 0 | 0 | 0.0 | 0.0 | 0.0 | 0.0 | 0.0 |
| Ohio | 5 | 6 | 3 | 3 | 0 | 0.0 | 0.1 | 0.0 | 0.0 | 0.0 |
| Oklahoma | 0 | 0 | 0 | 0 | 0 | 0.0 | 0.0 | 0.0 | 0.0 | 0.0 |
| Oregon | 0 | 0 | 1 | 0 | 1 | 0.0 | 0.0 | 0.0 | 0.0 | 0.0 |
| Pennsylvania | 0 | 0 | 0 | 0 | 0 | 0.0 | 0.0 | 0.0 | 0.0 | 0.0 |
| Rhode Island | 0 | 0 | 0 | 0 | 1 | 0.0 | 0.0 | 0.0 | 0.0 | 0.1 |
| South Carolina | 0 | 8 | 15 | 19 | 48 | 0.0 | 0.2 | 0.4 | 0.5 | 1.3 |
| South Dakota | 0 | 0 | 0 | 0 | 0 | 0.0 | 0.0 | 0.0 | 0.0 | 0.0 |
| Tennessee | 2 | 2 | 1 | 0 | 0 | 0.0 | 0.0 | 0.0 | 0.0 | 0.0 |
| Texas | 26 | 65 | 53 | 34 | 16 | 0.1 | 0.3 | 0.3 | 0.2 | 0.1 |
| Utah | 0 | 0 | 0 | 0 | 0 | 0.0 | 0.0 | 0.0 | 0.0 | 0.0 |
| Vermont | 0 | 0 | 0 | 0 | 0 | 0.0 | 0.0 | 0.0 | 0.0 | 0.0 |
| Virginia | 2 | 1 | 1 | 7 | 3 | 0.0 | 0.0 | 0.0 | 0.1 | 0.0 |
| Washington | 5 | 1 | 2 | 1 | 0 | 0.1 | 0.0 | 0.0 | 0.0 | 0.0 |
| West Virginia | 1 | 0 | 0 | 0 | 0 | 0.1 | 0.0 | 0.0 | 0.0 | 0.0 |
| Wisconsin | 3 | 2 | 0 | 3 | 4 | 0.1 | 0.0 | 0.0 | 0.1 | 0.1 |
| Wyoming | 0 | 0 | 1 | 1 | 1 | 0.0 | 0.0 | 0.2 | 0.2 | 0.2 |
| U.S. TOTAL[1] | 607 | 386 | 246 | 189 | 143 | 0.2 | 0.1 | 0.1 | 0.1 | 0.1 |
| Guam | 0 | 0 | 0 | 0 | 0 | 0.0 | 0.0 | 0.0 | 0.0 | 0.0 |
| Puerto Rico | 1 | 2 | 1 | 2 | 1 | 0.0 | 0.1 | 0.0 | 0.1 | 0.0 |
| Virgin Islands | 2 | 0 | 0 | 0 | 0 | 1.8 | 0.0 | 0.0 | 0.0 | 0.0 |
| OUTLYING AREAS | 3 | 2 | 1 | 2 | 1 | 0.1 | 0.1 | 0.0 | 0.0 | 0.0 |
| TOTAL | 610 | 388 | 247 | 191 | 144 | 0.2 | 0.1 | 0.1 | 0.1 | 0.1 |

[1]Includes cases reported by Washington, D.C.

*Source*: Centers for Disease Control and Prevention, U.S. Department of Health and Human Services. National Center for HIV, STD, and TB Prevention, Division of STD Prevention. *Sexually Transmitted Disease Surveillance 1999* (Atlanta, GA: CDC, 2000). http://www.cdc.gov/nchstp/dstd/Stats_Trends/1999Surveillance/99PDF/Surv99Master.pdf.

## Table D6.2. Chancroid—Reported Cases and Rates in Selected Cities of >200,000 Population Listed in Alphabetical Order: United States and Outlying Areas, 1995–1999

| | *Cases* | | | | | *Rates per 100,000 Population* | | | | |
|---|---|---|---|---|---|---|---|---|---|---|
| *City* | *1995* | *1996* | *1997* | *1998* | *1999* | *1995* | *1996* | *1997* | *1998* | *1999* |
| Akron, OH | 0 | 0 | 0 | 0 | 0 | 0.0 | 0.0 | 0.0 | 0.0 | 0.0 |
| Albuquerque, NM | 0 | 0 | 0 | 0 | 0 | 0.0 | 0.0 | 0.0 | 0.0 | 0.0 |
| Atlanta, GA | 0 | 0 | 1 | 1 | 0 | 0.0 | 0.0 | 0.1 | 0.1 | 0.0 |
| Austin, TX | 0 | 0 | 0 | 0 | 0 | 0.0 | 0.0 | 0.0 | 0.0 | 0.0 |
| Baltimore, MD | 0 | 1 | 0 | 0 | 0 | 0.0 | 0.1 | 0.0 | 0.0 | 0.0 |
| Birmingham, AL | 0 | 0 | 0 | 0 | 0 | 0.0 | 0.0 | 0.0 | 0.0 | 0.0 |
| Boston, MA | 2 | 0 | 3 | 0 | 0 | 0.4 | 0.0 | 0.5 | 0.0 | 0.0 |
| Buffalo, NY | 0 | 0 | 0 | 0 | 0 | 0.0 | 0.0 | 0.0 | 0.0 | 0.0 |
| Charlotte, NC | 3 | 4 | 1 | 0 | 1 | 0.5 | 0.7 | 0.2 | 0.0 | 0.2 |
| Chicago, IL | 21 | 20 | 5 | 0 | 0 | 0.7 | 0.7 | 0.2 | 0.0 | 0.0 |
| Cincinnati, OH | 1 | 0 | 0 | 0 | 0 | 0.1 | 0.0 | 0.0 | 0.0 | 0.0 |
| Cleveland, OH | 0 | 0 | 0 | 2 | 0 | 0.0 | 0.0 | 0.0 | 0.1 | 0.0 |
| Columbus, OH | 0 | 0 | 3 | 1 | 0 | 0.0 | 0.0 | 0.3 | 0.1 | 0.0 |
| Corpus Christi, TX | 1 | 0 | 0 | 0 | 1 | 0.3 | 0.0 | 0.0 | 0.0 | 0.3 |
| Dallas, TX | 12 | 13 | 13 | 6 | 4 | 0.6 | 0.7 | 0.6 | 0.3 | 0.2 |
| Dayton, OH | 1 | 1 | 0 | 0 | 0 | 0.2 | 0.2 | 0.0 | 0.0 | 0.0 |
| Denver, CO | 0 | 0 | 0 | 0 | 0 | 0.0 | 0.0 | 0.0 | 0.0 | 0.0 |
| Des Moines, IA | 0 | 0 | 0 | 0 | 0 | 0.0 | 0.0 | 0.0 | 0.0 | 0.0 |
| Detroit, MI | 0 | 0 | 0 | 0 | 0 | 0.0 | 0.0 | 0.0 | 0.0 | 0.0 |
| El Paso, TX | 0 | 1 | 2 | 4 | 0 | 0.0 | 0.1 | 0.3 | 0.6 | 0.0 |
| Fort Worth, TX | 0 | 0 | 1 | 0 | 2 | 0.0 | 0.0 | 0.1 | 0.0 | 0.1 |
| Honolulu, HI | 0 | 0 | 0 | 0 | 0 | 0.0 | 0.0 | 0.0 | 0.0 | 0.0 |
| Houston, TX | 0 | 25 | 23 | 20 | 7 | 0.0 | 0.8 | 0.7 | 0.6 | 0.2 |
| Indianapolis, IN | 0 | 0 | 0 | 0 | 0 | 0.0 | 0.0 | 0.0 | 0.0 | 0.0 |
| Jacksonville, FL | 0 | 0 | 0 | 0 | 0 | 0.0 | 0.0 | 0.0 | 0.0 | 0.0 |
| Jersey City, NJ | 0 | 0 | 0 | 0 | 0 | 0.0 | 0.0 | 0.0 | 0.0 | 0.0 |
| Kansas City, MO | 0 | 0 | 0 | 0 | 0 | 0.0 | 0.0 | 0.0 | 0.0 | 0.0 |
| Los Angeles, CA | 4 | 2 | 12 | 0 | 1 | 0.0 | 0.0 | 0.1 | 0.0 | 0.0 |
| Louisville, KY | 0 | 0 | 0 | 0 | 0 | 0.0 | 0.0 | 0.0 | 0.0 | 0.0 |
| Memphis, TN | 2 | 2 | 0 | 0 | 0 | 0.2 | 0.2 | 0.0 | 0.0 | 0.0 |
| Miami, FL | 0 | 0 | 0 | 0 | 0 | 0.0 | 0.0 | 0.0 | 0.0 | 0.0 |
| Milwaukee, WI | 0 | 1 | 0 | 2 | 2 | 0.0 | 0.1 | 0.0 | 0.2 | 0.2 |
| Minneapolis, MN | 0 | 0 | 0 | 0 | 1 | 0.0 | 0.0 | 0.0 | 0.0 | 0.3 |
| Nashville, TN | 0 | 0 | 0 | 0 | 0 | 0.0 | 0.0 | 0.0 | 0.0 | 0.0 |
| New Orleans, LA | 125 | 52 | 3 | 0 | 4 | 25.9 | 11.0 | 0.6 | 0.0 | 0.9 |
| New York City, NY | 334 | 181 | 119 | 82 | 39 | 4.6 | 2.5 | 1.6 | 1.1 | 0.5 |
| Newark, NJ | 1 | 0 | 0 | 0 | 0 | 0.3 | 0.0 | 0.0 | 0.0 | 0.0 |
| Norfolk, VA | 1 | 0 | 0 | 0 | 1 | 0.4 | 0.0 | 0.0 | 0.0 | 0.5 |
| Oakland, CA | 2 | 0 | 1 | 0 | 1 | 0.2 | 0.0 | 0.1 | 0.0 | 0.1 |
| Oklahoma City, OK | 0 | 0 | 0 | 0 | 0 | 0.0 | 0.0 | 0.0 | 0.0 | 0.0 |
| Omaha, NE | 0 | 0 | 0 | 0 | 0 | 0.0 | 0.0 | 0.0 | 0.0 | 0.0 |
| Philadelphia, PA | 0 | 0 | 0 | 0 | 0 | 0.0 | 0.0 | 0.0 | 0.0 | 0.0 |
| Phoenix, AZ | 0 | 1 | 0 | 2 | 0 | 0.0 | 0.0 | 0.0 | 0.1 | 0.0 |
| Pittsburgh, PA | 0 | 0 | 0 | 0 | 0 | 0.0 | 0.0 | 0.0 | 0.0 | 0.0 |
| Portland, OR | 0 | 0 | 0 | 0 | 0 | 0.0 | 0.0 | 0.0 | 0.0 | 0.0 |
| Richmond, VA | 0 | 0 | 0 | 0 | 0 | 0.0 | 0.0 | 0.0 | 0.0 | 0.0 |
| Rochester, NY | 0 | 0 | 0 | 0 | 0 | 0.0 | 0.0 | 0.0 | 0.0 | 0.0 |
| Sacramento, CA | 0 | 0 | 0 | 0 | 0 | 0.0 | 0.0 | 0.0 | 0.0 | 0.0 |
| San Antonio, TX | 0 | 0 | 0 | 0 | 0 | 0.0 | 0.0 | 0.0 | 0.0 | 0.0 |
| San Diego, CA | 2 | 2 | 0 | 0 | 0 | 0.1 | 0.1 | 0.0 | 0.0 | 0.0 |
| San Francisco, CA | 0 | 1 | 3 | 4 | 0 | 0.0 | 0.1 | 0.4 | 0.5 | 0.0 |
| San Jose, CA | 0 | 0 | 0 | 0 | 0 | 0.0 | 0.0 | 0.0 | 0.0 | 0.0 |
| Seattle, WA | 4 | 0 | 1 | 0 | 0 | 0.3 | 0.0 | 0.1 | 0.0 | 0.0 |
| St Louis, MO | 0 | 0 | 0 | 0 | 0 | 0.0 | 0.0 | 0.0 | 0.0 | 0.0 |
| St Paul, MN | 0 | 0 | 0 | 0 | 0 | 0.0 | 0.0 | 0.0 | 0.0 | 0.0 |
| St Petersburg, FL | 0 | 0 | 0 | 0 | 0 | 0.0 | 0.0 | 0.0 | 0.0 | 0.0 |
| Tampa, FL | 0 | 0 | 0 | 0 | 0 | 0.0 | 0.0 | 0.0 | 0.0 | 0.0 |
| Toledo, OH | 0 | 0 | 0 | 0 | 0 | 0.0 | 0.0 | 0.0 | 0.0 | 0.0 |
| Tucson, AZ | 0 | 1 | 0 | 0 | 0 | 0.0 | 0.1 | 0.0 | 0.0 | 0.0 |
| Tulsa, OK | 0 | 0 | 0 | 0 | 0 | 0.0 | 0.0 | 0.0 | 0.0 | 0.0 |
| Washington, DC | 0 | 0 | 0 | 0 | 0 | 0.0 | 0.0 | 0.0 | 0.0 | 0.0 |
| Wichita, KS | 0 | 1 | 0 | 0 | 0 | 0.0 | 0.2 | 0.0 | 0.0 | 0.0 |
| Yonkers, NY | 0 | 0 | 0 | 0 | 0 | 0.0 | 0.0 | 0.0 | 0.0 | 0.0 |
| U.S. CITY TOTAL | 516 | 309 | 191 | 124 | 64 | 0.7 | 0.4 | 0.3 | 0.2 | 0.1 |
| San Juan, PR | 0 | 1 | 0 | 1 | 1 | 0.0 | 0.1 | 0.0 | 0.1 | 0.1 |
| TOTAL | 516 | 310 | 191 | 125 | 65 | 0.7 | 0.4 | 0.3 | 0.2 | 0.1 |

*Source*: Centers for Disease Control and Prevention, U.S. Department of Health and Human Services. National Center for HIV, STD, and TB Prevention, Division of STD Prevention. *Sexually Transmitted Disease Surveillance 1999* (Atlanta, GA: CDC, 2000). http://www.cdc.gov/nchstp/dstd/Stats_Trends/99Surveillance/99PDF/Surv99Master.pdf.

## Table D6.3. Genital Herpes Simplex Virus Infections—Initial Visits to Physicians' Offices: United States, 1966–1999, and the Healthy People Year 2000 Objective

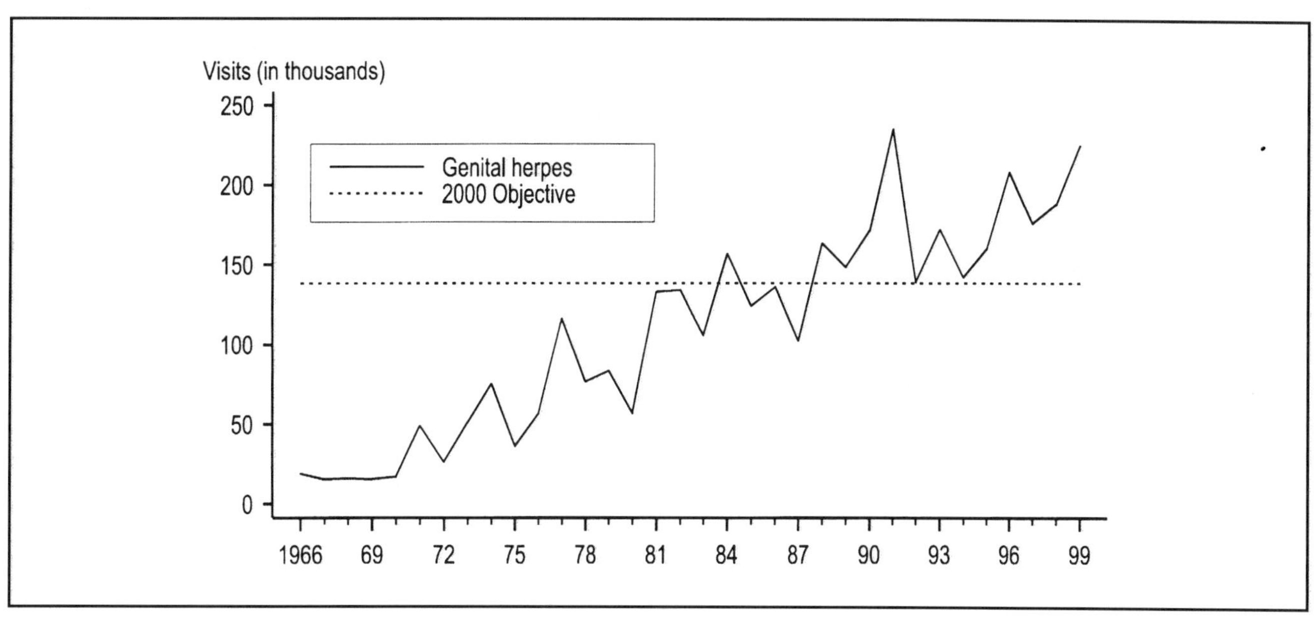


*Source*: Centers for Disease Control and Prevention, U.S. Department of Health and Human Services. National Center for HIV, STD, and TB Prevention, Division of STD Prevention. *Sexually Transmitted Disease Surveillance 1999* (Atlanta, GA: CDC, 2000). http://www.cdc.gov/nchstp/dstd/Stats_Trends/1999Surveillance/99PDF/Surv99Master.pdf.

## Table D6.4. Genital Herpes Simplex Virus Type 2—Percent Seroprevalence according to Age in NHANES* II (1976–1980) and NHANES III (1988–1994)

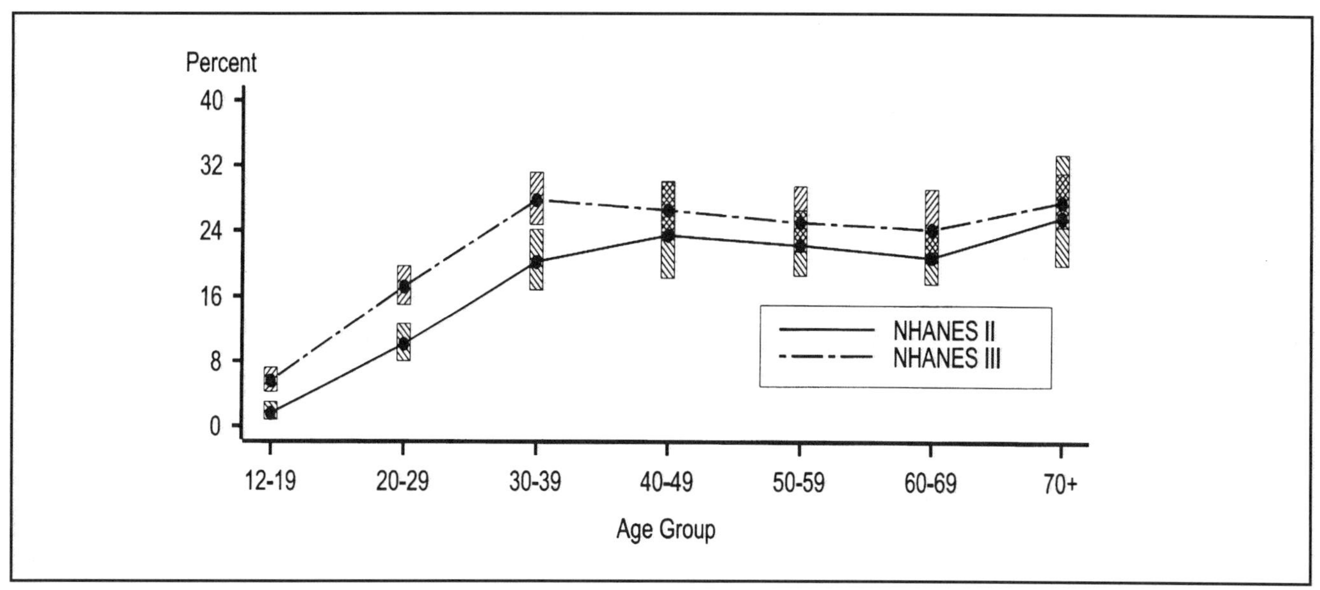


Note: Bars indicate 95% confidence intervals.

*National Health and Nutrition Examination Survey

*Source*: Centers for Disease Control and Prevention, U.S. Department of Health and Human Services. National Center for HIV, STD, and TB Prevention, Division of STD Prevention. *Sexually Transmitted Disease Surveillance 1999* (Atlanta, GA: CDC, 2000). http://www.cdc.gov/nchstp/dstd/Stats_Trends/1999Surveillance/99PDF/Surv99Master.pdf.

**Table D6.5. Human Papillomavirus (Genital Warts)—Initial Visits to Physicians' Offices: United States, 1966–1999, and the Healthy People Year 2000 Objective**

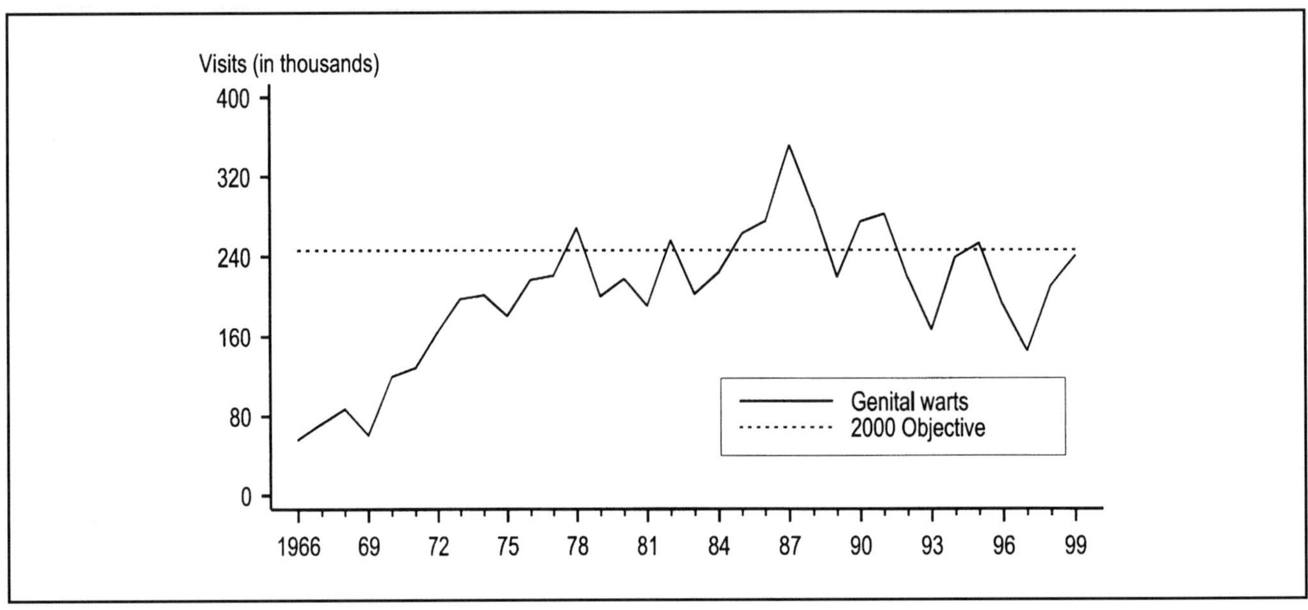


*Source*: Centers for Disease Control and Prevention, U.S. Department of Health and Human Services. National Center for HIV, STD, and TB Prevention, Division of STD Prevention. *Sexually Transmitted Disease Surveillance 1999* (Atlanta, GA: CDC, 2000). http://www.cdc.gov/nchstp/dstd/Stats_Trends/1999Surveillance/99PDF/Surv99Master.pdf.

**Table D6.6. Nonspecific Urethritis—Initial Visits to Physicians' Offices by Men: United States, 1966–1999**

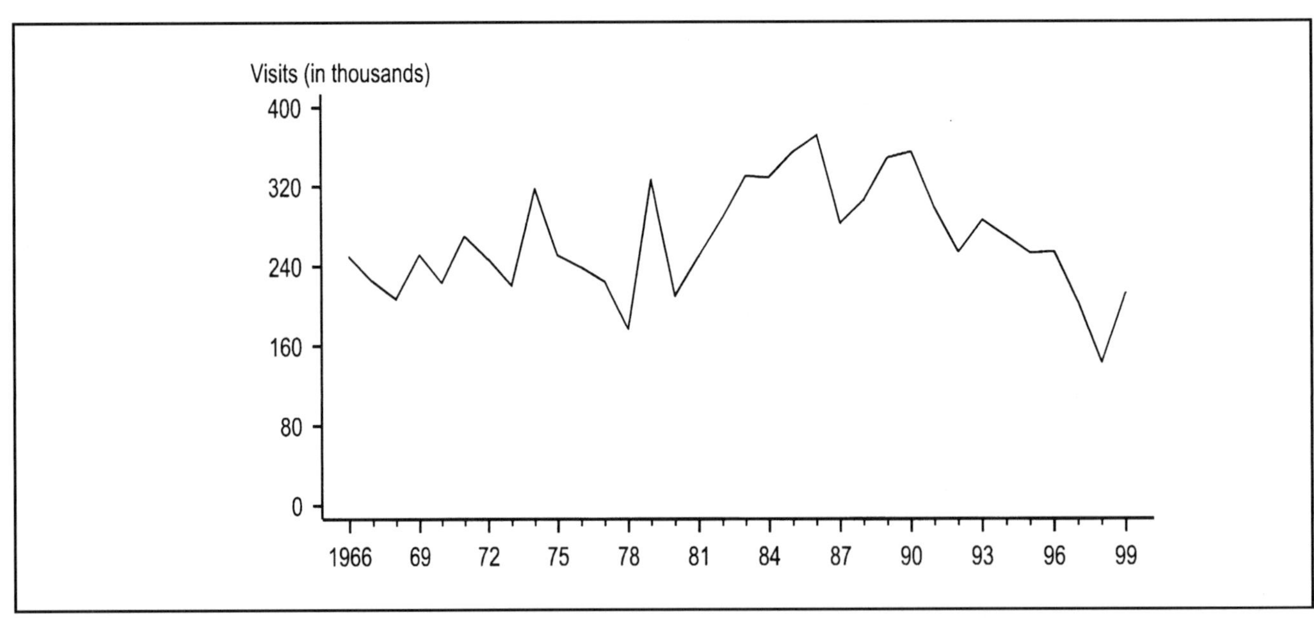


*Source*: Centers for Disease Control and Prevention, U.S. Department of Health and Human Services. National Center for HIV, STD, and TB Prevention, Division of STD Prevention. *Sexually Transmitted Disease Surveillance 1999* (Atlanta, GA: CDC, 2000). http://www.cdc.gov/nchstp/dstd/Stats_Trends/1999Surveillance/99PDF/Surv99Master.pdf.

**Table D6.7. Trichomonal and Other Vaginal Infections—Initial Visits to Physicians' Offices: United States, 1966–1999**

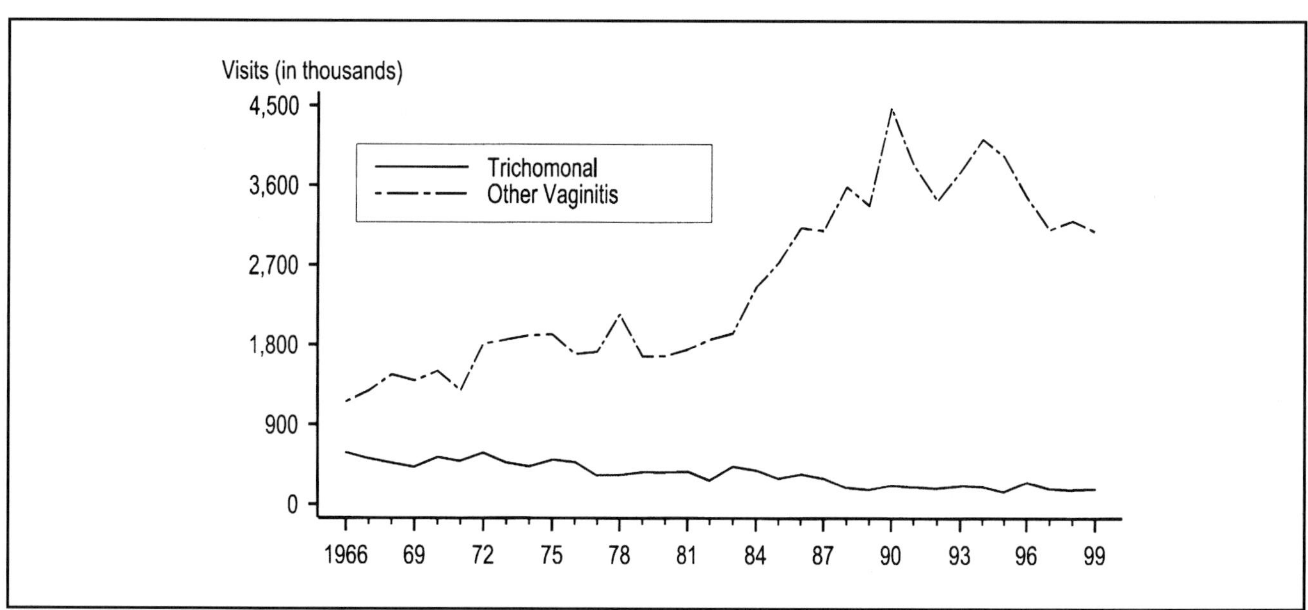


*Source*: Centers for Disease Control and Prevention, U.S. Department of Health and Human Services. National Center for HIV, STD, and TB Prevention, Division of STD Prevention. *Sexually Transmitted Disease Surveillance 1999* (Atlanta, GA: CDC, 2000). http://www.cdc.gov/nchstp/dstd/Stats_Trends/1999Surveillance/99PDF/Surv99Master.pdf.

# E. Tuberculosis

## OVERVIEW

One of the most prevalent infectious diseases in the world, especially in developing countries, tuberculosis (TB) is caused by the tubercle bacillus, *Mycobacterium tuberculosis*. TB commonly affects the respiratory system, but other parts of the body may become infected. Fish, amphibians, birds, and mammals are subject to the disease.

In the last several decades, tuberculosis decreased in incidence in the United States. However, two phenomena have caused increased public health concern about the disease: a great number of new cases have been reported in persons with HIV and/or AIDS, and there has been a rise in multidrug resistant TB (MDR-TB).

Immune deficiencies constitute one of many factors that increase the risk of developing TB. TB generally has a long latency period, and only about 10% of infected people with normal immunity ever experience TB. For people with immune deficiencies, however, active TB is much more common. Once infected with the TB bacillus, HIV-positive persons are 10 times more likely to develop active TB than are HIV-negative persons. It has also been shown that TB promotes HIV replication and increases viral load and possibly contributes toward HIV disease progression and mortality. For these reasons, the prevention and treatment of TB in HIV-positive persons remains a primary concern for those working with HIV/AIDS.

TB is considered multidrug resistant if it does not respond to two or more standard anti-TB drugs. MDR-TB usually occurs when treatment is interrupted, which allows mutations to occur that confer drug resistance. Resistance may also be the consequence of inadequate care and follow-up that result in undermedication for TB. However, primary infection with MDR-TB can occur as well. MDR-TB strains are difficult to treat with the existing range of medications. In most cases, MDR-TB has led to death in people with AIDS. MDR-TB has serious public health implications, because of rapid progression to life-threatening disease, efficient transmission to others, and delays in diagnosis.

## CASE DEFINITION

A chronic bacterial infection caused by *Mycobacterium tuberculosis*, TB is characterized pathologically by the formulation of granulomas. The most common site of infection is the lung, but other organs may be involved.

The clinical case definition for TB includes cases that meet the following criteria: a positive tuberculin skin test, other signs and symptoms compatible with tuberculosis (e.g., an abnormal, unstable chest radiograph or clinical evidence of current disease), treatment with two or more antituberculosis medications, and completed diagnostic evaluation.

## SYMPTOMS AND PATHOLOGIES

Tuberculosis is characterized pathologically by inflammatory infiltrations, formation of tubercles, caseation, necrosis, abscesses, fibrosis, and calcification. It most commonly affects the respiratory system, but other parts of the body such as gastrointestinal and genitourinary tracts, bones, joints, nervous system, lymph nodes, and skin may become infected.

Tuberculosis may occur in an acute generalized form (miliary tuberculosis) or in a chronic localized form. In humans, the primary infection usually consists of a localized lesion and regional adenitis, these constituting the primary complex. From this state, lesions may heal by fibrosis and calcification, and the disease may then exist in an arrested or inactive stage. Reactivation or exacerbation of the disease or reinfection gives rise to the chronic progressive form. Miliary tuberculosis, which spreads throughout the body via the bloodstream, may be fatal.

## DIAGNOSIS

Health care professionals verify TB cases by using the laboratory or clinical criteria for TB as defined in the document "Case Definitions for Infectious Conditions under Public Health Surveillance."[1] If all the criteria for a TB case are met, the TB case is then eligible for counting. When patients are diagnosed with TB but do not meet the case definition, reporting areas have the option of verifying TB cases based on provider diagnosis.

Laboratory criteria for diagnosis include isolation of *M. tuberculosis* from a clinical specimen, demonstration of *M. tuberculosis* from a clinical specimen by a nucleic acid amplification test, or demonstration of acid-fast bacilli in a clinical specimen when a culture has not been or cannot be obtained.

The tuberculin test determines the presence of tuberculosis infection based on positive reaction of subject to tuberculin, a soluble cell substance prepared from the tubercle bacillus. The test is performed using a special disposable instrument that contains multiple sharp points that penetrate the skin, introducing the tuberculin. Infected persons experience a local inflammatory reaction after 48 to 96 hours. The test is read in 48 to 72 hours. Tests do not reveal whether infection is active or inactive.

## TRANSMISSION

Three types of the tubercle bacillus exist: human, bovine (tuberculosis of cattle due to *Mycobacterium tuberculosis*), and avian (tuberculosis of birds, due to *Mycobacterium avium*). Humans may become infected by any of the three types, but in the United States the human type predominates. Infection usually results from contact with an infected person. TB is transmitted when a person with active TB coughs or sneezes, releasing microscopic particles containing live tubercle bacteria into the environment. When inhaled by another person, these particles may cause infection. Once infected, most people remain healthy and develop only latent infection. In this state they are neither sick nor infectious, but they do have the potential to become sick and infectious with active TB. To date, the immunological factors that allow latent TB infection to develop into active disease are unknown.

Although TB is spread through the air, infection usually occurs after prolonged exposure to someone with active TB. Documented TB outbreaks have been primarily associated with hospitals, clinics, nursing homes, prisons, shelters for the homeless, and other places where persons who may have TB congregate.

## TREATMENT

TB is treated with a combination of several antibiotics. For treating uncomplicated tuberculosis, a regimen of daily isoniazid (INH), pyrazinamide (PZA), and rifampin (RMP) for 2 months followed by 4 months of daily rifampin and isoniazid is effective. In this regimen, the medicines are self-administered. To ensure compliance and to help prevent the development of drug-resistant strains of the tubercle bacillus, it may be necessary for the health care worker to watch the patient take the medicine.

Twelve months of isoniazid (300 mg/day) is the present standard of care in the prevention of TB in HIV-positive individuals with a history of a positive TB skin test reaction, which marks latent as well as active disease. A short 2-month two-drug prevention regimen (450–600 mg/day rifampin plus pyrazinamide 20 mg/kg daily) that could have far-reaching implications in terms of both TB and HIV morbidity and mortality is under investigation. It is generally felt that any intervention to prevent TB reactivation through easier regimens that promote improved compliance or lend themselves to directly observed therapy is worth investigating.

## SURVEILLANCE

Sixty reporting areas (the 50 states, the District of Columbia, New York City, Puerto Rico, and other U.S. jurisdictions in the Pacific and the Caribbean) submit reports of TB cases to the Division of TB Elimination, CDC. There is a distinction between reporting TB cases to a health department and counting TB cases for determining incidence of disease. Throughout the year, clinics, hospitals, laboratories, and health care providers report TB cases and suspected cases to public health authorities. From these reports, the state or local TB control officer must determine which cases meet the current surveillance definition for TB disease. These verified TB cases are then reported to the CDC. CDC recommends that health care providers and laboratories be required to report all TB cases or suspected cases to state and local health departments based on the "Case Definition for Public Health Surveillance."[2] This notification is essential in order for TB programs to ensure case supervision, ensure completion of appropriate therapy, ensure completion of timely contact investigations, evaluate program effectiveness, and assess trends and characteristics of TB morbidity.

In January 1993, in conjunction with state and local health departments, CDC implemented an expanded surveillance system for TB to collect additional data to better monitor and target groups at risk for TB disease, to estimate and follow the extent of drug-resistant TB, and to evaluate outcomes of TB cases. Its "Report of a Verified Case of Tuberculosis" was revised to collect information on occupation, the initial drug regimen, human immunodeficiency virus (HIV) test results, history of substance abuse and homelessness, and residence in correctional or long-term care facilities at the time of diagnosis. Follow-up reports were added to collect drug susceptibility results for the initial *M. tuberculosis* isolate from patients with culture-positive disease and to evaluate the outcomes of TB therapy.

## TABLE OVERVIEW

**E1.1–E1.12. Trends** The first suite of tables presents TB data over time. E1.1 and E1.2 graph by 100,000 population and by U.S. and foreign-born persons respectively. E1.3 provides information on case counts and deaths from 1953 to 1999. E1.4–E1.8 present data for the past 10 years by selected demographic and clinical characteristics. E1.9 maps TB rates across the United States. The final tables (E1.10–E1.12) offer figures collected since implementation of the expanded system in 1993, including drug resistance and clinical outcomes.

During 1999, a total of 17,531 TB cases were reported to CDC from the 50 states and the District of Columbia, representing a 5% decrease from 1998 and a 34% decrease from 1992, when the number of cases peaked during the resurgence of TB in the United States. The national TB case rate also steadily decreased during this period. In 1999, 6% of cases were reported in children under 15 years old, 9% in persons aged 15–24 years, 35% in persons aged 25–44 years, 28% in persons aged 45–64 years, and 23% in persons aged 65 years and older. During 1992–1999, there was a decline in both the number of cases reported in each of these age groups and the respective TB cases.

The overall decrease in TB cases during 1992–1999 primarily reflected a 49% decrease in the number of cases among United States–born persons, with substantial declines in all age groups. In contrast, the total number of cases among foreign-born persons increased 4% during this period, reflecting a small increase among adults aged 25–44 years, a larger increase among adults aged 45 years or older, and a substantial decline among children aged less than 15 years. In terms of case rates, there was a 51% decrease in the case rate among United States–born persons (from 8.2 to 4.0 per 100,000), and there was a 15% decrease in the case rate among foreign-born persons (from 34.5 to 29.2 per 100,000).

**E2.1–E2.9. Case Rates by Selected Characteristics** The tables in this cluster present summary data by race, age, sex, and place of birth for 1999, the last complete year for which figures are available. Tables E2.1–E2.4 summarize total U.S. findings by demographic characteristic; tables E2.5–E2.9 break down information by state. The largest number of cases in 1999 occurred among African Americans, although Asians/Pacific Islanders had higher rates per 100,000. The rate among males was significantly higher than among females in all categories. Almost half the cases among the United States–born were those 45 years of age or older. In contrast, almost half of the cases among foreign born were in the 25–44 age group. The final table in the cluster permits state comparisons for 1999 and the six months of 2000. In 1999, 17 states had tuberculosis case rates of less than or equal to 3.5 cases per 100,000 population, the interim goal for the year 2000 established by the Advisory Committee (Council) for the Elimination of Tuberculosis (*MMWR* 1989;38 [Suppl.No. S-3]:1–25). Fifteen states and the District of Columbia had tuberculosis case rates that were higher than the 1999 national rate of 6.4 cases per 100,000 population.

**E3.1–E3.2. Cases by Form of the Disease** E3.1 presents figures by form of the disease; E3.2 breaks out cases by site of disease. In virtually all states, the pulmonary form made up more than 60% of the cases. The notable exception was in North Dakota, where the pulmonary and extrapulmonary forms both accounted for about 43% of cases. The most significant sites for extrapulmonary TB were the bones and the pleura, the thin membrane that covers the lungs.

**E4.1–E4.7. Cases by Subpopulation** The first two tables in this suite (E4.1–E4.2) offer data on cases in correctional and long-term residential facilities. The statistics are for residence at time of diagnosis. The next four tables (E4.3–E4.6) look at specific subgroups, the homeless, drug users, and cases by excess alcohol users. Statistics are for total cases and percentage of cases to total TB cases. Data are only for cases in which individuals have been homeless or using drugs within the past 12 months. The final table (E4.7) views TB cases by occupation. Over half of the cases for which a job status was known were unemployed.

**E5.1–E5.2. TB and HIV** The last suite of tables provides information on TB and HIV status over time and for 1999 by state. The information on HIV status for TB cases reported in 1999 is incomplete. Reasons for incomplete reporting of HIV test results to the national surveillance system include concerns about confidentiality, which may limit the exchange of data between TB and HIV/AIDS programs; laws and regulations in certain states and local jurisdictions that have been interpreted as prohibiting the HIV/AIDS program from sharing the HIV status of TB patients with the TB program or from reporting patients with TB and AIDS to the TB program; and reluctance by health care providers to report HIV test results to the TB surveillance program staff. In addition, health care providers may not offer counseling and HIV testing to some TB patients because of a lack of resources or of appropriately trained staff or because of the perception that selected patients are not at risk for HIV infection.

Reporting of HIV status has improved slowly since 1993, the year such information was first included on TB case reports submitted to the CDC. Nonetheless, data on the HIV infection status of reported TB cases in 1999 are not representative of all TB patients with HIV infection. HIV testing is performed after a patient receives counseling and gives informed consent. Since testing is voluntary, some TB patients may decline HIV testing. TB patients who are tested anonymously may choose not to share the results of HIV testing with their health care provider. TB patients managed in the private sector may receive confidential HIV testing, but results may not be reported to the TB program in the health department. In addition, many factors may influence HIV testing of TB patients, including the extent to which testing is targeted or routinely offered to specific groups and the availability of and access to HIV testing services.

## NOTES

1. Centers for Disease Control, "Case Definitions for Infectious Conditions under Public Health Surveillance," *MMWR* 46, no. RR-10 (1997): 40–41.
2. Ibid.

**Table E1.1. Tuberculosis (TB)—Reported Cases per 100.000 Population, by Year, United States, 1978–1998**

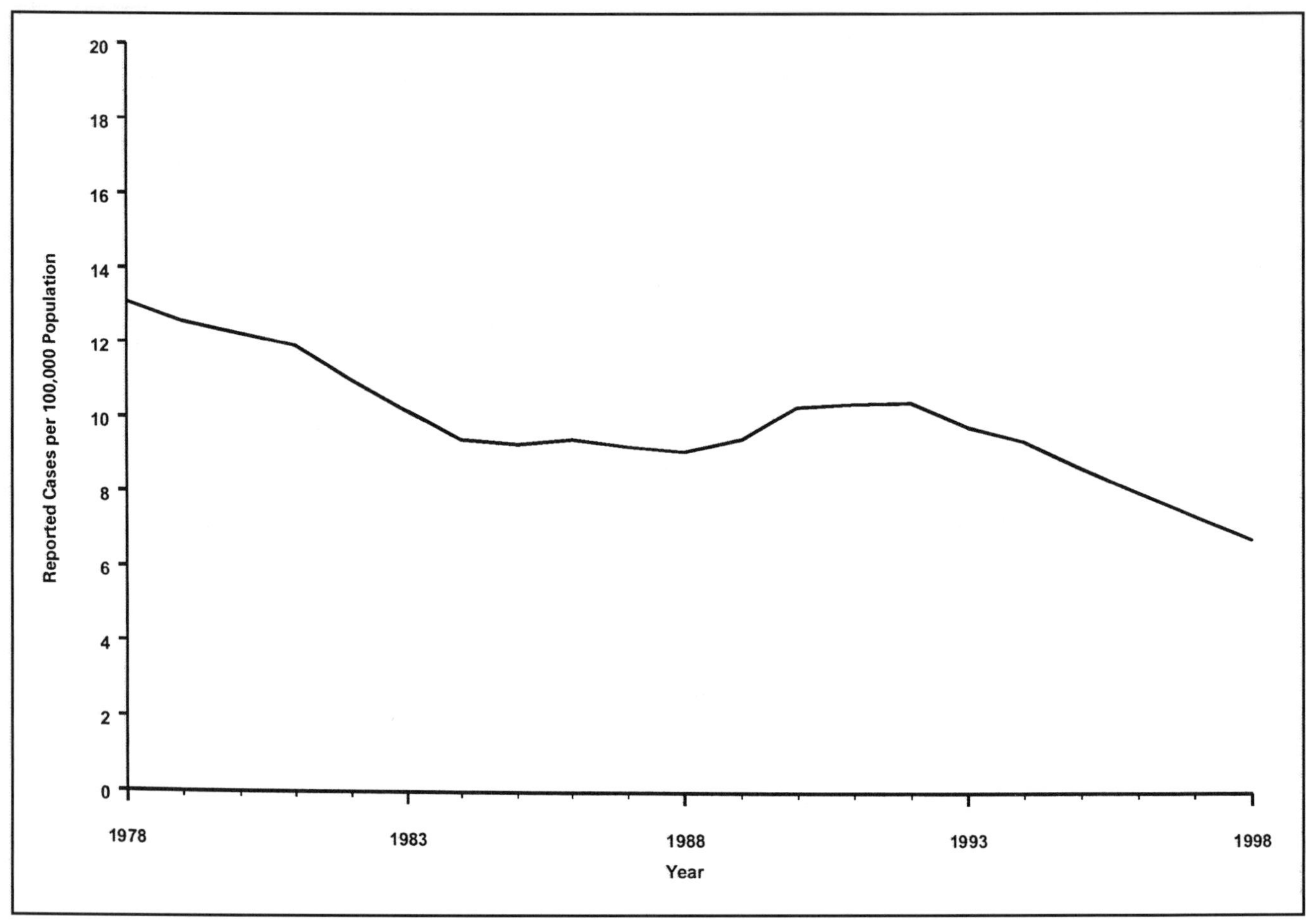


In 1998, a total of 18,361 cases of TB were reported to CDC, representing a 7.5% decrease from 1997.

*Source*: Center for Disease Control and Prevention. U.S. Department of Health and Human Services. *MMWR: Morbidity and Mortality Weekly Review Summary of Notifiable Disease, United States, 1999* 48 no. 53 (2001). http://www.cdc.gov/mmwr/PDF/wk/mm4853.pdf.

**Table E1.2. Tuberculosis (TB)—Reported Cases among U.S.- and foreign-born persons, by year, United States, 1986–1998**

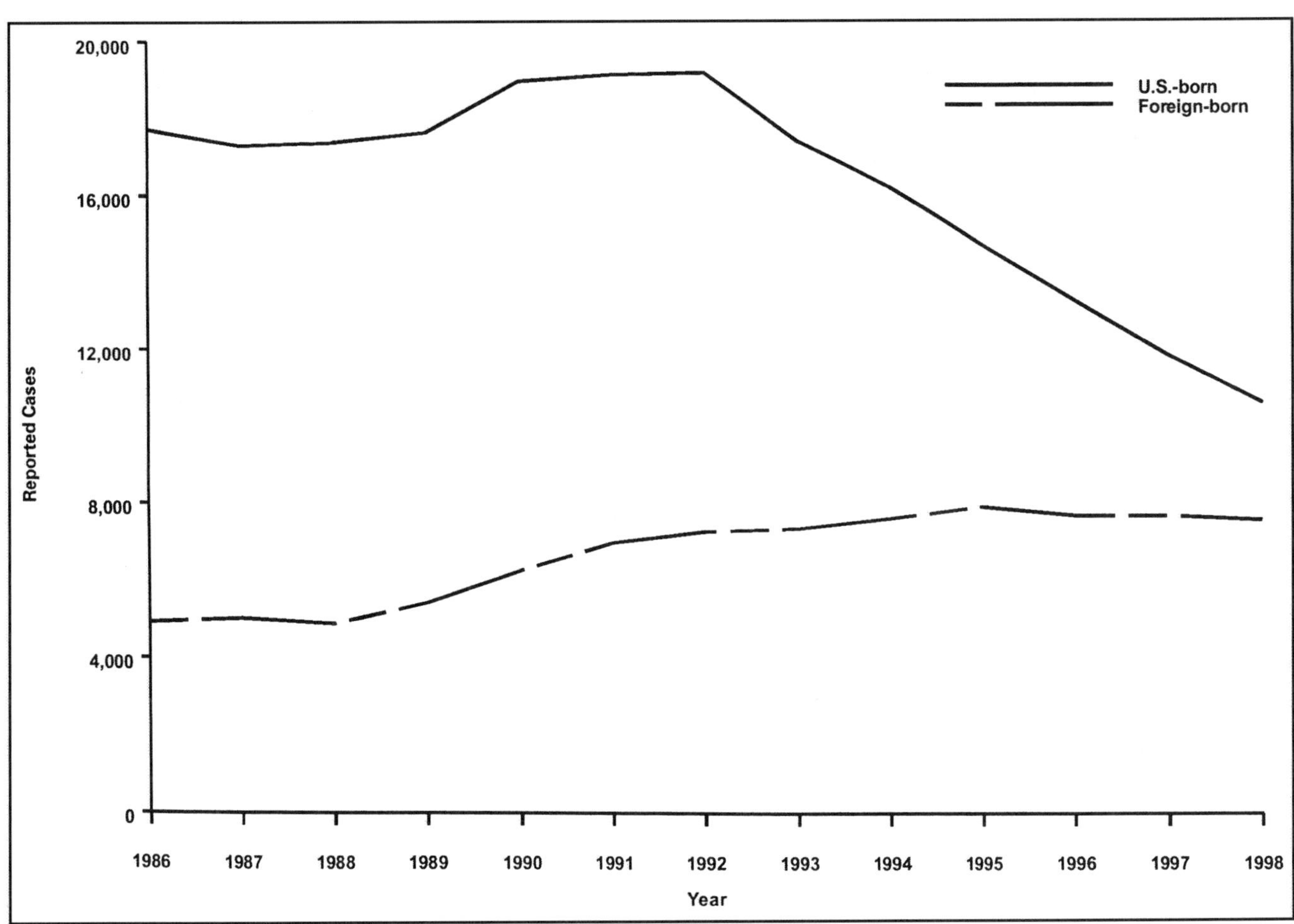


The number (and percentage) of TB cases among foreign-born persons in the United States has increased from 4,925 (22%) in 1986 to 7,591 (42%) in 1998. *Source*: Center for Disease Control and Prevention. U.S. Department of Health and Human Services. *MMWR: Morbidity and Mortality Weekly Review Summary of Notifiable Disease, United States, 1999* 48 no. 53 (2001). http://www.cdc.gov/mmwr/PDF/wk/mm4853.pdf.

**Table E1.3. Tuberculosis Cases and Case Rates per 100,000 Population, Deaths and Death Rates per 100,000 Population: United States, 1953–1999**

| | Tuberculosis Cases | | | | Tuberculosis Deaths | | | |
|---|---|---|---|---|---|---|---|---|
| | | | Percent Change | | | | Percent Change | |
| Year | Number | Rate[a] | Number | Rate | Number | Rate[a] | Number | Rate |
| 1953 | 84,304 | 53.0 | - - | - - | 19,707 | 12.4 | - - | - - |
| 1954 | 79,775 | 49.3 | -5.4 | - 7.0 | 16,527 | 10.2 | -16.1 | -17.7 |
| 1955 | 77,368 | 46.9 | -3.0 | - 4.9 | 15,016 | 9.1 | - 9.1 | -10.8 |
| 1956 | 69,895 | 41.6 | -9.7 | -11.0 | 14,137 | 8.4 | - 5.9 | - 7.7 |
| 1957 | 67,149 | 39.2 | -3.9 | - 5.8 | 13,390 | 7.8 | - 5.3 | - 7.1 |
| 1958 | 63,534 | 36.5 | -5.4 | - 6.9 | 12,417 | 7.1 | - 7.3 | - 9.0 |
| 1959 | 57,535 | 32.5 | -9.4 | -11.0 | 11,474 | 6.5 | - 7.6 | - 8.5 |
| 1960 | 55,494 | 30.8 | -3.5 | - 5.2 | 10,866 | 6.0 | - 5.3 | - 7.7 |
| 1961 | 53,726 | 29.4 | -3.2 | - 4.5 | 9,938 | 5.4 | - 8.5 | -10.0 |
| 1962 | 53,315 | 28.7 | -0.8 | - 2.4 | 9,506 | 5.1 | - 4.3 | - 5.6 |
| 1963 | 54,042 | 28.7 | +1.4 | 0.0 | 9,311 | 4.9 | - 2.1 | - 3.9 |
| 1964 | 50,874 | 26.6 | -5.9 | - 7.3 | 8,303 | 4.3 | -10.8 | -12.2 |
| 1965 | 49,016 | 25.3 | -3.7 | - 4.9 | 7,934 | 4.1 | - 4.4 | - 4.7 |
| 1966 | 47,767 | 24.4 | -2.5 | - 3.6 | 7,625 | 3.9 | - 3.9 | - 4.9 |
| 1967 | 45,647 | 23.1 | -4.4 | - 5.3 | 6,901 | 3.5 | - 9.5 | -10.3 |
| 1968 | 42,623 | 21.3 | -6.6 | - 7.8 | 6,292 | 3.1 | - 8.8 | -11.4 |
| 1969 | 39,120 | 19.4 | -8.2 | - 8.9 | 5,567 | 2.8 | -11.5 | - 9.7 |
| 1970 | 37,137 | 18.3 | -5.1 | - 5.7 | 5,217 | 2.6 | - 6.3 | - 7.1 |
| 1971 | 35,217 | 17.1 | -5.2 | - 6.6 | 4,501 | 2.2 | -13.7 | -15.4 |
| 1972 | 32,882 | 15.8 | -6.6 | - 7.6 | 4,376 | 2.1 | - 2.8 | - 4.5 |
| 1973 | 30,998 | 14.8 | -5.7 | - 6.3 | 3,875 | 1.8 | -11.4 | -14.5 |
| 1974 | 30,122 | 14.2 | -2.8 | - 4.1 | 3,513 | 1.7 | - 9.3 | - 5.6 |
| 1975 | 33,989 | 15.9 | -- | -- | 3,333 | 1.6 | - 5.1 | - 5.9 |
| 1976 | 32,105 | 15.0 | -5.5 | - 5.7 | 3,130 | 1.5 | - 6.1 | - 6.3 |
| 1977 | 30,145 | 13.9 | -6.1 | - 7.3 | 2,968 | 1.4 | - 5.2 | - 6.7 |
| 1978 | 28,521 | 13.1 | -5.4 | - 5.8 | 2,914 | 1.3 | - 1.8 | - 7.1 |
| 1979 | 27,669 | 12.6 | -3.0 | - 3.8 | 2,007 [b] | 0.9 [b] | -31.1 [b] | -30.8 [b] |
| 1980 | 27,749 | 12.3 | +0.3 | - 2.4 | 1,978 | 0.9 | - 1.4 | 0.0 |
| 1981 | 27,373 | 11.9 | -1.4 | - 3.3 | 1,937 | 0.8 | - 2.1 | -11.1 |
| 1982 | 25,520 | 11.0 | -6.8 | - 7.6 | 1,807 | 0.8 | - 6.7 | 0.0 |
| 1983 | 23,846 | 10.2 | -6.6 | - 7.3 | 1,779 | 0.8 | - 1.5 | 0.0 |
| 1984 | 22,255 | 9.4 | -6.7 | - 7.8 | 1,729 | 0.7 | - 2.8 | -12.5 |
| 1985 | 22,201 | 9.3 | -0.2 | - 1.1 | 1,752 | 0.7 | + 1.3 | 0.0 |
| 1986 | 22,768 | 9.4 | +2.6 | + 1.1 | 1,782 | 0.7 | + 1.7 | 0.0 |
| 1987 | 22,517 | 9.3 | -1.1 | - 1.1 | 1,755 | 0.7 | - 1.5 | 0.0 |
| 1988 | 22,436 | 9.1 | -0.4 | - 2.2 | 1,921 | 0.8 | + 9.5 | +14.3 |
| 1989 | 23,495 | 9.5 | +4.7 | + 4.4 | 1,970 | 0.8 | + 2.6 | 0.0 |
| 1990 | 25,701 | 10.3 | +9.4 | + 8.4 | 1,810 | 0.7 | - 8.1 | -12.5 |
| 1991 | 26,283 | 10.4 | +2.3 | + 1.0 | 1,713 | 0.7 | - 5.4 | 0.0 |
| 1992 | 26,673 | 10.5 | +1.5 | + 1.0 | 1,705 | 0.7 | - 0.5 | 0.0 |
| 1993 | 25,287 | 9.8 | -5.2 | - 6.7 | 1,631 | 0.6 | - 4.3 | -14.3 |
| 1994 | 24,361 | 9.4 | -3.7 | - 4.1 | 1,478 | 0.6 | - 9.4 | 0.0 |
| 1995 | 22,860 | 8.7 | -6.2 | - 7.4 | 1,336 | 0.5 | - 9.6 | -16.7 |
| 1996 | 21,337 | 8.0 | -6.7 | - 8.0 | 1,202 | 0.5 | -10.0 | 0.0 |
| 1997 | 19,851 | 7.4 | -7.0 | - 7.5 | 1,166 | 0.4 | -3.0 | -20.0 |
| 1998 | 18,361 | 6.8 | -7.5 | - 8.1 | 1,110 [c] | 0.4 [c] | -4.8 [c] | 0.0 [c] |
| 1999 | 17,531 | 6.4 | -4.5 | - 5.9 | ... | ... | ... | ... |

[a]Per 100,000 population.

[b]The large decrease in 1979 occurred because late effects of tuberculosis (e.g., bronchiectasis or fibrosis) and pleurisy with effusion (without mention of cause) are no longer included in tuberculosis deaths.

[c]Preliminary data obtained from National Center for Health Statistics (NCHS) *National Vital Statistics Reports, Vol. 47, No. 25, October 5, 1999.*

Ellipses indicate data not available.

Note: Case data after 1974 are not comparable to prior years due to changes in the surveillance case definitions which became effective in 1975.

*Source*: Centers for Disease Control and Prevention, U.S. Department of Health and Human Services. National Center for HIV, STD, and TB Prevention, Division of Tuberculosis Elimination. *Reported Tuberculosis in the United States, 1999* (Atlanta, GA: CDC, 2000). http://www.cdc.gov/nchstp/tb/surv/surv99/surv99.htm.

## Table E1.4. Tuberculosis Cases and Case Rates per 100,000 Population, by Age Group: United States, 1989–1999

| Year | Total Cases | 0 -14 | | | 15 - 24 | | | 25 - 44 | | | 45 - 64 | | | 65+ | | | Not Stated | |
|---|---|---|---|---|---|---|---|---|---|---|---|---|---|---|---|---|---|---|
| | | No. | (%) | Rate | No. | (%) | Rate | No. | (%) | Rate | No. | (%) | Rate | No. | (%) | Rate | No. | (%) |
| 1989 | 23,495 | 1,321 | (6) | 2.5 | 1,742 | (7) | 4.8 | 8,549 | (36) | 10.6 | 5,777 | (25) | 12.4 | 6,096 | (26) | 19.7 | 10 | (0) |
| 1990 | 25,701 | 1,596 | (6) | 3.0 | 1,867 | (7) | 5.1 | 9,730 | (38) | 12.0 | 6,365 | (25) | 13.7 | 6,115 | (24) | 19.6 | 28 | (0) |
| 1991 | 26,283 | 1,662 | (6) | 3.0 | 1,971 | (7) | 5.4 | 10,263 | (39) | 12.5 | 6,297 | (24) | 13.5 | 6,068 | (23) | 19.1 | 22 | (0) |
| 1992 | 26,673 | 1,707 | (6) | 3.1 | 1,974 | (7) | 5.5 | 10,444 | (39) | 12.7 | 6,487 | (24) | 13.4 | 6,025 | (23) | 18.7 | 36 | (0) |
| 1993 | 25,287 | 1,718 | (7) | 3.0 | 1,841 | (7) | 5.1 | 9,615 | (38) | 11.6 | 6,225 | (25) | 12.5 | 5,847 | (23) | 17.8 | 41 | (0) |
| 1994 | 24,361 | 1,695 | (7) | 3.0 | 1,825 | (7) | 5.1 | 9,106 | (37) | 11.0 | 6,141 | (25) | 12.1 | 5,546 | (23) | 16.7 | 48 | (0) |
| 1995 | 22,860 | 1,558 | (7) | 2.7 | 1,703 | (7) | 4.7 | 8,241 | (36) | 9.9 | 5,998 | (26) | 11.5 | 5,351 | (23) | 16.0 | 9 | (0) |
| 1996 | 21,337 | 1,372 | (6) | 2.4 | 1,656 | (8) | 4.6 | 7,604 | (36) | 9.1 | 5,588 | (26) | 10.4 | 5,103 | (24) | 15.1 | 14 | (0) |
| 1997 | 19,851 | 1,265 | (6) | 2.2 | 1,681 | (8) | 4.6 | 6,912 | (35) | 8.3 | 5,297 | (27) | 9.6 | 4,691 | (24) | 13.8 | 5 | (0) |
| 1998 | 18,361 | 1,082 | (6) | 1.9 | 1,548 | (8) | 4.2 | 6,365 | (35) | 7.6 | 4,973 | (27) | 8.7 | 4,393 | (24) | 12.8 | 0 | (0) |
| 1999 | 17,531 | 1,044 | (6) | 1.8 | 1,516 | (9) | 4.0 | 6,078 | (35) | 7.3 | 4,862 | (28) | 8.2 | 4,028 | (23) | 11.7 | 3 | (0) |

Note: Denominations for computing rates were based on official post-census estimates from the U.S. Census Bureau.
*Source*: Centers for Disease Control and Prevention, U.S. Department of Health and Human Services. National Center for HIV, STD, and TB Prevention, Division of Tuberculosis Elimination. *Reported Tuberculosis in the United States, 1999* (Atlanta, GA: CDC, 2000).

## Table E1.5. Tuberculosis Cases and Case Rates per 100,000 Population, by Race/Ethnicity: United States, 1989–1999

| Year | Total Cases | White, non-Hispanic | | | Black, non-Hispanic | | | Hispanic[a] | | | American Indian/ Alaskan Native | | | Asian/ Pacific Islander | | | Unknown/ Missing | |
|---|---|---|---|---|---|---|---|---|---|---|---|---|---|---|---|---|---|---|
| | | No. | (%) | Rate | No. | (%) | Rate | No. | (%) | Rate | No. | (%) | Rate | No. | (%) | Rate | No. | (%) |
| 1989 | 23,495 | 7,638 | (33) | 4.0 | 8,743 | (37) | 29.5 | 3,958 | (17) | 19.3 | 344 | (1) | 19.8 | 2,738 | (12) | 39.8 | 74 | (0) |
| 1990 | 25,701 | 7,836 | (30) | 4.2 | 9,634 | (37) | 33.0 | 4,809 | (19) | 21.5 | 361 | (1) | 20.1 | 3,004 | (12) | 43.1 | 57 | (0) |
| 1991 | 26,283 | 7,709 | (29) | 4.1 | 9,536 | (36) | 31.9 | 5,354 | (20) | 22.9 | 342 | (1) | 18.5 | 3,324 | (13) | 44.3 | 18 | (0) |
| 1992 | 26,673 | 7,618 | (29) | 4.0 | 9,623 | (36) | 31.7 | 5,437 | (20) | 22.4 | 299 | (1) | 16.2 | 3,649 | (14) | 46.3 | 47 | (0) |
| 1993 | 25,287 | 6,922 | (27) | 3.6 | 8,951 | (35) | 29.1 | 5,194 | (21) | 20.6 | 274 | (1) | 14.6 | 3,680 | (15) | 44.5 | 266 | (1) |
| 1994 | 24,361 | 6,494 | (27) | 3.4 | 8,345 | (34) | 26.8 | 5,074 | (21) | 19.5 | 332 | (1) | 17.4 | 3,821 | (16) | 45.3 | 295 | (1) |
| 1995 | 22,860 | 5,989 | (26) | 3.1 | 7,555 | (33) | 23.9 | 4,847 | (21) | 18.0 | 319 | (1) | 16.5 | 3,997 | (17) | 45.9 | 153 | (1) |
| 1996 | 21,337 | 5,506 | (26) | 2.8 | 7,106 | (33) | 22.3 | 4,533 | (21) | 16.0 | 284 | (1) | 14.5 | 3,814 | (18) | 41.6 | 94 | (0) |
| 1997 | 19,851 | 4,872 | (25) | 2.5 | 6,610 | (33) | 20.5 | 4,228 | (21) | 14.4 | 264 | (1) | 13.4 | 3,833 | (19) | 40.6 | 44 | (0) |
| 1998 | 18,361 | 4,495 | (24) | 2.3 | 5,831 | (32) | 17.8 | 4,099 | (22) | 13.6 | 253 | (1) | 12.6 | 3,623 | (20) | 36.6 | 60 | (0) |
| 1999 | 17,531 | 4,224 | (24) | 2.2 | 5,552 | (32) | 16.8 | 3,875 | (22) | 12.4 | 240 | (1) | 11.8 | 3,591 | (20) | 35.3 | 49 | (0) |

[a]Persons of Hispanic origin may be of any race.
Note: Denominations for computing rates were based on official post-census estimates from the U.S. Census Bureau.
*Source*: Centers for Disease Control and Prevention, U.S. Department of Health and Human Services. National Center for HIV, STD, and TB Prevention, Division of Tuberculosis Elimination. *Reported Tuberculosis in the United States, 1999* (Atlanta, GA: CDC, 2000).

## Table E1.6. Tuberculosis Cases and Case Rates per 100,000 Population, by Origin: United States, 1989–1999

| Year | Total Cases | U.S.-born Persons No. | U.S.-born Persons (%) | U.S.-born Persons Rate | Foreign-born Persons[a] No. | Foreign-born Persons[a] (%) | Foreign-born Persons[a] Rate | Unknown No. | Unknown (%) |
|---|---|---|---|---|---|---|---|---|---|
| 1989 | 23,495 | 17,646 | (75) | ... | 5,411 | (23) | ... | 438 | (2) |
| 1990 | 25,701 | 18,997 | (74) | 8.3 | 6,262 | (24) | 31.2 | 442 | (2) |
| 1991 | 26,283 | 19,161 | (73) | 8.2 | 6,982 | (27) | 33.9 | 140 | (1) |
| 1992 | 26,673 | 19,225 | (72) | 8.2 | 7,270 | (27) | 34.2 | 178 | (1) |
| 1993 | 25,287 | 17,464 | (69) | 7.4 | 7,354 | (29) | 33.6 | 469 | (2) |
| 1994 | 24,361 | 16,278 | (67) | 6.8 | 7,627 | (31) | 33.9 | 456 | (2) |
| 1995 | 22,860 | 14,772 | (65) | 6.1 | 7,930 | (35) | 34.2 | 158 | (1) |
| 1996 | 21,337 | 13,333 | (62) | 5.5 | 7,704 | (36) | 32.3 | 300 | (1) |
| 1997 | 19,851 | 11,898 | (60) | 4.9 | 7,702 | (39) | 31.2 | 251 | (1) |
| 1998 | 18,361 | 10,675 | (58) | 4.3 | 7,591 | (41) | 30.0 | 95 | (1) |
| 1999 | 17,531 | 9,809 | (56) | 4.0 | 7,553 | (43) | 29.2 | 169 | (1) |

[a]Includes persons from outside the United States, American Samoa, the Federated States of Micronesia, Guam, the Republic of the Marshall Islands, Midway Island, the Commonwealth of the Northern Mariana Islands, Puerto Rico, the Republic of Palau, U.S. Minor Outlying Islands, U.S. Miscellaneous Pacific Islands, and the U.S. Virgin Islands.

Ellipses indicate data not available.

Note: Denominations for computing rates were obtained from *Quarterly Estimates of the United States Foreign-born and Native Resident Populations: April 1, 1990, to July 1, 1999* (www.census.gov/population/estimates/nation/nativity/fbtab001.txt).

*Source*: Centers for Disease Control and Prevention, U.S. Department of Health and Human Services. National Center for HIV, STD, and TB Prevention, Division of Tuberculosis Elimination. *Reported Tuberculosis in the United States, 1999* (Atlanta, GA: CDC, 2000).

## Table E1.7. Tuberculosis Cases by Case Verification Criterion and by Site of Disease: United States, 1989–1999

| Year | Total Cases | Verification Criterion[a]: Positive Culture No. | (%) | Positive Smear No. | (%) | Clinical Case Definition No. | (%) | Provider Diagnosis No. | (%) | Site of Disease: Pulmonary[b] No. | (%) | Extra-pulmonary No. | (%) |
|---|---|---|---|---|---|---|---|---|---|---|---|---|---|
| 1989 | 23,495 | 19,483 | (83) | 351 | (1) | 2,475 | (11) | 1,186 | (5) | 19,639 | (84) | 3,835 | (16) |
| 1990 | 25,701 | 20,897 | (81) | 556 | (2) | 2,958 | (12) | 1,290 | (5) | 21,576 | (84) | 4,091 | (16) |
| 1991 | 26,283 | 21,417 | (81) | 388 | (1) | 2,992 | (11) | 1,486 | (6) | 21,937 | (83) | 4,327 | (16) |
| 1992 | 26,673 | 21,398 | (80) | 407 | (2) | 3,141 | (12) | 1,727 | (6) | 22,371 | (84) | 4,288 | (16) |
| 1993 | 25,287 | 20,081 | (79) | 309 | (1) | 2,994 | (12) | 1,903 | (8) | 21,255 | (84) | 3,995 | (16) |
| 1994 | 24,361 | 19,537 | (80) | 236 | (1) | 2,794 | (11) | 1,794 | (7) | 20,385 | (84) | 3,964 | (16) |
| 1995 | 22,860 | 18,292 | (80) | 220 | (1) | 2,664 | (12) | 1,684 | (7) | 18,991 | (83) | 3,860 | (17) |
| 1996 | 21,337 | 17,234 | (81) | 150 | (1) | 2,556 | (12) | 1,397 | (7) | 17,445 | (82) | 3,870 | (18) |
| 1997 | 19,851 | 16,015 | (81) | 177 | (1) | 2,355 | (12) | 1,304 | (7) | 16,285 | (82) | 3,554 | (18) |
| 1998 | 18,361 | 14,830 | (81) | 166 | (1) | 2,207 | (12) | 1,158 | (6) | 14,813 | (81) | 3,541 | (19) |
| 1999 | 17,531 | 13,997 | (80) | 176 | (1) | 2,058 | (12) | 1,300 | (7) | 14,083 | (80) | 3,438 | (20) |

[a]Based on the public health surveillance case definition for tuberculosis: CDC. Case definitions for infectious conditions under public health surveillance. *MMWR* 1997:46(No. RR-10):40-41. See Appendix B.

[b]Includes cases of both pulmonary and extrapulmonary disease and cases of miliary TB.

*Source*: Centers for Disease Control and Prevention, U.S. Department of Health and Human Services. National Center for HIV, STD, and TB Prevention, Division of Tuberculosis Elimination. *Reported Tuberculosis in the United States, 1999* (Atlanta, GA: CDC, 2000).

## Table E1.8. Pulmonary Tuberculosis Cases by Sputum Smear and Sputum Culture Results: United States, 1989–1999

| Year | Total Pulmonary Cases[a] | Sputum Smear Results | | | | | | Sputum Culture Results | | | | | |
|---|---|---|---|---|---|---|---|---|---|---|---|---|---|
| | | Positive | | Negative | | Not Done or Unknown | | Positive | | Negative | | Not Done or Unknown | |
| | | No. | (%) | No. | (%) | No. | (%) | No. | (%) | No. | (%) | No. | (%) |
| 1989 | 19,639 | 8,759 | (45) | 5,924 | (30) | 4,956 | (25) | 13,712 | (70) | 1,908 | (10) | 4,019 | (20) |
| 1990 | 21,576 | 9,391 | (44) | 6,865 | (32) | 5,320 | (25) | 14,816 | (69) | 2,124 | (10) | 4,636 | (21) |
| 1991 | 21,937 | 9,095 | (41) | 7,281 | (33) | 5,561 | (25) | 15,022 | (68) | 2,232 | (10) | 4,683 | (21) |
| 1992 | 22,371 | 8,975 | (40) | 7,413 | (33) | 5,983 | (27) | 15,124 | (68) | 2,476 | (11) | 4,771 | (21) |
| 1993 | 21,255 | 9,324 | (44) | 7,747 | (36) | 4,184 | (20) | 14,708 | (69) | 2,675 | (13) | 3,872 | (18) |
| 1994 | 20,385 | 8,845 | (43) | 7,770 | (38) | 3,770 | (18) | 14,080 | (69) | 2,618 | (13) | 3,687 | (18) |
| 1995 | 18,991 | 8,068 | (42) | 7,717 | (41) | 3,206 | (17) | 13,236 | (70) | 2,597 | (14) | 3,158 | (17) |
| 1996 | 17,445 | 7,449 | (43) | 7,337 | (42) | 2,659 | (15) | 12,232 | (70) | 2,507 | (14) | 2,706 | (16) |
| 1997 | 16,285 | 6,882 | (42) | 6,878 | (42) | 2,525 | (16) | 11,481 | (71) | 2,226 | (14) | 2,578 | (16) |
| 1998 | 14,813 | 6,630 | (45) | 6,016 | (41) | 2,167 | (15) | 10,472 | (71) | 2,101 | (14) | 2,240 | (15) |
| 1999 | 14,083 | 6,252 | (44) | 5,626 | (40) | 2,205 | (16) | 9,777 | (69) | 2,049 | (15) | 2,257 | (16) |

[a]Includes cases of both pulmonary and extrapulmonary disease and cases of miliary TB.

*Source*: Centers for Disease Control and Prevention. U.S. Department of Health and Human Services. National Center for HIV, STD, and TB Prevention, Division of Tuberculosis Elimination. *Reported Tuberculosis in the United States, 1999* (Atlanta, GA: CDC, 2000).

## Table E1.9. Tuberculosis (TB)—Reported Cases per 100,000 Population, United States and Territories, 1998

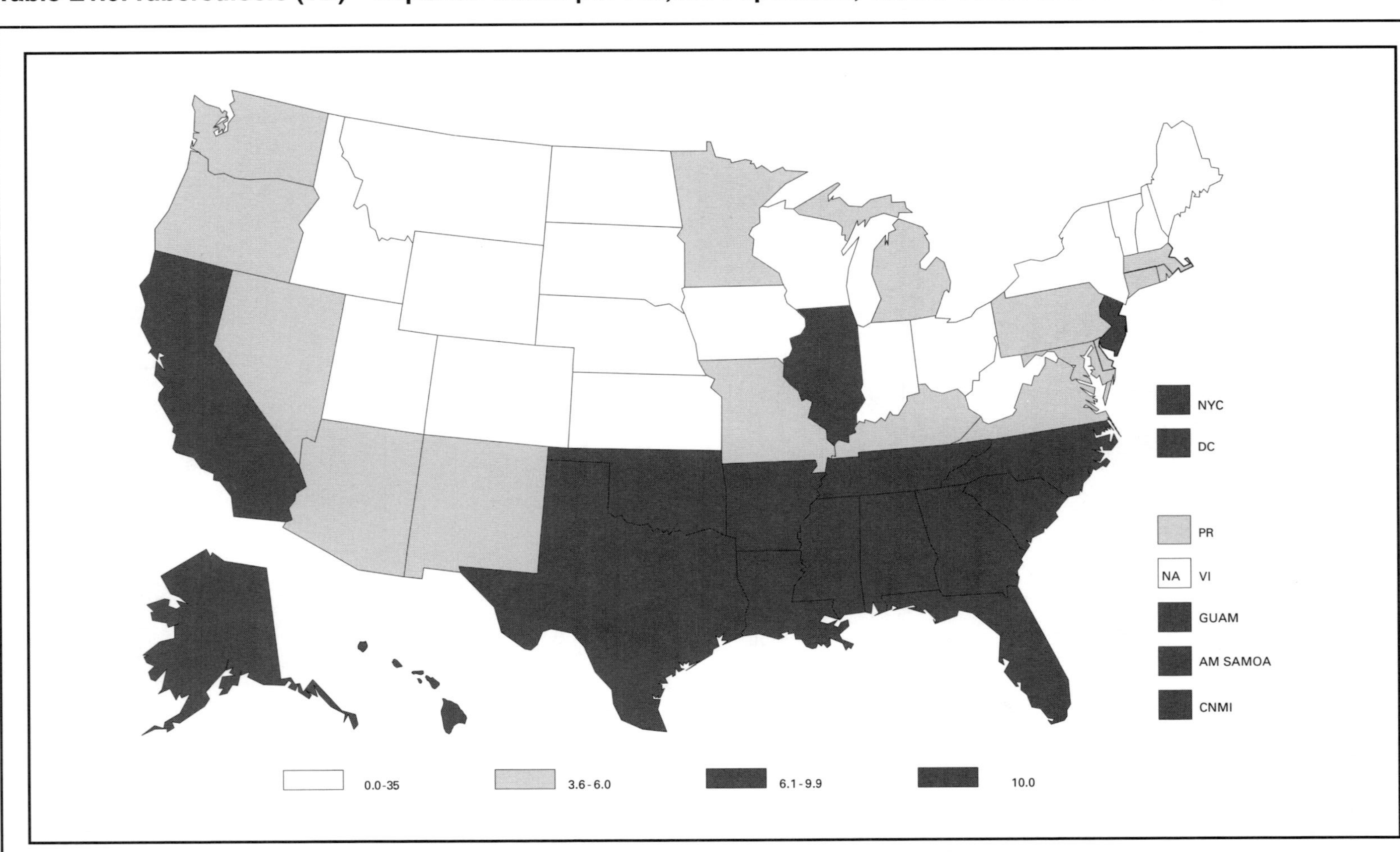


In 1998, a total of 19 states had TB rates of <3.5 cases per 100,000 population, which is the interim (i.e., year 2000) incidence target for the elimination of TB by the year 2010, established by CDC and the Advisory Council for the Elimination of Tuberculosis.

*Source*: Center for Disease Control and Prevention. U.S. Department of Health and Human Services. *MMWR: Morbidity and Mortality Weekly Review Summary of Notifiable Disease, United States, 1999* 48 no. 53 (2001). http://www.cdc.gov/mmwr/PDF/wk/mm4853.pdf.

## Table E1.10. Resistance to Isoniazid with or without Rifampin Resistance in Reported TB Cases with No Previous TB, by Origin: United States, 1993–1999

| | Resistant to Isoniazid[a] | | | | | | Resistant to Isoniazid and Rifampin[a] | | | | | |
|---|---|---|---|---|---|---|---|---|---|---|---|---|
| | Total Cases[b] | | U. S.-born | | Foreign-born[c] | | Total Cases[b] | | U. S.-born | | Foreign-born[c] | |
| Year | No. | (%) | No. | (%) | No. | (%) | No. | (%) | No. | (%) | No. | (%) |
| 1993 | 1,400 | (8.4) | 804 | (6.8) | 579 | (12.4) | 410 | (2.5) | 302 | (2.6) | 105 | (2.3) |
| 1994 | 1,355 | (8.3) | 709 | (6.5) | 632 | (12.1) | 352 | (2.2) | 238 | (2.2) | 109 | (2.1) |
| 1995 | 1,171 | (7.3) | 554 | (5.4) | 615 | (11.0) | 252 | (1.6) | 168 | (1.6) | 84 | (1.5) |
| 1996 | 1,134 | (7.4) | 492 | (5.2) | 638 | (11.3) | 205 | (1.3) | 103 | (1.1) | 101 | (1.8) |
| 1997 | 1,076 | (7.5) | 429 | (5.0) | 640 | (11.3) | 157 | (1.1) | 75 | (0.9) | 81 | (1.4) |
| 1998 | 1,012 | (7.6) | 366 | (4.8) | 644 | (11.4) | 127 | (1.0) | 52 | (0.7) | 74 | (1.3) |
| 1999 | 865 | (7.2) | 271 | (4.1) | 590 | (11.1) | 127 | (1.1) | 38 | (0.6) | 88 | (1.7) |

[a]Isolates may be resistant to other drugs.
[b]Includes persons of unknown country of birth.
[c]Includes persons from outside the United States, American Samoa, the Federated States of Micronesia, Guam, the Republic of the Marshall Islands, Midway Island, the Commonwealth of the Northern Mariana Islands, Puerto Rico, the Republic of Palau, U.S. Minor Outlying Islands, U.S. Miscellaneous Pacific Islands, and the U.S. Virgin Islands.
Note: Data for all years updated through May 3, 2000.
More than 85% of all cases in each group had drug susceptibility test results reported for an initial isolate.
*Source*: Centers for Disease Control and Prevention, U.S. Department of Health and Human Services. National Center for HIV, STD, and TB Prevention, Division of Tuberculosis Elimination. *Reported Tuberculosis in the United States, 1999* (Atlanta, GA: CDC, 2000).

## Table E1.11. Resistance to Isoniazid with or without Rifampin Resistance in Reported TB Cases with Previous TB, by Origin: United States, 1993–1999

| | Resistant to Isoniazid[a] | | | | | | Resistant to Isoniazid and Rifampin[a] | | | | | |
|---|---|---|---|---|---|---|---|---|---|---|---|---|
| | Total Cases[b] | | U. S.-born | | Foreign-born[c] | | Total Cases[b] | | U. S.-born | | Foreign-born[c] | |
| Year | No. | (%) | No. | (%) | No. | (%) | No. | (%) | No. | (%) | No. | (%) |
| 1993 | 164 | (16.6) | 85 | (12.6) | 76 | (25.2) | 75 | (7.6) | 30 | (4.5) | 45 | (15.0) |
| 1994 | 177 | (17.1) | 81 | (11.7) | 95 | (28.1) | 75 | (7.3) | 35 | (5.1) | 39 | (11.6) |
| 1995 | 168 | (17.6) | 77 | (13.0) | 91 | (25.1) | 70 | (7.3) | 28 | (4.7) | 42 | (11.6) |
| 1996 | 141 | (16.4) | 67 | (12.0) | 73 | (24.2) | 42 | (4.9) | 20 | (3.6) | 21 | (7.0) |
| 1997 | 108 | (14.9) | 35 | (8.0) | 73 | (25.6) | 42 | (5.8) | 11 | (2.5) | 31 | (10.9) |
| 1998 | 97 | (12.8) | 37 | (7.5) | 60 | (22.6) | 23 | (3.0) | 6 | (1.2) | 17 | (6.4) |
| 1999 | 80 | (12.2) | 27 | (7.2) | 51 | (18.3) | 25 | (3.8) | 6 | (1.6) | 19 | (6.8) |

[a]Isolates may be resistant to other drugs.
[b]Includes persons of unknown country of birth.
[c]Includes persons from outside the United States, American Samoa, the Federated States of Micronesia, Guam, the Republic of the Marshall Islands, Midway Island, the Commonwealth of the Northern Mariana Islands, Puerto Rico, the Republic of Palau, U.S. Minor Outlying Islands, U.S. Miscellaneous Pacific Islands, and the U.S. Virgin Islands.
Note: Data for all years updated through May 3, 2000.
More than 85% of all cases in each group had drug susceptibility test results reported for an initial isolate.
*Source*: Centers for Disease Control and Prevention, U.S. Department of Health and Human Services. National Center for HIV, STD, and TB Prevention, Division of Tuberculosis Elimination. *Reported Tuberculosis in the United States, 1999* (Atlanta, GA: CDC, 2000).

## Table E1.12. Percentage of Reported TB Cases by Initial Drug Regimen, Use of Directly Observed Therapy, and Completion of Therapy (COT): United States, 1993–1999

| | Initial Drug Regimen[a] | | | Directly Observed Therapy[c] | | Therapy ≤1 Year Indicated[d] | |
|---|---|---|---|---|---|---|---|
| Year | IR | IRZ | IRZ,E/S[b] | DOT Only | Both DOT and Self-Administered | COT ≤1 Year | COT |
| 1993 | 13.0 | 31.2 | 40.9 | 21.7 | 14.4 | 63.5 | 87.5 |
| 1994 | 7.0 | 23.3 | 56.3 | 28.1 | 20.5 | 68.4 | 87.8 |
| 1995 | 5.2 | 20.3 | 63.4 | 37.2 | 21.4 | 72.8 | 89.5 |
| 1996 | 4.1 | 17.5 | 67.9 | 42.4 | 22.4 | 75.5 | 90.2 |
| 1997 | 3.2 | 15.1 | 72.4 | 46.9 | 23.7 | 77.2 | 90.0 |
| 1998 | 2.6 | 12.9 | 74.6 | ... | ... | ... | ... |
| 1999 | 2.2 | 11.2 | 76.8 | ... | ... | ... | ... |

[a]Includes cases in persons alive at diagnosis.

[b]I=isoniazid; R=rifampin; Z=pyrazinamide; S=streptomycin. Excluding cases with no information on initial drug regimen, 1% were not started on any drugs, less than 1% were started on one drug, and approximately 10% had an initial multidrug regimen other than IR, IRZ, and IRZ,E/S.

[c]Includes cases in persons alive at diagnosis with initial drug regimen of one or more drugs prescribed.

[d]Includes cases in persons alive at diagnosis, with initial drug regimen of one or more drugs prescribed, who did not die during therapy. Excludes persons with initial isolate resistant to rifampin and pediatric (aged <15) cases with meningeal, bone or joint, or miliary disease. See Technical Notes (Appendix A) for description of COT calculation.

Ellipses indicate data not available.

Note: Data for all years updated through May 3, 2000.

*Source*: Centers for Disease Control and Prevention, U.S. Department of Health and Human Services. National Center for HIV, STD, and TB Prevention, Division of Tuberculosis Elimination. *Reported Tuberculosis in the United States, 1999* (Atlanta, GA: CDC, 2000).

## Table E2.1. Tuberculosis Cases, by Race/Ethnicity, Sex, and Age: United States, 1999

| Race/Ethnicity and Sex | All Ages | Age Group: Under 5 | 5 - 14 | 15 - 24 | 25 - 44 | 45 - 64 | 65+ | Not Stated |
|---|---|---|---|---|---|---|---|---|
| **Total Cases** | **17,531** | **605** | **439** | **1,516** | **6,078** | **4,862** | **4,028** | **3** |
| White, non-Hispanic | 4,224 | 76 | 52 | 117 | 1,020 | 1,263 | 1,694 | 2 |
| Male | 2,819 | 40 | 21 | 63 | 695 | 974 | 1,024 | 2 |
| Female | 1,405 | 36 | 31 | 54 | 325 | 289 | 670 | 0 |
| Unknown | 0 | 0 | 0 | 0 | 0 | 0 | 0 | 0 |
| Black, non-Hispanic | 5,552 | 195 | 151 | 432 | 2,198 | 1,688 | 888 | 0 |
| Male | 3,488 | 92 | 70 | 220 | 1,387 | 1,231 | 488 | 0 |
| Female | 2,063 | 103 | 81 | 212 | 811 | 456 | 400 | 0 |
| Unknown | 1 | 0 | 0 | 0 | 0 | 1 | 0 | 0 |
| Hispanic[a] | 3,875 | 250 | 181 | 569 | 1,462 | 870 | 543 | 0 |
| Male | 2,496 | 141 | 103 | 364 | 1,004 | 581 | 303 | 0 |
| Female | 1,379 | 109 | 78 | 205 | 458 | 289 | 240 | 0 |
| Unknown | 0 | 0 | 0 | 0 | 0 | 0 | 0 | 0 |
| American Indian/Alaskan Native | 240 | 12 | 5 | 10 | 72 | 83 | 57 | 1 |
| Male | 147 | 7 | 2 | 2 | 51 | 48 | 36 | 1 |
| Female | 93 | 5 | 3 | 8 | 21 | 35 | 21 | 0 |
| Unknown | 0 | 0 | 0 | 0 | 0 | 0 | 0 | 0 |
| Asian/Pacific Islander | 3,591 | 70 | 49 | 385 | 1,307 | 947 | 833 | 0 |
| Male | 1,966 | 37 | 26 | 177 | 667 | 535 | 524 | 0 |
| Female | 1,625 | 33 | 23 | 208 | 640 | 412 | 309 | 0 |
| Unknown | 0 | 0 | 0 | 0 | 0 | 0 | 0 | 0 |
| Not Stated | 49 | 2 | 1 | 3 | 19 | 11 | 13 | 0 |
| Male | 32 | 2 | 1 | 1 | 11 | 10 | 7 | 0 |
| Female | 17 | 0 | 0 | 2 | 8 | 1 | 6 | 0 |
| Unknown | 0 | 0 | 0 | 0 | 0 | 0 | 0 | 0 |

[a]Persons of Hispanic origin may be of any race.

*Source*: Centers for Disease Control and Prevention, U.S. Department of Health and Human Services. National Center for HIV, STD, and TB Prevention, Division of Tuberculosis Elimination. *Reported Tuberculosis in the United States, 1999* (Atlanta, GA: CDC, 2000).

## Table E2.2. Tuberculosis Case Rates per 100,000 Population, by Race/Ethnicity, Sex, and Age: United States, 1999

| Race/Ethnicity and Sex | All Ages | Age Group | | | | | |
|---|---|---|---|---|---|---|---|
| | | Under 5 | 5 - 14 | 15 - 24 | 25 - 44 | 45 - 64 | 65+ |
| **Total Cases** | **6.4** | **3.2** | **1.1** | **4.0** | **7.3** | **8.2** | **11.7** |
| White, non-Hispanic | 2.2 | 0.6 | 0.2 | 0.5 | 1.7 | 2.7 | 5.8 |
| Male | 2.9 | 0.7 | 0.2 | 0.5 | 2.4 | 4.3 | 8.5 |
| Female | 1.4 | 0.6 | 0.2 | 0.4 | 1.1 | 1.2 | 4.0 |
| Black, non-Hispanic | 16.8 | 7.5 | 2.6 | 7.9 | 21.2 | 28.1 | 31.9 |
| Male | 22.3 | 7.0 | 2.3 | 8.1 | 28.5 | 46.1 | 44.6 |
| Female | 11.8 | 8.0 | 2.8 | 7.8 | 14.8 | 13.7 | 23.6 |
| Hispanic[a] | 12.4 | 7.2 | 3.0 | 10.4 | 14.7 | 18.9 | 29.4 |
| Male | 15.8 | 8.0 | 3.4 | 12.8 | 19.6 | 26.4 | 39.0 |
| Female | 8.9 | 6.4 | 2.7 | 7.8 | 9.4 | 12.1 | 22.5 |
| American Indian/Alaskan Native | 11.8 | 7.3 | 1.3 | 2.8 | 11.8 | 23.3 | 38.8 |
| Male | 14.8 | 8.4 | 1.0 | 1.1 | 16.7 | 28.2 | 58.1 |
| Female | 9.0 | 6.2 | 1.6 | 4.5 | 6.9 | 18.7 | 24.7 |
| Asian/Pacific Islander | 35.3 | 8.4 | 3.1 | 26.0 | 37.5 | 46.5 | 108.2 |
| Male | 40.3 | 8.7 | 3.2 | 23.9 | 40.8 | 56.4 | 161.7 |
| Female | 30.6 | 8.0 | 3.0 | 28.1 | 34.5 | 37.9 | 69.3 |

[a]Persons of Hispanic origin may be of any race.

Note: Denominations for computing rates were obtained from *National Population Estimates for the 1990's: Monthly Postcensal Resident Population, by Single Years of Age, Sex, Race, and Hispanic Origin* (www.census.gov/population/estimates/nation/e90s/e9999rmp.txt).

*Source*: Centers for Disease Control and Prevention, U.S. Department of Health and Human Services. National Center for HIV, STD, and TB Prevention, Division of Tuberculosis Elimination. *Reported Tuberculosis in the United States, 1999* (Atlanta, GA: CDC, 2000).

## Table E2.3. Tuberculosis Cases, in U.S.-Born Persons, by Race/Ethnicity, Sex, and Age: United States, 1999

| Race/Ethnicity and Sex | All Ages | Age Group | | | | | | Not Stated |
|---|---|---|---|---|---|---|---|---|
| | | Under 5 | 5 - 14 | 15 - 24 | 25 - 44 | 45 - 64 | 65+ | |
| **Total Cases** | **9,809** | **508** | **259** | **453** | **2,939** | **3,021** | **2,626** | **3** |
| White, non-Hispanic | 3,637 | 65 | 38 | 68 | 841 | 1,116 | 1,507 | 2 |
| Male | 2,490 | 33 | 17 | 35 | 597 | 875 | 931 | 2 |
| Female | 1,147 | 32 | 21 | 33 | 244 | 241 | 576 | 0 |
| Unknown | 0 | 0 | 0 | 0 | 0 | 0 | 0 | 0 |
| Black, non-Hispanic | 4,593 | 183 | 106 | 238 | 1,692 | 1,529 | 845 | 0 |
| Male | 2,943 | 87 | 52 | 124 | 1,077 | 1,135 | 468 | 0 |
| Female | 1,649 | 96 | 54 | 114 | 615 | 393 | 377 | 0 |
| Unknown | 1 | 0 | 0 | 0 | 0 | 1 | 0 | 0 |
| Hispanic[a] | 1,127 | 202 | 94 | 101 | 292 | 267 | 171 | 0 |
| Male | 697 | 118 | 54 | 59 | 185 | 188 | 93 | 0 |
| Female | 430 | 84 | 40 | 42 | 107 | 79 | 78 | 0 |
| Unknown | 0 | 0 | 0 | 0 | 0 | 0 | 0 | 0 |
| American Indian/Alaskan Native | 234 | 12 | 4 | 9 | 70 | 83 | 55 | 1 |
| Male | 144 | 7 | 2 | 2 | 50 | 48 | 34 | 1 |
| Female | 90 | 5 | 2 | 7 | 20 | 35 | 21 | 0 |
| Unknown | 0 | 0 | 0 | 0 | 0 | 0 | 0 | 0 |
| Asian/Pacific Islander | 202 | 45 | 17 | 36 | 39 | 23 | 42 | 0 |
| Male | 104 | 23 | 11 | 13 | 18 | 10 | 29 | 0 |
| Female | 98 | 22 | 6 | 23 | 21 | 13 | 13 | 0 |
| Unknown | 0 | 0 | 0 | 0 | 0 | 0 | 0 | 0 |
| Not Stated | 16 | 1 | 0 | 1 | 5 | 3 | 6 | 0 |
| Male | 12 | 1 | 0 | 1 | 3 | 3 | 4 | 0 |
| Female | 4 | 0 | 0 | 0 | 2 | 0 | 2 | 0 |
| Unknown | 0 | 0 | 0 | 0 | 0 | 0 | 0 | 0 |

[a]Persons of Hispanic origin may be of any race.

*Source*: Centers for Disease Control and Prevention, U.S. Department of Health and Human Services. National Center for HIV, STD, and TB Prevention, Division of Tuberculosis Elimination. *Reported Tuberculosis in the United States, 1999* (Atlanta, GA: CDC, 2000).

## Table E2.4. Tuberculosis Cases in Foreign-Born Persons, by Race/Ethnicity, Sex, and Age: United States, 1999

| Race/Ethnicity and Sex | All Ages | Age Group | | | | | | Not Stated |
|---|---|---|---|---|---|---|---|---|
| | | Under 5 | 5 - 14 | 15 - 24 | 25 - 44 | 45 - 64 | 65+ | |
| **Total Cases** | **7,553** | **92** | **173** | **1,051** | **3,082** | **1,800** | **1,355** | **0** |
| White, non-Hispanic | 560 | 11 | 14 | 49 | 174 | 139 | 173 | 0 |
| Male | 310 | 7 | 4 | 28 | 94 | 92 | 85 | 0 |
| Female | 250 | 4 | 10 | 21 | 80 | 47 | 88 | 0 |
| Unknown | 0 | 0 | 0 | 0 | 0 | 0 | 0 | 0 |
| Black, non-Hispanic | 916 | 11 | 42 | 192 | 485 | 150 | 36 | 0 |
| Male | 519 | 5 | 16 | 94 | 297 | 88 | 19 | 0 |
| Female | 397 | 6 | 26 | 98 | 188 | 62 | 17 | 0 |
| Unknown | 0 | 0 | 0 | 0 | 0 | 0 | 0 | 0 |
| Hispanic[b] | 2,704 | 47 | 84 | 462 | 1,157 | 594 | 360 | 0 |
| Male | 1,766 | 22 | 49 | 301 | 806 | 386 | 202 | 0 |
| Female | 938 | 25 | 35 | 161 | 351 | 208 | 158 | 0 |
| Unknown | 0 | 0 | 0 | 0 | 0 | 0 | 0 | 0 |
| American Indian/Alaskan Native | 6 | 0 | 1 | 1 | 2 | 0 | 2 | 0 |
| Male | 3 | 0 | 0 | 0 | 1 | 0 | 2 | 0 |
| Female | 3 | 0 | 1 | 1 | 1 | 0 | 0 | 0 |
| Unknown | 0 | 0 | 0 | 0 | 0 | 0 | 0 | 0 |
| Asian/Pacific Islander | 3,355 | 22 | 31 | 347 | 1,259 | 915 | 781 | 0 |
| Male | 1,847 | 13 | 15 | 162 | 647 | 519 | 491 | 0 |
| Female | 1,508 | 9 | 16 | 185 | 612 | 396 | 290 | 0 |
| Unknown | 0 | 0 | 0 | 0 | 0 | 0 | 0 | 0 |
| Not Stated | 12 | 1 | 1 | 0 | 5 | 2 | 3 | 0 |
| Male | 7 | 1 | 1 | 0 | 2 | 2 | 1 | 0 |
| Female | 5 | 0 | 0 | 0 | 3 | 0 | 2 | 0 |
| Unknown | 0 | 0 | 0 | 0 | 0 | 0 | 0 | 0 |

[a]Includes persons born outside the United States, American Samoa, the Federated States of Micronesia, Guam, the Republic of the Marshall Islands, Midway Island, the Commonwealth of the Northern Mariana Islands, Puerto Rico, the Republic of Palau, U.S. Minor Outlying Islands, U.S. Miscellaneous Pacific Islands, and the U.S. Virgin Islands.

[b]Persons of Hispanic origin may be of any race.

*Source*: Centers for Disease Control and Prevention, U.S. Department of Health and Human Services. National Center for HIV, STD, and TB Prevention, Division of Tuberculosis Elimination. *Reported Tuberculosis in the United States, 1999* (Atlanta, GA: CDC, 2000).

## Table E2.5. Tuberculosis Cases, by Age Group: United States, 1999

| State | Total Cases | Under 5 | 5 - 14 | 15 - 24 | 25 - 44 | 45 - 64 | 65+ | Unknown or Missing |
|---|---|---|---|---|---|---|---|---|
| **United States** | **17,531** | **605** | **439** | **1,516** | **6,078** | **4,862** | **4,028** | **3** |
| Alabama | 314 | 8 | 1 | 13 | 80 | 102 | 110 | 0 |
| Alaska | 61 | 0 | 2 | 4 | 26 | 13 | 16 | 0 |
| Arizona | 262 | 7 | 2 | 26 | 99 | 59 | 69 | 0 |
| Arkansas | 181 | 13 | 9 | 8 | 32 | 47 | 72 | 0 |
| California | 3,606 | 153 | 116 | 334 | 1,161 | 975 | 867 | 0 |
| Colorado | 88 | 9 | 4 | 5 | 26 | 22 | 22 | 0 |
| Connecticut | 121 | 4 | 2 | 15 | 45 | 37 | 18 | 0 |
| Delaware | 34 | 0 | 2 | 0 | 15 | 6 | 11 | 0 |
| District of Columbia | 70 | 1 | 1 | 5 | 30 | 17 | 16 | 0 |
| Florida | 1,277 | 33 | 17 | 70 | 516 | 416 | 225 | 0 |
| Georgia | 665 | 38 | 22 | 67 | 251 | 191 | 96 | 0 |
| Hawaii | 184 | 0 | 4 | 19 | 46 | 57 | 58 | 0 |
| Idaho | 16 | 0 | 0 | 3 | 5 | 4 | 4 | 0 |
| Illinois | 825 | 26 | 22 | 57 | 295 | 242 | 183 | 0 |
| Indiana | 150 | 10 | 2 | 13 | 42 | 38 | 45 | 0 |
| Iowa | 58 | 2 | 1 | 3 | 30 | 9 | 13 | 0 |
| Kansas | 69 | 9 | 6 | 5 | 27 | 16 | 6 | 0 |
| Kentucky | 209 | 2 | 3 | 7 | 58 | 60 | 78 | 1 |
| Louisiana | 357 | 10 | 9 | 17 | 114 | 122 | 85 | 0 |
| Maine | 23 | 0 | 0 | 0 | 5 | 7 | 11 | 0 |
| Maryland | 294 | 8 | 6 | 32 | 109 | 71 | 68 | 0 |
| Massachusetts | 270 | 5 | 4 | 35 | 114 | 62 | 50 | 0 |
| Michigan | 351 | 14 | 10 | 22 | 112 | 99 | 94 | 0 |
| Minnesota | 201 | 4 | 15 | 59 | 67 | 38 | 18 | 0 |
| Mississippi | 215 | 12 | 7 | 12 | 45 | 62 | 77 | 0 |
| Missouri | 208 | 9 | 9 | 7 | 66 | 46 | 71 | 0 |
| Montana | 14 | 0 | 0 | 0 | 1 | 8 | 5 | 0 |
| Nebraska | 18 | 0 | 0 | 2 | 8 | 5 | 3 | 0 |
| Nevada | 93 | 3 | 2 | 8 | 25 | 36 | 17 | 2 |
| New Hampshire | 19 | 1 | 0 | 2 | 8 | 2 | 6 | 0 |
| New Jersey | 571 | 12 | 12 | 58 | 225 | 153 | 111 | 0 |
| New Mexico | 64 | 1 | 1 | 7 | 18 | 11 | 26 | 0 |
| New York | 1,837 | 43 | 49 | 163 | 814 | 476 | 292 | 0 |
| North Carolina | 488 | 15 | 5 | 51 | 165 | 139 | 113 | 0 |
| North Dakota | 7 | 0 | 0 | 1 | 0 | 3 | 3 | 0 |
| Ohio | 317 | 6 | 2 | 25 | 80 | 85 | 119 | 0 |
| Oklahoma | 208 | 14 | 7 | 20 | 70 | 54 | 43 | 0 |
| Oregon | 123 | 5 | 4 | 13 | 38 | 34 | 29 | 0 |
| Pennsylvania | 454 | 12 | 8 | 30 | 123 | 117 | 164 | 0 |
| Rhode Island | 53 | 3 | 4 | 7 | 11 | 15 | 13 | 0 |
| South Carolina | 315 | 7 | 6 | 19 | 107 | 101 | 75 | 0 |
| South Dakota | 21 | 0 | 1 | 1 | 6 | 8 | 5 | 0 |
| Tennessee | 382 | 16 | 4 | 21 | 118 | 102 | 121 | 0 |
| Texas | 1,649 | 67 | 42 | 158 | 594 | 494 | 294 | 0 |
| Utah | 40 | 1 | 2 | 3 | 10 | 13 | 11 | 0 |
| Vermont | 3 | 0 | 0 | 0 | 0 | 2 | 1 | 0 |
| Virginia | 334 | 9 | 4 | 40 | 114 | 79 | 88 | 0 |
| Washington | 258 | 9 | 6 | 37 | 82 | 71 | 53 | 0 |
| West Virginia | 41 | 0 | 0 | 0 | 3 | 17 | 21 | 0 |
| Wisconsin | 110 | 4 | 4 | 12 | 40 | 18 | 32 | 0 |
| Wyoming | 3 | 0 | 0 | 0 | 2 | 1 | 0 | 0 |
| American Samoa[a] | 4 | 0 | 0 | 1 | 0 | 2 | 1 | 0 |
| Fed. States of Micronesia[a] | ... | ... | ... | ... | ... | ... | ... | ... |
| Guam[a] | 69 | 0 | 1 | 4 | 21 | 36 | 7 | 0 |
| N. Mariana Islands[a] | 66 | 2 | 0 | 9 | 37 | 18 | 0 | 0 |
| Puerto Rico[a] | 200 | 3 | 1 | 14 | 67 | 68 | 47 | 0 |
| Republic of Palau[a] | 11 | 1 | 0 | 1 | 4 | 5 | 0 | 0 |
| U.S. Virgin Islands[a] | ... | ... | ... | ... | ... | ... | ... | ... |

[a]Not included in U.S. totals.

Ellipses indicate data not available.

*Source*: Centers for Disease Control and Prevention, U.S. Department of Health and Human Services. National Center for HIV, STD, and TB Prevention, Division of Tuberculosis Elimination. *Reported Tuberculosis in the United States, 1999* (Atlanta, GA: CDC, 2000).

## Table E2.6. Tuberculosis Cases, by Race/Ethnicity: United States, 1999

| State | Total Cases | White, non-Hispanic | Black, non-Hispanic | Hispanic[a] | American Indian or Alaskan Native | Asian or Pacific Islander | Unknown or Missing |
|---|---|---|---|---|---|---|---|
| **United States** | **17,531** | **4,224** | **5,552** | **3,875** | **240** | **3,591** | **49** |
| Alabama | 314 | 135 | 152 | 12 | 1 | 14 | 0 |
| Alaska | 61 | 5 | 0 | 2 | 41 | 13 | 0 |
| Arizona | 262 | 81 | 15 | 103 | 45 | 18 | 0 |
| Arkansas | 181 | 85 | 61 | 20 | 1 | 13 | 1 |
| California | 3,606 | 449 | 375 | 1,340 | 16 | 1,414 | 12 |
| Colorado | 88 | 26 | 13 | 29 | 1 | 19 | 0 |
| Connecticut | 121 | 26 | 35 | 30 | 0 | 30 | 0 |
| Delaware | 34 | 11 | 12 | 2 | 0 | 9 | 0 |
| District of Columbia | 70 | 6 | 53 | 7 | 0 | 4 | 0 |
| Florida | 1,277 | 374 | 620 | 209 | 1 | 72 | 1 |
| Georgia | 665 | 135 | 410 | 64 | 0 | 48 | 8 |
| Hawaii | 184 | 9 | 1 | 5 | 0 | 165 | 4 |
| Idaho | 16 | 8 | 0 | 4 | 3 | 1 | 0 |
| Illinois | 825 | 188 | 349 | 140 | 0 | 143 | 5 |
| Indiana | 150 | 75 | 40 | 20 | 1 | 14 | 0 |
| Iowa | 58 | 25 | 5 | 12 | 1 | 15 | 0 |
| Kansas | 69 | 17 | 10 | 28 | 0 | 14 | 0 |
| Kentucky | 209 | 150 | 38 | 13 | 0 | 8 | 0 |
| Louisiana | 357 | 126 | 201 | 9 | 1 | 18 | 2 |
| Maine | 23 | 16 | 2 | 0 | 0 | 5 | 0 |
| Maryland | 294 | 47 | 142 | 39 | 0 | 65 | 1 |
| Massachusetts | 270 | 75 | 74 | 35 | 0 | 86 | 0 |
| Michigan | 351 | 99 | 159 | 24 | 2 | 65 | 2 |
| Minnesota | 201 | 26 | 95 | 18 | 7 | 55 | 0 |
| Mississippi | 215 | 56 | 142 | 6 | 2 | 9 | 0 |
| Missouri | 208 | 81 | 92 | 8 | 2 | 24 | 1 |
| Montana | 14 | 6 | 0 | 0 | 8 | 0 | 0 |
| Nebraska | 18 | 7 | 2 | 4 | 1 | 4 | 0 |
| Nevada | 93 | 25 | 11 | 20 | 2 | 33 | 2 |
| New Hampshire | 19 | 11 | 1 | 1 | 0 | 5 | 1 |
| New Jersey | 571 | 96 | 196 | 130 | 0 | 149 | 0 |
| New Mexico | 64 | 8 | 0 | 31 | 24 | 1 | 0 |
| New York | 1,837 | 285 | 672 | 469 | 0 | 410 | 1 |
| North Carolina | 488 | 112 | 270 | 64 | 3 | 38 | 1 |
| North Dakota | 7 | 5 | 1 | 0 | 1 | 0 | 0 |
| Ohio | 317 | 131 | 136 | 19 | 1 | 29 | 1 |
| Oklahoma | 208 | 114 | 26 | 14 | 38 | 16 | 0 |
| Oregon | 123 | 44 | 9 | 26 | 3 | 41 | 0 |
| Pennsylvania | 454 | 171 | 137 | 30 | 0 | 111 | 5 |
| Rhode Island | 53 | 16 | 11 | 12 | 0 | 14 | 0 |
| South Carolina | 315 | 59 | 228 | 7 | 1 | 20 | 0 |
| South Dakota | 21 | 4 | 1 | 1 | 14 | 1 | 0 |
| Tennessee | 382 | 199 | 156 | 13 | 0 | 14 | 0 |
| Texas | 1,649 | 338 | 403 | 742 | 1 | 165 | 0 |
| Utah | 40 | 12 | 3 | 8 | 7 | 10 | 0 |
| Vermont | 3 | 2 | 0 | 0 | 0 | 1 | 0 |
| Virginia | 334 | 97 | 125 | 46 | 0 | 66 | 0 |
| Washington | 258 | 81 | 33 | 42 | 10 | 91 | 1 |
| West Virginia | 41 | 32 | 9 | 0 | 0 | 0 | 0 |
| Wisconsin | 110 | 37 | 26 | 15 | 1 | 31 | 0 |
| Wyoming | 3 | 1 | 0 | 2 | 0 | 0 | 0 |
| American Samoa[b] | 4 | 0 | 0 | 0 | 0 | 4 | 0 |
| Fed. States of Micronesia[b] | ... | ... | ... | ... | ... | ... | ... |
| Guam[b] | 69 | 0 | 0 | 0 | 0 | 64 | 5 |
| N. Mariana Islands[b] | 66 | 0 | 0 | 1 | 0 | 63 | 2 |
| Puerto Rico[b] | 200 | 0 | 0 | 199 | 0 | 0 | 1 |
| Republic of Palau[b] | 11 | 0 | 0 | 0 | 0 | 11 | 0 |
| U.S. Virgin Islands[b] | ... | ... | ... | ... | ... | ... | ... |

[a]Persons of Hispanic origin may be of any race.

[b]Not included in U.S. totals.

Ellipses indicate data not available.

*Source*: Centers for Disease Control and Prevention, U.S. Department of Health and Human Services. National Center for HIV, STD, and TB Prevention, Division of Tuberculosis Elimination. *Reported Tuberculosis in the United States, 1999* (Atlanta, GA: CDC, 2000).

## Table E2.7. Tuberculosis Cases, U.S.-born Persons and Foreign-born Persons: United States, 1999

| State | Total Cases | U.S.-born Persons No. | U.S.-born Persons % | Foreign-born Persons[a] No. | Foreign-born Persons[a] % | Unknown No. | Unknown % |
|---|---|---|---|---|---|---|---|
| **United States** | **17,531** | **9,809** | **56.0** | **7,553** | **43.1** | **169** | **1.0** |
| Alabama | 314 | 287 | 91.4 | 26 | 8.3 | 1 | 0.3 |
| Alaska | 61 | 46 | 75.4 | 14 | 23.0 | 1 | 1.6 |
| Arizona | 262 | 154 | 58.8 | 107 | 40.8 | 1 | 0.4 |
| Arkansas | 181 | 159 | 87.8 | 16 | 8.8 | 6 | 3.3 |
| California | 3,606 | 1,074 | 29.8 | 2,503 | 69.4 | 29 | 0.8 |
| Colorado | 88 | 41 | 46.6 | 47 | 53.4 | 0 | 0.0 |
| Connecticut | 121 | 46 | 38.0 | 74 | 61.2 | 1 | 0.8 |
| Delaware | 34 | 20 | 58.8 | 14 | 41.2 | 0 | 0.0 |
| District of Columbia | 70 | 48 | 68.6 | 22 | 31.4 | 0 | 0.0 |
| Florida | 1,277 | 834 | 65.3 | 442 | 34.6 | 1 | 0.1 |
| Georgia | 665 | 520 | 78.2 | 136 | 20.5 | 9 | 1.4 |
| Hawaii | 184 | 46 | 25.0 | 137 | 74.5 | 1 | 0.5 |
| Idaho | 16 | 11 | 68.8 | 5 | 31.3 | 0 | 0.0 |
| Illinois | 825 | 547 | 66.3 | 264 | 32.0 | 14 | 1.7 |
| Indiana | 150 | 113 | 75.3 | 36 | 24.0 | 1 | 0.7 |
| Iowa | 58 | 20 | 34.5 | 38 | 65.5 | 0 | 0.0 |
| Kansas | 69 | 40 | 58.0 | 28 | 40.6 | 1 | 1.4 |
| Kentucky | 209 | 188 | 90.0 | 21 | 10.0 | 0 | 0.0 |
| Louisiana | 357 | 323 | 90.5 | 30 | 8.4 | 4 | 1.1 |
| Maine | 23 | 16 | 69.6 | 7 | 30.4 | 0 | 0.0 |
| Maryland | 294 | 140 | 47.6 | 154 | 52.4 | 0 | 0.0 |
| Massachusetts | 270 | 83 | 30.7 | 187 | 69.3 | 0 | 0.0 |
| Michigan | 351 | 251 | 71.5 | 99 | 28.2 | 1 | 0.3 |
| Minnesota | 201 | 46 | 22.9 | 155 | 77.1 | 0 | 0.0 |
| Mississippi | 215 | 202 | 94.0 | 13 | 6.0 | 0 | 0.0 |
| Missouri | 208 | 169 | 81.3 | 38 | 18.3 | 1 | 0.5 |
| Montana | 14 | 14 | 100.0 | 0 | 0.0 | 0 | 0.0 |
| Nebraska | 18 | 9 | 50.0 | 9 | 50.0 | 0 | 0.0 |
| Nevada | 93 | 40 | 43.0 | 52 | 55.9 | 1 | 1.1 |
| New Hampshire | 19 | 12 | 63.2 | 7 | 36.8 | 0 | 0.0 |
| New Jersey | 571 | 245 | 42.9 | 324 | 56.7 | 2 | 0.4 |
| New Mexico | 64 | 45 | 70.3 | 19 | 29.7 | 0 | 0.0 |
| New York | 1,837 | 774 | 42.1 | 988 | 53.8 | 75 | 4.1 |
| North Carolina | 488 | 386 | 79.1 | 101 | 20.7 | 1 | 0.2 |
| North Dakota | 7 | 6 | 85.7 | 1 | 14.3 | 0 | 0.0 |
| Ohio | 317 | 241 | 76.0 | 74 | 23.3 | 2 | 0.6 |
| Oklahoma | 208 | 176 | 84.6 | 32 | 15.4 | 0 | 0.0 |
| Oregon | 123 | 52 | 42.3 | 71 | 57.7 | 0 | 0.0 |
| Pennsylvania | 454 | 300 | 66.1 | 145 | 31.9 | 9 | 2.0 |
| Rhode Island | 53 | 26 | 49.1 | 27 | 50.9 | 0 | 0.0 |
| South Carolina | 315 | 292 | 92.7 | 23 | 7.3 | 0 | 0.0 |
| South Dakota | 21 | 17 | 81.0 | 4 | 19.0 | 0 | 0.0 |
| Tennessee | 382 | 341 | 89.3 | 41 | 10.7 | 0 | 0.0 |
| Texas | 1,649 | 994 | 60.3 | 648 | 39.3 | 7 | 0.4 |
| Utah | 40 | 21 | 52.5 | 19 | 47.5 | 0 | 0.0 |
| Vermont | 3 | 2 | 66.7 | 1 | 33.3 | 0 | 0.0 |
| Virginia | 334 | 179 | 53.6 | 155 | 46.4 | 0 | 0.0 |
| Washington | 258 | 108 | 41.9 | 150 | 58.1 | 0 | 0.0 |
| West Virginia | 41 | 41 | 100.0 | 0 | 0.0 | 0 | 0.0 |
| Wisconsin | 110 | 62 | 56.4 | 48 | 43.6 | 0 | 0.0 |
| Wyoming | 3 | 2 | 66.7 | 1 | 33.3 | 0 | 0.0 |

[a]Includes persons born outside the United States, American Samoa, the Federated States of Micronesia, Guam, the Republic of the Marshall Islands, Midway Island, the Commonwealth of the Northern Mariana Islands, Puerto Rico, the Republic of Palau, U.S. Minor Outlying Islands, U.S. Miscellaneous Pacific Islands, and the U.S. Virgin Islands.

*Source*: Centers for Disease Control and Prevention, U.S. Department of Health and Human Services. National Center for HIV, STD, and TB Prevention, Division of Tuberculosis Elimination. *Reported Tuberculosis in the United States, 1999* (Atlanta, GA: CDC, 2000).

## Table E2.8. Tuberculosis Cases in Foreign-born Persons,[a] by Country of Origin: United States, 1999

| | | Country of Origin | | | | | | | | |
|---|---|---|---|---|---|---|---|---|---|---|
| State | Total Cases | Mexico | Philippines | Vietnam | India | Rep. of China | Haiti | Rep. of Korea | All Others[b] | Unknown or Missing |
| **United States** | **7,553** | **1,753** | **913** | **721** | **557** | **366** | **284** | **220** | **2,736** | **3** |
| Alabama | 26 | 5 | 2 | 3 | 3 | 0 | 0 | 2 | 11 | 0 |
| Alaska | 14 | 1 | 8 | 0 | 1 | 0 | 0 | 2 | 2 | 0 |
| Arizona | 107 | 67 | 9 | 3 | 5 | 0 | 0 | 0 | 23 | 0 |
| Arkansas | 16 | 5 | 0 | 3 | 1 | 1 | 0 | 0 | 6 | 0 |
| California | 2,503 | 820 | 487 | 346 | 90 | 142 | 2 | 81 | 533 | 2 |
| Colorado | 47 | 14 | 0 | 7 | 7 | 0 | 0 | 0 | 19 | 0 |
| Connecticut | 74 | 1 | 9 | 4 | 9 | 2 | 4 | 0 | 45 | 0 |
| Delaware | 14 | 2 | 2 | 0 | 1 | 0 | 2 | 0 | 7 | 0 |
| District of Columbia | 22 | 1 | 2 | 1 | 1 | 0 | 0 | 0 | 17 | 0 |
| Florida | 442 | 45 | 20 | 18 | 16 | 8 | 142 | 5 | 188 | 0 |
| Georgia | 136 | 32 | 2 | 17 | 13 | 3 | 0 | 4 | 65 | 0 |
| Hawaii | 137 | 1 | 103 | 4 | 0 | 8 | 0 | 9 | 12 | 0 |
| Idaho | 5 | 4 | 0 | 0 | 0 | 0 | 0 | 0 | 1 | 0 |
| Illinois | 264 | 81 | 33 | 10 | 49 | 8 | 1 | 14 | 68 | 0 |
| Indiana | 36 | 11 | 3 | 3 | 3 | 1 | 0 | 0 | 15 | 0 |
| Iowa | 38 | 9 | 1 | 6 | 4 | 0 | 0 | 1 | 17 | 0 |
| Kansas | 28 | 12 | 3 | 2 | 4 | 0 | 0 | 0 | 7 | 0 |
| Kentucky | 21 | 8 | 2 | 1 | 5 | 0 | 0 | 0 | 5 | 0 |
| Louisiana | 30 | 2 | 4 | 8 | 1 | 1 | 1 | 1 | 12 | 0 |
| Maine | 7 | 0 | 0 | 3 | 1 | 0 | 0 | 0 | 3 | 0 |
| Maryland | 154 | 7 | 13 | 11 | 15 | 3 | 5 | 16 | 84 | 0 |
| Massachusetts | 187 | 2 | 3 | 28 | 18 | 15 | 18 | 1 | 102 | 0 |
| Michigan | 99 | 6 | 9 | 8 | 27 | 12 | 0 | 4 | 33 | 0 |
| Minnesota | 155 | 11 | 3 | 12 | 9 | 10 | 1 | 1 | 108 | 0 |
| Mississippi | 13 | 2 | 5 | 1 | 2 | 0 | 0 | 0 | 3 | 0 |
| Missouri | 38 | 3 | 4 | 5 | 4 | 4 | 0 | 2 | 16 | 0 |
| Montana | 0 | 0 | 0 | 0 | 0 | 0 | 0 | 0 | 0 | 0 |
| Nebraska | 9 | 2 | 0 | 2 | 0 | 0 | 0 | 1 | 4 | 0 |
| Nevada | 52 | 14 | 28 | 2 | 1 | 0 | 0 | 0 | 7 | 0 |
| New Hampshire | 7 | 0 | 1 | 1 | 2 | 0 | 0 | 0 | 3 | 0 |
| New Jersey | 324 | 19 | 27 | 8 | 82 | 10 | 25 | 10 | 143 | 0 |
| New Mexico | 19 | 17 | 0 | 0 | 1 | 0 | 0 | 0 | 1 | 0 |
| New York | 988 | 47 | 38 | 18 | 62 | 101 | 74 | 28 | 620 | 0 |
| North Carolina | 101 | 40 | 4 | 8 | 4 | 1 | 2 | 2 | 40 | 0 |
| North Dakota | 1 | 0 | 0 | 0 | 0 | 0 | 0 | 0 | 1 | 0 |
| Ohio | 74 | 4 | 0 | 6 | 8 | 3 | 1 | 3 | 48 | 1 |
| Oklahoma | 32 | 7 | 1 | 4 | 4 | 1 | 0 | 0 | 15 | 0 |
| Oregon | 71 | 21 | 6 | 14 | 4 | 1 | 0 | 1 | 24 | 0 |
| Pennsylvania | 145 | 5 | 9 | 27 | 34 | 9 | 4 | 7 | 50 | 0 |
| Rhode Island | 27 | 1 | 1 | 0 | 0 | 4 | 1 | 0 | 20 | 0 |
| South Carolina | 23 | 2 | 2 | 3 | 7 | 1 | 0 | 2 | 6 | 0 |
| South Dakota | 4 | 1 | 1 | 0 | 0 | 0 | 0 | 0 | 2 | 0 |
| Tennessee | 41 | 8 | 4 | 5 | 5 | 0 | 0 | 0 | 19 | 0 |
| Texas | 648 | 364 | 20 | 70 | 29 | 5 | 1 | 10 | 149 | 0 |
| Utah | 19 | 5 | 1 | 3 | 0 | 1 | 0 | 0 | 9 | 0 |
| Vermont | 1 | 0 | 0 | 0 | 0 | 0 | 0 | 0 | 1 | 0 |
| Virginia | 155 | 5 | 18 | 17 | 10 | 3 | 0 | 8 | 94 | 0 |
| Washington | 150 | 27 | 21 | 27 | 8 | 5 | 0 | 5 | 57 | 0 |
| West Virginia | 0 | 0 | 0 | 0 | 0 | 0 | 0 | 0 | 0 | 0 |
| Wisconsin | 48 | 11 | 4 | 2 | 7 | 3 | 0 | 0 | 21 | 0 |
| Wyoming | 1 | 1 | 0 | 0 | 0 | 0 | 0 | 0 | 0 | 0 |

[a]Includes persons from outside the United States, American Samoa, the Federated States of Micronesia, Guam, the Republic of the Marshall Islands, Midway Island, the Commonwealth of the Northern Mariana Islands, Puerto Rico, the Republic of Palau, U.S. Minor Outlying Islands, U.S. Miscellaneous Pacific Islands, and the U.S. Virgin Islands.

[b]Includes 145 countries.

*Source*: Centers for Disease Control and Prevention, U.S. Department of Health and Human Services. National Center for HIV, STD, and TB Prevention, Division of Tuberculosis Elimination. *Reported Tuberculosis in the United States, 1999* (Atlanta, GA: CDC, 2000).

## Table E2.9. Tuberculosis Cases and Case Rates per 100,000 Population: United States, 2000 and 1999

| State | Cases 2000 | Cases 1999 | Case Rates 2000 | Case Rates 1999 | Rank According to Rate 2000 | Rank According to Rate 1999 | April 1, 2000 Census Population |
|---|---|---|---|---|---|---|---|
| **United States** | **16,377** | **17,531** | **5.8** | **6.4** | **--** | **--** | **281,421,906** |
| Alabama | 310 | 314 | 7.0 | 7.2 | 11 | 11 | 4,447,100 |
| Alaska | 108 | 61 | 17.2 | 9.8 | 1 | 4 | 626,932 |
| Arizona | 261 | 262 | 5.1 | 5.5 | 18 | 19 | 5,130,632 |
| Arkansas | 199 | 181 | 7.4 | 7.1 | 6 | 12 | 2,673,400 |
| California | 3,297 | 3,606 | 9.7 | 10.9 | 3 | 2 | 33,871,648 |
| Colorado | 97 | 88 | 2.3 | 2.2 | 38 | 39 | 4,301,261 |
| Connecticut | 105 | 121 | 3.1 | 3.7 | 31 | 31 | 3,405,565 |
| Delaware | 28 | 34 | 3.6 | 4.5 | 28 | 24 | 783,600 |
| District of Columbia(a) | 85 | 70 | 14.9 | 13.5 | -- | -- | 572,059 |
| Florida | 1,171 | 1,277 | 7.3 | 8.5 | 8 | 6 | 15,982,378 |
| Georgia | 703 | 665 | 8.6 | 8.5 | 5 | 5 | 8,186,453 |
| Hawaii | 136 | 184 | 11.2 | 15.5 | 2 | 1 | 1,211,537 |
| Idaho | 16 | 16 | 1.2 | 1.3 | 47 | 46 | 1,293,953 |
| Illinois | 743 | 825 | 6.0 | 6.8 | 15 | 15 | 12,419,293 |
| Indiana | 145 | 150 | 2.4 | 2.5 | 36 | 37 | 6,080,485 |
| Iowa | 40 | 58 | 1.4 | 2.0 | 46 | 41 | 2,926,324 |
| Kansas | 77 | 69 | 2.9 | 2.6 | 34 | 36 | 2,688,418 |
| Kentucky | 147 | 209 | 3.6 | 5.3 | 26 | 21 | 4,041,769 |
| Louisiana | 331 | 357 | 7.4 | 8.2 | 7 | 8 | 4,468,976 |
| Maine | 24 | 23 | 1.9 | 1.8 | 41 | 43 | 1,274,923 |
| Maryland | 282 | 294 | 5.3 | 5.7 | 17 | 18 | 5,296,486 |
| Massachusetts | 285 | 270 | 4.5 | 4.4 | 21 | 26 | 6,349,097 |
| Michigan | 287 | 351 | 2.9 | 3.6 | 33 | 33 | 9,938,444 |
| Minnesota | 178 | 201 | 3.6 | 4.2 | 27 | 27 | 4,919,479 |
| Mississippi | 173 | 215 | 6.1 | 7.8 | 14 | 10 | 2,844,658 |
| Missouri | 211 | 208 | 3.8 | 3.8 | 25 | 28 | 5,595,211 |
| Montana | 21 | 14 | 2.3 | 1.6 | 37 | 44 | 902,195 |
| Nebraska | 24 | 18 | 1.4 | 1.1 | 45 | 48 | 1,711,263 |
| Nevada | 96 | 93 | 4.8 | 5.1 | 19 | 22 | 1,998,257 |
| New Hampshire | 22 | 19 | 1.8 | 1.6 | 43 | 45 | 1,235,786 |
| New Jersey | 565 | 571 | 6.7 | 7.0 | 13 | 13 | 8,414,350 |
| New Mexico | 46 | 64 | 2.5 | 3.7 | 35 | 32 | 1,819,046 |
| New York | 1,744 | 1,837 | 9.2 | 10.1 | 4 | 3 | 18,976,457 |
| North Carolina | 447 | 488 | 5.6 | 6.4 | 16 | 16 | 8,049,313 |
| North Dakota | 5 | 7 | 0.8 | 1.1 | 49 | 47 | 642,200 |
| Ohio | 340 | 317 | 3.0 | 2.8 | 32 | 35 | 11,353,140 |
| Oklahoma | 154 | 208 | 4.5 | 6.2 | 22 | 17 | 3,450,654 |
| Oregon | 119 | 123 | 3.5 | 3.7 | 29 | 30 | 3,421,399 |
| Pennsylvania | 383 | 454 | 3.1 | 3.8 | 30 | 29 | 12,281,054 |
| Rhode Island | 49 | 53 | 4.7 | 5.3 | 20 | 20 | 1,048,319 |
| South Carolina | 286 | 315 | 7.1 | 8.1 | 10 | 9 | 4,012,012 |
| South Dakota | 16 | 21 | 2.1 | 2.9 | 40 | 34 | 754,844 |
| Tennessee | 383 | 382 | 6.7 | 7.0 | 12 | 14 | 5,689,283 |
| Texas | 1,506 | 1,649 | 7.2 | 8.2 | 9 | 7 | 20,851,820 |
| Utah | 49 | 40 | 2.2 | 1.9 | 39 | 42 | 2,233,169 |
| Vermont | 4 | 3 | 0.7 | 0.5 | 50 | 50 | 608,827 |
| Virginia | 292 | 334 | 4.1 | 4.9 | 24 | 23 | 7,078,515 |
| Washington | 258 | 258 | 4.4 | 4.5 | 23 | 25 | 5,894,121 |
| West Virginia | 33 | 41 | 1.8 | 2.3 | 42 | 38 | 1,808,344 |
| Wisconsin | 92 | 110 | 1.7 | 2.1 | 44 | 40 | 5,363,675 |
| Wyoming | 4 | 3 | 0.8 | 0.6 | 48 | 49 | 493,782 |
| American Samoa(a,b) | ... | 4 | ... | 6.3 | -- | -- | ... |
| Fed. States of Micronesia(a,b) | ... | ... | ... | ... | -- | -- | ... |
| Guam(a,b) | 54 | 69 | ... | 45.4 | -- | -- | ... |
| N. Mariana Islands(a,b) | 75 | 66 | ... | 95.4 | -- | -- | ... |
| Puerto Rico(a,b) | 174 | 200 | 4.6 | 5.1 | -- | -- | 3,808,610 |
| Republic of Palau(a,b) | ... | 11 | ... | 59.7 | -- | -- | ... |
| U.S. Virgin Islands(a,b) | ... | ... | ... | ... | -- | -- | ... |

(a)Not ranked with the states.

(b)Not included in U.S. totals.

Ellipses indicate data not available.

Note: Denominators for computing 2000 rates for the states, District of Columbia, and Puerto Rico were obtained from the U.S. Census Bureau *(http://www.census.gov/population/www/cen2000/respop.html).* April 1, 2000 populations not yet available for other jurisdictions.

*Source*: Centers for Disease Control and Prevention, U.S. Department of Health and Human Services. National Center for HIV, STD, and TB Prevention, Division of Tuberculosis Elimination. Web site for *Reported Tuberculosis in the United States, 2000.* http://www.cdc.gov/nchstp/tb/surv/surv2000/pdfs/st2000.pdf.

## Table E3.1. Tuberculosis Cases, by Form of Disease: United States, 1999

| State | Total Cases | Pulmonary[a] No. | Pulmonary[a] % | Extrapulmonary[b] No. | Extrapulmonary[b] % | Cases with Both Pulmonary and Extrapulmonary Disease: Total[c] No. | Total[c] % | Miliary No. |
|---|---|---|---|---|---|---|---|---|
| **United States** | **17,531** | **12,761** | **72.8** | **3,438** | **19.6** | **1,322** | **7.5** | **321** |
| Alabama | 314 | 257 | 81.8 | 42 | 13.4 | 15 | 4.8 | 0 |
| Alaska | 61 | 51 | 83.6 | 7 | 11.5 | 3 | 4.9 | 0 |
| Arizona | 262 | 215 | 82.1 | 27 | 10.3 | 20 | 7.6 | 6 |
| Arkansas | 181 | 151 | 83.4 | 16 | 8.8 | 14 | 7.7 | 2 |
| California | 3,606 | 2,629 | 72.9 | 721 | 20.0 | 253 | 7.0 | 67 |
| Colorado | 88 | 54 | 61.4 | 23 | 26.1 | 11 | 12.5 | 4 |
| Connecticut | 121 | 79 | 65.3 | 33 | 27.3 | 9 | 7.4 | 3 |
| Delaware | 34 | 25 | 73.5 | 3 | 8.8 | 6 | 17.6 | 2 |
| District of Columbia | 70 | 60 | 85.7 | 9 | 12.9 | 1 | 1.4 | 0 |
| Florida | 1,277 | 1,005 | 78.7 | 203 | 15.9 | 69 | 5.4 | 18 |
| Georgia | 665 | 508 | 76.4 | 113 | 17.0 | 43 | 6.5 | 9 |
| Hawaii | 184 | 156 | 84.8 | 24 | 13.0 | 4 | 2.2 | 0 |
| Idaho | 16 | 12 | 75.0 | 1 | 6.3 | 3 | 18.8 | 2 |
| Illinois | 825 | 617 | 74.8 | 182 | 22.1 | 26 | 3.2 | 8 |
| Indiana | 150 | 119 | 79.3 | 26 | 17.3 | 5 | 3.3 | 3 |
| Iowa | 58 | 39 | 67.2 | 18 | 31.0 | 1 | 1.7 | 1 |
| Kansas | 69 | 44 | 63.8 | 18 | 26.1 | 7 | 10.1 | 0 |
| Kentucky | 209 | 176 | 84.2 | 25 | 12.0 | 8 | 3.8 | 2 |
| Louisiana | 357 | 297 | 83.2 | 43 | 12.0 | 17 | 4.8 | 2 |
| Maine | 23 | 14 | 60.9 | 9 | 39.1 | 0 | 0.0 | 0 |
| Maryland | 294 | 196 | 66.7 | 67 | 22.8 | 31 | 10.5 | 17 |
| Massachusetts | 270 | 150 | 55.6 | 89 | 33.0 | 31 | 11.5 | 15 |
| Michigan | 351 | 234 | 66.7 | 83 | 23.6 | 33 | 9.4 | 3 |
| Minnesota | 201 | 129 | 64.2 | 55 | 27.4 | 17 | 8.5 | 5 |
| Mississippi | 215 | 176 | 81.9 | 35 | 16.3 | 4 | 1.9 | 0 |
| Missouri | 208 | 157 | 75.5 | 37 | 17.8 | 14 | 6.7 | 2 |
| Montana | 14 | 10 | 71.4 | 4 | 28.6 | 0 | 0.0 | 0 |
| Nebraska | 18 | 11 | 61.1 | 7 | 38.9 | 0 | 0.0 | 0 |
| Nevada | 93 | 77 | 82.8 | 15 | 16.1 | 1 | 1.1 | 0 |
| New Hampshire | 19 | 14 | 73.7 | 3 | 15.8 | 2 | 10.5 | 0 |
| New Jersey | 571 | 376 | 65.8 | 141 | 24.7 | 54 | 9.5 | 11 |
| New Mexico | 64 | 46 | 71.9 | 7 | 10.9 | 11 | 17.2 | 1 |
| New York | 1,837 | 1,235 | 67.2 | 373 | 20.3 | 228 | 12.4 | 45 |
| North Carolina | 488 | 377 | 77.3 | 85 | 17.4 | 26 | 5.3 | 14 |
| North Dakota | 7 | 3 | 42.9 | 3 | 42.9 | 1 | 14.3 | 0 |
| Ohio | 317 | 216 | 68.1 | 81 | 25.6 | 19 | 6.0 | 8 |
| Oklahoma | 208 | 157 | 75.5 | 39 | 18.8 | 12 | 5.8 | 3 |
| Oregon | 123 | 80 | 65.0 | 32 | 26.0 | 11 | 8.9 | 4 |
| Pennsylvania | 454 | 314 | 69.2 | 106 | 23.3 | 33 | 7.3 | 9 |
| Rhode Island | 53 | 30 | 56.6 | 19 | 35.8 | 4 | 7.5 | 2 |
| South Carolina | 315 | 203 | 64.4 | 67 | 21.3 | 45 | 14.3 | 16 |
| South Dakota | 21 | 13 | 61.9 | 6 | 28.6 | 2 | 9.5 | 0 |
| Tennessee | 382 | 279 | 73.0 | 60 | 15.7 | 43 | 11.3 | 7 |
| Texas | 1,649 | 1,218 | 73.9 | 306 | 18.6 | 124 | 7.5 | 17 |
| Utah | 40 | 23 | 57.5 | 12 | 30.0 | 5 | 12.5 | 1 |
| Vermont | 3 | 1 | 33.3 | 1 | 33.3 | 1 | 33.3 | 1 |
| Virginia | 334 | 252 | 75.4 | 71 | 21.3 | 11 | 3.3 | 2 |
| Washington | 258 | 163 | 63.2 | 60 | 23.3 | 35 | 13.6 | 6 |
| West Virginia | 41 | 34 | 82.9 | 5 | 12.2 | 1 | 2.4 | 1 |
| Wisconsin | 110 | 77 | 70.0 | 26 | 23.6 | 7 | 6.4 | 1 |
| Wyoming | 3 | 2 | 66.7 | 0 | 0.0 | 1 | 33.3 | 1 |
| American Samoa[d] | 4 | 3 | 75.0 | 1 | 25.0 | 0 | 0.0 | 0 |
| Fed. States of Micronesia[d] | ... | ... | ... | ... | ... | ... | ... | ... |
| Guam[d] | 69 | 64 | 92.8 | 3 | 4.3 | 2 | 2.9 | 2 |
| N. Mariana Islands[d] | 66 | 55 | 83.3 | 5 | 7.6 | 6 | 9.1 | 1 |
| Puerto Rico[d] | 200 | 172 | 86.0 | 22 | 11.0 | 6 | 3.0 | 2 |
| Republic of Palau[d] | 11 | 9 | 81.8 | 2 | 18.2 | 0 | 0.0 | 0 |
| U.S. Virgin Islands[d] | ... | ... | ... | ... | ... | ... | ... | ... |

[a]Includes cases with pulmonary listed as major site of disease and no additional site of disease.

[b]Includes cases with pleural, lymphatic, bone and/or joint, meningeal, peritoneal, or other site, excluding pulmonary, listed as major site of disease.

[c]Includes miliary cases.

[d]Not included in U.S. totals.

Ellipses indicate data not available.

Note: 10 (0.1%) cases had missing and/or unknown site of disease.

*Source*: Centers for Disease Control and Prevention, U.S. Department of Health and Human Services. National Center for HIV, STD, and TB Prevention, Division of Tuberculosis Elimination. *Reported Tuberculosis in the United States, 1999* (Atlanta, GA: CDC, 2000).

## Table E3.2. Extrapulmonary Tuberculosis Cases, by Site of Disease: United States, 1999

| State | Total Extra-pulmonary Cases | Site of Disease | | | | | | |
|---|---|---|---|---|---|---|---|---|
| | | Pleural | Lymphatic | Bone and/ or Joint | Genito-urinary | Meningeal | Peritoneal | Other |
| **United States** | **3,438** | **727** | **1,385** | **376** | **217** | **171** | **136** | **426** |
| Alabama | 42 | 18 | 7 | 7 | 1 | 3 | 0 | 6 |
| Alaska | 7 | 0 | 4 | 0 | 0 | 0 | 1 | 2 |
| Arizona | 27 | 6 | 8 | 6 | 3 | 0 | 1 | 3 |
| Arkansas | 16 | 8 | 6 | 0 | 1 | 0 | 0 | 1 |
| California | 721 | 128 | 319 | 87 | 55 | 31 | 33 | 68 |
| Colorado | 23 | 2 | 14 | 2 | 0 | 1 | 1 | 3 |
| Connecticut | 33 | 5 | 12 | 4 | 3 | 3 | 3 | 3 |
| Delaware | 3 | 1 | 0 | 0 | 2 | 0 | 0 | 0 |
| District of Columbia | 9 | 0 | 5 | 2 | 1 | 0 | 0 | 1 |
| Florida | 203 | 38 | 77 | 19 | 12 | 9 | 7 | 41 |
| Georgia | 113 | 28 | 37 | 8 | 3 | 12 | 4 | 21 |
| Hawaii | 24 | 4 | 6 | 4 | 4 | 1 | 0 | 5 |
| Idaho | 1 | 0 | 0 | 0 | 0 | 0 | 0 | 1 |
| Illinois | 182 | 46 | 64 | 25 | 12 | 8 | 6 | 21 |
| Indiana | 26 | 9 | 8 | 0 | 1 | 3 | 0 | 5 |
| Iowa | 18 | 5 | 7 | 2 | 3 | 0 | 0 | 1 |
| Kansas | 18 | 3 | 6 | 1 | 0 | 1 | 2 | 5 |
| Kentucky | 25 | 7 | 5 | 6 | 4 | 0 | 1 | 2 |
| Louisiana | 43 | 11 | 14 | 5 | 2 | 1 | 2 | 8 |
| Maine | 9 | 0 | 1 | 4 | 2 | 0 | 0 | 2 |
| Maryland | 67 | 16 | 29 | 6 | 4 | 2 | 7 | 3 |
| Massachusetts | 89 | 13 | 50 | 9 | 4 | 0 | 1 | 12 |
| Michigan | 83 | 21 | 33 | 10 | 2 | 3 | 6 | 8 |
| Minnesota | 55 | 10 | 26 | 7 | 0 | 2 | 4 | 6 |
| Mississippi | 35 | 14 | 8 | 2 | 0 | 5 | 1 | 5 |
| Missouri | 37 | 10 | 11 | 6 | 4 | 2 | 1 | 3 |
| Montana | 4 | 2 | 0 | 1 | 0 | 0 | 0 | 1 |
| Nebraska | 7 | 0 | 5 | 0 | 0 | 0 | 0 | 2 |
| Nevada | 15 | 3 | 6 | 2 | 0 | 1 | 1 | 2 |
| New Hampshire | 3 | 0 | 1 | 0 | 1 | 0 | 0 | 1 |
| New Jersey | 141 | 17 | 76 | 21 | 8 | 2 | 4 | 13 |
| New Mexico | 7 | 4 | 2 | 1 | 0 | 0 | 0 | 0 |
| New York | 373 | 64 | 167 | 40 | 19 | 26 | 15 | 42 |
| North Carolina | 85 | 30 | 19 | 10 | 5 | 7 | 3 | 11 |
| North Dakota | 3 | 1 | 0 | 0 | 1 | 0 | 0 | 1 |
| Ohio | 81 | 16 | 26 | 12 | 4 | 4 | 3 | 16 |
| Oklahoma | 39 | 7 | 22 | 3 | 0 | 2 | 2 | 3 |
| Oregon | 32 | 3 | 12 | 6 | 4 | 1 | 2 | 4 |
| Pennsylvania | 106 | 21 | 47 | 9 | 11 | 3 | 3 | 12 |
| Rhode Island | 19 | 1 | 11 | 0 | 0 | 0 | 0 | 7 |
| South Carolina | 67 | 28 | 18 | 2 | 4 | 1 | 3 | 11 |
| South Dakota | 6 | 1 | 0 | 0 | 1 | 2 | 2 | 0 |
| Tennessee | 60 | 19 | 18 | 2 | 3 | 5 | 3 | 10 |
| Texas | 306 | 73 | 117 | 29 | 19 | 23 | 9 | 36 |
| Utah | 12 | 1 | 5 | 1 | 2 | 0 | 1 | 2 |
| Vermont | 1 | 0 | 1 | 0 | 0 | 0 | 0 | 0 |
| Virginia | 71 | 18 | 37 | 2 | 3 | 5 | 2 | 4 |
| Washington | 60 | 12 | 29 | 8 | 2 | 1 | 2 | 6 |
| West Virginia | 5 | 0 | 0 | 1 | 3 | 0 | 0 | 1 |
| Wisconsin | 26 | 3 | 9 | 4 | 4 | 1 | 0 | 5 |
| Wyoming | 0 | 0 | 0 | 0 | 0 | 0 | 0 | 0 |
| American Samoa[a] | 1 | 0 | 1 | 0 | 0 | 0 | 0 | 0 |
| Fed. States of Micronesia[a] | ... | ... | ... | ... | ... | ... | ... | ... |
| Guam[a] | 3 | 2 | 1 | 0 | 0 | 0 | 0 | 0 |
| N. Mariana Islands[a] | 5 | 1 | 4 | 0 | 0 | 0 | 0 | 0 |
| Puerto Rico[a] | 22 | 9 | 7 | 3 | 1 | 0 | 0 | 2 |
| Republic of Palau[a] | 2 | 0 | 0 | 1 | 1 | 0 | 0 | 0 |
| U.S. Virgin Islands[a] | ... | ... | ... | ... | ... | ... | ... | ... |

[a]Not included in U.S. totals.

Ellipses indicate data not available.

*Source*: Centers for Disease Control and Prevention, U.S. Department of Health and Human Services. National Center for HIV, STD, and TB Prevention, Division of Tuberculosis Elimination. *Reported Tuberculosis in the United States, 1999* (Atlanta, GA: CDC, 2000).

## Table E4.1. Tuberculosis Cases in Residents of Correctional Facilities: 59 Reporting Areas, 1999

| Reporting Area | Total Cases | Cases with Information on Residence in Correctional Facilities No. | % | Percent of Cases in Residents of Correctional Facilities[a] |
|---|---|---|---|---|
| **United States** | **17,531** | **17,462** | **99.6** | **3.3** |
| Alabama | 314 | 314 | 100.0 | 2.2 |
| Alaska | 61 | 61 | 100.0 | 1.6 |
| Arizona | 262 | 262 | 100.0 | 6.9 |
| Arkansas | 181 | 180 | 99.4 | 5.0 |
| California | 3,606 | 3,597 | 99.8 | 3.3 |
| Colorado | 88 | 88 | 100.0 | 0.0 |
| Connecticut | 121 | 120 | 99.2 | 1.7 |
| Delaware | 34 | 33 | 97.1 | 0.0 |
| District of Columbia | 70 | 70 | 100.0 | 4.3 |
| Florida | 1,277 | 1,277 | 100.0 | 3.7 |
| Georgia | 665 | 652 | 98.0 | 3.2 |
| Hawaii | 184 | 181 | 98.4 | 2.8 |
| Idaho | 16 | 16 | 100.0 | 6.3 |
| Illinois | 825 | 818 | 99.2 | 2.2 |
| Indiana | 150 | 147 | 98.0 | 1.4 |
| Iowa | 58 | 54 | 93.1 | 0.0 |
| Kansas | 69 | 68 | 98.6 | 1.5 |
| Kentucky | 209 | 209 | 100.0 | 4.8 |
| Louisiana | 357 | 355 | 99.4 | 2.5 |
| Maine | 23 | 23 | 100.0 | 0.0 |
| Maryland | 294 | 294 | 100.0 | 2.7 |
| Massachusetts | 270 | 270 | 100.0 | 0.4 |
| Michigan | 351 | 351 | 100.0 | 2.3 |
| Minnesota | 201 | 201 | 100.0 | 2.0 |
| Mississippi | 215 | 215 | 100.0 | 1.4 |
| Missouri | 208 | 205 | 98.6 | 3.4 |
| Montana | 14 | 14 | 100.0 | 0.0 |
| Nebraska | 18 | 18 | 100.0 | 0.0 |
| Nevada | 93 | 92 | 98.9 | 5.4 |
| New Hampshire | 19 | 19 | 100.0 | 0.0 |
| New Jersey | 571 | 571 | 100.0 | 1.2 |
| New Mexico | 64 | 64 | 100.0 | 1.6 |
| New York State[b] | 377 | 376 | 99.7 | 5.9 |
| New York City | 1,460 | 1,460 | 100.0 | 2.8 |
| North Carolina | 488 | 488 | 100.0 | 2.3 |
| North Dakota | 7 | 7 | 100.0 | 0.0 |
| Ohio | 317 | 315 | 99.4 | 2.2 |
| Oklahoma | 208 | 208 | 100.0 | 6.7 |
| Oregon | 123 | 122 | 99.2 | 0.8 |
| Pennsylvania | 454 | 440 | 96.9 | 1.8 |
| Rhode Island | 53 | 52 | 98.1 | 1.9 |
| South Carolina | 315 | 314 | 99.7 | 7.6 |
| South Dakota | 21 | 21 | 100.0 | 0.0 |
| Tennessee | 382 | 382 | 100.0 | 3.4 |
| Texas | 1,649 | 1,649 | 100.0 | 6.2 |
| Utah | 40 | 40 | 100.0 | 2.5 |
| Vermont | 3 | 3 | 100.0 | 0.0 |
| Virginia | 334 | 334 | 100.0 | 2.1 |
| Washington | 258 | 258 | 100.0 | 1.6 |
| West Virginia | 41 | 41 | 100.0 | 0.0 |
| Wisconsin | 110 | 110 | 100.0 | 2.7 |
| Wyoming | 3 | 3 | 100.0 | 33.3 |
| American Samoa[c] | 4 | 4 | 100.0 | 0.0 |
| Fed. States of Micronesia[c] | ... | ... | ... | ... |
| Guam[c] | 69 | 69 | 100.0 | 1.4 |
| N. Mariana Islands[c] | 66 | 66 | 100.0 | 1.5 |
| Puerto Rico[c] | 200 | 200 | 100.0 | 6.5 |
| Republic of Palau[c] | 11 | 11 | 100.0 | 18.2 |
| U.S. Virgin Islands[c] | ... | ... | ... | ... |

[a]Resident of correctional facility at time of diagnosis. Percentage for U.S. based on 52 reporting areas (50 states, New York City, and the District of Columbia). Percentages shown only for reporting areas with information reported for >75% of cases.

[b]Excludes New York City.

[c]Not included in U.S. totals.

Ellipses indicate data not available.

*Source*: Centers for Disease Control and Prevention, U.S. Department of Health and Human Services. National Center for HIV, STD, and TB Prevention, Division of Tuberculosis Elimination. *Reported Tuberculosis in the United States, 1999* (Atlanta, GA: CDC, 2000).

## Table E4.2. Tuberculosis Cases in Residents of Long-Term Care Facilities: 59 Reporting Areas, 1999

| Reporting Area | Total Cases | Cases with Information on Residence in Long-term Care Facilities No. | % | Percent of Cases in Residents of Long-term Care Facilities[a] |
|---|---|---|---|---|
| **United States** | **17,531** | **17,466** | **99.6** | **3.0** |
| Alabama | 314 | 314 | 100.0 | 5.4 |
| Alaska | 61 | 61 | 100.0 | 0.0 |
| Arizona | 262 | 262 | 100.0 | 2.7 |
| Arkansas | 181 | 179 | 98.9 | 8.9 |
| California | 3,606 | 3,599 | 99.8 | 2.1 |
| Colorado | 88 | 88 | 100.0 | 3.4 |
| Connecticut | 121 | 120 | 99.2 | 2.5 |
| Delaware | 34 | 34 | 100.0 | 2.9 |
| District of Columbia | 70 | 70 | 100.0 | 4.3 |
| Florida | 1,277 | 1,277 | 100.0 | 2.0 |
| Georgia | 665 | 651 | 97.9 | 2.5 |
| Hawaii | 184 | 184 | 100.0 | 1.1 |
| Idaho | 16 | 16 | 100.0 | 6.3 |
| Illinois | 825 | 816 | 98.9 | 4.4 |
| Indiana | 150 | 149 | 99.3 | 2.7 |
| Iowa | 58 | 52 | 89.7 | 1.9 |
| Kansas | 69 | 68 | 98.6 | 5.9 |
| Kentucky | 209 | 209 | 100.0 | 9.1 |
| Louisiana | 357 | 355 | 99.4 | 2.8 |
| Maine | 23 | 23 | 100.0 | 17.4 |
| Maryland | 294 | 293 | 99.7 | 2.4 |
| Massachusetts | 270 | 270 | 100.0 | 3.7 |
| Michigan | 351 | 351 | 100.0 | 2.6 |
| Minnesota | 201 | 201 | 100.0 | 1.0 |
| Mississippi | 215 | 215 | 100.0 | 3.7 |
| Missouri | 208 | 205 | 98.6 | 8.8 |
| Montana | 14 | 14 | 100.0 | 7.1 |
| Nebraska | 18 | 18 | 100.0 | 5.6 |
| Nevada | 93 | 92 | 98.9 | 0.0 |
| New Hampshire | 19 | 19 | 100.0 | 5.3 |
| New Jersey | 571 | 571 | 100.0 | 2.1 |
| New Mexico | 64 | 64 | 100.0 | 3.1 |
| New York State[b] | 377 | 377 | 100.0 | 4.2 |
| New York City | 1,460 | 1,458 | 99.9 | 1.4 |
| North Carolina | 488 | 488 | 100.0 | 4.9 |
| North Dakota | 7 | 7 | 100.0 | 14.3 |
| Ohio | 317 | 315 | 99.4 | 5.7 |
| Oklahoma | 208 | 208 | 100.0 | 2.4 |
| Oregon | 123 | 122 | 99.2 | 9.0 |
| Pennsylvania | 454 | 445 | 98.0 | 6.1 |
| Rhode Island | 53 | 52 | 98.1 | 1.9 |
| South Carolina | 315 | 314 | 99.7 | 2.5 |
| South Dakota | 21 | 21 | 100.0 | 9.5 |
| Tennessee | 382 | 381 | 99.7 | 3.4 |
| Texas | 1,649 | 1,649 | 100.0 | 2.5 |
| Utah | 40 | 40 | 100.0 | 2.5 |
| Vermont | 3 | 3 | 100.0 | 0.0 |
| Virginia | 334 | 334 | 100.0 | 1.8 |
| Washington | 258 | 258 | 100.0 | 3.1 |
| West Virginia | 41 | 41 | 100.0 | 0.0 |
| Wisconsin | 110 | 110 | 100.0 | 4.5 |
| Wyoming | 3 | 3 | 100.0 | 0.0 |
| American Samoa[c] | 4 | 4 | 100.0 | 0.0 |
| Fed. States of Micronesia[c] | ... | ... | ... | ... |
| Guam[c] | 69 | 69 | 100.0 | 0.0 |
| N. Mariana Islands[c] | 66 | 66 | 100.0 | 0.0 |
| Puerto Rico[c] | 200 | 200 | 100.0 | 3.0 |
| Republic of Palau[c] | 11 | 11 | 100.0 | 0.0 |
| U.S. Virgin Islands[c] | ... | ... | ... | ... |

[a]Resident of long-term care facility at time of diagnosis. Percentage for U.S. based on 52 reporting areas (50 states, New York City, and the District of Columbia). Percentages shown only for reporting areas with information reported for >75% of cases.

[b]Excludes New York City.

[c]Not included in U.S. totals.

Ellipses indicate data not available.

*Source*: Centers for Disease Control and Prevention, U.S. Department of Health and Human Services. National Center for HIV, STD, and TB Prevention, Division of Tuberculosis Elimination. *Reported Tuberculosis in the United States, 1999* (Atlanta, GA: CDC, 2000).

## Table E4.3. Tuberculosis Cases by Homeless Status: 59 Reporting Areas, 1999

| Reporting Area | Total Cases | Cases with Information on Homeless Status No. | Cases with Information on Homeless Status % | Percent of Cases in Homeless Persons[a] |
|---|---|---|---|---|
| **United States** | **17,531** | **16,808** | **95.9** | **6.3** |
| Alabama | 314 | 312 | 99.4 | 3.8 |
| Alaska | 61 | 61 | 100.0 | 3.3 |
| Arizona | 262 | 258 | 98.5 | 14.0 |
| Arkansas | 181 | 180 | 75.0 | 3.9 |
| California | 3,606 | 3,554 | 98.6 | 6.6 |
| Colorado | 88 | 88 | 100.0 | 12.5 |
| Connecticut | 121 | 119 | 98.3 | 9.2 |
| Delaware | 34 | 34 | 100.0 | 2.9 |
| District of Columbia | 70 | 70 | 100.0 | 14.3 |
| Florida | 1,277 | 1,276 | 99.9 | 8.7 |
| Georgia | 665 | 632 | 95.0 | 7.0 |
| Hawaii | 184 | 184 | 100.0 | 0.0 |
| Idaho | 16 | 15 | 93.8 | 6.7 |
| Illinois | 825 | 796 | 96.5 | 6.7 |
| Indiana | 150 | 133 | 88.7 | 3.0 |
| Iowa | 58 | 48 | 82.8 | 6.3 |
| Kansas | 69 | 64 | 92.8 | 1.6 |
| Kentucky | 209 | 205 | 98.1 | 12.2 |
| Louisiana | 357 | 350 | 98.0 | 5.7 |
| Maine | 23 | 23 | 100.0 | 8.7 |
| Maryland | 294 | 293 | 99.7 | 3.1 |
| Massachusetts | 270 | 269 | 99.6 | 4.5 |
| Michigan | 351 | 342 | 97.4 | 3.5 |
| Minnesota | 201 | 201 | 100.0 | 3.0 |
| Mississippi | 215 | 215 | 100.0 | 1.4 |
| Missouri | 208 | 197 | 94.7 | 14.2 |
| Montana | 14 | 14 | 100.0 | 35.7 |
| Nebraska | 18 | 18 | 100.0 | 11.1 |
| Nevada | 93 | 92 | 98.9 | 8.7 |
| New Hampshire | 19 | 18 | 94.7 | 0.0 |
| New Jersey | 571 | 571 | 100.0 | 5.3 |
| New Mexico | 64 | 64 | 100.0 | 7.8 |
| New York State[b] | 377 | 372 | 98.7 | 1.9 |
| New York City | 1,460 | 987 | 67.6 | -- |
| North Carolina | 488 | 486 | 99.6 | 7.0 |
| North Dakota | 7 | 6 | 85.7 | 16.7 |
| Ohio | 317 | 313 | 98.7 | 7.3 |
| Oklahoma | 208 | 208 | 100.0 | 11.1 |
| Oregon | 123 | 121 | 98.4 | 10.7 |
| Pennsylvania | 454 | 423 | 93.2 | 2.1 |
| Rhode Island | 53 | 52 | 98.1 | 0.0 |
| South Carolina | 315 | 314 | 99.7 | 3.8 |
| South Dakota | 21 | 21 | 100.0 | 14.3 |
| Tennessee | 382 | 376 | 98.4 | 7.4 |
| Texas | 1,649 | 1,649 | 100.0 | 6.6 |
| Utah | 40 | 40 | 100.0 | 17.5 |
| Vermont | 3 | 3 | 100.0 | 0.0 |
| Virginia | 334 | 334 | 100.0 | 2.7 |
| Washington | 258 | 257 | 99.6 | 6.2 |
| West Virginia | 41 | 37 | 90.2 | 13.5 |
| Wisconsin | 110 | 110 | 100.0 | 4.5 |
| Wyoming | 3 | 3 | 100.0 | 0.0 |
| American Samoa[c] | 4 | 4 | 100.0 | 0.0 |
| Fed. States of Micronesia[c] | ... | ... | ... | ... |
| Guam[c] | 69 | 69 | 100.0 | 0.0 |
| N. Mariana Islands[c] | 66 | 66 | 100.0 | 0.0 |
| Puerto Rico[c] | 200 | 200 | 100.0 | 3.0 |
| Republic of Palau[c] | 11 | 11 | 100.0 | 0.0 |
| U.S. Virgin Islands[c] | ... | ... | ... | ... |

[a]Homeless within past 12 months. Percentage for U.S. based on 52 reporting areas (50 states, New York City, and the District of Columbia). Percentages shown only for reporting areas with information reported for >75% of cases.

[b]Excludes New York City.

[c]Not included in U.S. totals.

Ellipses indicate data not available.

*Source*: Centers for Disease Control and Prevention, U.S. Department of Health and Human Services. National Center for HIV, STD, and TB Prevention, Division of Tuberculosis Elimination. *Reported Tuberculosis in the United States, 1999* (Atlanta, GA: CDC, 2000).

## Table E4.4. Tuberculosis Cases by Injecting Drug Use: 59 Reporting Areas, 1999

| Reporting Area | Total Cases | Cases with Information on Injecting Drug Use | | Percent of Cases in Injecting Drug Users[a] |
|---|---|---|---|---|
| | | No. | % | |
| **United States** | **17,531** | **16,331** | **93.2** | **2.6** |
| Alabama | 314 | 280 | 89.2 | 1.8 |
| Alaska | 61 | 50 | 82.0 | 0.0 |
| Arizona | 262 | 251 | 95.8 | 4.0 |
| Arkansas | 181 | 176 | 97.2 | 0.0 |
| California | 3,606 | 3,438 | 95.3 | 2.7 |
| Colorado | 88 | 87 | 98.9 | 1.1 |
| Connecticut | 121 | 112 | 92.6 | 3.6 |
| Delaware | 34 | 34 | 100.0 | 0.0 |
| District of Columbia | 70 | 67 | 95.7 | 6.0 |
| Florida | 1,277 | 1,218 | 95.4 | 1.7 |
| Georgia | 665 | 517 | 77.7 | 1.4 |
| Hawaii | 184 | 165 | 89.7 | 0.6 |
| Idaho | 16 | 14 | 87.5 | 0.0 |
| Illinois | 825 | 648 | 78.5 | 4.5 |
| Indiana | 150 | 138 | 92.0 | 2.9 |
| Iowa | 58 | 25 | 43.1 | -- |
| Kansas | 69 | 60 | 87.0 | 3.3 |
| Kentucky | 209 | 199 | 95.2 | 1.5 |
| Louisiana | 357 | 325 | 91.0 | 5.8 |
| Maine | 23 | 22 | 95.7 | 0.0 |
| Maryland | 294 | 285 | 96.9 | 3.9 |
| Massachusetts | 270 | 237 | 87.8 | 2.5 |
| Michigan | 351 | 331 | 94.3 | 1.8 |
| Minnesota | 201 | 200 | 99.5 | 1.0 |
| Mississippi | 215 | 215 | 100.0 | 0.5 |
| Missouri | 208 | 192 | 92.3 | 3.1 |
| Montana | 14 | 14 | 100.0 | 14.3 |
| Nebraska | 18 | 18 | 100.0 | 0.0 |
| Nevada | 93 | 92 | 98.9 | 1.1 |
| New Hampshire | 19 | 18 | 94.7 | 0.0 |
| New Jersey | 571 | 567 | 99.3 | 5.3 |
| New Mexico | 64 | 60 | 93.8 | 0.0 |
| New York State[b] | 377 | 356 | 94.4 | 0.8 |
| New York City | 1,460 | 1,320 | 90.4 | 3.2 |
| North Carolina | 488 | 482 | 98.8 | 0.4 |
| North Dakota | 7 | 5 | 71.4 | -- |
| Ohio | 317 | 293 | 92.4 | 1.7 |
| Oklahoma | 208 | 206 | 99.0 | 5.8 |
| Oregon | 123 | 117 | 95.1 | 1.7 |
| Pennsylvania | 454 | 370 | 81.5 | 5.7 |
| Rhode Island | 53 | 52 | 98.1 | 1.9 |
| South Carolina | 315 | 285 | 90.5 | 0.7 |
| South Dakota | 21 | 21 | 100.0 | 0.0 |
| Tennessee | 382 | 370 | 96.9 | 1.9 |
| Texas | 1,649 | 1,632 | 99.0 | 3.1 |
| Utah | 40 | 39 | 97.5 | 5.1 |
| Vermont | 3 | 1 | 33.3 | -- |
| Virginia | 334 | 334 | 100.0 | 0.3 |
| Washington | 258 | 253 | 98.1 | 1.6 |
| West Virginia | 41 | 30 | 73.2 | -- |
| Wisconsin | 110 | 108 | 98.2 | 2.8 |
| Wyoming | 3 | 2 | 66.7 | -- |
| American Samoa[c] | 4 | 4 | 100.0 | 0.0 |
| Fed. States of Micronesia[c] | ... | ... | ... | ... |
| Guam[c] | 69 | 67 | 97.1 | 0.0 |
| N. Mariana Islands[c] | 66 | 66 | 100.0 | 0.0 |
| Puerto Rico[c] | 200 | 198 | 99.0 | 19.2 |
| Republic of Palau[c] | 11 | 7 | 63.6 | -- |
| U.S. Virgin Islands[c] | ... | ... | ... | ... |

[a]Injecting drug use within past 12 months. Percentage for U.S. based on 52 reporting areas (50 states, New York City, and the District of Columbia). Percentages shown only for reporting areas with information reported for >75% of cases.

[b]Excludes New York City.

[c]Not included in U.S. totals.

Ellipses indicate data not available.

*Source*: Centers for Disease Control and Prevention, U.S. Department of Health and Human Services. National Center for HIV, STD, and TB Prevention, Division of Tuberculosis Elimination. *Reported Tuberculosis in the United States, 1999* (Atlanta, GA: CDC, 2000).

## Table E4.5. Tuberculosis Cases by Noninjecting Drug Use: 59 Reporting Areas, 1999

| Reporting Area | Total Cases | Cases with Information on Noninjecting Drug Use | | Percent of Cases in Noninjecting Drug Users[a] |
|---|---|---|---|---|
| | | No. | % | |
| **United States** | **17,531** | **16,232** | **92.6** | **7.1** |
| Alabama | 314 | 275 | 87.6 | 5.1 |
| Alaska | 61 | 50 | 82.0 | 12.0 |
| Arizona | 262 | 250 | 95.4 | 8.0 |
| Arkansas | 181 | 176 | 97.2 | 0.6 |
| California | 3,606 | 3,425 | 95.0 | 6.7 |
| Colorado | 88 | 87 | 98.9 | 5.7 |
| Connecticut | 121 | 109 | 90.1 | 6.4 |
| Delaware | 34 | 33 | 97.1 | 0.0 |
| District of Columbia | 70 | 67 | 95.7 | 11.9 |
| Florida | 1,277 | 1,218 | 95.4 | 12.2 |
| Georgia | 665 | 514 | 77.3 | 11.3 |
| Hawaii | 184 | 164 | 89.1 | 0.0 |
| Idaho | 16 | 13 | 81.3 | 7.7 |
| Illinois | 825 | 635 | 77.0 | 10.2 |
| Indiana | 150 | 136 | 90.7 | 3.7 |
| Iowa | 58 | 23 | 39.7 | -- |
| Kansas | 69 | 63 | 91.3 | 9.5 |
| Kentucky | 209 | 198 | 94.7 | 7.6 |
| Louisiana | 357 | 323 | 90.5 | 13.0 |
| Maine | 23 | 22 | 95.7 | 0.0 |
| Maryland | 294 | 280 | 95.2 | 6.1 |
| Massachusetts | 270 | 233 | 86.3 | 3.9 |
| Michigan | 351 | 329 | 93.7 | 4.6 |
| Minnesota | 201 | 199 | 99.0 | 3.5 |
| Mississippi | 215 | 214 | 99.5 | 5.6 |
| Missouri | 208 | 192 | 92.3 | 9.9 |
| Montana | 14 | 14 | 100.0 | 21.4 |
| Nebraska | 18 | 18 | 100.0 | 0.0 |
| Nevada | 93 | 91 | 97.8 | 1.1 |
| New Hampshire | 19 | 18 | 94.7 | 0.0 |
| New Jersey | 571 | 566 | 99.1 | 7.4 |
| New Mexico | 64 | 60 | 93.8 | 0.0 |
| New York State[b] | 377 | 352 | 93.4 | 4.3 |
| New York City | 1,460 | 1,318 | 90.3 | 8.7 |
| North Carolina | 488 | 473 | 96.9 | 10.6 |
| North Dakota | 7 | 5 | 71.4 | -- |
| Ohio | 317 | 289 | 91.2 | 7.3 |
| Oklahoma | 208 | 205 | 98.6 | 4.9 |
| Oregon | 123 | 113 | 91.9 | 6.2 |
| Pennsylvania | 454 | 359 | 79.1 | 5.8 |
| Rhode Island | 53 | 52 | 98.1 | 5.8 |
| South Carolina | 315 | 283 | 89.8 | 8.5 |
| South Dakota | 21 | 21 | 100.0 | 0.0 |
| Tennessee | 382 | 370 | 96.9 | 8.6 |
| Texas | 1,649 | 1,632 | 99.0 | 5.0 |
| Utah | 40 | 39 | 97.5 | 7.7 |
| Vermont | 3 | 1 | 33.3 | -- |
| Virginia | 334 | 334 | 100.0 | 0.9 |
| Washington | 258 | 250 | 96.9 | 2.8 |
| West Virginia | 41 | 31 | 75.6 | 3.2 |
| Wisconsin | 110 | 108 | 98.2 | 4.6 |
| Wyoming | 3 | 2 | 66.7 | -- |
| American Samoa[c] | 4 | 4 | 100.0 | 0.0 |
| Fed. States of Micronesia[c] | ... | ... | ... | ... |
| Guam[c] | 69 | 65 | 94.2 | 1.5 |
| N. Mariana Islands[c] | 66 | 66 | 100.0 | 0.0 |
| Puerto Rico[c] | 200 | 198 | 99.0 | 16.2 |
| Republic of Palau[c] | 11 | 8 | 72.7 | -- |
| U.S. Virgin Islands[c] | ... | ... | ... | ... |

[a]Noninjecting drug use within past 12 months. Percentage for U.S. based on 52 reporting areas (50 states, New York City, and the District of Columbia). Percentages shown only for reporting areas with information reported for >75% of cases.

[b]Excludes New York City.

[c]Not included in U.S. totals.

Ellipses indicate data not available.

*Source*: Centers for Disease Control and Prevention, U.S. Department of Health and Human Services. National Center for HIV, STD, and TB Prevention, Division of Tuberculosis Elimination. *Reported Tuberculosis in the United States, 1999* (Atlanta, GA: CDC, 2000).

## Table E4.6. Tuberculosis Cases by Excess Alcohol Use: 59 Reporting Areas, 1999

| Reporting Area | Total Cases | Cases with Information on Excess Alcohol Use | | Percent of Cases in Persons with Excess Alcohol Use[a] |
|---|---|---|---|---|
| | | No. | % | |
| **United States** | **17,531** | **16,328** | **93.1** | **15.5** |
| Alabama | 314 | 278 | 88.5 | 18.3 |
| Alaska | 61 | 55 | 90.2 | 43.6 |
| Arizona | 262 | 252 | 96.2 | 21.0 |
| Arkansas | 181 | 177 | 97.8 | 10.2 |
| California | 3,606 | 3,433 | 95.2 | 12.2 |
| Colorado | 88 | 88 | 100.0 | 8.0 |
| Connecticut | 121 | 110 | 90.9 | 13.6 |
| Delaware | 34 | 33 | 97.1 | 9.1 |
| District of Columbia | 70 | 67 | 95.7 | 19.4 |
| Florida | 1,277 | 1,218 | 95.4 | 24.3 |
| Georgia | 665 | 532 | 80.0 | 19.4 |
| Hawaii | 184 | 172 | 93.5 | 6.4 |
| Idaho | 16 | 16 | 100.0 | 37.5 |
| Illinois | 825 | 636 | 77.1 | 20.6 |
| Indiana | 150 | 140 | 93.3 | 3.6 |
| Iowa | 58 | 27 | 46.6 | -- |
| Kansas | 69 | 63 | 91.3 | 17.5 |
| Kentucky | 209 | 201 | 96.2 | 18.9 |
| Louisiana | 357 | 320 | 89.6 | 27.8 |
| Maine | 23 | 22 | 95.7 | 0.0 |
| Maryland | 294 | 284 | 96.6 | 8.5 |
| Massachusetts | 270 | 232 | 85.9 | 7.8 |
| Michigan | 351 | 326 | 92.9 | 8.3 |
| Minnesota | 201 | 198 | 98.5 | 9.1 |
| Mississippi | 215 | 215 | 100.0 | 25.6 |
| Missouri | 208 | 191 | 91.8 | 20.9 |
| Montana | 14 | 14 | 100.0 | 42.9 |
| Nebraska | 18 | 18 | 100.0 | 5.6 |
| Nevada | 93 | 92 | 98.9 | 8.7 |
| New Hampshire | 19 | 19 | 100.0 | 10.5 |
| New Jersey | 571 | 568 | 99.5 | 14.1 |
| New Mexico | 64 | 60 | 93.8 | 16.7 |
| New York State[b] | 377 | 353 | 93.6 | 8.2 |
| New York City | 1,460 | 1,321 | 90.5 | 12.3 |
| North Carolina | 488 | 475 | 97.3 | 27.2 |
| North Dakota | 7 | 5 | 71.4 | -- |
| Ohio | 317 | 295 | 93.1 | 15.6 |
| Oklahoma | 208 | 206 | 99.0 | 14.6 |
| Oregon | 123 | 114 | 92.7 | 15.8 |
| Pennsylvania | 454 | 363 | 80.0 | 13.8 |
| Rhode Island | 53 | 52 | 98.1 | 7.7 |
| South Carolina | 315 | 287 | 91.1 | 27.9 |
| South Dakota | 21 | 21 | 100.0 | 38.1 |
| Tennessee | 382 | 366 | 95.8 | 18.3 |
| Texas | 1,649 | 1,636 | 99.2 | 15.3 |
| Utah | 40 | 39 | 97.5 | 20.5 |
| Vermont | 3 | 2 | 66.7 | -- |
| Virginia | 334 | 334 | 100.0 | 3.6 |
| Washington | 258 | 253 | 98.1 | 7.5 |
| West Virginia | 41 | 37 | 90.2 | 29.7 |
| Wisconsin | 110 | 110 | 100.0 | 13.6 |
| Wyoming | 3 | 2 | 66.7 | -- |
| American Samoa[c] | 4 | 3 | 75.0 | 0.0 |
| Fed. States of Micronesia[c] | ... | ... | ... | ... |
| Guam[c] | 69 | 64 | 92.8 | 3.1 |
| N. Mariana Islands[c] | 66 | 65 | 98.5 | 13.8 |
| Puerto Rico[c] | 200 | 198 | 99.0 | 15.7 |
| Republic of Palau[c] | 11 | 7 | 63.6 | -- |
| U.S. Virgin Islands[c] | ... | ... | ... | ... |

[a]Excess alcohol use within past 12 months. Percentage for U.S. based on 52 reporting areas (50 states, New York City, and the District of Columbia). Percentages shown only for reporting areas with information reported for >75% of cases.

[b]Excludes New York City.

[c]Not included in U.S. totals.

Ellipses indicate data not available.

*Source*: Centers for Disease Control and Prevention, U.S. Department of Health and Human Services. National Center for HIV, STD, and TB Prevention, Division of Tuberculosis Elimination. *Reported Tuberculosis in the United States, 1999* (Atlanta, GA: CDC, 2000).

## Table E4.7. Tuberculosis Cases by Occupation: 59 Reporting Areas, 1999

| Reporting Area | Total Cases | Cases with Information on Occupation | | Percent of Cases by Occupation[a] | | | | | |
|---|---|---|---|---|---|---|---|---|---|
| | | No. | % | Unemployed Past 24 Mos. | Health Care Worker | Correctional Employee | Migrant Worker | Other Occupation | Multiple Occupations |
| **United States** | **17,531** | **16,223** | **92.5** | **58.2** | **2.6** | **0.1** | **1.1** | **37.8** | **0.2** |
| Alabama | 314 | 308 | 98.1 | 64.0 | 2.6 | 0.0 | 0.3 | 33.1 | 0.0 |
| Alaska | 61 | 34 | 55.7 | -- | -- | -- | -- | -- | -- |
| Arizona | 262 | 253 | 96.6 | 59.7 | 0.4 | 0.0 | 2.0 | 37.9 | 0.0 |
| Arkansas | 181 | 168 | 92.8 | 75.6 | 3.6 | 0.6 | 0.0 | 20.2 | 0.0 |
| California | 3,606 | 3,430 | 95.1 | 59.4 | 2.1 | 0.2 | 1.8 | 36.5 | 0.1 |
| Colorado | 88 | 88 | 100.0 | 62.5 | 2.3 | 0.0 | 0.0 | 35.2 | 0.0 |
| Connecticut | 121 | 107 | 88.4 | 52.3 | 4.7 | 0.0 | 0.0 | 43.0 | 0.0 |
| Delaware | 34 | 33 | 97.1 | 48.5 | 3.0 | 0.0 | 6.1 | 42.4 | 0.0 |
| District of Columbia | 70 | 70 | 100.0 | 81.4 | 0.0 | 0.0 | 0.0 | 18.6 | 0.0 |
| Florida | 1,277 | 1,245 | 97.5 | 48.9 | 2.1 | 0.2 | 3.3 | 45.1 | 0.5 |
| Georgia | 665 | 554 | 83.3 | 52.3 | 1.4 | 0.4 | 1.8 | 44.0 | 0.0 |
| Hawaii | 184 | 171 | 92.9 | 65.5 | 1.2 | 0.6 | 0.6 | 32.2 | 0.0 |
| Idaho | 16 | 16 | 100.0 | 62.5 | 0.0 | 0.0 | 12.5 | 25.0 | 0.0 |
| Illinois | 825 | 706 | 85.6 | 58.8 | 3.7 | 0.1 | 0.7 | 36.5 | 0.1 |
| Indiana | 150 | 115 | 76.7 | 56.5 | 4.3 | 0.0 | 0.0 | 39.1 | 0.0 |
| Iowa | 58 | 40 | 69.0 | -- | -- | -- | -- | -- | -- |
| Kansas | 69 | 53 | 76.8 | 58.5 | 1.9 | 0.0 | 0.0 | 39.6 | 0.0 |
| Kentucky | 209 | 202 | 96.7 | 63.4 | 3.0 | 0.0 | 3.5 | 30.2 | 0.0 |
| Louisiana | 357 | 329 | 92.2 | 59.3 | 2.7 | 0.0 | 0.0 | 38.0 | 0.0 |
| Maine | 23 | 23 | 100.0 | 65.2 | 4.3 | 0.0 | 0.0 | 30.4 | 0.0 |
| Maryland | 294 | 281 | 95.6 | 56.6 | 3.6 | 0.0 | 0.0 | 39.9 | 0.0 |
| Massachusetts | 270 | 254 | 94.1 | 53.5 | 3.1 | 0.0 | 0.0 | 43.3 | 0.0 |
| Michigan | 351 | 234 | 66.7 | -- | -- | -- | -- | -- | -- |
| Minnesota | 201 | 196 | 97.5 | 59.2 | 5.1 | 0.0 | 1.0 | 34.7 | 0.0 |
| Mississippi | 215 | 213 | 99.1 | 66.2 | 1.4 | 0.5 | 0.9 | 30.5 | 0.5 |
| Missouri | 208 | 190 | 91.3 | 61.1 | 3.7 | 0.0 | 0.0 | 35.3 | 0.0 |
| Montana | 14 | 14 | 100.0 | 71.4 | 0.0 | 0.0 | 0.0 | 28.6 | 0.0 |
| Nebraska | 18 | 18 | 100.0 | 38.9 | 0.0 | 0.0 | 0.0 | 61.1 | 0.0 |
| Nevada | 93 | 90 | 96.8 | 63.3 | 0.0 | 0.0 | 0.0 | 36.7 | 0.0 |
| New Hampshire | 19 | 19 | 100.0 | 42.1 | 5.3 | 0.0 | 0.0 | 52.6 | 0.0 |
| New Jersey | 571 | 570 | 99.8 | 60.2 | 2.5 | 0.0 | 0.5 | 36.3 | 0.5 |
| New Mexico | 64 | 59 | 92.2 | 55.9 | 1.7 | 0.0 | 1.7 | 40.7 | 0.0 |
| New York State[b] | 377 | 348 | 92.3 | 57.5 | 4.0 | 0.3 | 0.6 | 37.4 | 0.3 |
| New York City | 1,460 | 1,289 | 88.3 | 65.6 | 2.9 | 0.2 | 0.0 | 31.3 | 0.1 |
| North Carolina | 488 | 473 | 96.9 | 51.8 | 2.7 | 0.4 | 1.7 | 42.9 | 0.4 |
| North Dakota | 7 | 5 | 71.4 | -- | -- | -- | -- | -- | -- |
| Ohio | 317 | 298 | 94.0 | 64.4 | 3.4 | 0.3 | 0.7 | 31.2 | 0.0 |
| Oklahoma | 208 | 205 | 98.6 | 50.7 | 2.0 | 0.5 | 0.0 | 46.8 | 0.0 |
| Oregon | 123 | 116 | 94.3 | 52.6 | 6.0 | 0.0 | 3.4 | 37.1 | 0.9 |
| Pennsylvania | 454 | 371 | 81.7 | 67.4 | 4.6 | 0.0 | 0.0 | 28.0 | 0.0 |
| Rhode Island | 53 | 52 | 98.1 | 71.2 | 3.8 | 0.0 | 0.0 | 25.0 | 0.0 |
| South Carolina | 315 | 292 | 92.7 | 59.9 | 1.4 | 0.0 | 1.7 | 36.3 | 0.7 |
| South Dakota | 21 | 21 | 100.0 | 71.4 | 9.5 | 0.0 | 0.0 | 19.0 | 0.0 |
| Tennessee | 382 | 358 | 93.7 | 63.7 | 2.0 | 0.0 | 0.0 | 34.4 | 0.0 |
| Texas | 1,649 | 1,538 | 93.3 | 59.8 | 2.1 | 0.1 | 0.7 | 37.1 | 0.2 |
| Utah | 40 | 40 | 100.0 | 67.5 | 2.5 | 0.0 | 0.0 | 30.0 | 0.0 |
| Vermont | 3 | 3 | 100.0 | 33.3 | 0.0 | 0.0 | 0.0 | 66.7 | 0.0 |
| Virginia | 334 | 334 | 100.0 | 36.8 | 3.6 | 0.0 | 0.0 | 59.3 | 0.3 |
| Washington | 258 | 246 | 95.3 | 22.8 | 2.0 | 0.0 | 2.0 | 72.8 | 0.4 |
| West Virginia | 41 | 41 | 100.0 | 87.8 | 0.0 | 0.0 | 0.0 | 12.2 | 0.0 |
| Wisconsin | 110 | 108 | 98.2 | 48.1 | 2.8 | 0.0 | 0.9 | 48.1 | 0.0 |
| Wyoming | 3 | 2 | 66.7 | -- | -- | -- | -- | -- | -- |
| American Samoa[c] | 4 | 3 | 75.0 | 66.7 | 0.0 | 0.0 | 0.0 | 33.3 | 0.0 |
| Fed. States of Micronesia[c] | ... | ... | ... | ... | ... | ... | ... | ... | ... |
| Guam[c] | 69 | 45 | 65.2 | -- | -- | -- | -- | -- | -- |
| N. Mariana Islands[c] | 66 | 66 | 100.0 | 12.1 | 0.0 | 0.0 | 0.0 | 87.9 | 0.0 |
| Puerto Rico[c] | 200 | 199 | 99.5 | 86.9 | 1.0 | 1.0 | 0.0 | 11.1 | 0.0 |
| Republic of Palau[c] | 11 | 8 | 72.7 | -- | -- | -- | -- | -- | -- |
| U.S. Virgin Islands[c] | ... | ... | ... | ... | ... | ... | ... | ... | ... |

[a]Occupation within past 12 months. Percentage for U.S. based on 52 reporting areas (50 states, New York City, and the District of Columbia). Percentages shown only for reporting areas with information reported for >75% of cases.

[b]Excludes New York City.

[c]Not included in U.S. totals.

Ellipses indicate data not available.

*Source*: Centers for Disease Control and Prevention, U.S. Department of Health and Human Services. National Center for HIV, STD, and TB Prevention, Division of Tuberculosis Elimination. *Reported Tuberculosis in the United States, 1999* (Atlanta, GA: CDC, 2000).

## Table E5.1. Number and Percentage of Reported TB Cases with HIV Test Results and with HIV Coinfection, by Age Group: United States, 1993–1998

| Year | 25-44 Years Old | | | | All Ages | | | |
|---|---|---|---|---|---|---|---|---|
| | HIV Test Results[a] | | HIV Positive[b] | | HIV Test Results[a] | | HIV Positive[b] | |
| | No. | (%) | No. | (%) | No. | (%) | No. | (%) |
| 1993 | 4,372 | (46) | 2,786 | (29) | 7,447 | (30) | 3,678 | (15) |
| 1994 | 4,432 | (49) | 2,659 | (29) | 7,869 | (33) | 3,588 | (15) |
| 1995 | 4,266 | (52) | 2,167 | (26) | 8,168 | (36) | 3,031 | (13) |
| 1996 | 4,328 | (57) | 1,856 | (25) | 8,757 | (41) | 2,615 | (12) |
| 1997 | 4,106 | (60) | 1,466 | (21) | 8,715 | (44) | 2,084 | (11) |
| 1998 | 3,837 | (60) | 1,239 | (20) | 8,229 | (45) | 1,824 | (10) |

[a]Rhode Island reported HIV test results during 1998. HIV test results were not reported from California.
California did provide HIV status for TB cases reported during 1993-1998 in persons also reported with AIDS (i.e., HIV-positive). Includes cases with positive, negative, or indeterminate HIV test results and California cases also reported with AIDS. Percentages based on all reported TB cases.
[b]Indicates cases with HIV-positive test results and California cases also reported with AIDS. Percentages based on all reported TB cases.
Note: Data for all years updated through May 3, 2000.
*Source*: Centers for Disease Control and Prevention, U.S. Department of Health and Human Services. National Center for HIV, STD, and TB Prevention, Division of Tuberculosis Elimination. *Reported Tuberculosis in the United States, 1999* (Atlanta, GA: CDC, 2000).

## Table E5.2. Tuberculosis Cases, Aged 25–44, by HIV Status: 59 Reporting Areas, 1999

| Reporting Area | Total Cases | Cases with Information on HIV Status[a] No. | Cases with Information on HIV Status[a] % | Percent of Cases in HIV-Positive Persons[b] |
|---|---|---|---|---|
| **United States** | **6,078** | **3,475** | **57.2** | -- |
| Alabama | 80 | 73 | 91.3 | 11.0 |
| Alaska | 26 | 15 | 57.7 | -- |
| Arizona | 99 | 83 | 83.8 | 12.0 |
| Arkansas | 32 | 25 | 78.1 | 8.0 |
| California | 1,161 | ... | ... | ... |
| Colorado | 26 | 23 | 88.5 | 8.7 |
| Connecticut | 45 | 32 | 71.1 | -- |
| Delaware | 15 | 11 | 73.3 | -- |
| District of Columbia | 30 | 30 | 100.0 | 43.3 |
| Florida | 516 | 444 | 86.0 | 44.1 |
| Georgia | 251 | 193 | 76.9 | 35.8 |
| Hawaii | 46 | 3 | 6.5 | -- |
| Idaho | 5 | 4 | 80.0 | 0.0 |
| Illinois | 295 | 110 | 37.3 | -- |
| Indiana | 42 | 13 | 31.0 | -- |
| Iowa | 30 | 12 | 40.0 | -- |
| Kansas | 27 | 18 | 66.7 | -- |
| Kentucky | 58 | 42 | 72.4 | -- |
| Louisiana | 114 | 101 | 88.6 | 24.8 |
| Maine | 5 | 0 | 0.0 | -- |
| Maryland | 109 | 89 | 81.7 | 21.3 |
| Massachusetts | 114 | 58 | 50.9 | -- |
| Michigan | 112 | 39 | 34.8 | -- |
| Minnesota | 67 | 44 | 65.7 | -- |
| Mississippi | 45 | 44 | 97.8 | 6.8 |
| Missouri | 66 | 55 | 83.3 | 10.9 |
| Montana | 1 | 1 | 100.0 | 0.0 |
| Nebraska | 8 | 2 | 25.0 | -- |
| Nevada | 25 | 25 | 100.0 | 16.0 |
| New Hampshire | 8 | 5 | 62.5 | -- |
| New Jersey | 225 | 126 | 56.0 | -- |
| New Mexico | 18 | 12 | 66.7 | -- |
| New York State[c] | 143 | 84 | 58.7 | -- |
| New York City | 671 | 506 | 75.4 | 42.5 |
| North Carolina | 165 | 149 | 90.3 | 24.2 |
| North Dakota | 0 | 0 | 0.0 | -- |
| Ohio | 80 | 49 | 61.3 | -- |
| Oklahoma | 70 | 29 | 41.4 | -- |
| Oregon | 38 | 32 | 84.2 | 12.5 |
| Pennsylvania | 123 | 57 | 46.3 | -- |
| Rhode Island | 11 | 3 | 27.3 | -- |
| South Carolina | 107 | 100 | 93.5 | 35.0 |
| South Dakota | 6 | 5 | 83.3 | 0.0 |
| Tennessee | 118 | 94 | 79.7 | 25.5 |
| Texas | 594 | 448 | 75.4 | 30.1 |
| Utah | 10 | 10 | 100.0 | 30.0 |
| Vermont | 0 | 0 | 0.0 | -- |
| Virginia | 114 | 81 | 71.1 | -- |
| Washington | 82 | 57 | 69.5 | -- |
| West Virginia | 3 | 3 | 100.0 | 0.0 |
| Wisconsin | 40 | 34 | 85.0 | 5.9 |
| Wyoming | 2 | 2 | 100.0 | 0.0 |
| American Samoa[d] | 0 | 0 | 0.0 | -- |
| Fed. States of Micronesia[d] | ... | ... | ... | ... |
| Guam[d] | 21 | 4 | 19.0 | -- |
| N. Mariana Islands[d] | 37 | 35 | 94.6 | 2.9 |
| Puerto Rico[d] | 67 | 54 | 80.6 | 77.8 |
| Republic of Palau[d] | 4 | 2 | 50.0 | -- |
| U.S. Virgin Islands[d] | ... | ... | ... | ... |

[a]Includes only those cases with negative, positive, and indeterminate HIV test results.

[b]Percentages shown only for reporting areas with information reported for >75% of cases.

[c]Excludes New York City.

[d]Not included in U.S. totals.

Ellipses indicate data not available.

*Source*: Centers for Disease Control and Prevention, U.S. Department of Health and Human Services. National Center for HIV, STD, and TB Prevention, Division of Tuberculosis Elimination. *Reported Tuberculosis in the United States, 1999* (Atlanta, GA: CDC, 2000).

# F. Foodborne Diseases

## OVERVIEW

Hardly a day passes without news media coverage of one or another foodborne illness, and now there are new fears, that terrorists may tamper with America's food supply. Many bacteria (e.g., *Campylobacter pylori, Escherichia coli* O157:H7, *Salmonella enteritidis*), and viruses (e.g., caliciviruses) cause foodborne illnesses. New pathogens continue to emerge (e.g., *Salmonella typhimurium* DT104, *Salmonella enteritidis* phage type 4). Older conditions also continue to reemerge (e.g., salmonellosis from pet reptiles). Resistance of foodborne pathogens to antimicrobial agents is increasing. Some of the more significant illnesses include amebiasis, botulism, cryptosporidiosis, gastroenteritis, giardiasis, listeriosis, Norwalk-like viruses, salmonellosis, and trichinosis.

Interest in the role of food and milk in outbreaks of intestinal illness has been the basis for public health action for over half a century. The reporting of foodborne diseases in the United States began over 60 years ago, when state and territorial health officers,

> concerned about the high morbidity and mortality caused by typhoid fever and infantile diarrhea, recommended cases of "enteric fever" be investigated and reported. The purpose of the investigation and reporting of these cases was to obtain information regarding the role of food, milk and water in outbreaks of intestinal illness as the basis for public health action. Beginning in 1925, the Public Health Service published summaries of outbreaks of gastrointestinal illness attributed to milk. In 1938, it added summaries of outbreaks caused by all foods. These early surveillance efforts led to the enactment of important public health measures (e.g., the Pasteurized Milk Ordinance) that led to decreased incidence of enteric diseases, particularly those transmitted by milk and water.[1]

A foodborne disease outbreak (FBDO) is defined as the occurrence of two or more cases of a similar illness resulting from the ingestion of a common food. Before 1992, three exceptions existed to this definition; only one case of botulism, marine-toxin intoxication, or chemical intoxication was required to constitute an FBDO if the etiology for that type of FBDO was confirmed. This definition was changed in 1992; currently, two or more cases are required to constitute an outbreak.

## SYMPTOMS AND PATHOLOGIES

More than 250 foodborne diseases have been described. Symptoms vary widely depending on etiologic agent. Gastrointestinal symptoms are the most common, such as pain, nausea, vomiting, and serious diarrhea. The development of muscular symptoms often follows, as does fluid volume deficit. Sometimes infections cause no symptoms. Long-term consequences of infection also vary from disease to disease, as do pathologies.

## DIAGNOSIS

Laboratory or clinical guidelines for confirming an FBDO outbreak vary for bacterial, chemical, parasitic, and viral agents. Outbreaks of unknown etiology are divided into four subgroups according to incubation period of their illness: $<1$ hour (probably chemical poisoning), 1–7 hours (probably *Staphylococcus aureus* or *Bacillus cereus* food poisoning), 8–14 hours (other agents), and greater than or equal to 15 hours (other agents).

## TRANSMISSION

Foodborne diseases are caused by the ingestion of contaminated food, with or without subsequent spread from person to person by the fecal-oral route. All persons are at risk; infants, the elderly, and the immunocompromised are at greatest risk of serious illness and death. Contamination may stem from the consumption of food that has not been cooked sufficiently to kill infection-causing agents, the consumption of unpasteurized milk and juice, and swimming in or drinking sewage-contaminated water. Organisms in diarrheal stools of infected persons can also be passed from one person to another if hygiene or handwashing habits are inadequate.

Outbreak investigations are a critical means of identifying new and emerging pathogens as well as maintaining awareness about ongoing problems. However, the pathogen is not identified in many outbreaks because of delayed or incomplete laboratory investigation, inadequate laboratory capacity, or inability to recognize a pathogen as a cause of foodborne disease. Prompt and thorough investigations of foodborne outbreaks aid in the timely identification of etiologic agents and lead to appropriate prevention and control measures.

## SURVEILLANCE

The CDC currently maintains two types of foodborne disease surveillance systems—one "passive," one "active." Under its passive system, begun in 1973, state and local public health departments have primary responsibility for identifying, investigating, and reporting foodborne disease outbreaks (FBDOs). Clinical laboratories report FBDOs to state health departments, which in turn report to CDC. At the regional and national levels, surveillance data provide an indication of the etiologic agents, vehicles of transmission, and contributing factors associated with FBDOs and help direct public health actions to reduce illness and death caused by FBDOs. This passive system has significant limitations. Only a fraction of the most common foodborne illnesses are routinely reported to CDC, because of the complex reporting system.

In the mid-1990s the CDC established the Foodborne Diseases Active Surveillance Network (FoodNet), an active surveillance system. Under this system public health officials frequently contact laboratory directors to find new cases of foodborne diseases and report these cases electronically to CDC. In addition, FoodNet is designed to monitor each of the events that occurs along the foodborne diseases pyramid[2] and thereby allow more accurate and precise estimates and interpretation of the burden of foodborne diseases over time. FoodNet is a collaborative project of the CDC, the U.S. Department of Agriculture (USDA), the Food and Drug Administration (FDA), and several states. In 1995, FoodNet surveillance began in five locations: California, Connecticut, Georgia, Minnesota, and Oregon. Each year the surveillance area, or catchment, has expanded, with the inclusion of additional counties or additional sites (New York and Maryland in 1998, Tennessee in 2000, and Colorado in 2001). The total population of the current catchment, as of October 5, 2000, was 25.4 million persons, or 10% of the United States population.

Information is being collected on every laboratory-diagnosed case of bacterial pathogens including *Campylobacter, Escherichia coli* O157, *Listeria monocytogenes, Salmonella, Shigella, Yersinia enterocolitica*, and *Vibrio* and on parasitic organisms including *Cryptosporidium* and *Cyclospora* infections among residents of the catchment areas of the nine EIP sites. In addition to collecting laboratory-diagnosed cases of foodborne pathogens, investigators at FoodNet sites began active surveillance for hemolytic uremic syndrome (HUS) (a serious complication of *E. coli* O157 infection), Guillain-Barre syndrome (a serious complication of *Campylobacter* infection) and toxoplasmosis. The result is a comprehensive and timely database of foodborne illness in a well-defined population. FoodNet provides a network for responding to new and emerging foodborne diseases of national importance, monitoring the burden of foodborne diseases, and identifying the sources of specific foodborne diseases.

Foodborne disease surveillance has served three purposes: (1) disease prevention and control; (2) knowledge of disease causation; and (3) administrative guidance. Resulting prevention and control measures include the early identification and removal of contaminated products from the commercial market, the correction of faulty food-preparation practices in food-service establishments and in the home, and the identification and appropriate treatment of human carriers of foodborne pathogens. Despite the fact that the pathogen is not identified in many outbreaks because of delayed or incomplete laboratory investigation, inadequate laboratory capacity, or inability to recognize a pathogen as a cause of foodborne disease, outbreak investigations are considered a critical means of identifying new and emerging pathogens as well as maintaining awareness about ongoing problems. The information derived from investigations of FBDOs enables assessment of trends over time in the prevalence of outbreaks caused by specific etiologic agents, food vehicles, and common errors in food handling. This information provides the basis for regulatory and other changes to improve food safety.

The CDC's system has several limitations. First, the system excludes outbreaks that occur on cruise ships; outbreaks in which food was eaten outside the United States, even if the illness occurred within the United States; and outbreaks that are traced to water intended for drinking. A second limitation is the classification of outbreaks by only one food vehicle. The CDC also does not include FBDOs in the surveillance system if the route of transmission from the contaminated food to the infected persons is indirect. Finally, there are no standard criteria for classifying a death as being FBDO-related. This determination is made by the reporting agency.

From 1951 through 1960, the National Office of Vital Statistics reviewed reports of outbreaks of foodborne illness and published annual summaries in *Public Health Reports*. In 1961, CDC—then the Communicable Disease Center—assumed responsibility for publishing reports concerning foodborne illness. During 1961–1965, CDC discontinued publication of annual reviews but reported pertinent statistics and detailed individual investigations in *MMWR: Morbidity and Mortality Weekly Report*.

In 1966, the present system of surveillance of foodborne and waterborne diseases began with the incorporation of all reports of enteric-disease outbreaks attributed to microbial or chemical contamination of food or water into an annual summary. Since 1978, because of increasing interest and activity in waterborne disease surveillance, foodborne and waterborne disease outbreaks have been reported in separate annual summaries. Summaries of foodborne disease outbreaks (FBDOs) have been published for the years 1983–1987, 1988–1992, and 1993–1997.[3]

## TABLE OVERVIEW

**F1.1–F1.6. Foodborne Diseases by Etiology** This suite of tables shows the number of reported foodborne-disease outbreaks, cases, and death by etiology for 1993 through 1997, the most recent data available. The CDC tables do not isolate data for foodborne disease caused by infectious agents. The tables in this section also include outbreaks and cases traced to chemical agents as well. F1.1 provides totals for the 5-year period; F1.2–F1.6 provide totals for each of the 5 years. During 1993–1997, a total of 2,751 outbreaks of foodborne disease were reported. These outbreaks caused a reported 86,058 persons to become ill. Among outbreaks for which the etiology was determined, bacterial pathogens caused the largest percentage of outbreaks (75%) and the largest percentage of cases (86%). *Salmonella* serotype *enteritis* accounted for the largest number of outbreaks, cases, and deaths; most of these outbreaks were attributed to eating eggs.

**F2.1–F2.5. Foodborne Diseases by Etiology and Month of Occurrence** The next suite of tables shows the number of reported foodborne-disease outbreaks by etiology and month of occurrence for each of the five years between 1993 and 1997. Again, these tables include data on chemical as well as infectious agents. A large portion of the outbreaks occurred from May through November in each of the years included.

**F3.1–F3.5. Foodborne Diseases by Place Where Food Was Eaten** The focus of the next cluster is the place where food was eaten, such as private residence; delicatessen, cafeteria, or restaurant; school; picnic; church; or camp. Primary residences and delicatessens/restaurants account for most outbreaks.

**F4.1–F4.5. Vehicle of Transmission** This cluster offers data on the food source of disease, either individual food items (e.g., milk or eggs) or food categories (e.g., ice cream or multitype vehicles). The value of the data is limited because the CDC identifies only one food vehicle per outbreak.

**F5.1–F5.5. Etiology and Contributing Factors** This cluster presents data on outbreaks by etiology and contributing factors, such as improper holding temperatures, inadequate cooking, contaminated equipment, food from unsafe source, or poor personal hygiene, for 1993 through 1997. Improper holding temperature is the largest contributing factor, followed by poor personal hygiene.

**F6.1–F6.10. Significant Foodborne Diseases** The last cluster in this chapter presents maps and graphs on seven significant foodborne diseases: botulism, Cryptosporidiosis, *E. coli*, hemoloytic uremic syndrome, *salmonella*, Salmoneilosis, *Shigella*, Shigellosis and trichinosis.

## NOTES

1. Sonja J. Olsen et al., "Surveillance for Foodborne-Disease Outbreaks—United States, 1993–1997," *Morbidity and Mortality Weekly Report* 49, no. SS-1 (March 2000): 2.
2. The burden of foodborne diseases pyramid consists of 7 layers or components—exposures in the general population; person becomes ill; person seeks care; specimen obtained; lab tests for organism; culture-confirmed case; reported to health department/CDC. *See* http://www.cdc.gov/foodnet/what_is.htm
3. Centers for Disease Control and Prevention, "Foodborne Disease Outbreaks, 5-Year Summary, 1983–1987," *MMWR: Morbidity and Mortality Weekly Report* 39, no. SS-1 (1990): 15–57; Centers for Disease Control and Prevention, "Surveillance for Foodborne-Disease Outbreaks—United States, 1988–1992," *MMWR: Morbidity and Mortality Weekly Report* 45, no. SS-5 (1996): 1–66; Centers for Disease Control and Prevention, "Surveillance for Foodborne-Disease Outbreaks—United States, 1993–1997," *MMWR: Morbidity and Mortality Weekly Report* 49, no. SS-1 (2000): 1–64.

**Table F1.1. Number of Reported Foodborne-Disease Outbreaks, Cases, and Deaths, by Etiology—United States,* 1993–1997†**

| Etiology | Outbreaks No. | Outbreaks (%) | Cases No. | Cases (%) | Deaths No. | Deaths (%) |
|---|---|---|---|---|---|---|
| **Bacterial** | | | | | | |
| *Bacillus cereus* | 14 | ( 0.5) | 691 | ( 0.8) | 0 | ( 0.0) |
| *Brucella* | 1 | ( 0.0) | 19 | ( 0.0) | 0 | ( 0.0) |
| *Campylobacter* | 25 | ( 0.9) | 539 | ( 0.6) | 1 | ( 3.4) |
| *Clostridium botulinum* | 13 | ( 0.5) | 56 | ( 0.1) | 1 | ( 3.4) |
| *Clostridium perfringens* | 57 | ( 2.1) | 2,772 | ( 3.2) | 0 | ( 0.0) |
| *Escherichia coli* | 84 | ( 3.1) | 3,260 | ( 3.8) | 8 | ( 27.6) |
| *Listeria monocytogenes* | 3 | ( 0.1) | 100 | ( 0.1) | 2 | ( 6.9) |
| *Salmonella* | 357 | ( 13.0) | 32,610 | ( 37.9) | 13 | ( 44.8) |
| *Shigella* | 43 | ( 1.6) | 1,555 | ( 1.8) | 0 | ( 0.0) |
| *Staphylococcus aureus* | 42 | ( 1.5) | 1,413 | ( 1.6) | 1 | ( 3.4) |
| *Streptococcus*, group A | 1 | ( 0.0) | 122 | ( 0.1) | 0 | ( 0.0) |
| *Streptococcus*, other | 1 | ( 0.0) | 6 | ( 0.0) | 0 | ( 0.0) |
| *Vibrio cholerae* | 1 | ( 0.0) | 2 | ( 0.0) | 0 | ( 0.0) |
| *Vibrio parahaemolyticus* | 5 | ( 0.2) | 40 | ( 0.0) | 0 | ( 0.0) |
| *Yersinia enterocolitica* | 2 | ( 0.1) | 27 | ( 0.0) | 1 | ( 3.4) |
| Other bacterial | 6 | ( 0.2) | 609 | ( 0.7) | 1 | ( 3.4) |
| **Total bacterial** | **655** | **( 23.8)** | **43,821** | **( 50.9)** | **28** | **( 96.6)** |
| **Chemical** | | | | | | |
| Ciguatoxin | 60 | ( 2.2) | 205 | ( 0.2) | 0 | ( 0.0) |
| Heavy metals | 4 | ( 0.1) | 17 | ( 0.0) | 0 | ( 0.0) |
| Monosodium glutamate | 1 | ( 0.0) | 2 | ( 0.0) | 0 | ( 0.0) |
| Mushroom poisoning | 7 | ( 0.3) | 21 | ( 0.0) | 0 | ( 0.0) |
| Scombrotoxin | 69 | ( 2.5) | 297 | ( 0.3) | 0 | ( 0.0) |
| Shellfish | 1 | ( 0.0) | 3 | ( 0.0) | 0 | ( 0.0) |
| Other chemical | 6 | ( 0.2) | 31 | ( 0.0) | 0 | ( 0.0) |
| **Total chemical** | **148** | **( 5.4)** | **576** | **( 0.7)** | **0** | **( 0.0)** |
| **Parasitic** | | | | | | |
| *Giardia lamblia* | 4 | ( 0.1) | 45 | ( 0.1) | 0 | ( 0.0) |
| *Trichinella spiralis* | 2 | ( 0.1) | 19 | ( 0.0) | 0 | ( 0.0) |
| Other parasitic | 13 | ( 0.5) | 2,261 | ( 2.6) | 0 | ( 0.0) |
| **Total parasitic** | **19** | **( 0.7)** | **2,325** | **( 2.7)** | **0** | **( 0.0)** |
| **Viral** | | | | | | |
| Hepatitis A | 23 | ( 0.8) | 729 | ( 0.8) | 0 | ( 0.0) |
| Norwalk | 9 | ( 0.3) | 1,233 | ( 1.4) | 0 | ( 0.0) |
| Other viral | 24 | ( 0.9) | 2,104 | ( 2.4) | 0 | ( 0.0) |
| **Total viral** | **56** | **( 2.0)** | **4,066** | **( 4.7)** | **0** | **( 0.0)** |
| **Confirmed etiology** | 878 | ( 31.9) | 50,788 | ( 59.0) | 28 | ( 96.6) |
| **Unknown etiology** | 1,873 | ( 68.1) | 35,270 | ( 41.0) | 1 | ( 3.4) |
| **Total 1993–1997** | **2,751** | **(100.0)** | **86,058** | **(100.0)** | **29** | **(100.0)** |

*Includes Guam, Puerto Rico, and the U.S. Virgin Islands.

†Totals might vary by <1% from summed components because of rounding.

*Source*: Center for Disease Control and Prevention, U.S. Department of Health and Human Services. *MMWR: Morbidity and Mortality Weekly Review CDC Surveillance Summaries Surveillance for Foodborne-Disease Outbreaks United States, 1993–1997* 49 No. SS-1 (2000). http://www.cdc.gov/mmwr/PDF/ss/ss4901.pdf.

**Table F1.2. Number of Reported Foodborne-Disease Outbreaks, Cases, and Deaths, by Etiology—United States,* 1993†**

| | Outbreaks | | Cases | | Deaths | |
|---|---|---|---|---|---|---|
| **Etiology** | **No.** | **(%)** | **No.** | **(%)** | **No.** | **(%)** |
| **Bacterial** | | | | | | |
| *Bacillus cereus* | 4 | ( 0.8) | 188 | ( 1.1) | 0 | ( 0.0) |
| *Campylobacter* | 6 | ( 1.2) | 110 | ( 0.6) | 0 | ( 0.0) |
| *Clostridium botulinum* | 5 | ( 1.0) | 17 | ( 0.1) | 1 | ( 11.1) |
| *Clostridium perfringens* | 15 | ( 3.1) | 534 | ( 3.1) | 0 | ( 0.0) |
| *Escherichia coli* | 15 | ( 3.1) | 1,340 | ( 7.7) | 5 | ( 55.6) |
| *Salmonella* | 68 | ( 13.9) | 7,122 | ( 40.8) | 1 | ( 11.1) |
| *Shigella* | 9 | ( 1.8) | 338 | ( 1.9) | 0 | ( 0.0) |
| *Staphylococcus aureus* | 7 | ( 1.4) | 355 | ( 2.0) | 1 | ( 11.1) |
| *Streptococcus*, other | 1 | ( 0.2) | 6 | ( 0.0) | 0 | ( 0.0) |
| *Vibrio parahaemolyticus* | 1 | ( 0.2) | 4 | ( 0.0) | 0 | ( 0.0) |
| Other bacterial | 4 | ( 0.8) | 388 | ( 2.2) | 1 | ( 11.1) |
| **Total bacterial** | **135** | **( 27.6)** | **10,402** | **( 59.5)** | **9** | **(100.0)** |
| **Chemical** | | | | | | |
| Ciguatoxin | 13 | ( 2.7) | 44 | ( 0.3) | 0 | ( 0.0) |
| Heavy metals | 1 | ( 0.2) | 6 | ( 0.0) | 0 | ( 0.0) |
| Mushroom poisoning | 1 | ( 0.2) | 2 | ( 0.0) | 0 | ( 0.0) |
| Scombrotoxin | 5 | ( 1.0) | 21 | ( 0.1) | 0 | ( 0.0) |
| Other chemical | 1 | ( 0.2) | 2 | ( 0.0) | 0 | ( 0.0) |
| **Total chemical** | **21** | **( 4.3)** | **75** | **( 0.4)** | **0** | **( 0.0)** |
| **Parasitic** | | | | | | |
| *Trichinella spiralis* | 1 | ( 0.2) | 10 | ( 0.1) | 0 | ( 0.0) |
| Other parasitic | 1 | ( 0.2) | 6 | ( 0.0) | 0 | ( 0.0) |
| **Total parasitic** | **2** | **( 0.4)** | **16** | **( 0.1)** | **0** | **( 0.0)** |
| **Viral** | | | | | | |
| Hepatitis A | 5 | ( 1.0) | 81 | ( 0.5) | 0 | ( 0.0) |
| Norwalk | 1 | ( 0.2) | 45 | ( 0.3) | 0 | ( 0.0) |
| Other viral | 4 | ( 0.8) | 631 | ( 3.6) | 0 | ( 0.0) |
| **Total viral** | **10** | **( 2.0)** | **757** | **( 4.3)** | **0** | **( 0.0)** |
| **Confirmed etiology** | 168 | ( 34.4) | 11,250 | ( 64.4) | 9 | (100.0) |
| **Unknown etiology** | 321 | ( 65.6) | 6,227 | ( 35.6) | 0 | ( 0.0) |
| **Total 1993** | **489** | **(100.0)** | **17,477** | **(100.0)** | **9** | **(100.0)** |

*Includes Guam, Puerto Rico, and the U.S. Virgin Islands.

†Totals might vary by <1% from summed components because of rounding.

*Source*: Center for Disease Control and Prevention. U.S. Department of Health and Human Services. *MMWR: Morbidity and Mortality Weekly Review CDC Surveillance Summaries Surveillance for Foodborne-Disease Outbreaks United States, 1993–1997* 49 No. SS-1 (2000). http://www.cdc.gov/mmwr/PDF/ss/ss4901.pdf.

**Table F1.3. Number of Reported Foodborne-Disease Outbreaks, Cases, and Deaths, by Etiology—United States;* 1994†**

| | Outbreaks | | Cases | | Deaths | |
|---|---|---|---|---|---|---|
| **Etiology** | **No.** | **(%)** | **No.** | **(%)** | **No.** | **(%)** |
| **Bacterial** | | | | | | |
| *Bacillus cereus* | 3 | ( 0.5) | 19 | ( 0.1) | 0 | ( 0.0) |
| *Campylobacter* | 6 | ( 0.9) | 97 | ( 0.6) | 0 | ( 0.0) |
| *Clostridium botulinum* | 3 | ( 0.5) | 27 | ( 0.2) | 0 | ( 0.0) |
| *Clostridium perfringens* | 12 | ( 1.8) | 517 | ( 3.2) | 0 | ( 0.0) |
| *Escherichia coli* | 25 | ( 3.8) | 902 | ( 5.6) | 0 | ( 0.0) |
| *Listeria monocytogenes* | 3 | ( 0.5) | 100 | ( 0.6) | 2 | ( 66.7) |
| *Salmonella* | 70 | ( 10.7) | 2,858 | ( 17.6) | 1 | ( 33.3) |
| *Shigella* | 11 | ( 1.7) | 534 | ( 3.3) | 0 | ( 0.0) |
| *Staphylococcus aureus* | 13 | ( 2.0) | 421 | ( 2.6) | 0 | ( 0.0) |
| *Vibrio cholerae* | 1 | ( 0.2) | 2 | ( 0.0) | 0 | ( 0.0) |
| *Yersinia enterocolitica* | 1 | ( 0.2) | 10 | ( 0.0) | 0 | ( 0.0) |
| **Total bacterial** | **148** | **( 22.7)** | **5,487** | **( 33.8)** | **3** | **(100.0)** |
| **Chemical** | | | | | | |
| Ciguatoxin | 11 | ( 1.7) | 54 | ( 0.3) | 0 | ( 0.0) |
| Heavy metals | 2 | ( 0.3) | 8 | ( 0.0) | 0 | ( 0.0) |
| Monosodium glutamate | 1 | ( 0.2) | 2 | ( 0.0) | 0 | ( 0.0) |
| Scombrotoxin | 21 | ( 3.2) | 83 | ( 0.5) | 0 | ( 0.0) |
| Other chemical | 2 | ( 0.3) | 14 | ( 0.1) | 0 | ( 0.0) |
| **Total chemical** | **37** | **( 5.7)** | **161** | **( 1.0)** | **0** | **( 0.0)** |
| **Parasitic** | | | | | | |
| *Giardia lamblia* | 2 | ( 0.3) | 22 | ( 0.1) | 0 | ( 0.0) |
| **Viral** | | | | | | |
| Hepatitis A | 6 | ( 0.9) | 310 | ( 1.9) | 0 | ( 0.0) |
| Norwalk | 1 | ( 0.2) | 34 | ( 0.2) | 0 | ( 0.0) |
| Other viral | 3 | ( 0.5) | 268 | ( 1.7) | 0 | ( 0.0) |
| **Total viral** | **10** | **( 1.6)** | **612** | **( 3.8)** | **0** | **( 0.0)** |
| **Confirmed etiology** | 197 | ( 30.2) | 6,282 | ( 38.7) | 3 | (100.0) |
| **Unknown etiology** | 456 | ( 69.8) | 9,952 | ( 61.3) | 0 | ( 0.0) |
| **Total 1994** | **653** | **(100.0)** | **16,234** | **(100.0)** | **3** | **(100.0)** |

*Includes Guam, Puerto Rico, and the U.S. Virgin Islands.

†Totals might vary by <1% from summed components because of rounding.

*Source*: Center for Disease Control and Prevention. U.S. Department of Health and Human Services. *MMWR: Morbidity and Mortality Weekly Review CDC Surveillance Summaries Surveillance for Foodborne-Disease Outbreaks United States, 1993–1997* 49 No. SS-1 (2000). http://www.cdc.gov/mmwr/PDF/ss/ss4901.pdf.

**Table F1.4. Number of Reported Foodborne-Disease Outbreaks, Cases, and Deaths, by Etiology—United States;* 1995†**

| Etiology | Outbreaks No. | Outbreaks (%) | Cases No. | Cases (%) | Deaths No. | Deaths (%) |
|---|---|---|---|---|---|---|
| **Bacterial** | | | | | | |
| *Bacillus cereus* | 2 | ( 0.3) | 24 | ( 0.1) | 0 | ( 0.0) |
| *Campylobacter* | 6 | ( 1.0) | 127 | ( 0.7) | 0 | ( 0.0) |
| *Clostridium botulinum* | 2 | ( 0.3) | 6 | ( 0.0) | 0 | ( 0.0) |
| *Clostridium perfringens* | 14 | ( 2.2) | 455 | ( 2.6) | 0 | ( 0.0) |
| *Escherichia coli* | 25 | ( 4.0) | 393 | ( 2.2) | 1 | ( 9.1) |
| *Salmonella* | 90 | ( 14.3) | 8,449 | ( 47.5) | 9 | ( 81.8) |
| *Shigella* | 7 | ( 1.1) | 259 | ( 1.5) | 0 | ( 0.0) |
| *Staphylococcus aureus* | 6 | ( 1.0) | 66 | ( 0.4) | 0 | ( 0.0) |
| *Yersina enterocolitica* | 1 | ( 0.2) | 17 | ( 0.1) | 1 | ( 9.1) |
| Other bacterial | 2 | ( 0.3) | 221 | ( 1.2) | 0 | ( 0.0) |
| **Total bacterial** | **155** | **( 24.7)** | **10,017** | **( 56.3)** | **11** | **(100.0)** |
| **Chemical** | | | | | | |
| Ciguatoxin | 10 | ( 1.6) | 27 | ( 0.2) | 0 | ( 0.0) |
| Heavy metals | 1 | ( 0.2) | 3 | ( 0.0) | 0 | ( 0.0) |
| Scombrotoxin | 16 | ( 2.5) | 91 | ( 0.5) | 0 | ( 0.0) |
| Other chemical | 2 | ( 0.3) | 12 | ( 0.1) | 0 | ( 0.0) |
| **Total chemical** | **29** | **( 4.6)** | **133** | **( 0.7)** | **0** | **( 0.0)** |
| **Parasitic** | | | | | | |
| *Trichinella spiralis* | 1 | ( 0.2) | 9 | ( 0.1) | 0 | ( 0.0) |
| **Viral** | | | | | | |
| Hepatitis A | 4 | ( 0.6) | 38 | ( 0.2) | 0 | ( 0.0) |
| Norwalk | 4 | ( 0.6) | 433 | ( 2.4) | 0 | ( 0.0) |
| Other viral | 1 | ( 0.2) | 41 | ( 0.2) | 0 | ( 0.0) |
| **Total viral** | **9** | **( 1.4)** | **512** | **( 2.9)** | **0** | **( 0.0)** |
| **Confirmed etiology** | 194 | ( 30.9) | 10,671 | ( 59.9) | 11 | (100.0) |
| **Unknown etiology** | 434 | ( 69.1) | 7,129 | ( 40.1) | 0 | ( 0.0) |
| **Total 1995** | **628** | **(100.0)** | **17,800** | **(100.0)** | **11** | **(100.0)** |

*Includes Guam, Puerto Rico, and the U.S. Virgin Islands.

†Totals might vary by <1% from summed components because of rounding.

*Source*: Center for Disease Control and Prevention. U.S. Department of Health and Human Services. *MMWR: Morbidity and Mortality Weekly Review CDC Surveillance Summaries Surveillance for Foodborne-Disease Outbreaks United States, 1993–1997* 49 no. SS-1 (2000). http://www.cdc.gov/mmwr/PDF/ss/ss4901.pdf.

**Table F1.5. Number of Reported Foodborne-Disease Outbreaks, Cases, and Deaths, by Etiology—United States;* 1996†**

| | Outbreaks | | Cases | | Deaths | |
|---|---|---|---|---|---|---|
| **Etiology** | **No.** | **(%)** | **No.** | **(%)** | **No.** | **(%)** |
| **Bacterial** | | | | | | |
| *Bacillus cereus* | 1 | ( 0.2) | 22 | ( 0.1) | 0 | ( 0.0) |
| *Brucella* | 1 | ( 0.2) | 19 | ( 0.1) | 0 | ( 0.0) |
| *Campylobacter* | 5 | ( 1.0) | 101 | ( 0.4) | 0 | ( 0.0) |
| *Clostridium botulinum* | 2 | ( 0.4) | 4 | ( 0.0) | 0 | ( 0.0) |
| *Clostridium perfringens* | 10 | ( 2.1) | 1,011 | ( 4.5) | 0 | ( 0.0) |
| *Escherichia coli* | 11 | ( 2.3) | 325 | ( 1.4) | 1 | ( 25.0) |
| *Salmonella* | 69 | ( 14.5) | 12,450 | ( 55.1) | 2 | ( 50.0) |
| *Shigella* | 6 | ( 1.3) | 109 | ( 0.5) | 0 | ( 0.0) |
| *Staphylococcus aureus* | 7 | ( 1.5) | 178 | ( 0.8) | 0 | ( 0.0) |
| **Total bacterial** | **112** | **( 23.5)** | **14,219** | **( 62.9)** | **3** | **( 75.0)** |
| **Chemical** | | | | | | |
| Ciguatoxin | 9 | ( 1.9) | 32 | ( 0.1) | 0 | ( 0.0) |
| Mushroom poisoning | 3 | ( 0.6) | 10 | ( 0.0) | 0 | ( 0.0) |
| Scombrotoxin | 12 | ( 2.5) | 37 | ( 0.2) | 0 | ( 0.0) |
| Shellfish | 1 | ( 0.2) | 3 | ( 0.0) | 0 | ( 0.0) |
| Other chemical | 1 | ( 0.2) | 3 | ( 0.0) | 0 | ( 0.0) |
| **Total chemical** | **26** | **( 5.5)** | **85** | **( 0.4)** | **0** | **( 0.0)** |
| **Parasitic** | | | | | | |
| *Giardia lamblia* | 1 | ( 0.2) | 6 | ( 0.0) | 0 | ( 0.0) |
| Other parasitic | 2 | ( 0.4) | 1,582 | ( 7.0) | 0 | ( 0.0) |
| **Total parasitic** | **3** | **( 0.6)** | **1,588** | **( 7.0)** | **0** | **( 0.0)** |
| **Viral** | | | | | | |
| Hepatitis A | 5 | ( 1.0) | 126 | ( 0.6) | 0 | ( 0.0) |
| Norwalk | 3 | ( 0.6) | 721 | ( 3.2) | 0 | ( 0.0) |
| Other viral | 2 | ( 0.4) | 573 | ( 2.5) | 0 | ( 0.0) |
| **Total viral** | **10** | **( 2.1)** | **1,420** | **( 6.3)** | **0** | **( 0.0)** |
| **Confirmed etiology** | 151 | ( 31.7) | 17,312 | ( 76.6) | 3 | ( 75.0) |
| **Unknown etiology** | 326 | ( 68.3) | 5,295 | ( 23.4) | 1 | ( 25.0) |
| **Total 1996** | **477** | **(100.0)** | **22,607** | **(100.0)** | **4** | **(100.0)** |

*Includes Guam, Puerto Rico, and the U.S. Virgin Islands.
†Totals might vary by <1% from summed components because of rounding.
*Source*: Center for Disease Control and Prevention. U.S. Department of Health and Human Services. *MMWR: Morbidity and Mortality Weekly Review CDC Surveillance Summaries Surveillance for Foodborne-Disease Outbreaks United States, 1993–1997* 49 no. SS-1 (2000). http://www.cdc.gov/mmwr/PDF/ss/ss4901.pdf.

**Table F1.6. Number of Reported Foodborne-Disease Outbreaks, Cases, and Deaths, by Etiology—United States;* 1997†**

| Etiology | Outbreaks | | Cases | | Deaths | |
|---|---|---|---|---|---|---|
| | No. | (%) | No. | (%) | No. | (%) |
| **Bacterial** | | | | | | |
| *Bacillus cereus* | 4 | ( 0.8) | 438 | ( 3.7) | 0 | ( 0.0) |
| *Campylobacter* | 2 | ( 0.4) | 104 | ( 0.9) | 1 | ( 50.0) |
| *Clostridium botulinum* | 1 | ( 0.2) | 2 | ( 0.0) | 0 | ( 0.0) |
| *Clostridium perfringens* | 6 | ( 1.2) | 255 | ( 2.1) | 0 | ( 0.0) |
| *Escherichia coli* | 8 | ( 1.6) | 300 | ( 2.5) | 1 | ( 50.0) |
| *Salmonella* | 60 | ( 11.9) | 1,731 | ( 14.5) | 0 | ( 0.0) |
| *Shigella* | 10 | ( 2.0) | 315 | ( 2.6) | 0 | ( 0.0) |
| *Staphylococcus aureus* | 9 | ( 1.8) | 393 | ( 3.3) | 0 | ( 0.0) |
| *Streptococcus*, group A | 1 | ( 0.2) | 122 | ( 1.0) | 0 | ( 0.0) |
| *Vibrio parahaemolyticus* | 4 | ( 0.8) | 36 | ( 0.3) | 0 | ( 0.0) |
| **Total bacterial** | **105** | **( 20.8)** | **3,696** | **( 31.0)** | **2** | **(100.0)** |
| **Chemical** | | | | | | |
| Ciguatoxin | 17 | ( 3.4) | 48 | ( 0.4) | 0 | ( 0.0) |
| Mushroom poisoning | 3 | ( 0.6) | 9 | ( 0.1) | 0 | ( 0.0) |
| Scombrotoxin | 15 | ( 3.0) | 65 | ( 0.5) | 0 | ( 0.0) |
| **Total chemical** | **35** | **( 6.9)** | **122** | **( 1.0)** | **0** | **( 0.0)** |
| **Parasitic** | | | | | | |
| *Giardia lamblia* | 1 | ( 0.2) | 17 | ( 0.1) | 0 | ( 0.0) |
| Other parasitic | 10 | ( 2.0) | 673 | ( 5.6) | 0 | ( 0.0) |
| **Total parasitic** | **11** | **( 2.2)** | **690** | **( 5.8)** | **0** | **( 0.0)** |
| **Viral** | | | | | | |
| Hepatitis A | 3 | ( 0.6) | 174 | ( 1.5) | 0 | ( 0.0) |
| Other viral | 14 | ( 2.8) | 591 | ( 4.9) | 0 | ( 0.0) |
| **Total viral** | **17** | **( 3.4)** | **765** | **( 6.4)** | **0** | **( 0.0)** |
| **Confirmed etiology** | 168 | ( 33.3) | 5,273 | ( 44.2) | 2 | (100.0) |
| **Unknown etiology** | 336 | ( 66.7) | 6,667 | ( 55.8) | 0 | ( 0.0) |
| **Total 1997** | **504** | **(100.0)** | **11,940** | **(100.0)** | **2** | **(100.0)** |

*Includes Guam, Puerto Rico, and the U.S. Virgin Islands.

†Totals might vary by <1% from summed components because of rounding.

*Source*: Center for Disease Control and Prevention. U.S. Department of Health and Human Services. *MMWR: Morbidity and Mortality Weekly Review CDC Surveillance Summaries Surveillance for Foodborne-Disease Outbreaks United States, 1993–1997* 49 no. SS-1 (2000). http://www.cdc.gov/mmwr/PDF/ss/ss4901.pdf.

**Table F2.1. Number of Reported Foodborne-Disease Outbreaks, by Etiology and Month of Occurrence—United States;* 1993**

| Etiology | Month of occurrence | | | | | | | | | | | | Total |
|---|---|---|---|---|---|---|---|---|---|---|---|---|---|
| | Jan | Feb | Mar | Apr | May | Jun | Jul | Aug | Sep | Oct | Nov | Dec | |
| **Bacterial** | | | | | | | | | | | | | |
| *Bacillus cereus* | — | — | — | 1 | — | — | 2 | 1 | — | — | — | — | 4 |
| *Campylobacter* | — | — | — | — | — | — | — | 1 | 2 | 1 | 2 | — | 6 |
| *Clostridium botulinum* | — | — | — | — | 1 | — | 1 | — | 1 | 1 | 1 | — | 5 |
| *Clostridium perfringens* | — | 1 | 4 | 3 | — | 1 | 1 | 1 | — | 2 | 1 | 1 | 15 |
| *Escherichia coli* | 1 | — | 2 | 2 | — | — | 4 | 1 | 3 | 1 | 1 | — | 15 |
| *Salmonella* | 5 | 4 | 7 | 4 | 7 | 4 | 8 | 3 | 15 | 5 | 4 | 2 | 68 |
| *Shigella* | 1 | — | — | 2 | 1 | 1 | — | 1 | 3 | — | — | — | 9 |
| *Staphylococcus aureus* | 1 | — | 1 | — | 1 | 2 | — | — | 1 | — | 1 | — | 7 |
| *Streptococcus*, other | — | — | — | — | — | — | 1 | — | — | — | — | — | 1 |
| *Vibrio parahaemolyticus* | — | — | — | — | 1 | — | — | — | — | — | — | — | 1 |
| Other bacterial | — | — | 1 | 1 | — | — | 1 | 1 | — | — | — | — | 4 |
| **Total bacterial** | **8** | **5** | **15** | **13** | **11** | **8** | **18** | **9** | **25** | **10** | **10** | **3** | **135** |
| **Chemical** | | | | | | | | | | | | | |
| Ciguatoxin | — | 1 | — | 1 | 3 | 1 | 1 | 3 | 2 | — | 1 | — | 13 |
| Heavy metals | — | — | 1 | — | — | — | — | — | — | — | — | — | 1 |
| Mushroom poisoning | — | — | — | — | — | — | — | — | 1 | — | — | — | 1 |
| Scombrotoxin | — | 2 | — | — | — | — | 2 | — | 1 | — | — | — | 5 |
| Other chemical | — | — | — | — | 1 | — | — | — | — | — | — | — | 1 |
| **Total chemical** | **—** | **3** | **1** | **1** | **4** | **1** | **3** | **3** | **4** | **—** | **1** | **—** | **21** |
| **Parasitic** | | | | | | | | | | | | | |
| *Trichinella spiralis* | — | — | — | — | — | — | — | — | — | 1 | — | — | 1 |
| Other parasitic | — | — | — | 1 | — | — | — | — | — | — | — | — | 1 |
| **Total parasitic** | **—** | **—** | **—** | **1** | **—** | **—** | **—** | **—** | **—** | **1** | **—** | **—** | **2** |
| **Viral** | | | | | | | | | | | | | |
| Hepatitis A | — | 1 | — | — | — | — | 1 | 1 | — | — | 2 | — | 5 |
| Norwalk | — | — | — | — | — | — | — | — | — | — | 1 | — | 1 |
| Other viral | 1 | — | — | — | — | — | — | — | — | — | 2 | 1 | 4 |
| **Total viral** | **1** | **1** | **—** | **—** | **—** | **—** | **1** | **1** | **—** | **—** | **5** | **1** | **10** |
| **Confirmed etiology** | 9 | 9 | 16 | 15 | 15 | 9 | 22 | 13 | 29 | 11 | 16 | 4 | **168** |
| **Unknown etiology** | 20 | 13 | 28 | 27 | 39 | 33 | 26 | 23 | 22 | 22 | 30 | 38 | **321** |
| **Total 1993** | **29** | **22** | **44** | **42** | **54** | **42** | **48** | **36** | **51** | **33** | **46** | **42** | **489** |

*Includes Guam, Puerto Rico, and the U.S. Virgin Islands.

*Source*: Center for Disease Control and Prevention. U.S. Department of Health and Human Services. *MMWR: Morbidity and Mortality Weekly Review CDC Surveillance Summaries Surveillance for Foodborne-Disease Outbreaks United States, 1993–1997* 49 no. SS-1 (2000). http://www.cdc.gov/mmwr/PDF/ss/ss4901.pdf.

**Table F2.2. Number of Reported Foodborne-Disease Outbreaks, by Etiology and Month of Occurrence—United States,* 1994**

| Etiology | Month of occurrence | | | | | | | | | | | | Total |
|---|---|---|---|---|---|---|---|---|---|---|---|---|---|
| | Jan | Feb | Mar | Apr | May | Jun | Jul | Aug | Sep | Oct | Nov | Dec | |
| **Bacterial** | | | | | | | | | | | | | |
| *Bacillus cereus* | — | — | — | — | 1 | — | — | 1 | 1 | — | — | — | **3** |
| *Campylobacter* | — | — | — | — | — | 3 | 1 | 1 | — | — | 1 | — | **6** |
| *Clostridium botulinum* | — | — | — | 1 | — | 1 | — | 1 | — | — | — | — | **3** |
| *Clostridium perfringens* | 1 | — | 1 | 1 | — | 4 | — | — | — | 1 | 1 | 3 | **12** |
| *Escherichia coli* | 1 | 2 | — | 1 | 1 | 7 | 4 | — | 5 | 1 | 3 | — | **25** |
| *Listeria monocytogenes* | — | — | — | — | — | 1 | — | — | — | 2 | — | — | **3** |
| *Salmonella* | 1 | — | 1 | 4 | 8 | 6 | 11 | 13 | 6 | 9 | 6 | 5 | **70** |
| *Shigella* | — | — | 2 | — | — | 4 | 2 | — | — | — | 3 | — | **11** |
| *Staphylococcus aureus* | — | — | — | — | 2 | 3 | — | 2 | 1 | — | 2 | 3 | **13** |
| *Vibrio cholera* | — | — | — | — | — | — | — | — | — | — | — | 1 | **1** |
| *Yersinia enterocolitica* | — | — | — | — | — | — | — | — | — | 1 | — | — | **1** |
| **Total bacterial** | **3** | **2** | **4** | **7** | **12** | **29** | **18** | **18** | **13** | **14** | **16** | **12** | **148** |
| **Chemical** | | | | | | | | | | | | | |
| Ciguatoxin | — | — | — | 1 | 4 | 3 | — | 2 | — | 1 | — | — | **11** |
| Heavy metals | — | — | — | — | — | — | — | 1 | — | — | — | 1 | **2** |
| Monosodium glutamate | — | — | — | — | 1 | — | — | — | — | — | — | — | **1** |
| Scombrotoxin | 2 | 2 | 1 | 1 | 2 | — | — | 3 | 3 | 4 | 2 | 1 | **21** |
| Other chemical | — | — | 2 | — | — | — | — | — | — | — | — | — | **2** |
| **Total chemical** | **2** | **2** | **3** | **2** | **7** | **3** | **—** | **6** | **3** | **5** | **2** | **2** | **37** |
| **Parasitic** | | | | | | | | | | | | | |
| *Giardia lamblia* | — | — | — | — | — | — | 2 | — | — | — | — | — | **2** |
| **Viral** | | | | | | | | | | | | | |
| Hepatitis A | — | — | — | 1 | 1 | 1 | — | 1 | 1 | 1 | — | — | **6** |
| Norwalk | — | 1 | — | — | — | — | — | — | — | — | — | — | **1** |
| Other viral | — | 1 | — | — | — | — | — | — | — | — | — | 2 | **3** |
| **Total viral** | **—** | **2** | **—** | **1** | **1** | **1** | **—** | **1** | **1** | **1** | **—** | **2** | **10** |
| **Confirmed etiology** | 5 | 6 | 7 | 10 | 20 | 33 | 20 | 25 | 17 | 20 | 18 | 16 | **197** |
| **Unknown etiology** | 17 | 32 | 33 | 46 | 55 | 33 | 35 | 34 | 31 | 38 | 36 | 66 | **456** |
| **Total 1994** | **22** | **38** | **40** | **56** | **75** | **66** | **55** | **59** | **48** | **58** | **54** | **82** | **653** |

*Includes Guam, Puerto Rico, and the U.S. Virgin Islands.

*Source*: Center for Disease Control and Prevention. U.S. Department of Health and Human Services. *MMWR: Morbidity and Mortality Weekly Review CDC Surveillance Summaries Surveillance for Foodborne-Disease Outbreaks United States, 1993–1997* 49 no. SS-1 (2000). http://www.cdc.gov/mmwr/PDF/ss/ss4901.pdf.

**Table F2.3. Number of Reported Foodborne-Disease Outbreaks, by Etiology and Month of Occurrence—United States;* 1995**

| | Month of occurrence | | | | | | | | | | | | |
|---|---|---|---|---|---|---|---|---|---|---|---|---|---|
| **Etiology** | **Jan** | **Feb** | **Mar** | **Apr** | **May** | **Jun** | **Jul** | **Aug** | **Sep** | **Oct** | **Nov** | **Dec** | **Total** |
| **Bacterial** | | | | | | | | | | | | | |
| *Bacillus cereus* | — | — | — | — | — | — | — | 1 | — | 1 | — | — | **2** |
| *Campylobacter* | — | — | — | — | — | 1 | 2 | — | 1 | 2 | — | — | **6** |
| *Clostridium botulinum* | — | — | — | — | — | — | — | 1 | 1 | — | — | — | **2** |
| *Clostridium perfringens* | 1 | 1 | 1 | 2 | 2 | — | — | — | 1 | 1 | 4 | 1 | **14** |
| *Escherichia coli* | — | — | — | 1 | 2 | 4 | 6 | 4 | 2 | 2 | 3 | 1 | **25** |
| *Salmonella* | 7 | 3 | 4 | 6 | 7 | 9 | 12 | 19 | 9 | 8 | 3 | 3 | **90** |
| *Shigella* | 1 | 1 | 2 | 2 | — | — | 1 | — | — | — | — | — | **7** |
| *Staphylococcus aureus* | — | — | — | — | — | — | 2 | — | — | 2 | — | 2 | **6** |
| *Yersinia enterocolitica* | — | — | — | — | — | — | — | — | — | — | 1 | — | **1** |
| Other bacterial | — | — | — | — | 1 | — | — | 1 | — | — | — | — | **2** |
| **Total bacterial** | **9** | **5** | **7** | **11** | **12** | **14** | **23** | **26** | **14** | **16** | **11** | **7** | **155** |
| **Chemical** | | | | | | | | | | | | | |
| Ciguatoxin | 1 | — | 2 | — | — | 1 | 1 | 2 | 2 | — | — | 1 | **10** |
| Heavy metals | — | — | — | — | — | — | — | — | 1 | — | — | — | **1** |
| Scombrotoxin | 1 | 1 | 2 | 1 | 2 | — | 1 | 1 | 1 | 2 | 4 | — | **16** |
| Other chemical | — | — | — | — | — | — | 1 | — | — | — | — | 1 | **2** |
| **Total chemical** | **2** | **1** | **4** | **1** | **2** | **1** | **3** | **3** | **4** | **2** | **4** | **2** | **29** |
| **Parasitic** | | | | | | | | | | | | | |
| *Trichinella spiralis* | 1 | — | — | — | — | — | — | — | — | — | — | — | **1** |
| **Viral** | | | | | | | | | | | | | |
| Hepatitis A | — | — | — | 1 | 1 | — | — | — | 1 | 1 | — | — | **4** |
| Norwalk | 1 | — | — | 1 | — | — | — | — | 1 | — | — | 1 | **4** |
| Other viral | — | — | — | 1 | — | — | — | — | — | — | — | — | **1** |
| **Total viral** | **1** | **—** | **—** | **3** | **1** | **—** | **—** | **—** | **2** | **1** | **—** | **1** | **9** |
| **Confirmed etiology** | 13 | 6 | 11 | 15 | 15 | 15 | 26 | 29 | 20 | 19 | 15 | 10 | **194** |
| **Unknown etiology** | 34 | 30 | 41 | 44 | 49 | 36 | 36 | 30 | 18 | 34 | 45 | 37 | **434** |
| **Total 1995** | **47** | **36** | **52** | **59** | **64** | **51** | **62** | **59** | **38** | **53** | **60** | **47** | **628** |

*Includes Guam, Puerto Rico, and the U.S. Virgin Islands.

*Source*: Center for Disease Control and Prevention. U.S. Department of Health and Human Services. *MMWR: Morbidity and Mortality Weekly Review CDC Surveillance Summaries Surveillance for Foodborne-Disease Outbreaks United States, 1993–1997* 49 no. SS-1 (2000). http://www.cdc.gov/mmwr/PDF/ss/ss4901.pdf.

**Table F2.4. Number of Reported Foodborne-Disease Outbreaks, by Etiology and Month of Occurrence—United States,* 1996**

| Etiology | Month of occurrence | | | | | | | | | | | | Total |
|---|---|---|---|---|---|---|---|---|---|---|---|---|---|
| | Jan | Feb | Mar | Apr | May | Jun | Jul | Aug | Sep | Oct | Nov | Dec | |
| **Bacterial** | | | | | | | | | | | | | |
| *Bacillus cereus* | — | — | 1 | — | — | — | — | — | — | — | — | — | **1** |
| *Brucella* | — | — | — | — | — | — | — | — | — | — | 1 | — | **1** |
| *Campylobacter* | — | — | 1 | — | — | 2 | — | 1 | — | — | 1 | — | **5** |
| *Clostridium botulinum* | — | — | — | — | 1 | 1 | — | — | — | — | — | — | **2** |
| *Clostridium perfringens* | — | 1 | — | 2 | 1 | — | 1 | — | — | — | 3 | 2 | **10** |
| *Escherichia coli* | — | — | — | — | 3 | 3 | — | — | 2 | 3 | — | — | **11** |
| *Salmonella* | 3 | 4 | 4 | 2 | 5 | 12 | 12 | 10 | 4 | 4 | 4 | 5 | **69** |
| *Shigella* | 1 | — | — | — | 2 | — | 1 | 2 | — | — | — | — | **6** |
| *Staphylococcus aureus* | — | 2 | — | — | — | — | — | 1 | 1 | 2 | 1 | — | **7** |
| **Total bacterial** | **4** | **7** | **6** | **4** | **12** | **18** | **14** | **14** | **7** | **9** | **10** | **7** | **112** |
| **Chemical** | | | | | | | | | | | | | |
| Ciguatoxin | — | 3 | — | 1 | 1 | — | 1 | 1 | 1 | 1 | — | — | **9** |
| Mushroom poisoning | — | 1 | — | — | — | — | — | — | — | — | — | 2 | **3** |
| Scombotoxin | 1 | 1 | — | 1 | — | 1 | 1 | 3 | 1 | 2 | — | 1 | **12** |
| Shellfish | — | — | — | — | — | — | — | 1 | — | — | — | — | **1** |
| Other chemical | — | — | — | 1 | — | — | — | — | — | — | — | — | **1** |
| **Total chemical** | **1** | **5** | **—** | **3** | **1** | **1** | **2** | **5** | **2** | **3** | **—** | **3** | **26** |
| **Parasitic** | | | | | | | | | | | | | |
| *Giardia lamblia* | — | — | — | — | — | — | — | — | 1 | — | — | — | **1** |
| Other parasitic | — | — | — | — | 1 | — | — | — | 1 | — | — | — | **2** |
| **Total parasitic** | **—** | **—** | **—** | **—** | **1** | **—** | **—** | **—** | **2** | **—** | **—** | **—** | **3** |
| **Viral** | | | | | | | | | | | | | |
| Hepatitis A | 2 | — | — | — | — | — | — | — | — | — | 3 | — | **5** |
| Norwalk | — | 1 | 2 | — | — | — | — | — | — | — | — | — | **3** |
| Other viral | — | — | — | — | 1 | — | — | — | — | — | — | 1 | **2** |
| **Total viral** | **2** | **1** | **2** | **—** | **1** | **—** | **—** | **—** | **—** | **—** | **3** | **1** | **10** |
| **Confirmed etiology** | 7 | 13 | 8 | 7 | 15 | 19 | 16 | 19 | 11 | 12 | 13 | 11 | **151** |
| **Unknown etiology** | 27 | 21 | 27 | 33 | 36 | 37 | 27 | 29 | 24 | 14 | 30 | 21 | **326** |
| **Total 1996** | **34** | **34** | **35** | **40** | **51** | **56** | **43** | **48** | **35** | **26** | **43** | **32** | **477** |

*Includes Guam, Puerto Rico, and the U.S. Virgin Islands.

*Source*: Center for Disease Control and Prevention. U.S. Department of Health and Human Services. *MMWR: Morbidity and Mortality Weekly Review CDC Surveillance Summaries Surveillance for Foodborne-Disease Outbreaks United States, 1993–1997* 49 No. SS-1 (2000). http://www.cdc.gov/mmwr/PDF/ss/ss4901.pdf.

**Table F2.5. Number of Reported Foodborne-Disease Outbreaks, by Etiology and Month of Occurrence—United States;* 1997**

| | Month of occurrence | | | | | | | | | | | | |
|---|---|---|---|---|---|---|---|---|---|---|---|---|---|
| **Etiology** | **Jan** | **Feb** | **Mar** | **Apr** | **May** | **Jun** | **Jul** | **Aug** | **Sep** | **Oct** | **Nov** | **Dec** | **Total** |
| **Bacterial** | | | | | | | | | | | | | |
| *Bacillus cereus* | — | — | 1 | — | — | — | — | — | 1 | — | — | 2 | **4** |
| *Campylobacter* | — | — | 1 | — | — | — | — | 1 | — | — | — | — | **2** |
| *Clostridium botulinum* | — | 1 | — | — | — | — | — | — | — | — | — | — | **1** |
| *Clostridium perfringens* | 1 | — | 1 | 3 | — | 1 | — | — | — | — | — | — | **6** |
| *Escherichia coli* | — | — | 1 | 2 | — | 4 | — | — | — | — | — | 1 | **8** |
| *Salmonella* | 5 | 5 | 3 | 2 | 5 | 6 | 5 | 10 | 6 | 2 | 11 | — | **60** |
| *Shigella* | — | — | — | 1 | — | — | 1 | 3 | 2 | — | 2 | 1 | **10** |
| *Staphylococcus aureus* | — | — | — | — | 1 | — | — | 3 | 2 | — | 2 | 1 | **9** |
| *Streptococcus, group A* | — | — | — | — | — | — | — | — | — | 1 | — | — | **1** |
| *Vibrio parahaemolyticus* | — | — | — | — | — | — | 1 | 1 | 2 | — | — | — | **4** |
| **Total bacterial** | **6** | **6** | **7** | **8** | **6** | **11** | **7** | **18** | **13** | **3** | **15** | **5** | **105** |
| **Chemical** | | | | | | | | | | | | | |
| Ciguatoxin | 2 | 1 | — | — | 2 | 1 | 1 | 1 | 6 | — | 3 | — | **17** |
| Mushroom poisoning | 1 | — | — | — | — | — | — | 1 | — | — | 1 | — | **3** |
| Scombrotoxin | — | — | 1 | — | 3 | 3 | — | 1 | 3 | 2 | — | 2 | **15** |
| **Total chemical** | **3** | **1** | **1** | **—** | **5** | **4** | **1** | **3** | **9** | **2** | **4** | **2** | **35** |
| **Parasitic** | | | | | | | | | | | | | |
| *Giardia lamblia* | — | — | 1 | — | — | — | — | — | — | — | — | — | **1** |
| Other parasitic | — | — | 1 | 2 | 4 | — | 1 | — | — | 1 | — | 1 | **10** |
| **Total parasitic** | **—** | **—** | **2** | **2** | **4** | **—** | **1** | **—** | **—** | **1** | **—** | **1** | **11** |
| **Viral** | | | | | | | | | | | | | |
| Hepatitis A | — | — | 1 | — | — | 1 | 1 | — | — | — | — | — | **3** |
| Other viral | 3 | 1 | 2 | 1 | — | 1 | 2 | — | — | 1 | 2 | 1 | **14** |
| **Total viral** | **3** | **1** | **3** | **1** | **—** | **2** | **3** | **—** | **—** | **1** | **2** | **1** | **17** |
| **Confirmed etiology** | 12 | 8 | 13 | 11 | 15 | 17 | 12 | 21 | 22 | 7 | 21 | 9 | **168** |
| **Unknown etiology** | 29 | 23 | 37 | 38 | 33 | 32 | 16 | 30 | 14 | 31 | 26 | 27 | **336** |
| **Total 1997** | **41** | **31** | **50** | **49** | **48** | **49** | **28** | **51** | **36** | **38** | **47** | **36** | **504** |

*Includes Guam, Puerto Rico, and the U.S. Virgin Islands.

*Source*: Center for Disease Control and Prevention. U.S. Department of Health and Human Services. *MMWR: Morbidity and Mortality Weekly Review CDC Surveillance Summaries Surveillance for Foodborne-Disease Outbreaks United States, 1993–1997* 49 No. SS-1 (2000). http://www.cdc.gov/mmwr/PDF/ss/ss4901.pdf.

**Table F3.1. Number of Reported Foodborne-Disease Outbreaks, by Etiology and Place Where Food was Eaten—United States,* 1993**

| Etiology | Place where food was eaten | | | | | | | | | |
|---|---|---|---|---|---|---|---|---|---|---|
| | Private residence | Delicatessen, cafeteria, or restaurant | School | Picnic | Church | Camp | Other | Known place | Unknown place | Total |
| **Bacterial** | | | | | | | | | | |
| *Bacillus cereus* | — | 1 | — | — | — | — | 3 | 4 | — | **4** |
| *Campylobacter* | — | 4 | — | — | — | — | 2 | 6 | — | **6** |
| *Clostridium botulinum* | 4 | — | — | — | — | — | — | 4 | 1 | **5** |
| *Clostridium perfringens* | 2 | 6 | — | 1 | 1 | — | 5 | 15 | — | **15** |
| *Escherichia coli* | 1 | 4 | — | 1 | 1 | — | 8 | 15 | — | **15** |
| *Salmonella* | 9 | 26 | 2 | — | 4 | 2 | 24 | 67 | 1 | **68** |
| *Shigella* | 2 | 4 | — | — | — | — | 3 | 9 | — | **9** |
| *Staphylococcus aureus* | — | 1 | 2 | — | — | — | 4 | 7 | — | **7** |
| *Streptococcus*, other | 1 | — | — | — | — | — | — | 1 | — | **1** |
| *Vibrio parahaemolyticus* | — | — | — | — | — | — | — | — | 1 | **1** |
| Other bacterial | 1 | 2 | — | — | — | — | 1 | 4 | — | **4** |
| **Total bacterial** | **20** | **48** | **4** | **2** | **6** | **2** | **50** | **132** | **3** | **135** |
| **Chemical** | | | | | | | | | | |
| Ciguatoxin | 11 | 1 | — | — | — | — | — | 12 | 1 | **13** |
| Heavy metals | — | — | — | — | — | — | 1 | 1 | — | **1** |
| Mushroom poisoning | 1 | — | — | — | — | — | — | 1 | — | **1** |
| Scombrotoxin | 1 | 4 | — | — | — | — | — | 5 | — | **5** |
| Other chemical | — | 1 | — | — | — | — | — | 1 | — | **1** |
| **Total chemical** | **13** | **6** | **—** | **—** | **—** | **—** | **1** | **20** | **1** | **21** |
| **Parasitic** | | | | | | | | | | |
| *Trichinella spiralis* | — | — | — | — | — | — | 1 | 1 | — | **1** |
| Other parasitic | 1 | — | — | — | — | — | — | 1 | — | **1** |
| **Total parasitic** | **1** | **—** | **—** | **—** | **—** | **—** | **1** | **2** | **—** | **2** |
| **Viral** | | | | | | | | | | |
| Hepatitis A | — | 2 | — | 1 | — | — | 2 | 5 | — | **5** |
| Norwalk | — | — | — | — | — | — | 1 | 1 | — | **1** |
| Other viral | — | — | 1 | — | — | — | 3 | 4 | — | **4** |
| **Total viral** | **—** | **2** | **1** | **1** | **—** | **—** | **6** | **10** | **—** | **10** |
| **Confirmed etiology** | 34 | 56 | 5 | 3 | 6 | 2 | 58 | 164 | 4 | **168** |
| **Unknown etiology** | 53 | 168 | 9 | 7 | 8 | 3 | 68 | 316 | 5 | **321** |
| **Total 1993** | **87** | **224** | **14** | **10** | **14** | **5** | **126** | **480** | **9** | **489** |

*Includes Guam, Puerto Rico, and the U.S. Virgin Islands.

*Source*: Center for Disease Control and Prevention. U.S. Department of Health and Human Services. *MMWR: Morbidity and Mortality Weekly Review CDC Surveillance Summaries Surveillance for Foodborne-Disease Outbreaks United States, 1993–1997* 49 No. SS-1 (2000). http://www.cdc.gov/mmwr/PDF/ss/ss4901.pdf.

**Table F3.2. Number of Reported Foodborne-Disease Outbreaks, by Etiology and Place Where Food was Eaten—United States,* 1994**

| | Place where food was eaten | | | | | | | | | |
|---|---|---|---|---|---|---|---|---|---|---|
| **Etiology** | **Private residence** | **Delicatessen, cafeteria, or restaurant** | **School** | **Picnic** | **Church** | **Camp** | **Other** | **Known place** | **Unknown place** | **Total** |
| **Bacterial** | | | | | | | | | | |
| *Bacillus cereus* | — | 1 | — | — | — | — | 2 | 3 | — | **3** |
| *Campylobacter* | 1 | 3 | 1 | 1 | — | — | — | 6 | — | **6** |
| *Clostridium botulinum* | 1 | 1 | — | — | — | — | 1 | 2 | — | **3** |
| *Clostridium perfringens* | — | 4 | 2 | 1 | — | — | 5 | 12 | — | **12** |
| *Escherichia coli* | 8 | 2 | 1 | — | — | 2 | 9 | 22 | 3 | **25** |
| *Listeria monocytogenes* | — | — | — | — | — | — | 2 | 2 | 1 | **3** |
| *Salmonella* | 8 | 26 | 2 | — | 4 | 2 | 26 | 68 | 2 | **70** |
| *Shigella* | 3 | 4 | 2 | — | — | — | 2 | 11 | — | **11** |
| *Staphylococcus aureus* | 2 | 3 | 1 | — | — | — | 7 | 13 | — | **13** |
| *Vibrio cholera* | 1 | — | — | — | — | — | — | 1 | — | **1** |
| *Yersinia enterocolitica* | 1 | — | — | — | — | — | — | 1 | — | **1** |
| **Total bacterial** | **25** | **44** | **9** | **2** | **4** | **4** | **54** | **141** | **6** | **148** |
| **Chemical** | | | | | | | | | | |
| Ciguatoxin | 8 | 2 | — | — | 1 | — | — | 11 | — | **11** |
| Heavy metals | 1 | — | — | — | — | — | 1 | 2 | — | **2** |
| Monosodium gluatamate | — | 1 | — | — | — | — | — | 1 | — | **1** |
| Scombrotoxin | 6 | 11 | — | — | — | — | 4 | 21 | — | **21** |
| Other chemical | 1 | — | — | — | — | — | 1 | 2 | — | **2** |
| **Total chemical** | **16** | **14** | **—** | **—** | **1** | **—** | **6** | **37** | **—** | **37** |
| **Parasitic** | | | | | | | | | | |
| *Giardia lamblia* | 1 | 1 | — | — | — | — | — | 2 | — | **2** |
| **Viral** | | | | | | | | | | |
| Hepatitis A | — | 2 | — | — | — | — | 4 | 6 | — | **6** |
| Norwalk | 1 | — | — | — | — | — | — | 1 | — | **1** |
| Other viral | 1 | — | — | — | — | — | 2 | 3 | — | **3** |
| **Total viral** | **2** | **2** | **—** | **—** | **—** | **—** | **6** | **10** | **—** | **10** |
| **Confirmed etiology** | 44 | 61 | 9 | 2 | 5 | 4 | 66 | 191 | 6 | **197** |
| **Unknown etiology** | 86 | 198 | 20 | 5 | 9 | 4 | 119 | 441 | 15 | **456** |
| **Total 1994** | **130** | **259** | **29** | **7** | **14** | **8** | **185** | **632** | **21** | **653** |

*Includes Guam, Puerto Rico, and the U.S. Virgin Islands.

*Source*: Center for Disease Control and Prevention. U.S. Department of Health and Human Services. *MMWR: Morbidity and Mortality Weekly Review CDC Surveillance Summaries Surveillance for Foodborne-Disease Outbreaks United States, 1993–1997* 49 no. SS-1 (2000). http://www.cdc.gov/mmwr/PDF/ss/ss4901.pdf.

**Table F3.3. Number of Reported Foodborne-Disease Outbreaks, by Etiology and Place Where Food was Eaten—United States,* 1995**

| | Place where food was eaten | | | | | | | | | |
|---|---|---|---|---|---|---|---|---|---|---|
| **Etiology** | **Private residence** | **Delicatessen, cafeteria, or restaurant** | **School** | **Picnic** | **Church** | **Camp** | **Other** | **Known place** | **Unknown place** | **Total** |
| **Bacterial** | | | | | | | | | | |
| *Bacillus cereus* | 1 | 1 | — | — | — | — | — | 2 | — | **2** |
| *Campylobacter* | 2 | — | — | — | 1 | 1 | 2 | 6 | — | **6** |
| *Clostridium botulinum* | 2 | — | — | — | — | — | — | 2 | — | **2** |
| *Clostridium perfringens* | 1 | 8 | — | — | 1 | — | 4 | 14 | — | **14** |
| *Escherichia coli* | 8 | 3 | — | — | 4 | 3 | 6 | 24 | 1 | **25** |
| *Salmonella* | 21 | 35 | — | 1 | 2 | — | 29 | 88 | 2 | **90** |
| *Shigella* | — | 4 | — | — | 1 | — | 2 | 7 | — | **7** |
| *Staphylococcus aureus* | 1 | 2 | 1 | — | — | — | 2 | 6 | — | **6** |
| *Yersinia enterocolitica* | 1 | — | — | — | — | — | — | 1 | — | **1** |
| Other bacterial | — | — | — | — | — | — | 2 | 2 | — | **2** |
| **Total bacterial** | **37** | **53** | **1** | **1** | **9** | **4** | **47** | **152** | **3** | **155** |
| **Chemical** | | | | | | | | | | |
| Ciguatoxin | 10 | — | — | — | — | — | — | 10 | — | **10** |
| Heavy metals | — | 1 | — | — | — | — | — | 1 | — | **1** |
| Scombrotoxin | 5 | 9 | — | — | — | — | 2 | 16 | — | **16** |
| Other chemical | — | 1 | — | — | — | — | 1 | 2 | — | **2** |
| **Total chemical** | **15** | **11** | **—** | **—** | **—** | **—** | **3** | **29** | **—** | **29** |
| **Parasitic** | | | | | | | | | | |
| *Trichinella spiralis* | 1 | — | — | — | — | — | — | 1 | — | **1** |
| **Viral** | | | | | | | | | | |
| Hepatitis A | 1 | 2 | — | — | — | — | 1 | 4 | — | **4** |
| Norwalk | — | — | — | — | — | — | 3 | 3 | 1 | **4** |
| Other viral | — | — | — | — | — | — | 1 | 1 | — | **1** |
| **Total viral** | **1** | **2** | **—** | **—** | **—** | **—** | **5** | **8** | **1** | **9** |
| **Confirmed etiology** | 54 | 66 | 1 | 1 | 9 | 4 | 55 | 190 | 4 | **194** |
| **Unknown etiology** | 93 | 222 | 7 | 2 | 7 | 6 | 74 | 411 | 23 | **434** |
| **Total 1995** | **147** | **288** | **8** | **3** | **16** | **10** | **129** | **600** | **27** | **628** |

*Includes Guam, Puerto Rico, and the U.S. Virgin Islands.

*Source*: Center for Disease Control and Prevention. U.S. Department of Health and Human Services. *MMWR: Morbidity and Mortality Weekly Review CDC Surveillance Summaries Surveillance for Foodborne-Disease Outbreaks United States, 1993–1997* 49 no. SS-1 (2000). http://www.cdc.gov/mmwr/PDF/ss/ss4901.pdf.

**Table F3.4. Number of Reported Foodborne-Disease Outbreaks, by Etiology and Place Where Food was Eaten—United States;* 1996**

| | Place where food was eaten | | | | | | | | | |
|---|---|---|---|---|---|---|---|---|---|---|
| Etiology | Private residence | Delicatessen, cafeteria, or restaurant | School | Picnic | Church | Camp | Other | Knwon place | Unknown place | Total |
| **Bacterial** | | | | | | | | | | |
| *Bacillus cereus* | — | — | 1 | — | — | — | — | 1 | — | **1** |
| *Brucella* | — | — | — | — | — | — | 1 | 1 | — | **1** |
| *Campylobacter* | — | 2 | 1 | — | 1 | — | 1 | 5 | — | **5** |
| *Clostridium botulinum* | 2 | — | — | — | — | — | — | 2 | — | **2** |
| *Clostridium perfringens* | — | 3 | 3 | — | — | — | 4 | 10 | — | **10** |
| *Escherichia coli* | 3 | 3 | — | 1 | — | — | 2 | 9 | 2 | **11** |
| *Salmonella* | 11 | 26 | 4 | 4 | 3 | — | 17 | 65 | 4 | **69** |
| *Shigella* | — | 4 | — | — | — | — | 2 | 6 | — | **6** |
| *Staphylococcus aureus* | 2 | 1 | 3 | — | — | — | 1 | 7 | — | **7** |
| **Total bacterial** | **18** | **39** | **12** | **5** | **4** | **—** | **28** | **106** | **6** | **112** |
| **Chemical** | | | | | | | | | | |
| Ciguatoxin | 8 | — | — | — | — | 1 | — | 9 | — | **9** |
| Mushroom poisoning | 2 | — | — | — | — | — | 1 | 3 | — | **3** |
| Scombrotoxin | 2 | 8 | — | — | — | — | 2 | 12 | — | **12** |
| Shellfish | 1 | — | — | — | — | — | — | 1 | — | **1** |
| Other chemical | — | — | — | — | — | — | 1 | 1 | — | **1** |
| **Total chemical** | **13** | **8** | **—** | **—** | **—** | **1** | **4** | **26** | **—** | **26** |
| **Parasitic** | | | | | | | | | | |
| *Giardia lamblia* | — | — | — | — | — | — | 1 | 1 | — | **1** |
| Other parasitic | — | — | — | — | — | — | 1 | 1 | 1 | **2** |
| **Total parasitic** | **—** | **—** | **—** | **—** | **—** | **—** | **2** | **2** | **1** | **3** |
| **Viral** | | | | | | | | | | |
| Hepatitis A | 1 | 1 | — | — | — | — | 2 | 4 | 1 | **5** |
| Norwalk | — | 1 | — | — | — | — | 2 | 3 | — | **3** |
| Other viral | — | — | — | — | — | — | 2 | 2 | — | **2** |
| **Total viral** | **1** | **2** | **—** | **—** | **—** | **—** | **6** | **9** | **1** | **10** |
| **Confirmed etiology** | 32 | 49 | 12 | 5 | 4 | 1 | 40 | 143 | 8 | **151** |
| **Unknown etiology** | 76 | 149 | 11 | 3 | 5 | 2 | 69 | 315 | 11 | **326** |
| **Total 1996** | **108** | **198** | **23** | **8** | **9** | **3** | **109** | **458** | **19** | **477** |

*Includes Guam, Puerto Rico, and the U.S. Virgin Islands.

*Source*: Center for Disease Control and Prevention. U.S. Department of Health and Human Services. *MMWR: Morbidity and Mortality Weekly Review CDC Surveillance Summaries Surveillance for Foodborne-Disease Outbreaks United States, 1993–1997* 49 no. SS-1 (2000). http://www.cdc.gov/mmwr/PDF/ss/ss4901.pdf.

**Table F3.5. Number of Reported Foodborne-Disease Outbreaks, by Etiology and Place Where Food Was Eaten—United States,* 1997**

| Etiology | Place where food was eaten | | | | | | | | | |
|---|---|---|---|---|---|---|---|---|---|---|
| | Private residence | Delicatessen, cafeteria, or restaurant | School | Picnic | Church | Camp | Other | Known place | Unknown place | Total |
| **Bacterial** | | | | | | | | | | |
| *Bacillus cereus* | 2 | — | — | — | 1 | — | 1 | 4 | — | **4** |
| *Campylobacter* | — | — | — | — | — | — | 1 | 1 | 1 | **2** |
| *Clostridium botulinum* | 1 | — | — | — | — | — | — | 1 | — | **1** |
| *Clostridium perfringens* | — | 2 | — | — | — | — | 4 | 6 | — | **6** |
| *Escherichia coli* | — | 2 | — | — | — | — | 5 | 7 | 1 | **8** |
| *Salmonella* | 18 | 24 | 2 | 1 | 3 | 1 | 10 | 59 | 1 | **60** |
| *Shigella* | 3 | 5 | — | — | — | — | 2 | 10 | — | **10** |
| *Staphylococcus aureus* | 2 | — | 2 | 1 | — | — | 4 | 9 | — | **9** |
| *Streptococcus,* group A | — | — | 1 | — | — | — | — | 1 | — | **1** |
| *Vibrio parahaemolyticus* | 1 | 2 | — | — | — | — | 1 | 4 | — | **4** |
| **Total bacterial** | **27** | **35** | **5** | **2** | **4** | **1** | **28** | **102** | **3** | **105** |
| **Chemical** | | | | | | | | | | |
| Ciguatoxin | 13 | 3 | — | — | — | — | 1 | 17 | — | **17** |
| Mushroom poisoning | — | 1 | — | — | — | — | 1 | 2 | 1 | **3** |
| Scombrotoxin | 5 | 8 | — | — | — | — | 2 | 15 | — | **15** |
| **Total chemical** | **18** | **12** | **—** | **—** | **—** | **—** | **4** | **34** | **1** | **35** |
| **Parasitic** | | | | | | | | | | |
| *Giardia lamblia* | — | 1 | — | — | — | — | — | 1 | — | **1** |
| Other parasitic | — | 2 | — | — | — | — | 8 | 10 | — | **10** |
| **Total parasitic** | **—** | **3** | **—** | **—** | **—** | **—** | **8** | **11** | **—** | **11** |
| **Viral** | | | | | | | | | | |
| Hepatitis A | 1 | 1 | 1 | — | — | — | — | 3 | — | **3** |
| Other viral | 3 | 4 | — | — | 2 | — | 5 | 14 | — | **14** |
| **Total viral** | **4** | **5** | **1** | **—** | **2** | **—** | **5** | **17** | **—** | **17** |
| **Confirmed etiology** | 49 | 55 | 6 | 2 | 6 | 1 | 45 | 164 | 4 | **168** |
| **Unknown etiology** | 64 | 161 | 11 | 4 | 4 | 3 | 70 | 317 | 19 | **336** |
| **Total 1997** | **113** | **216** | **17** | **6** | **10** | **4** | **115** | **481** | **23** | **504** |

*Includes Guam, Puerto Rico, and the U.S. Virgin Islands.

*Source*: Center for Disease Control and Prevention. U.S. Department of Health and Human Services. *MMWR: Morbidity and Mortality Weekly Review CDC Surveillance Summaries Surveillance for Foodborne-Disease Outbreaks United States, 1993–1997* 49 no. SS-1 (2000). http://www.cdc.gov/mmwr/PDF/ss/ss4901.pdf.

**Table F4.1. Number of Reported Foodborne-Disease Outbreaks, Cases, and Deaths, by Vehicle of Transmission—United States;* 1993†**

| | Outbreaks | | Cases | | Deaths | |
|---|---|---|---|---|---|---|
| **Vehicle of transmission** | **No.** | **(%)** | **No.** | **(%)** | **No.** | **(%)** |
| Beef | 16 | ( 3.3) | 1,368 | ( 7.8) | 4 | ( 44.4) |
| Pork | 3 | ( 0.6) | 95 | ( 0.5) | 0 | ( 0.0) |
| Chicken | 5 | ( 1.0) | 157 | ( 0.9) | 0 | ( 0.0) |
| Turkey | 1 | ( 0.2) | 10 | ( 0.1) | 0 | ( 0.0) |
| Other/unknown meat | 3 | ( 0.6) | 167 | ( 1.0) | 1 | ( 11.1) |
| Shellfish | 7 | ( 1.4) | 657 | ( 3.8) | 0 | ( 0.0) |
| Other fish | 24 | ( 4.9) | 187 | ( 1.1) | 0 | ( 0.0) |
| Milk | 2 | ( 0.4) | 28 | ( 0.2) | 0 | ( 0.0) |
| Cheese | 2 | ( 0.4) | 20 | ( 0.1) | 1 | ( 11.1) |
| Eggs | 4 | ( 0.8) | 71 | ( 0.4) | 0 | ( 0.0) |
| Ice cream | 3 | ( 0.6) | 32 | ( 0.2) | 0 | ( 0.0) |
| Other/unknown dairy | 2 | ( 0.4) | 41 | ( 0.2) | 0 | ( 0.0) |
| Baked foods | 4 | ( 0.8) | 182 | ( 1.0) | 0 | ( 0.0) |
| Fruits and vegetables | 12 | ( 2.5) | 4,213 | ( 24.1) | 0 | ( 0.0) |
| Mushrooms | 1 | ( 0.2) | 2 | ( 0.0) | 0 | ( 0.0) |
| Potato salad | 1 | ( 0.2) | 24 | ( 0.1) | 0 | ( 0.0) |
| Poultry, fish, and egg salads | 4 | ( 0.8) | 287 | ( 1.6) | 0 | ( 0.0) |
| Other salad | 18 | ( 3.7) | 1,060 | ( 6.1) | 0 | ( 0.0) |
| Chinese food | 4 | ( 0.8) | 52 | ( 0.3) | 0 | ( 0.0) |
| Mexican food | 7 | ( 1.4) | 192 | ( 1.1) | 0 | ( 0.0) |
| Carbonated drink | 2 | ( 0.4) | 31 | ( 0.2) | 0 | ( 0.0) |
| Multiple vehicles | 51 | ( 10.4) | 3,363 | ( 19.2) | 1 | ( 11.1) |
| **Known vehicle** | 176 | ( 36.0) | 12,239 | ( 70.0) | 7 | ( 77.8) |
| **Unknown vehicle** | 313 | ( 64.0) | 5,238 | ( 30.0) | 2 | ( 22.2) |
| **Total 1993** | **489** | **(100.0)** | **17,477** | **(100.0)** | **9** | **(100.0)** |

*Includes Guam, Puerto Rico, and the U.S. Virgin Islands.
†Totals might vary by <1% from summed components because of rounding.
*Source*: Center for Disease Control and Prevention. U.S. Department of Health and Human Services. *MMWR: Morbidity and Mortality Weekly Review CDC Surveillance Summaries Surveillance for Foodborne-Disease Outbreaks United States, 1993–1997* 49 no. SS-1 (2000). http://www.cdc.gov/mmwr/PDF/ss/ss4901.pdf.

**Table F4.2. Number of Reported Foodborne-Disease Outbreaks, Cases, and Deaths, by Vehicle of Transmission—United States,* 1994†**

| | Outbreaks | | Cases | | Deaths | |
|---|---|---|---|---|---|---|
| **Vehicle of transmission** | **No.** | **(%)** | **No.** | **(%)** | **No.** | **(%)** |
| Beef | 22 | ( 3.4) | 871 | ( 5.4) | 0 | ( 0.0) |
| Ham | 4 | ( 0.6) | 119 | ( 0.7) | 0 | ( 0.0) |
| Pork | 3 | ( 0.5) | 56 | ( 0.3) | 0 | ( 0.0) |
| Chicken | 4 | ( 0.6) | 165 | ( 1.0) | 0 | ( 0.0) |
| Turkey | 12 | ( 1.8) | 418 | ( 2.6) | 0 | ( 0.0) |
| Other/unknown meat | 6 | ( 0.9) | 175 | ( 1.1) | 1 | ( 33.3) |
| Shellfish | 12 | ( 1.8) | 220 | ( 1.4) | 0 | ( 0.0) |
| Other fish | 35 | ( 5.4) | 150 | ( 0.9) | 0 | ( 0.0) |
| Milk | 3 | ( 0.5) | 105 | ( 0.6) | 0 | ( 0.0) |
| Cheese | 1 | ( 0.2) | 5 | ( 0.0) | 0 | ( 0.0) |
| Eggs | 3 | ( 0.5) | 36 | ( 0.2) | 0 | ( 0.0) |
| Ice cream | 5 | ( 0.8) | 919 | ( 5.7) | 0 | ( 0.0) |
| Baked foods | 12 | ( 1.8) | 328 | ( 2.0) | 0 | ( 0.0) |
| Fruits and vegetables | 17 | ( 2.6) | 1,311 | ( 8.1) | 0 | ( 0.0) |
| Potato salad | 8 | ( 1.2) | 266 | ( 1.6) | 2 | ( 66.7) |
| Other salad | 19 | ( 2.9) | 1,093 | ( 6.7) | 0 | ( 0.0) |
| Chinese food | 2 | ( 0.3) | 42 | ( 0.3) | 0 | ( 0.0) |
| Mexican food | 6 | ( 0.9) | 309 | ( 1.9) | 0 | ( 0.0) |
| Carbonated drink | 1 | ( 0.2) | 11 | ( 0.1) | 0 | ( 0.0) |
| Nondairy beverage | 5 | ( 0.8) | 101 | ( 0.6) | 0 | ( 0.0) |
| Multiple vehicles | 74 | ( 11.3) | 3,224 | ( 19.9) | 0 | ( 0.0) |
| **Known vehicle** | 254 | ( 38.9) | 9,924 | ( 61.1) | 3 | (100.0) |
| **Unknown vehicle** | 399 | ( 61.1) | 6,310 | ( 38.9) | 0 | ( 0.0) |
| **Total 1994** | **653** | **(100.0)** | **16,234** | **(100.0)** | **3** | **(100.0)** |

*Includes Guam, Puerto Rico, and the U.S. Virgin Islands.

†Totals might vary by <1% from summed components because of rounding.

*Source*: Center for Disease Control and Prevention. U.S. Department of Health and Human Services. *MMWR: Morbidity and Mortality Weekly Review CDC Surveillance Summaries Surveillance for Foodborne-Disease Outbreaks United States, 1993–1997* 49 no. SS-1 (2000). http://www.cdc.gov/mmwr/PDF/ss/ss4901.pdf.

## Table F4.3. Number of Reported Foodborne-Disease Outbreaks, Cases, and Deaths, by Vehicle of Transmission—United States;* 1995†

| | Outbreaks | | Cases | | Deaths | |
|---|---|---|---|---|---|---|
| **Vehicle of transmission** | **No.** | **(%)** | **No.** | **(%)** | **No.** | **(%)** |
| Beef | 14 | ( 2.2) | 437 | ( 2.5) | 0 | ( 0.0) |
| Pork | 4 | ( 0.6) | 322 | ( 1.8) | 1 | ( 9.1) |
| Sausage | 1 | ( 0.2) | 12 | ( 0.1) | 0 | ( 0.0) |
| Chicken | 6 | ( 1.0) | 220 | ( 1.2) | 0 | ( 0.0) |
| Turkey | 3 | ( 0.5) | 46 | ( 0.3) | 0 | ( 0.0) |
| Other/unknown meat | 7 | ( 1.1) | 107 | ( 0.6) | 0 | ( 0.0) |
| Shellfish | 12 | ( 1.9) | 428 | ( 2.4) | 0 | ( 0.0) |
| Other fish | 31 | ( 4.9) | 146 | ( 0.8) | 0 | ( 0.0) |
| Milk | 1 | ( 0.2) | 3 | ( 0.0) | 0 | ( 0.0) |
| Cheese | 1 | ( 0.2) | 9 | ( 0.1) | 0 | ( 0.0) |
| Eggs | 6 | ( 1.0) | 103 | ( 0.6) | 3 | ( 27.3) |
| Ice cream | 1 | ( 0.2) | 60 | ( 0.3) | 0 | ( 0.0) |
| Baked foods | 9 | ( 1.4) | 193 | ( 1.1) | 0 | ( 0.0) |
| Fruits and vegetables | 9 | ( 1.4) | 4,307 | ( 24.2) | 0 | ( 0.0) |
| Potato salad | 1 | ( 0.2) | 11 | ( 0.1) | 0 | ( 0.0) |
| Poultry, fish, and egg salads | 4 | ( 0.6) | 162 | ( 0.9) | 0 | ( 0.0) |
| Other salad | 21 | ( 3.3) | 662 | ( 3.7) | 0 | ( 0.0) |
| Chinese food | 3 | ( 0.5) | 53 | ( 0.3) | 0 | ( 0.0) |
| Mexican food | 7 | ( 1.1) | 216 | ( 1.2) | 0 | ( 0.0) |
| Carbonated drink | 1 | ( 0.2) | 3 | ( 0.0) | 0 | ( 0.0) |
| Nondairy beverage | 6 | ( 1.0) | 302 | ( 1.7) | 0 | ( 0.0) |
| Multiple vehicles | 60 | ( 9.6) | 3,642 | ( 20.5) | 0 | ( 0.0) |
| **Known vehicle** | 208 | ( 33.1) | 11,444 | ( 64.3) | 4 | ( 36.4) |
| **Unknown vehicle** | 420 | ( 66.9) | 6,356 | ( 35.7) | 7 | ( 63.6) |
| **Total 1995** | **628** | **(100.0)** | **17,800** | **(100.0)** | **11** | **(100.0)** |

*Includes Guam, Puerto Rico, and the U.S. Virgin Islands.
†Totals might vary by <1% from summed components because of rounding.
*Source*: Center for Disease Control and Prevention. U.S. Department of Health and Human Services. *MMWR: Morbidity and Mortality Weekly Review CDC Surveillance Summaries Surveillance for Foodborne-Disease Outbreaks United States, 1993–1997* 49 no. SS-1 (2000). http://www.cdc.gov/mmwr/PDF/ss/ss4901.pdf.

**Table F4.4. Number of Reported Foodborne-Disease Outbreaks, Cases, and Deaths, by Vehicle of Transmission—United States;* 1996†**

| | Outbreaks | | Cases | | Deaths | |
|---|---|---|---|---|---|---|
| **Vehicle of transmission** | **No.** | **(%)** | **No.** | **(%)** | **No.** | **(%)** |
| Beef | 7 | ( 1.5) | 227 | ( 1.0) | 0 | ( 0.0) |
| Ham | 4 | ( 0.8) | 89 | ( 0.4) | 0 | ( 0.0) |
| Pork | 2 | ( 0.4) | 115 | ( 0.5) | 0 | ( 0.0) |
| Chicken | 6 | ( 1.3) | 315 | ( 1.4) | 0 | ( 0.0) |
| Turkey | 3 | ( 0.6) | 187 | ( 0.8) | 0 | ( 0.0) |
| Other/unknown meat | 1 | ( 0.2) | 59 | ( 0.3) | 0 | ( 0.0) |
| Shellfish | 5 | ( 1.0) | 514 | ( 2.3) | 0 | ( 0.0) |
| Other fish | 24 | ( 5.0) | 105 | ( 0.5) | 0 | ( 0.0) |
| Milk | 2 | ( 0.4) | 48 | ( 0.2) | 0 | ( 0.0) |
| Eggs | 3 | ( 0.6) | 66 | ( 0.3) | 0 | ( 0.0) |
| Ice cream | 6 | ( 1.3) | 183 | ( 0.8) | 0 | ( 0.0) |
| Other/unknown dairy | 2 | ( 0.4) | 31 | ( 0.1) | 0 | ( 0.0) |
| Baked foods | 6 | ( 1.3) | 81 | ( 0.4) | 0 | ( 0.0) |
| Fruits and vegetables | 13 | ( 2.7) | 1,807 | ( 8.0) | 1 | ( 25.0) |
| Mushrooms | 3 | ( 0.6) | 10 | ( 0.0) | 0 | ( 0.0) |
| Potato salad | 1 | ( 0.2) | 12 | ( 0.1) | 0 | ( 0.0) |
| Poultry, fish, and egg salads | 7 | ( 1.5) | 789 | ( 3.5) | 0 | ( 0.0) |
| Other salad | 18 | ( 3.8) | 628 | ( 2.8) | 0 | ( 0.0) |
| Mexican food | 3 | ( 0.6) | 196 | ( 0.9) | 0 | ( 0.0) |
| Nondairy beverage | 6 | ( 1.3) | 140 | ( 0.6) | 0 | ( 0.0) |
| Multiple vehicles | 38 | ( 8.0) | 12,692 | ( 56.1) | 0 | ( 0.0) |
| **Known vehicle** | 160 | ( 33.5) | 18,294 | ( 80.9) | 1 | ( 25.0) |
| **Unknown vehicle** | 317 | ( 66.5) | 4,313 | ( 19.1) | 3 | ( 75.0) |
| **Total 1996** | **477** | **(100.0)** | **22,607** | **(100.0)** | **4** | **(100.0)** |

*Includes Guam, Puerto Rico, and the U.S. Virgin Islands.

†Totals might vary by <1% from summed components because of rounding.

*Source*: Center for Disease Control and Prevention. U.S. Department of Health and Human Services. *MMWR: Morbidity and Mortality Weekly Review CDC Surveillance Summaries Surveillance for Foodborne-Disease Outbreaks United States, 1993–1997* 49 no. SS-1 (2000). http://www.cdc.gov/mmwr/PDF/ss/ss4901.pdf.

**Table F4.5. Number of Reported Foodborne-Disease Outbreaks, Cases, and Deaths, by Vehicle of Transmission—United States;* 1997†**

| | Outbreaks | | Cases | | Deaths | |
|---|---|---|---|---|---|---|
| **Vehicle of transmission** | **No.** | **(%)** | **No.** | **(%)** | **No.** | **(%)** |
| Beef | 7 | ( 1.4) | 302 | ( 2.5) | 0 | ( 0.0) |
| Ham | 4 | ( 0.8) | 85 | ( 0.7) | 0 | ( 0.0) |
| Pork | 2 | ( 0.4) | 50 | ( 0.4) | 0 | ( 0.0) |
| Sausage | 1 | ( 0.2) | 45 | ( 0.4) | 0 | ( 0.0) |
| Chicken | 9 | ( 1.8) | 256 | ( 2.1) | 0 | ( 0.0) |
| Turkey | 3 | ( 0.6) | 97 | ( 0.8) | 0 | ( 0.0) |
| Other/unknown meat | 5 | ( 1.0) | 137 | ( 1.1) | 0 | ( 0.0) |
| Shellfish | 11 | ( 2.2) | 49 | ( 0.4) | 0 | ( 0.0) |
| Other fish | 26 | ( 5.2) | 108 | ( 0.9) | 0 | ( 0.0) |
| Milk | 2 | ( 0.4) | 23 | ( 0.2) | 0 | ( 0.0) |
| Eggs | 3 | ( 0.6) | 91 | ( 0.8) | 0 | ( 0.0) |
| Baked foods | 4 | ( 0.8) | 69 | ( 0.6) | 0 | ( 0.0) |
| Fruits and vegetables | 15 | ( 3.0) | 719 | ( 6.0) | 1 | ( 50.0) |
| Potato salad | 3 | ( 0.6) | 242 | ( 2.0) | 0 | ( 0.0) |
| Poultry, fish, and egg salads | 1 | ( 0.2) | 143 | ( 1.2) | 0 | ( 0.0) |
| Other salad | 21 | ( 4.2) | 1,104 | ( 9.2) | 0 | ( 0.0) |
| Chinese food | 1 | ( 0.2) | 16 | ( 0.1) | 0 | ( 0.0) |
| Mexican food | 9 | ( 1.8) | 701 | ( 5.9) | 0 | ( 0.0) |
| Nondairy beverage | 3 | ( 0.6) | 63 | ( 0.5) | 0 | ( 0.0) |
| Multiple vehicles | 39 | ( 7.7) | 2,707 | ( 22.7) | 0 | ( 0.0) |
| **Known vehicle** | 169 | ( 33.5) | 7,007 | ( 58.7) | 1 | ( 50.0) |
| **Unknown vehicle** | 335 | ( 66.5) | 4,933 | ( 41.3) | 1 | ( 50.0) |
| **Total 1997** | **504** | **(100.0)** | **11,940** | **(100.0)** | **2** | **(100.0)** |

*Includes Guam, Puerto Rico, and the U.S. Virgin Islands.

†Totals might vary by <1% from summed components because of rounding.

*Source*: Center for Disease Control and Prevention. U.S. Department of Health and Human Services. *MMWR: Morbidity and Mortality Weekly Review CDC Surveillance Summaries Surveillance for Foodborne-Disease Outbreaks United States, 1993–1997* 49 no. SS-1 (2000). http://www.cdc.gov/mmwr/PDF/ss/ss4901.pdf.

**Table F5.1. Number of Reported Foodborne-Disease Outbreaks, by Etiology and Contributing Factors—United States;* 1993**

| Etiology | Contributing factors | | | | | | Outbreaks in which factors reported | Total |
|---|---|---|---|---|---|---|---|---|
| | Improper holding temperatures | Inadequate cooking | Contaminated equipment | Food from unsafe source | Poor personal hygiene | Other | | |
| **Bacterial** | | | | | | | | |
| *Bacillus cereus* | 3 | 1 | 1 | — | — | 1 | 4 | **4** |
| *Campylobacter* | 2 | — | 3 | — | — | 1 | 3 | **6** |
| *Clostridium botulinum* | 3 | — | — | — | — | 2 | 4 | **5** |
| *Clostridium perfringens* | 12 | 2 | — | — | 2 | 3 | 12 | **15** |
| *Escherichia coli* | 2 | 5 | 1 | 3 | 1 | 4 | 9 | **15** |
| *Salmonella* | 35 | 22 | 15 | 10 | 11 | 5 | 52 | **68** |
| *Shigella* | — | — | — | — | 5 | — | 5 | **9** |
| *Staphylococcus aureus* | 5 | 1 | 2 | 2 | 3 | 1 | 6 | **7** |
| *Streptococcus*, other | 1 | — | — | — | — | — | 1 | **1** |
| *Vibrio parahaemolyticus* | — | — | — | — | — | — | — | **1** |
| Other bacterial | 4 | 1 | 1 | — | — | — | 4 | **4** |
| **Total bacterial** | **67** | **32** | **23** | **15** | **22** | **17** | **100** | **135** |
| **Chemical** | | | | | | | | |
| Ciguatoxin | — | — | — | 4 | — | 2 | 6 | **13** |
| Heavy metals | — | — | — | — | — | — | — | **1** |
| Mushroom poisoning | — | — | — | 1 | — | — | 1 | **1** |
| Scombrotoxin | 4 | 1 | 1 | 1 | — | — | 4 | **5** |
| Other chemical | — | — | 1 | — | — | 1 | 1 | **1** |
| **Total chemical** | **4** | **1** | **2** | **6** | **—** | **3** | **12** | **21** |
| **Parasitic** | | | | | | | | |
| *Trichinella spiralis* | — | — | — | — | — | — | — | **1** |
| Other parasitic | — | — | — | — | — | — | — | **1** |
| **Total parasitic** | **—** | **—** | **—** | **—** | **—** | **—** | **—** | **2** |
| **Viral** | | | | | | | | |
| Hepatitis A | 1 | — | — | — | 4 | 1 | 5 | **5** |
| Norwalk | — | 1 | — | 1 | — | — | 1 | **1** |
| Other viral | 1 | 1 | 1 | 2 | 1 | — | 4 | **4** |
| **Total viral** | **2** | **2** | **1** | **3** | **5** | **1** | **10** | **10** |
| **Confirmed etiology** | 73 | 35 | 26 | 24 | 27 | 21 | 122 | **168** |
| **Unknown etiology** | 135 | 24 | 54 | 9 | 55 | 46 | 187 | **321** |
| **Total 1993** | **208** | **59** | **80** | **33** | **82** | **67** | **309** | **489** |

*Includes Guam, Puerto Rico, and the U.S. Virgin Islands.

*Source*: Center for Disease Control and Prevention. U.S. Department of Health and Human Services. *MMWR: Morbidity and Mortality Weekly Review CDC Surveillance Summaries Surveillance for Foodborne-Disease Outbreaks United States, 1993–1997* 49 no. SS-1 (2000). http://www.cdc.gov/mmwr/PDF/ss/ss4901.pdf.

**Table F5.2. Number of Reported Foodborne-Disease Outbreaks, by Etiology and Contributing Factors—United States;* 1994**

| Etiology | Contributing factors | | | | | | Outbreaks in which factors reported | Total |
|---|---|---|---|---|---|---|---|---|
| | Improper holding temperatures | Inadequate cooking | Contaminated equipment | Food from unsafe source | Poor personal hygiene | Other | | |
| **Bacterial** | | | | | | | | |
| *Bacillus cereus* | 3 | 1 | — | — | — | — | 3 | **3** |
| *Campylobacter* | 3 | 1 | 5 | — | 5 | 3 | 6 | **6** |
| *Clostridium botulinum* | 2 | — | — | 1 | — | — | 3 | **3** |
| *Clostridium perfringens* | 11 | 1 | 1 | — | — | 2 | 11 | **12** |
| *Escherichia coli* | 2 | 3 | 4 | 4 | 1 | 3 | 12 | **25** |
| *Listeria monocytogenes* | 1 | — | 1 | — | — | 1 | 2 | **3** |
| *Salmonella* | 23 | 24 | 18 | 6 | 16 | 8 | 50 | **70** |
| *Shigella* | — | — | — | 2 | 5 | — | 7 | **11** |
| *Staphylococcus aureus* | 10 | — | 2 | 1 | 2 | 2 | 11 | **13** |
| *Vibrio cholera* | — | — | — | — | — | — | 0 | **1** |
| *Yersinia enterocolitica* | — | — | 1 | — | 1 | — | 1 | **1** |
| **Total bacterial** | **55** | **30** | **32** | **14** | **30** | **19** | **106** | **148** |
| **Chemical** | | | | | | | | |
| Ciguatoxin | 1 | — | — | 5 | — | 1 | 6 | **11** |
| Heavy metals | — | — | 1 | — | — | 1 | 2 | **2** |
| Monosodium glutamate | — | — | — | — | — | 1 | 1 | **1** |
| Scombrotoxin | 12 | — | — | 5 | — | 1 | 15 | **21** |
| Other chemical | — | — | — | 2 | — | — | 2 | **2** |
| **Total chemical** | **13** | **—** | **1** | **12** | **—** | **4** | **26** | **37** |
| **Parasitic** | | | | | | | | |
| *Giardia lamblia* | — | — | — | — | — | — | 0 | **2** |
| **Viral** | | | | | | | | |
| Hepatitis A | — | — | — | — | 6 | — | 6 | **6** |
| Norwalk | — | — | — | — | — | — | 0 | **1** |
| Other viral | — | 2 | — | 1 | 1 | — | 3 | **3** |
| **Total viral** | **—** | **2** | **—** | **1** | **7** | **—** | **9** | **10** |
| **Confirmed etiology** | 68 | 32 | 33 | 27 | 37 | 23 | 141 | **197** |
| **Unknown etiology** | 149 | 28 | 66 | 15 | 87 | 42 | 237 | **456** |
| **Total 1994** | **217** | **60** | **99** | **42** | **124** | **65** | **378** | **653** |

*Includes Guam, Puerto Rico, and the U.S. Virgin Islands.

*Source*: Center for Disease Control and Prevention. U.S. Department of Health and Human Services. *MMWR: Morbidity and Mortality Weekly Review CDC Surveillance Summaries Surveillance for Foodborne-Disease Outbreaks United States, 1993–1997* 49 no. SS-1 (2000). http://www.cdc.gov/mmwr/PDF/ss/ss4901.pdf.

**Table F5.3. Number of Reported Foodborne-Disease Outbreaks, by Etiology and Contributing Factors—United States;* 1995**

| Etiology | Contributing factors | | | | | | Outbreaks in which factors reported | Total |
|---|---|---|---|---|---|---|---|---|
| | Improper holding temperatures | Inadequate cooking | Contaminated equipment | Food from unsafe source | Poor personal hygiene | Other | | |
| **Bacterial** | | | | | | | | |
| *Bacillus cereus* | 1 | — | 1 | — | 1 | — | 1 | **2** |
| *Campylobacter* | 2 | 3 | 1 | 1 | 1 | 1 | 4 | **6** |
| *Clostridium botulinum* | — | — | — | 1 | — | — | 1 | **2** |
| *Clostridium perfringens* | 12 | 4 | 3 | — | 3 | 2 | 12 | **14** |
| *Escherichia coli* | 3 | 8 | 2 | 1 | 2 | 4 | 11 | **25** |
| *Salmonella* | 40 | 26 | 18 | 11 | 16 | 17 | 66 | **90** |
| *Shigella* | 1 | — | — | 1 | 2 | — | 3 | **7** |
| *Staphylococcus aureus* | 5 | 1 | 1 | — | 3 | — | 5 | **6** |
| *Yersinia enterocolitica* | — | — | 1 | — | — | — | 1 | **1** |
| Other bacterial | 1 | — | — | — | 1 | — | 1 | **2** |
| **Total bacterial** | **65** | **42** | **27** | **15** | **29** | **24** | **105** | **155** |
| **Chemical** | | | | | | | | |
| Ciguatoxin | — | — | — | 7 | — | 2 | 8 | **10** |
| Heavy metals | — | — | — | — | — | 1 | 1 | **1** |
| Scombrotoxin | 11 | — | — | 4 | — | — | 13 | **16** |
| Other chemical | — | — | — | — | — | 1 | 1 | **2** |
| **Total chemical** | **11** | **—** | **—** | **11** | **—** | **4** | **23** | **29** |
| **Parasitic** | | | | | | | | |
| *Trichinella spiralis* | — | 1 | — | — | — | — | 1 | **1** |
| **Viral** | | | | | | | | |
| Hepatitis A | — | — | — | — | 2 | — | 2 | **4** |
| Norwalk | — | — | — | 1 | 2 | — | 3 | **4** |
| Other viral | — | — | — | — | — | — | 0 | **1** |
| **Total viral** | **—** | **—** | **—** | **1** | **4** | **—** | **5** | **9** |
| **Confirmed etiology** | 76 | 43 | 27 | 27 | 33 | 28 | 134 | **194** |
| **Unknown etiology** | 134 | 20 | 48 | 8 | 61 | 34 | 211 | **434** |
| **Total 1995** | **210** | **63** | **75** | **35** | **94** | **62** | **345** | **628** |

*Includes Guam, Puerto Rico, and the U.S. Virgin Islands.

*Source*: Center for Disease Control and Prevention. U.S. Department of Health and Human Services. *MMWR: Morbidity and Mortality Weekly Review CDC Surveillance Summaries Surveillance for Foodborne-Disease Outbreaks United States, 1993–1997* 49 no. SS-1 (2000). http://www.cdc.gov/mmwr/PDF/ss/ss4901.pdf.

**Table F5.4. Number of Reported Foodborne-Disease Outbreaks, by Etiology and Contributing Factors—United States,* 1996**

| | Contributing factors | | | | | | | |
|---|---|---|---|---|---|---|---|---|
| **Etiology** | **Improper holding temperatures** | **Inadequate cooking** | **Contaminated equipment** | **Food from unsafe source** | **Poor personal hygiene** | **Other** | **Outbreaks in which factors reported** | **Total** |
| **Bacterial** | | | | | | | | |
| *Bacillus cereus* | — | — | — | — | — | — | — | **1** |
| *Brucella* | — | — | — | — | — | — | — | **1** |
| *Campylobacter* | — | 1 | — | 1 | 1 | — | 3 | **5** |
| *Clostridium botulinum* | 1 | — | — | — | — | — | 1 | **2** |
| *Clostridium perfringens* | 6 | 4 | 1 | — | — | 3 | 6 | **10** |
| *Escherichia coli* | — | 1 | 1 | 3 | 2 | — | 5 | **11** |
| *Salmonella* | 23 | 17 | 11 | 4 | 10 | 16 | 41 | **69** |
| *Shigella* | — | 1 | — | — | 3 | — | 3 | **6** |
| *Staphylococcus aureus* | 2 | — | 1 | — | 2 | — | 3 | **7** |
| **Total bacterial** | **32** | **24** | **14** | **8** | **18** | **19** | **62** | **112** |
| **Chemical** | | | | | | | | |
| Ciguatoxin | 1 | — | — | 6 | — | 3 | 6 | **9** |
| Mushroom poisoning | — | — | — | 1 | — | — | 1 | **3** |
| Scombrotoxin | 7 | 1 | — | 1 | — | — | 8 | **12** |
| Shellfish | — | — | — | 1 | — | 1 | 1 | **1** |
| Other chemical | — | — | — | — | — | — | — | **1** |
| **Total chemical** | **8** | **1** | **—** | **9** | **—** | **4** | **16** | **26** |
| **Parasitic** | | | | | | | | |
| *Giardia lamblia* | — | — | — | — | 1 | 1 | 1 | **1** |
| Other parasitic | — | — | — | 1 | — | — | 1 | **2** |
| **Total parasitic** | **—** | **—** | **—** | **1** | **1** | **1** | **2** | **3** |
| **Viral** | | | | | | | | |
| Hepatitis A | — | 1 | — | 1 | 2 | — | 3 | **5** |
| Norwalk | — | 1 | — | 1 | 2 | — | 3 | **3** |
| Other viral | — | — | — | 1 | — | — | 1 | **2** |
| **Total viral** | **—** | **2** | **—** | **3** | **4** | **—** | **7** | **10** |
| **Confirmed etiology** | 40 | 27 | 14 | 21 | 23 | 24 | 87 | **151** |
| **Unknown etiology** | 109 | 17 | 46 | 3 | 67 | 21 | 173 | **326** |
| **Total 1996** | **149** | **44** | **60** | **24** | **90** | **45** | **260** | **477** |

*Includes Guam, Puerto Rico, and the U.S. Virgin Islands.

*Source*: Center for Disease Control and Prevention. U.S. Department of Health and Human Services. *MMWR: Morbidity and Mortality Weekly Review CDC Surveillance Summaries Surveillance for Foodborne-Disease Outbreaks United States, 1993–1997* 49 no. SS-1 (2000). http://www.cdc.gov/mmwr/PDF/ss/ss4901.pdf.

**Table F5.5. Number of Reported Foodborne-Disease Outbreaks, by Etiology and Contributing Factors—United States;* 1997**

| Etiology | Contributing factors | | | | | | Outbreaks in which factors reported | Total |
|---|---|---|---|---|---|---|---|---|
| | Improper holding temperatures | Inadequate cooking | Contaminated equipment | Food from unsafe source | Poor personal hygiene | Other | | |
| **Bacterial** | | | | | | | | |
| *Bacillus cereus* | 4 | 1 | — | — | 1 | — | 4 | **4** |
| *Campylobacter* | — | — | 2 | — | 1 | — | 2 | **2** |
| *Clostridium botulinum* | — | 1 | — | 1 | — | — | 1 | **1** |
| *Clostridium perfringens* | 5 | 2 | — | — | — | 1 | 5 | **6** |
| *Escherichia coli* | 1 | 2 | — | — | — | — | 2 | **8** |
| *Salmonella* | 32 | 23 | 16 | 2 | 17 | 7 | 46 | **60** |
| *Shigella* | 3 | — | 1 | — | 4 | 1 | 6 | **10** |
| *Staphylococcus aureus* | 3 | 1 | — | 1 | 2 | 1 | 5 | **9** |
| *Streptococcus*, group A | 1 | — | — | — | 1 | — | 1 | **1** |
| *Vibrio parahaemolyticus* | 1 | 1 | 1 | 1 | — | — | 2 | **4** |
| **Total bacterial** | **50** | **31** | **20** | **5** | **26** | **10** | **74** | **105** |
| **Chemical** | | | | | | | | |
| Ciguatoxin | — | — | — | 3 | — | 8 | 9 | **17** |
| Mushroom poisoning | — | — | — | 1 | — | 1 | 2 | **3** |
| Scombrotoxin | 4 | — | 1 | — | 1 | 1 | 6 | **15** |
| **Total chemical** | **4** | **—** | **1** | **4** | **1** | **10** | **17** | **35** |
| **Parasitic** | | | | | | | | |
| *Giardia lamblia* | — | — | 1 | — | 1 | — | 1 | **1** |
| Other parasitic | — | — | — | 3 | — | 2 | 4 | **10** |
| **Total parasitic** | **—** | **—** | **1** | **3** | **1** | **2** | **5** | **11** |
| **Viral** | | | | | | | | |
| Hepatitis A | — | — | — | — | 1 | — | 1 | **3** |
| Other viral | 1 | — | 1 | 1 | 5 | 2 | 6 | **14** |
| **Total viral** | **1** | **—** | **1** | **1** | **6** | **2** | **7** | **17** |
| **Confirmed etiology** | 55 | 31 | 23 | 13 | 34 | 24 | 103 | **168** |
| **Unknown etiology** | 99 | 17 | 63 | 6 | 66 | 19 | 163 | **336** |
| **Total 1997** | **154** | **48** | **86** | **19** | **100** | **43** | **266** | **504** |

*Includes Guam, Puerto Rico, and the U.S. Virgin Islands.

*Source*: Center for Disease Control and Prevention. U.S. Department of Health and Human Services. *MMWR: Morbidity and Mortality Weekly Review CDC Surveillance Summaries Surveillance for Foodborne-Disease Outbreaks United States, 1993–1997* 49 no. SS-1 (2000). http://www.cdc.gov/mmwr/PDF/ss/ss4901.pdf.

**Table F6.1. Botulism (Foodborne)—Reported Cases, by Year, United States, 1978–1998**

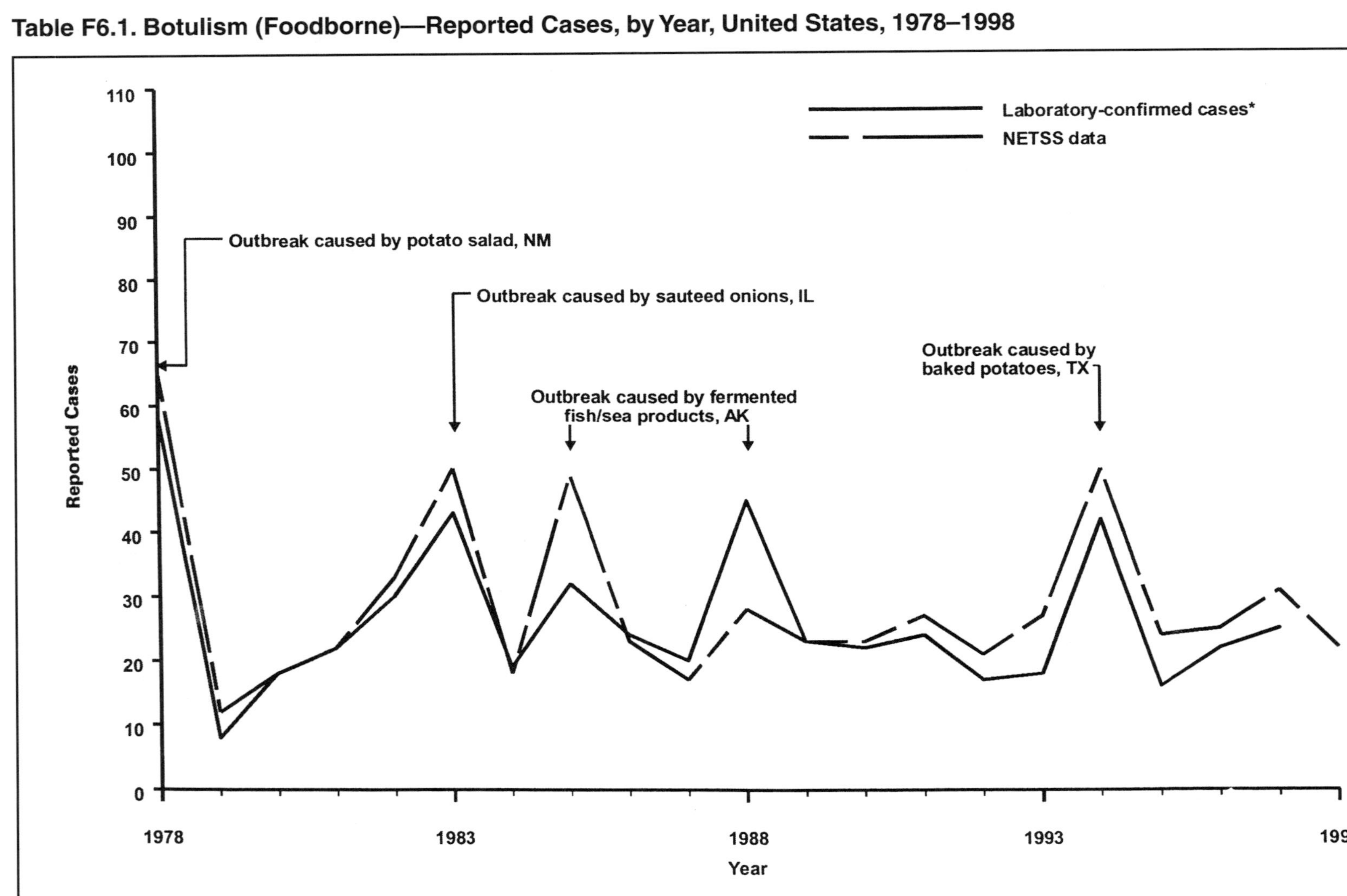


*Data from annual survey of state epidemiologists and directors of state public health laboratories. Data are not yet available for 1998.

Although outbreaks of foodborne botulism occur infrequently, they can rapidly kill many affected persons. Such outbreaks require prompt and effective communication among clinicians and public health officials.

*Source*: Center for Disease Control and Prevention. U.S. Department of Health and Human Services. *MMWR: Morbidity and Mortality Weekly Review Summary of Notifiable Disease, United States, 1999* 48 no. 53 (2001). http://www.cdc.gov/mmwr/PDF/wk/mm4853.pdf.

**Table F6.2. Botulism (Infant)—Reported Cases, by Year, United States, 1978–1998**

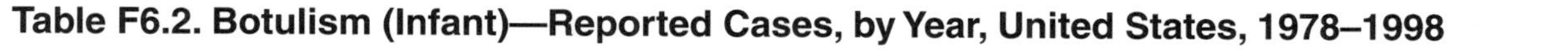

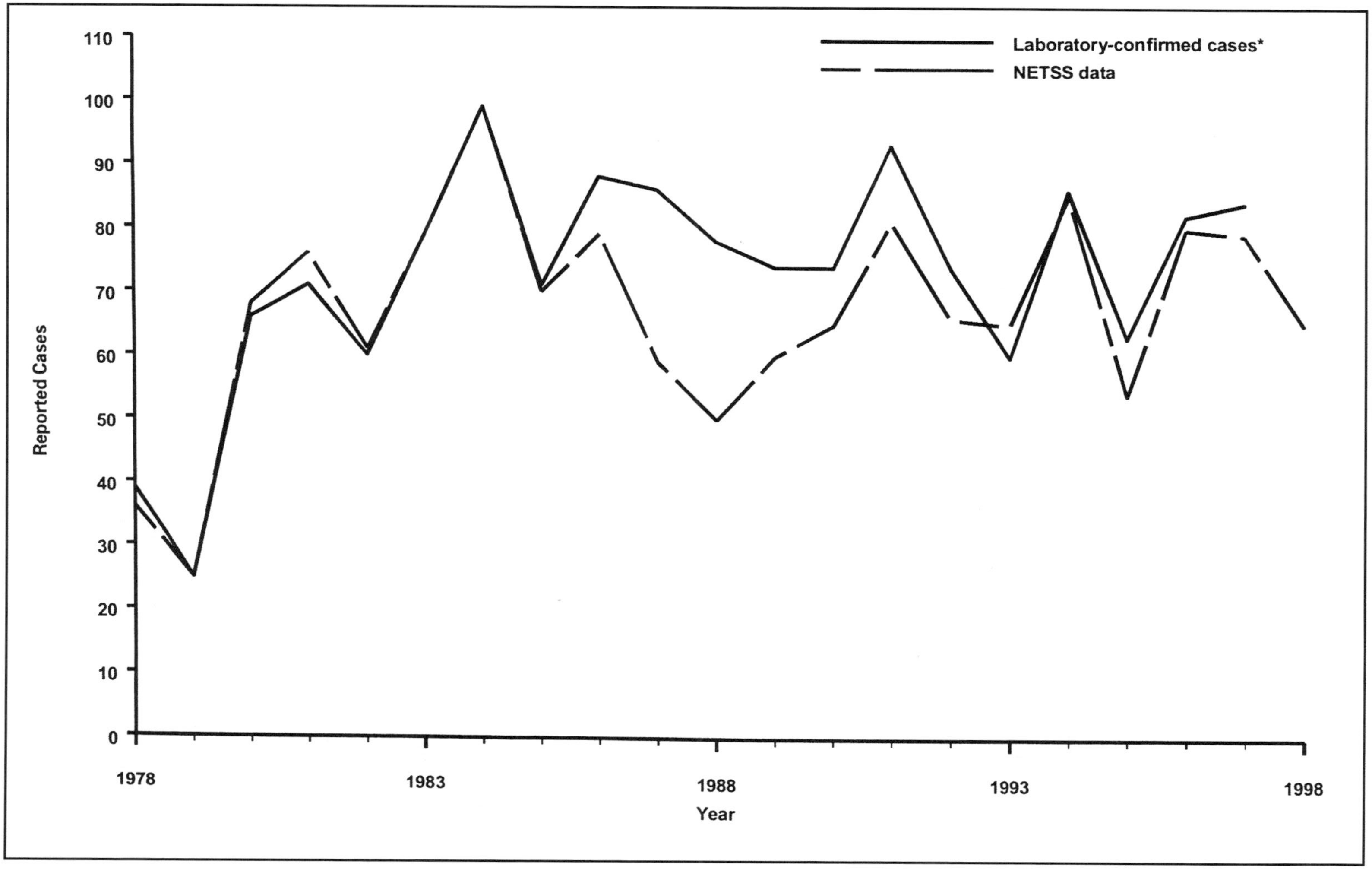

*Data from annual survey of state epidemiologists and directors of state public health laboratories. Data are not yet available for 1998.

In the United States, approximately one third of the reported cases of infant botulism occur in California.

*Source*: Center for Disease Control and Prevention. U.S. Department of Health and Human Services. *MMWR: Morbidity and Mortality Weekly Review Summary of Notifiable Disease, United States, 1999* 48 no. 53 (2001). http://www.cdc.gov/mmwr/PDF/wk/mm4853.pdf.

## Table F6.3. Cryptosporidiosis—Reported Cases per 100,000 Population, United States and Territories, 1999

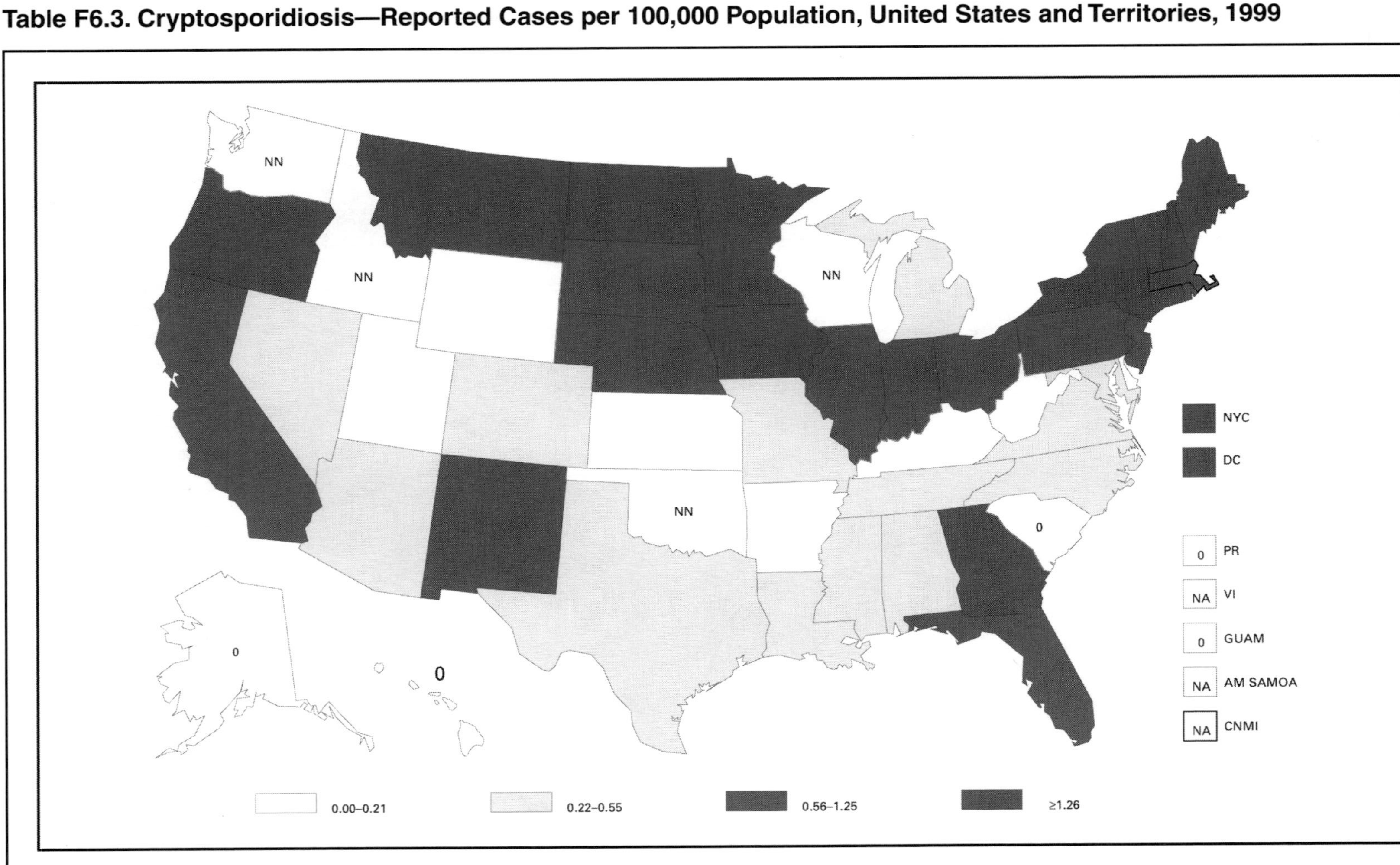


In 1999, *Cryptosporidium* infection was geographically widespread. Waterborne (i.e., from drinking or recreational water) and foodborne outbreaks were reported from Florida, Massachusetts, Minnesota, and Wisconsin. Cases primarily occur in the late summer and early fall and are most prevalent among children aged 1–9 years and adults aged 30–49 years. Case detection and reporting rates can be higher in states that participate in CDC's FoodNet or Emerging Infectious Diseases Program. States participating in 1999 included California, Connecticut, Georgia, Maryland, Minnesota, New York, and Oregon.

*Source*: Center for Disease Control and Prevention. U.S. Department of Health and Human Services. *MMWR: Morbidity and Mortality Weekly Review Summary of Notifiable Disease, United States, 1999* 48 no. 53 (2001). http://www.cdc.gov/mmwr/PDF/wk/mm4853.pdf.

## Table F6.4. *Escherichia Coli* 0157:H7—Reported Cases, United States and Territories, 1999

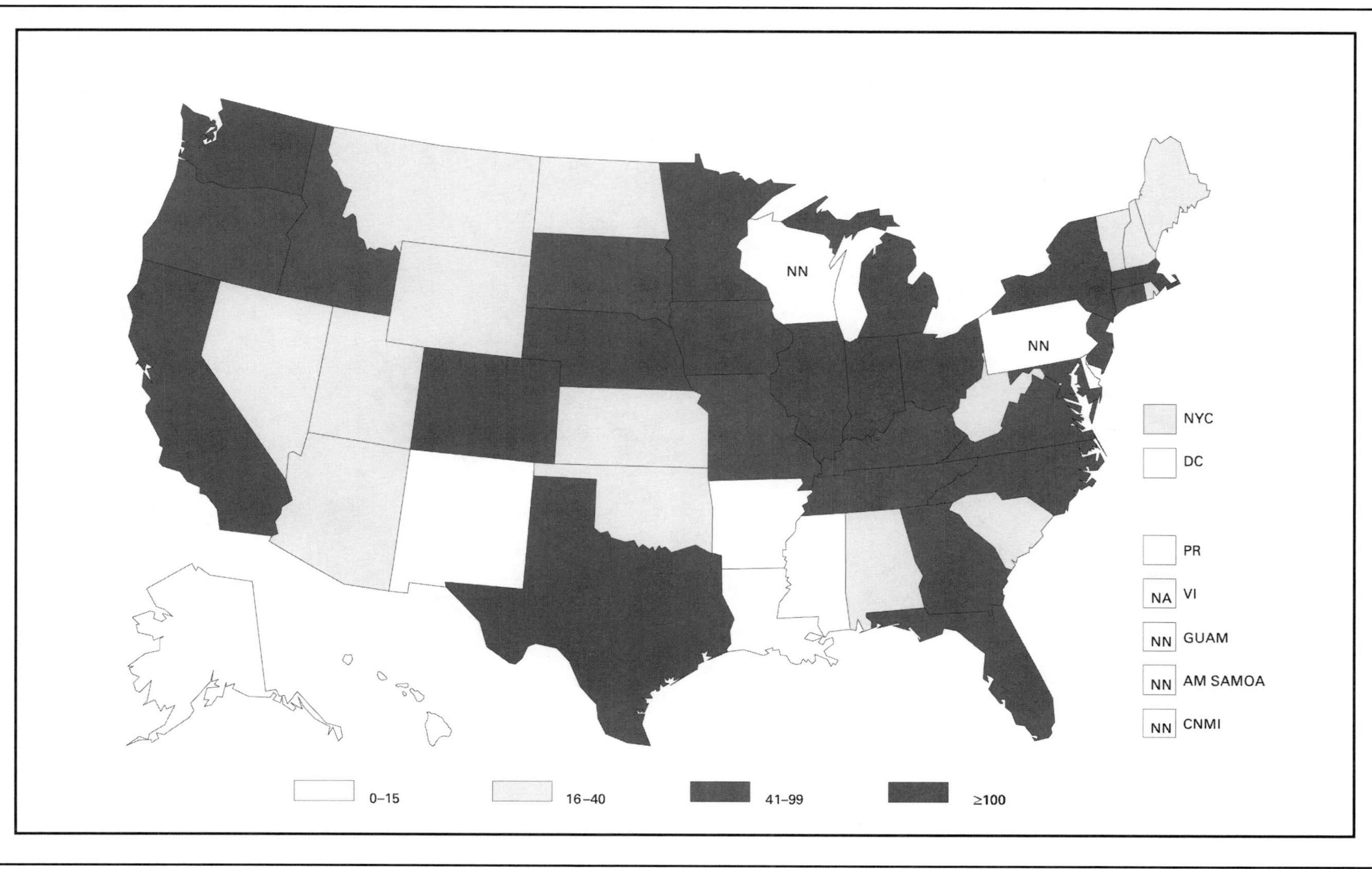


The number of states in which *Escherichia coli* O157:H7 infection is a notifiable disease increased to 48 in 1999. However, because <60% of clinical laboratories routinely test all stool specimens—or even all bloody stool specimens—for *E. coli* O157:H7, many infections are not recognized or reported.

*Source*: Center for Disease Control and Prevention. U.S. Department of Health and Human Services. *MMWR: Morbidity and Mortality Weekly Review Summary of Notifiable Disease, United States, 1999* 48 no. 53 (2001). http://www.cdc.gov/mmwr/PDF/wk/mm4853.pdf.

## Table F6.5. Hemolytic Uremic Syndrome, Postdiarrheal—Reported Cases, United States and Territories, 1999

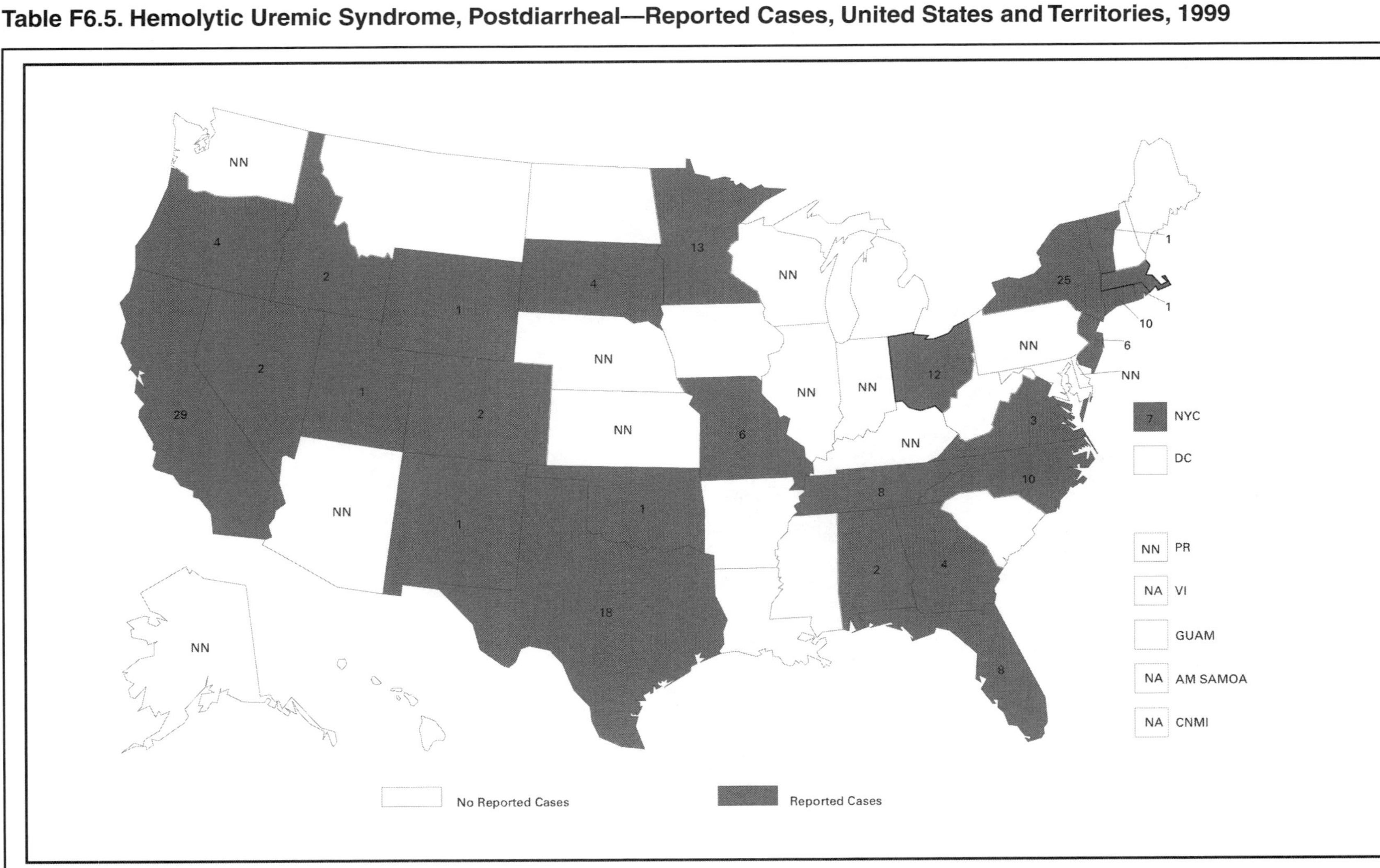


In the United States, most cases of postdiarrheal hemolytic uremic syndrome are caused by infection with *Escherichia coli* O157:H7 or other *E. coli* bacteria that produce Shiga toxin.

*Source*: Center for Disease Control and Prevention. U.S. Department of Health and Human Services. *MMWR: Morbidity and Mortality Weekly Review Summary of Notifiable Diseases, United States, 1999* 48 no. 53 (2001). http://www.cdc.gov/mmwr/PDF/wk/mm4853.pdf.

## Table F6.6. *Salmonella*—Reported Isolates, by Serotype and Year,* United States, 1974–1999

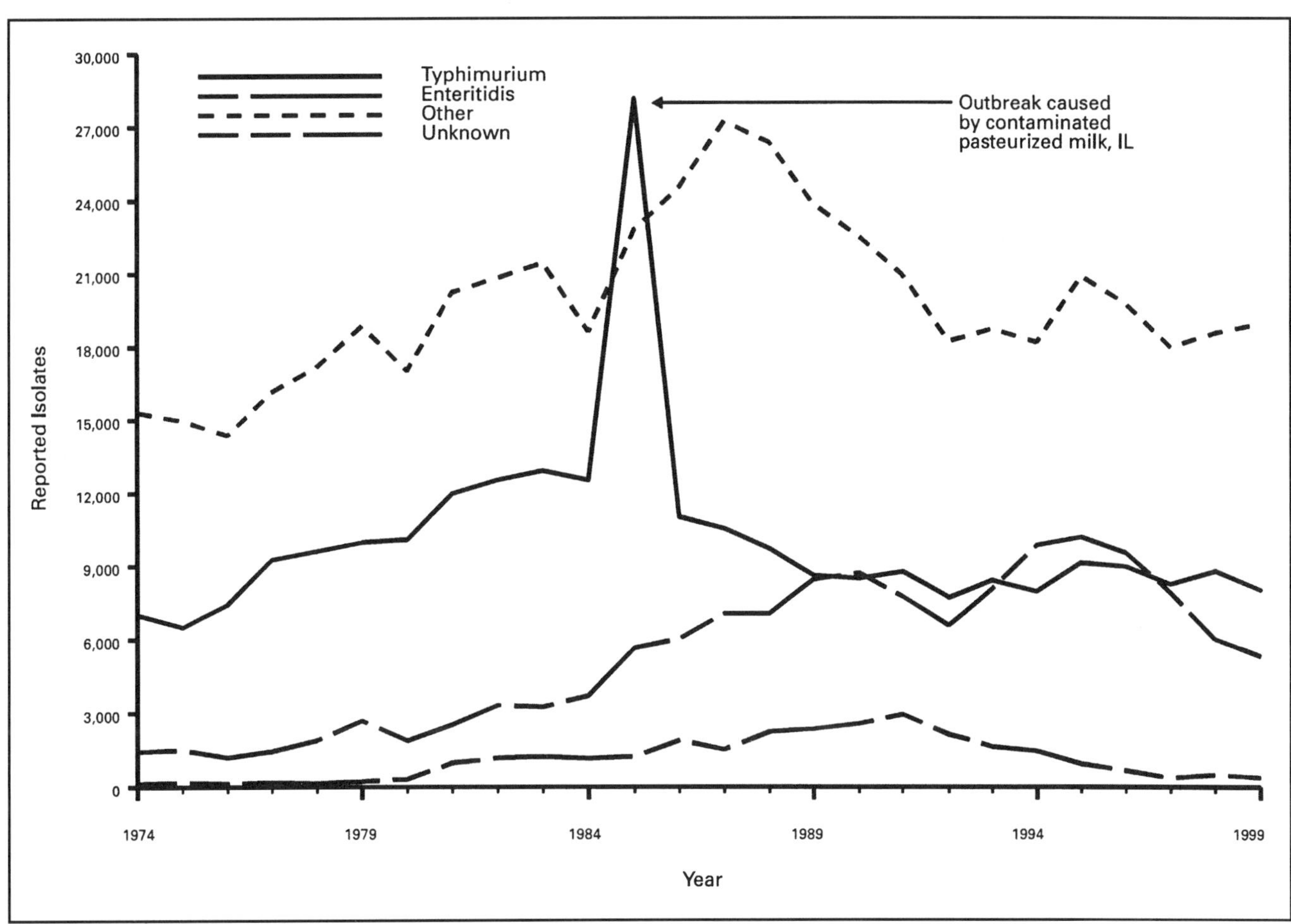


*Data from Public Health Laboratory Information System (PHLIS).

A multiple-resistant strain of *Salmonella* serotype Typhimurium accounts for approximately 30% of the Typhimurium isolates in the United States. The continued decline in *Salmonella* serotype Enteritidis could be associated with expanded farm-to-table control programs.

*Source*: Center for Disease Control and Prevention. U.S. Department of Health and Human Services. *MMWR: Morbidity and Mortality Weekly Review Summary of Notifiable Diseases, United States, 1999* 48 no. 53 (2001). http://www.cdc.gov/mmwr/PDF/wk/mm4853.pdf.

## Table F6.7. Salmonellosis—Reported Cases, per 100,000 Population, by Year, United States, 1969–1999

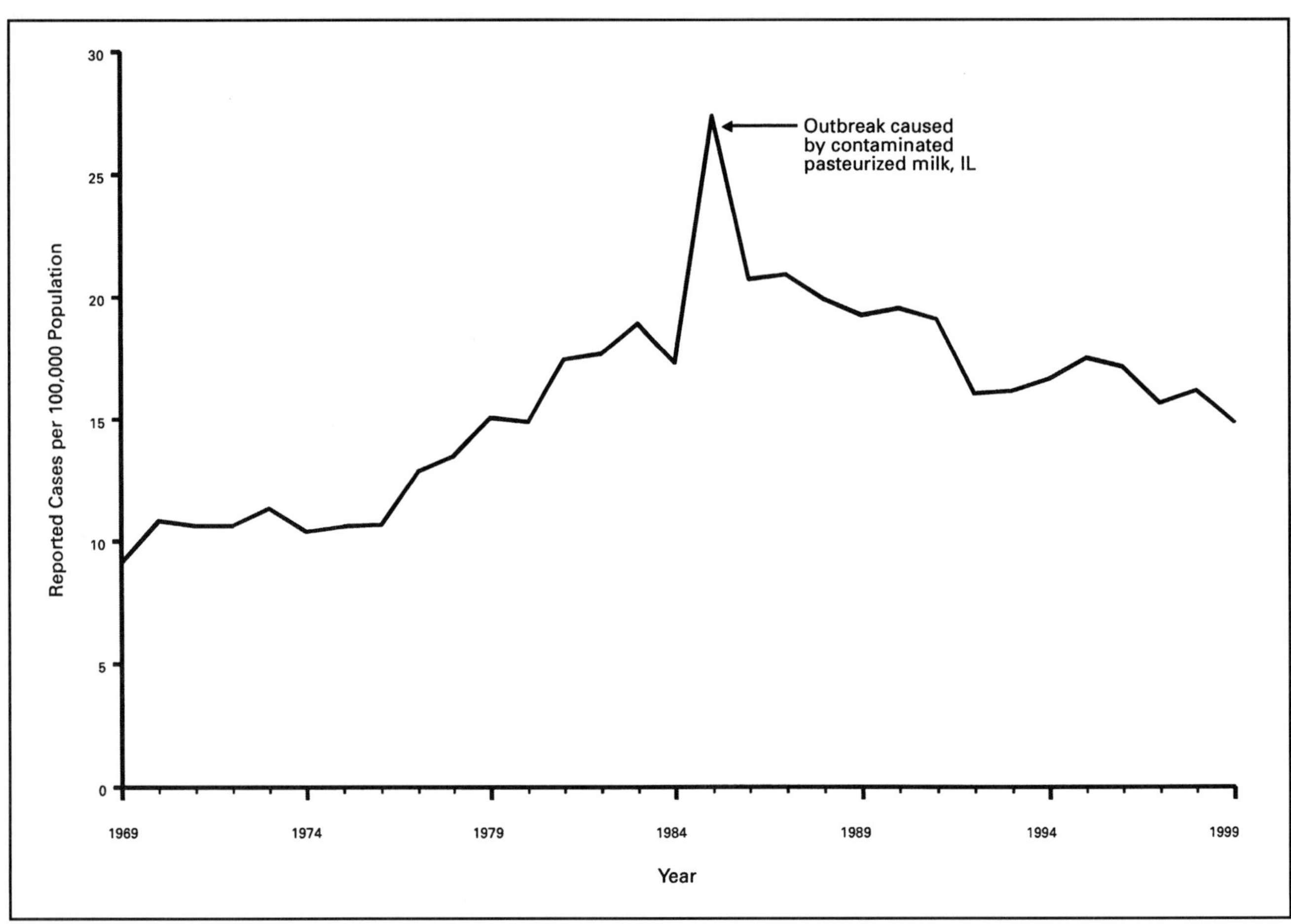


In 1999, *Salmonella* serotypes Typhimurium and Enteritidis accounted for 41% of all reported laboratory-confirmed human salmonellosis cases.
*Source*: Center for Disease Control and Prevention. U.S. Department of Health and Human Services. *MMWR: Morbidity and Mortality Weekly Review Summary of Notifiable Diseases, United States, 1999* 48 no. 53 (2001). http://www.cdc.gov/mmwr/PDF/wk/mm4853.pdf.

# Table F6.8. *Shigella*—Reported Isolates, by Species and Year,* United States, 1974–1999

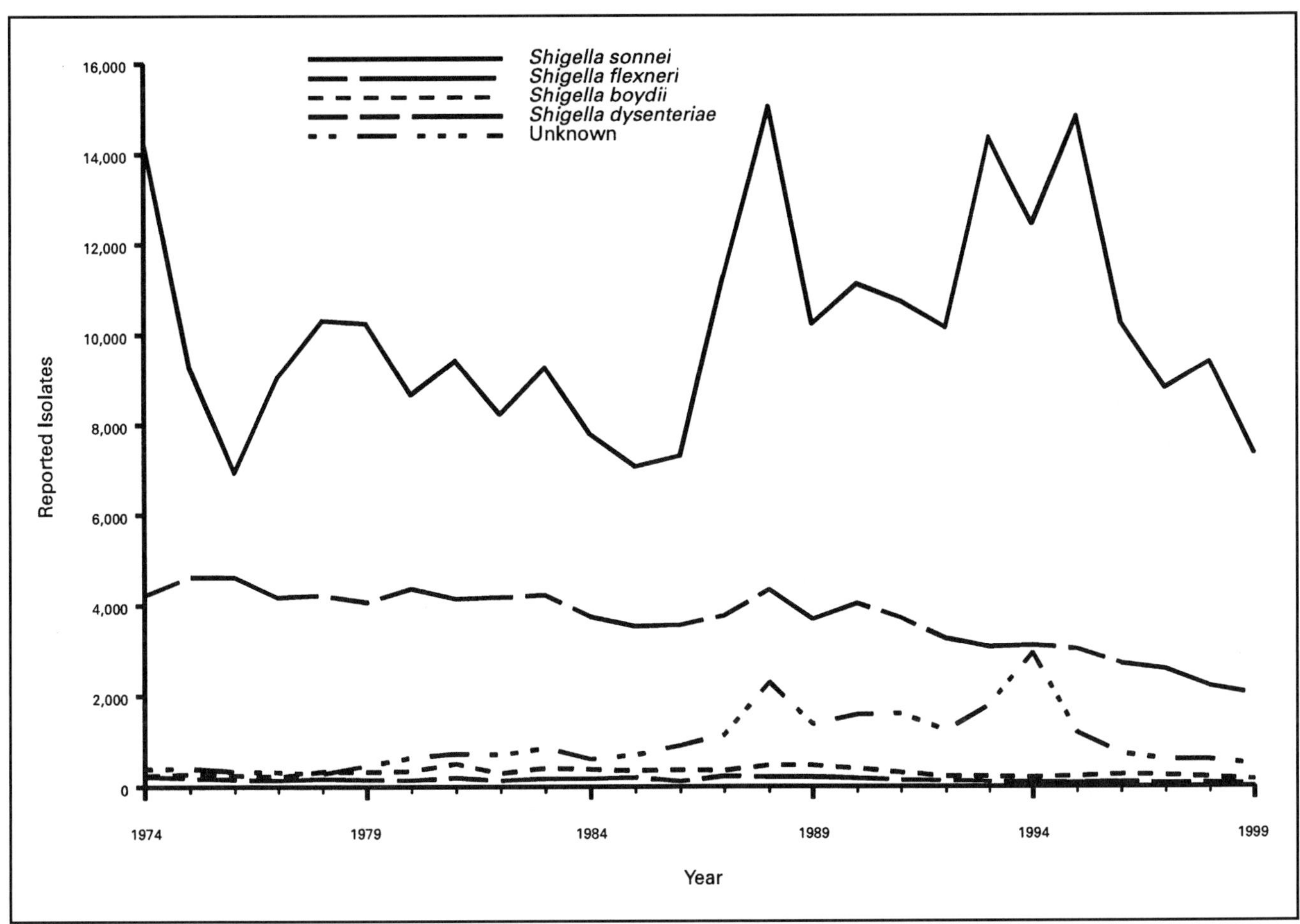


*Data from Public Health Laboratory Information System (PHLIS).

In recent years, reported isolations of *Shigella* have gradually decreased.

*Source*: Center for Disease Control and Prevention. U.S. Department of Health and Human Services. *MMWR: Morbidity and Mortality Weekly Review Summary of Notifiable Diseases, United States, 1999* 48 no. 53 (2001). http://www.cdc.gov/mmwr/PDF/wk/mm4853.pdf.

**Table F6.9. Shigellosis—Reported Cases, per 100,000 Population, by Year, United States, 1969–1999**

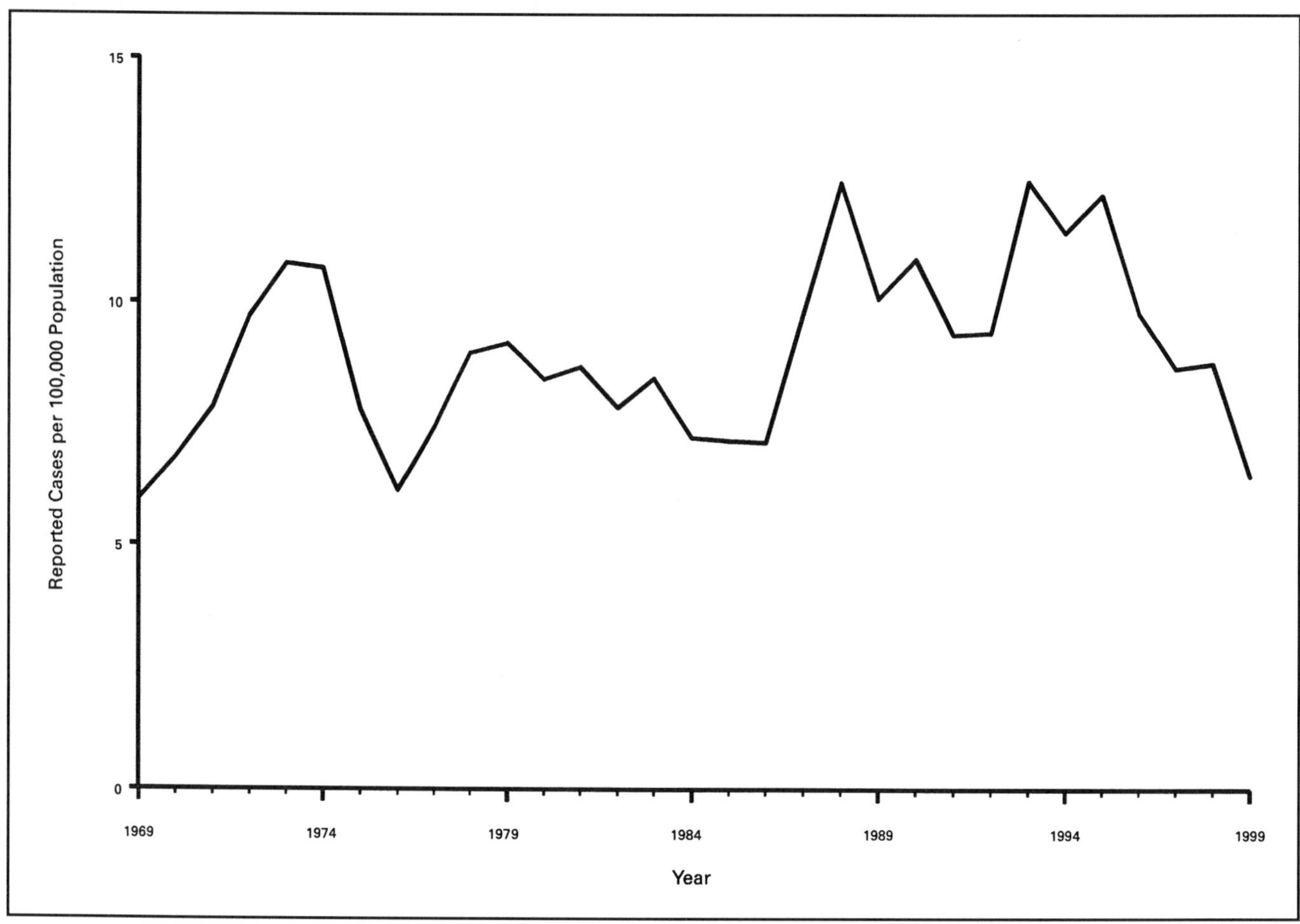


Although the incidence of shigellosis has decreased in recent years, prolonged and extensive *Shigella sonnei* outbreaks continue to occur in child care settings. *Source*: Center for Disease Control and Prevention, U.S. Department of Health and Human Services. *MMWR: Morbidity and Mortality Weekly Review Summary of Notifiable Diseases, United States, 1999* 48 no. 53 (2001). http://www.cdc.gov/mmwr/PDF/wk/mm4853.pdf.

## Table F6.10. Trichinosis—Reported Cases, by Year, United States, 1969–1999

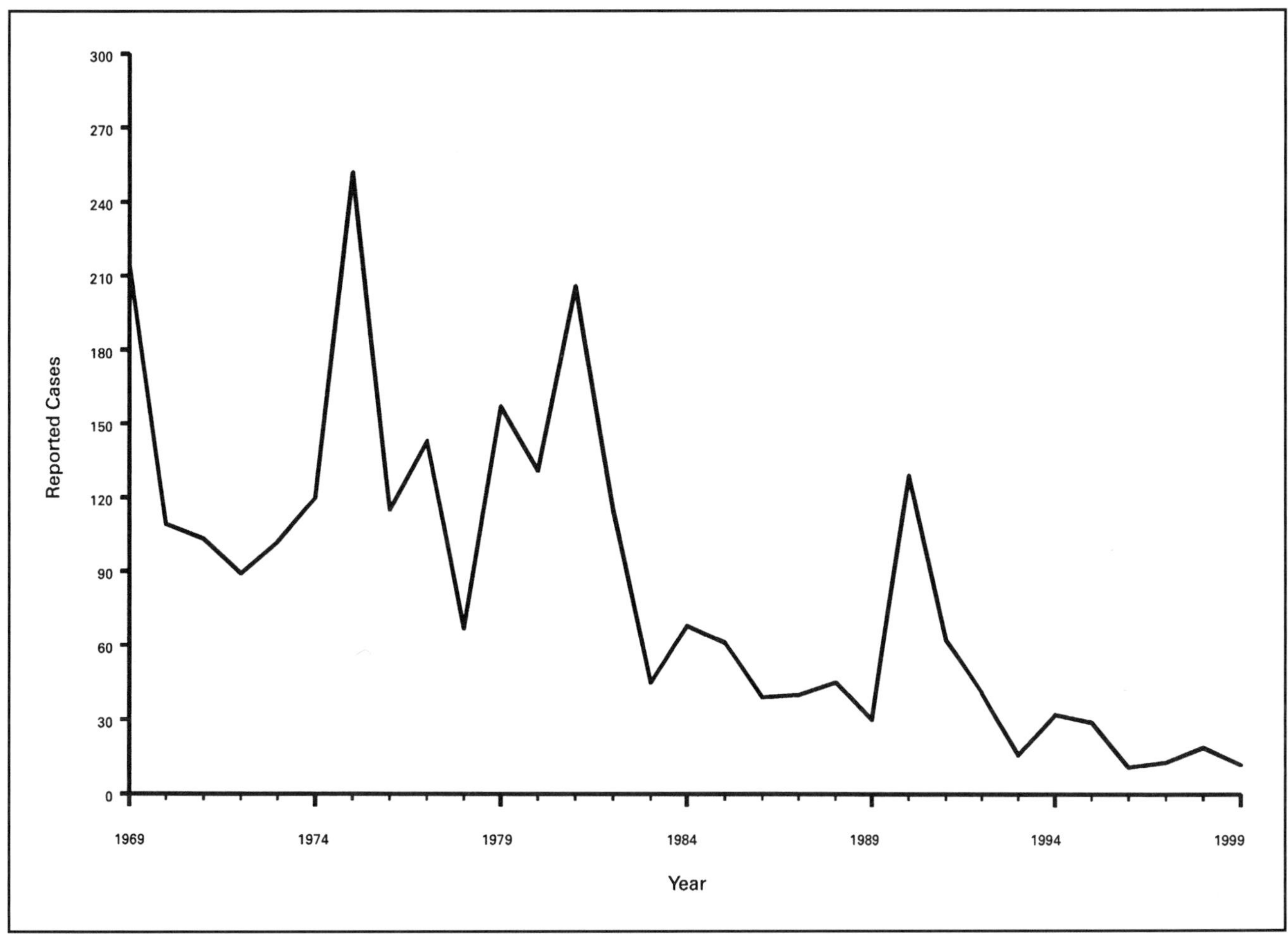


In 1999, a total of 12 cases of trichinosis was reported in the United States. Cases have declined in recent years, with numbers reported at <50 since 1993. *Source*: Center for Disease Control and Prevention, U.S. Department of Health and Human Services. *MMWR: Morbidity and Mortality Weekly Review Summary of Notifiable Diseases, United States, 1999*. 48 no. 53 (2001). http://www.cdc.gov/mmwr/PDF/wk/mm4853.pdf.

# G. Waterborne Diseases

## OVERVIEW

Like food, water can carry germs that cause illness. Two of the more important—and insidious—disease pathways are drinking and "recreational water," such as swimming pools, waterparks, lakes, rivers, and the ocean. These germs may cause serious infections, particularly in immunocompromised individuals.

Interest in environmental hazards and health effects has, it seems, never been higher. Indeed, the adequacy of current regulations for water treatment and monitoring of water quality is often the focus of both public and legislative scrutiny. Interest in the role of water—as with the role of food and milk in outbreaks of intestinal illness—has also been the basis for public health action for over half a century. Today, the public health importance of the timely identification of an outbreak's etiologic agent and the correctable source(s) of water contamination cannot be overstated. Rapid recognition and control of waterborne diseases is as important as it was when reporting began more than 60 years ago.[1]

## SYMPTOMS AND COURSES OF ILLNESS

Because waterborne diseases stem from a variety of known and unknown etiologic agents, they do not exhibit similar symptoms or courses of illness. Incubation periods, duration, and symptom complexes, for example, are generally consistent with individual viral syndromes.

## DIAGNOSIS

The surveillance system for waterborne disease outbreaks (WBDOs) resembles that used for foodborne-disease outbreaks and differs from other systems in that the unit of analysis is an outbreak rather than an individual case of a particular disease. Two criteria must be met for an event to be defined as a WBDO. First, at least two persons must have experienced a similar illness after ingestion of water intended for drinking or after exposure to water used for recreational purposes. Second, epidemiological evidence must implicate water as the probable source of illness. The stipulation that at least two persons must be ill is waived for single cases of laboratory-confirmed primary amebic meningoencephalitis and for single cases of chemical poisoning (if water quality data indicate contamination by the chemical). The identification of the etiologic agents of outbreaks is critical because agents newly associated with WBDOs could require new methods of control. Trends in the incidence of WBDOs caused by various etiologic agents can lead to changes in polices or resource allotment.

## TRANSMISSION

Waterborne diseases are caused by a variety of microbial contaminants known or anticipated to occur in both drinking and recreational water and possibly needing regulation. These include, for example, viruses (e.g., Norwalk-like virus), bacteria (e.g., *E. coli, Shigella sonnei*, etc.), and parasites (e.g., *Cryptosporidium, Giardia, Naegleria*). Transmission varies according to the etiologic agent and the specifics of each case.

## TREATMENT

Treatment varies depending on the specific etiologic agent and a variety of other factors; for example, whether the outbreak involves serious illness or whether there is an outbreak of acute disease.

## SURVEILLANCE

The reporting of WBDOs is voluntary in the United States. Since 1971, CDC, the U. S. Environmental Protection Agency (EPA), and the Council of State and Territorial Epidemiologists have maintained a collaborative surveillance program for collection and periodic reporting of data on the occurrence and causes of waterborne disease outbreaks. The surveillance system includes data about outbreaks associated with water intended for drinking and also about those associated with recreational water.

State, territorial, and local public health agencies have the primary responsibility for detecting and investigating WBDOs and voluntarily reporting them to CDC on a standard form. CDC annually requests reports from state and territorial epidemiologists or from persons designated as WBDO surveillance coordinators. When needed, additional information regarding water quality and treatment is obtained from the state's drinking water agency.

National statistics on outbreaks associated with water intended for drinking have been available since 1920.[2] In 1966, the present system of surveillance of foodborne and waterborne diseases began with the incorporation of all reports of enteric-disease outbreaks attributed to microbial or chemical contamination of food or water into an annual summary. Because of increasing interest and activity in waterborne disease surveillance, WBDOs have been reported separately since 1978. The CDC began publishing the summaries in 1991.[3]

The goals of the waterborne-disease surveillance efforts of CDC and EPA are to

> a) characterize the epidemiology of waterborne diseases; b) identify the etiologic agents that caused WBDOs and determine why the outbreaks occurred; c) train public health personnel to detect and investigate WBDO; and d) collaborate with local, state, federal, and international agencies on initiatives to prevent waterborne diseases.[4]

The data gathered through surveillance are useful for identifying major deficiencies in providing safe drinking and recreational water. Surveillance information also influences research priorities and can lead to improved water-quality regulations.

There are several considerations to bear in mind regarding waterborne-disease surveillance data. First note that not all WBDOs are recognized, investigated, and reported to CDC or EPA, and the extent to which WBDOs are unrecognized and underreported is unknown. To date, there is no national quick-response notification system through which public health officials and health-care providers can share provisional data on WBDOs. Thus, data on WBDOs probably underestimate the true incidence of WBDOs.

Second is the likelihood that

> individual cases of illness will be detected, epidemiologically linked, and associated with water varies considerably among locales and is dependent on many factors. These factors include: a) public awareness, b) the likelihood that persons who are ill will consult the same rather than different health-care providers, c) availability and extent of laboratory testing, d) local requirements for reporting cases of particular diseases, and e) the surveillance and investigative activities of state and local health and environmental agencies.[5]

Third, recognition of WBDOs is also dependent on certain outbreak characteristics. Outbreaks involving serious illness are most likely to receive the attention of health authorities, and outbreaks of acute diseases are more readily identified than those associated with disease from chronic, low-level exposure to an agent. Additionally, recreational water outbreaks that result from persons congregating in one venue and then dispersing into a wide area could be difficult to document. Also, outbreaks associated with community water systems are more likely to be recognized than those associated with noncommunity systems because the latter serve mostly nonresidential areas and transient populations. Finally, outbreaks associated with individual systems are the most likely to be underreported because they generally involve few persons.

Last, the identification of the etiologic agent of a WBDO depends on the timely recognition of the outbreak so that appropriate clinical and environmental samples can be obtained. Numerous factors influence whether or not the etiologic agent is identified. These include the practices of investigators' laboratories, the fact that the water-quality data collected vary widely among outbreak investigations, the influence of large outbreaks on the relative proportion of cases of waterborne diseases attributed to a particular agent, and the method and accuracy of the approximation of the number of reported cases.

## TABLE OVERVIEW

**G1. Classification of Investigations of Waterborne-Disease Outbreaks** This surveillance system classifies WBDOs according to the strength of the epidemiologic and water-quality data implicating water as the source of the outbreak. The classification numbers (i.e., Classes I–IV) are based on the epidemiologic and water-quality data provided on the outbreak form. Epidemiologic data are weighted more heavily than water-quality data. A classification of I means that adequate epidemiologic and water-quality data were reported but does not necessarily imply that the investigation was optimal. Classifications II–IV do not necessarily imply that the investigations were flawed; the circumstances of each outbreak differ, and not all outbreaks can or should be rigorously investigated.

**G2.1–G2.4. Waterborne Disease and Drinking Water** The first tables in this suite (G2.1 and G2.2) present an overview of waterborne-disease outbreaks associated with drinking water in the United States during 1997 and 1998, the last years for which data are available. G2.3 provides data on waterborne-disease outbreaks by etiologic agent and type of water system. G2.4 provides data by type of deficiency (e.g., untreated surface water, untreated groundwater, inadequate treatment).

The data in these tables may underestimate outbreaks because the CDC data includes only instances in which waterborne diseases were the primary cause of the outbreak. The figures do not include occurrences in which these diseases may have been a secondary factor. In addition, the CDC does not classify outbreaks caused by contamination of water or ice at the point of use as WBDOs. Instead the CDC reports them as foodborne-disease outbreaks.

During 1997–1998, 13 states reported outbreaks associated with drinking water: seven in 1997, 10 in 1998. Seven (41.2%) of the 17 outbreaks were assigned to Class I based on epidemiologic and water-quality data; none were Class II or Class IV, and 10 (58.8%) were Class III. These outbreaks caused an estimated 2,038 persons to become ill. No deaths were attributed to these outbreaks. Outbreaks are listed by state and are tabulated by the etiologic agent and by the type of water system. Outbreaks occurred in a variety of settings, including cabins, campgrounds, country clubs, fairgrounds, group homes, private homes, restaurants, trailer parks, and treatment plants. Lakes, springs, surface water, and wells were cited as different sources of water involved.

The microbe or chemical that caused the outbreak was identified for 12 (70.6%) of the 17 outbreaks; 15 (88.2%) were linked to groundwater sources. Of the 10 outbreaks with known infectious etiology, 6 (60.0%) were caused by parasites and 4 (40.0%) by bacteria.

Eight (47.1%) of the 17 WBDOs were associated with community systems, 5 (29.4%) with noncommunity systems, and 4 (23.5%) with individual water systems. Only two (11.8%) of the outbreaks were associated with surface water systems. Three (37.5%) of the eight outbreaks associated with community water systems were caused by problems at water treatment plants, three (37.5%) were the result of problems in the water distribution systems and plumbing of individual facilities, and two (25.0%) were associated with contaminated, untreated groundwater. All five of the outbreaks in noncommunity systems were associated with groundwater systems. Two (40.0%) of the five outbreaks were caused by contamination in the distribution system. All four outbreaks in individual water systems were associated with groundwater systems. Outbreaks caused by *Giardia, Cryptosporidium*, and *E. coli* O157:H7 were reported in untreated well systems; an outbreak of unknown etiology was associated with inadequate chlorination of well water.

**G3.1–G3.4. Waterborne Disease and Recreational Water** The last cluster of tables presents data on diseases attributed to recreational water exposure. As in the case of drinking water, the number of outbreaks may be underestimated. Thirty-two outbreaks from 18 states were attributed to this source and affected an estimated 2,128 persons. Seven outbreaks were reported for 1997 and 25 for 1998. Eighteen (56.3%) of the 32 were outbreaks of gastroenteritis, and 4 (12.5%) were single cases of primary amebic meningoencephalitis caused by *Naegleria fowleri*, all of which were fatal. The etiologic agent was identified for 29 (90.6%) of the 32 outbreaks, with one death associated with an *Escherichia coli* O157:H7 outbreak. Ten (55.6%) of the 18 gastroenteritis outbreaks were associated with treated pools or ornamental fountains. Of the 8 outbreaks of dermatitis, 7 (87.5%) were associated with hot tubs, pools, or springs.

## NOTES

1. *See* Foodborne Diseases.
2. G.F. Craun, ed., *Waterborne Diseases in the United States* (Boca Raton, FL: CRC Press, 1986).
3. Center for Disease Control, "Waterborne Disease Outbreaks, 1989–1990," *Morbidity and Mortality Weekly Review* 40, no. SS-3 (1991): 1–21; Center for Disease Control, "Surveillance for Waterborne-Disease Outbreaks—United States, 1991–1992," *Morbidity and Mortality Weekly Review* 42, no. SS-5 (1993): 1–22; Center for Disease Control, "Surveillance for Waterborne-Disease Outbreaks—United States, 1993–1994," Center for Disease Control, "Surveillance for Waterborne-Disease Outbreaks—United States, 1995–1996," *MMWR* 47, no. SS-5 (1998): 1– ; Center for Disease Control, "Surveillance for Waterborne-Disease Outbreaks—United States, 1997–1998," *MMWR* 49, no. SS-4 (2000): 1– .
4. Rachel S. Barwick et al., "Surveillance for Waterborne Disease Outbreaks—United States, 1997–1998," *Morbidity and Mortality Weekly Report* 49, no. SS-4 (2000): 2.
5. Ibid., pp. 12–13.

Center for Disease Control and Prevention. U.S. Department of Health and Human Services. *Waterborne Disease Outbreaks, 1989–1990* 40 no. SS-3 (1990).

Center for Disease Control and Prevention. U.S. Department of Health and Human Services. *MMWR: Morbidity and Mortality Weekly Review CDC Surveillance Summaries Surveillance for Waterborne-Disease Outbreaks—United States, 1991–1992* 42 no. SS-5 (1993): 1–22.

Center for Disease Control and Prevention. U.S. Department of Health and Human Services. *MMWR: Morbidity and Mortality Weekly Review CDC Surveillance Summaries Surveillance for Waterborne-Disease Outbreaks—United States, 1993–1994* 45 no. SS-1 (1996).

Center for Disease Control and Prevention. U.S. Department of Health and Human Services. *MMWR: Morbidity and Mortality Weekly Review CDC Surveillance Summaries Surveillance for Waterborne-Disease Outbreaks—United States, 1995–1996* 47 no. SS-5 (1998).

Center for Disease Control and Prevention. U.S. Department of Health and Human Services. *MMWR: Morbidity and Mortality Weekly Review CDC Surveillance Summaries Surveillance for Waterborne-Disease Outbreaks—United States, 1997–1998* 49 no. SS-4 (2000).

## Table G1. Classification of Investigations of Waterborne-Disease Outbreaks—United States*

| Class† | Epidemiologic data | Water-quality data |
|---|---|---|
| I | Adequate§<br>a) Data were provided regarding exposed and unexposed persons; and<br>b) relative risk or odds ratio was ≥2, or the p-value was <0.05. | Provided and adequate<br>(Historical information or laboratory data [e.g., chlorinator malfunction or a water main break, no detectable free-chlorine residual, or the presence of coliforms in the water]) |
| II | Adequate | Not provided or inadequate<br>(e.g., stating that a lake was crowded) |
| III | Provided, but limited<br>a) Epidemiologic data provided did not meet the criteria for Class I; or<br>b) the claim was made that ill persons had no exposures in common besides water, but no data were provided. | Provided and adequate |
| IV | Provided, but limited | Not provided or inadequate |

*Outbreaks of *Pseudomonas* dermatitis and single cases of primary amebic meningoencephalitis or illness resulting from chemical poisoning are not classified according to this scheme.

†Based on the epidemiologic and water-quality data provided on CDC form 52.12.

§Adequate data were provided to implicate water as the source of the outbreak.

*Source*: Center for Disease Control and Prevention. U.S. Department of Health and Human Services. *MMWR: Morbidity and Mortality Weekly Review CDC Surveillance Summaries Surveillance for Waterborne-Disease Outbreaks United States, 1997–1998* 49 no. SS-4 (2000). http://www.cdc.gov/mmwr/PDF/ss/ss4904.pdf.

## Table G2.1. Waterborne-Disease Outbreaks Associated with Drinking Water—United States, 1997 (n = 7)*

| State | Month | Class† | Etiologic agent | No. of cases | Type of system§ | Deficiency¶ | Source | Setting |
|---|---|---|---|---|---|---|---|---|
| Colorado | Jul | III | AGI** | 9 | NCom | 3 | Spring | Cabins |
| Florida | Mar | III | Copper poisoning | 2 | Com | 4 | Well | Restaurant |
| New Mexico | Jul | I | AGI†† | 123 | NCom | 4 | Well | Country club |
| New York | Jun | I | *Giardia intestinalis* | 50 | Com | 3 | Lake | Community |
| Oregon | Jun | III | *G. intestinalis* | 100 | NCom | 4 | Well/spring | Campground |
| South Dakota | May | I | AGI | 16 | NCom | 3 | Well | Campground |
| Washington | Sep | III | *Escherichia coli* O157:H7 | 4 | NCom | 3 | Well | Trailer park |

*An outbreak is defined as a) at least two persons experiencing a similar illness after ingestion of drinking water and b) epidemiologic evidence that implicate water as the probable source of the illness.

†Based on the epidemiologic and water-quality data provided on CDC form 52.12.

§Com=community; NCom=noncommunity. Community and noncommunity water systems are public water systems that serve >15 service connections or an average of >25 residents for >60 days/year. A community water system serves year-round residents of a community, subdivision, or mobile home park with >15 service connections or an average of >25 residents. A noncommunity water system can be nontransient or transient. Nontransient systems serve >25 of the same persons for >6 months of the year (e.g., factories or schools), whereas transient systems do not (e.g., restaurants, highway rest stations, or parks).

¶1-untreated surface water; 2=untreated groundwater; 3=treatment deficiency (e.g., cross-connection, contamination of water mains during construction or repair, and contamination of a storage facility); and 5=unknown or miscellaneous deficiency (e.g., contaminated bottled water).

**Acute gastrointestinal illness of unknown etiology.

††Eleven persons had stool specimens that tested positive for *E. coli* O86:H11; one stool specimen was also positive for *Giardia.*

*Source*: Center for Disease Control and Prevention. U.S. Department of Health and Human Services. *MMWR: Morbidity and Mortality Weekly Review CDC Surveillance Summaries Surveillance for Waterborne-Disease Outbreaks United States, 1997–1998* 49 no. SS-4 (2000). http://www.cdc.gov/mmwr/PDF/ss/ss4904.pdf.

## Table G2.2. Waterborne-Disease Outbreaks Associated with Drinking Water—United States, 1998 (n = 10)*

| State | Month | Class[†] | Etiologic agent | No. of cases | Type of system[§] | Deficiency[¶] | Source | Setting |
|---|---|---|---|---|---|---|---|---|
| Florida | May | III | *Giardia intestinalis* | 7 | Com | 2 | Well | Community |
| Florida | Sep | III | Copper poisoning | 35 | Com | 3 | Well | Community |
| Florida | Dec | III | *G. intestinalis* | 2 | Ind | 2 | Well | House |
| Illinois | May | III | *Escherichia coli* O157:H7 | 3 | Ind | 2 | Well | House |
| Minnesota | Aug | I | *Shigella sonnei* | 83 | Com | 4 | Well | Fairgrounds |
| Montana | Jul | III | AGI** | 5 | Ind | 3 | Well | Home |
| New Mexico | Jul | I | *Cryptosporidium parvum*[††] | 32 | Ind | 5 | Well | Group home |
| Ohio | Oct | III | AGI[§§] | 10 | Com | 4 | Surface[¶¶] | Treatment plant |
| Texas | Jul | I | *C. parvum**** | 1400 | Com | 3 | Well | Subdivision |
| Wyoming | Jun | I | *E. coli* O157:H7 | 157 | Com | 2 | Well/spring | Community |

*An outbreak is defined as a) at least two persons experiencing a similar illness after ingestion of drinking water and b) epidemiologic evidence that implicate water as the probable source of the illness.
[†]Based on the epidemiologic and water-quality data provided on CDC form 52.12.
[§]Com=community; Ind=Individual. A community water system serves year-round residents of a community, subdivision, or mobile home park with >15 service connections or an average of >25 residents for >60 days/year. Individual water systems are small systems that are not owned or operated by a water utility and that serve <15 connections or <25 persons.
[¶]1-untreated surface water; 2=untreated groundwater; 3=treatment deficiency (e.g., temporary interruption of distinction, chronically inadequate disinfection, and inadequate or no filtration); 4=distribution system deficiency (e.g., cross-connection, contamination of water mains during construction or repair, and contamination of a storage facility); and 5=unknown or miscellaneous deficiency (e.g., contaminated bottled water).
**Acute gastrointestinal illness of unknown etiology.
[††]Nine persons had stool specimens that tested positive only for *Cryptosporidium,* and one person had a specimen that was also positive for *Blastocystis hominis.*
[§§]One person had a stool specimen that was positive for *B. hominis.*
[¶¶]Surface water from an unknown source.
***Eighty-nine persons had stool specimens that tested positive only for *Cryptosporidium,* and one person had a specimen that tested positive only for *Giardia.* None of the specimens were positive for both organisms.
*Source*: Center for Disease Control and Prevention. U.S. Department of Health and Human Services. *MMWR: Morbidity and Mortality Weekly Review CDC Surveillance Summaries Surveillance for Waterborne-Disease Outbreaks United States, 1997–1998* 49 no. SS-4 (2000). http://www.cdc.gov/mmwr/PDF/ss/ss4904.pdf.

## Table G2.3. Waterborne-Disease Outbreaks Associated with Drinking Water, by Etiologic Agent and Type of Water System—United States, 1997–1998 (n = 17)

| | Type of water system* | | | | | | | |
|---|---|---|---|---|---|---|---|---|
| | Community | | Noncommunity | | Individual | | Total | |
| Etiologic agent | Outbreaks | Cases | Outbreaks | Cases | Outbreaks | Cases | Outbreaks | Cases |
| AGI[†] | 1 | 10 | 3 | 148 | 1 | 5 | 5 | 163 |
| Copper | 2 | 37 | 0 | 0 | 0 | 0 | 2 | 37 |
| *Cryptosporidium parvum* | 1 | 1,400 | 0 | 0 | 1 | 32 | 2 | 1,432 |
| *Escherichia coli* O157:H7 | 1 | 157 | 1 | 4 | 1 | 3 | 3 | 164 |
| *Giardia intestinalis* | 2 | 57 | 1 | 100 | 1 | 2 | 4 | 159 |
| *Shigella sonnei* | 1 | 83 | 0 | 0 | 0 | 0 | 1 | 83 |
| **Total (%)** | **8 (47.1%)** | **1,744 (85.6%)** | **5 (29.4%)** | **252 (12.4%)** | **4 (23.5%)** | **42 (2.1%)** | **17 (100.0%)** | **2,038 (100.0%)** |

*Community and noncommunity water systems are public water systems that serve >15 service connections or an average of >25 residents for >60 days/year. A community water system serves year-round residents of a community, subdivision, or mobile home park with >15 service connections or an average of >25 residents. A noncommunity water system can be nontransient or transient. Nontransient systems serve >25 of the same persons for >6 months of the year (e.g., factories or schools), whereas transient systems do not (e.g., restaurants, highway rest stations, or parks). Individual water systems are small systems not owned or operated by a water utility that serve <15 connections or <25 persons.
[†]Acute gastrointestinal illness of unknown etiology.
*Source*: Center for Disease Control and Prevention. U.S. Department of Health and Human Services. *MMWR: Morbidity and Mortality Weekly Review CDC Surveillance Summaries Surveillance for Waterborne-Disease Outbreaks United States, 1997–1998* 49 no. SS-4 (2000). http://www.cdc.gov/mmwr/PDF/ss/ss4904.pdf.

## Table G2.4. Waterborne-Disease Outbreaks Associated with Drinking Water, by Type of Deficiency and Type of Water System—United States, 1997–1998 (n = 17)

| | Type of water system* | | | | | | | |
|---|---|---|---|---|---|---|---|---|
| | Community | | Noncommunity | | Individual | | Total | |
| Type of deficiency† | Outbreaks | (%) | Outbreaks | (%) | Outbreaks | (%) | Outbreaks | (%) |
| Untreated surface water | 0 | (0.0) | 0 | (0.0) | 0 | (0.0) | 0 | (0.0) |
| Untreated groundwater | 2 | (25.0) | 0 | (0.0) | 2 | (50.0) | 4 | (23.5) |
| Inadequate treatment | 3 | (37.5) | 3 | (60.0) | 1 | (25.0) | 7 | (41.2) |
| Distribution system | 3 | (37.5) | 2 | (40.0) | 0 | (0.0) | 5 | (29.4) |
| Miscellaneous or unknown | 0 | (0.0) | 0 | (0.0) | 1 | (25.0) | 1 | (5.9) |
| **Total** | **8** | **(100.0)** | **5** | **(100.0)** | **4** | **(100.0)** | **17** | **(100.0)** |

*Community and noncommunity water systems are public water systems that serve >15 service connections or an average of >25 residents for >60 days/year. A community water system serves year-round residents of a community, subdivision, or mobile home park with >15 service connections or an average of >25 residents. A noncommunity water system can be nontransient or transient. Nontransient systems serve >25 of the same persons for >6 months of the year (e.g., factories or schools), whereas transient systems do not (e.g., restaurants, highway rest stations, or parks). Individual water systems are small systems not owned or operated by a water utility that serve <15 connections or <25 persons.

†1-untreated surface water; 2=untreated groundwater; 3=treatment deficiency (e.g., temporary interruption of distinction, chronically inadequate disinfection, and inadequate or no filtration); 4=distribution system deficiency (e.g., cross-connection, contamination of water mains during construction or repair, and contamination of a storage facility); and 5=unknown or miscellaneous deficiency (e.g., contaminated bottled water).

*Source*: Center for Disease Control and Prevention. U.S. Department of Health and Human Services. *MMWR: Morbidity and Mortality Weekly Review CDC Surveillance Summaries Surveillance for Waterborne-Disease Outbreaks United States, 1997–1998* 49 no. SS-4 (2000). http://www.cdc.gov/mmwr/PDF/ss/ss4904.pdf.

## Table G3.1. Waterborne-Disease Outbreaks of Gastroenteritis Associated with Recreational water—United States, 1997 (n = 3)

| State | Month | Class* | Etiologic agent | Illness | No. of cases | Source | Setting |
|---|---|---|---|---|---|---|---|
| Massachusetts | Jul | III | *Shigella sonnei* | Gastroenteritis | 9 | Pool/fountain | Public park |
| Minnesota | Jul | II | *Cryptosporidium parvum* | Gastroenteritis | 369 | Fountain | Zoo |
| Missouri | Jul | I | *Escherichia coli* O157:H7 | Gastroenteritis | 8 | Lake | Resort |

*Based on the epidemiologic and water-quality data provided on CDC form 52.12.

*Source*: Center for Disease Control and Prevention. U.S. Department of Health and Human Services. *MMWR: Morbidity and Mortality Weekly Review CDC Surveillance Summaries Surveillance for Waterborne-Disease Outbreaks United States, 1997–1998* 49 no. SS-4 (2000). http://www.cdc.gov/mmwr/PDF/ss/ss4904.pdf.

## Table G3.2. Waterborne-Disease Outbreaks of Gastroenteritis Associated with Recreational Water—United States, 1998 (n = 15)

| State | Month | Class* | Etiologic agent | Illness | No. of cases | Source | Setting |
|---|---|---|---|---|---|---|---|
| Florida | Jul | IV | *Cryptosporidium parvum* | Gastroenteritis | 7 | Pool | Day care center |
| Georgia | Jun | I | *Escherichia coli* O157:H7 | Gastroenteritis | 26 | Pool | Water park |
| Maine | Aug | I | AGI† | Gastroenteritis | 650 | Lake | Campground |
| Minnesota | Apr | IV | *C. parvum* | Gastroenteritis | 45 | Pool | Swim club |
| Minnesota | Jul | IV | *E. coli* O157:H7 | Gastroenteritis | 5 | Lake | Beach |
| Minnesota | Jul | IV | *C. parvum* | Gastroenteritis | 7 | Pool | Community pool |
| Ohio | Jul | III | NLV§ | Gastroenteritis | 30 | Lake | Campground |
| Oregon | Aug | II | *C. parvum* | Gastroenteritis | 69 | Pool | Community pool |
| Pennsylvania | Jul | III | *C. parvum* | Gastroenteritis | 8 | Lake | State park |
| Washington | Jul | II | AGI | Gastroenteritis | 41 | Lake | Children's camp |
| Washington | Jul | III | AGI | Gastroenteritis | 248 | Lake | Park |
| Wisconsin | Jun | I | NLV | Gastroenteritis | 18 | Lake | Public beach |
| Wisconsin | Jun | III | *C. parvum* | Gastroenteritis | 12 | Pool | Community pool |
| Wisconsin | Jul | III | *C. parvum* | Gastroenteritis | 9 | Pool | Community pool |
| Wisconsin | Jul | IV | *C. parvum* | Gastroenteritis | 12 | Pool | Community pool |

*Based on the epidemiologic and water-quality data provided on CDC form 52.12.
†Acute gastrointestinal illness of unknown etiology.
§Norwalk-like virus.
*Source*: Center for Disease Control and Prevention. U.S. Department of Health and Human Services. *MMWR: Morbidity and Mortality Weekly Review CDC Surveillance Summaries Surveillance for Waterborne-Disease Outbreaks United States, 1997–1998* 49 no. SS-4 (2000). http://www.cdc.gov/mmwr/PDF/ss/ss4904.pdf.

## Table G3.3. Waterborne-Disease Outbreaks of Meningoencephalitis, Leptospirosis, and Pontiac Fever Associated with Recreational Water—United States, 1998 (n = 6)

| State | Month | Class* | Etiologic agent | Illness | No. of cases | Source | Setting |
|---|---|---|---|---|---|---|---|
| Florida | Aug | NA† | *Naegleria* | Meningoencephalitis | 1 | Stream | Drainage canal |
| Illinois | Jun | I | *Leptospira* | Leptospirosis | 375 | Lake | Triathalon |
| Oklahoma | Aug | NA | *Naegleria* | Meningoencephalitis | 1 | Lake | Lake |
| Texas | Jul | NA | *Naegleria* | Meningoencephalitis | 1 | Lake | Lake |
| Texas | Aug | NA | *Naegleria* | Meningoencephalitis | 1 | River | River |
| Wisconsin | Jan | I | *Legionellae* | Pontiac fever | 45 | Whirlpool | Hotel |

*Based on the epidemiologic and water-quality data provided on CDC form 52.12.
†Not applicable.
*Source*: Center for Disease Control and Prevention. U.S. Department of Health and Human Services. *MMWR: Morbidity and Mortality Weekly Review CDC Surveillance Summaries Surveillance for Waterborne-Disease Outbreaks United States, 1997–1998* 49 no. SS-4 (2000). http://www.cdc.gov/mmwr/PDF/ss/ss4904.pdf.

## Table G3.4. Waterborne-Disease Outbreaks of Dermatitis Associated with Recreational Water—United States, 1997–1998 (n = 8)

| State | Year | Month | Class* | Etiologic agent | No. of cases | Source | Setting |
|---|---|---|---|---|---|---|---|
| Alaska | 1998 | Jun | NA† | *Pseudomonas aeruginosa*§ | 50 | Spring | Resort |
| Arkansas | 1997 | Jan | NA | *P. aeruginosa*¶ | 12 | Pool and hot tub | Hotel |
| Indiana | 1997 | Feb | NA | *P. aeruginosa*§ | 42 | Pool | Hotel |
| Maine | 1997 | Jan | NA | *P. aeruginosa*¶ | 3 | Hot tub | Hotel |
| Maryland | 1998 | Feb | NA | *P. aeruginosa*¶ | 7 | Hot tub | Hotel |
| Oregon | 1997 | Jul | IV | *Schistosoma spindale*¶ | 2 | Lake | Campground |
| Wisconsin | 1998 | Feb | NA | *P. aeruginosa*§ | 8 | Pool | Hotel |
| Wisconsin | 1998 | Feb | NA | *P. aeruginos*¶ | 3 | Hot tub | Hotel |

*Based on the epidemiologic and water-quality data provided on CDC form 52.12.

†Not applicable.

§Laboratory-confirmed case.

¶Suspended case based on clinical syndrome.

*Source*: Center for Disease Control and Prevention. U.S. Department of Health and Human Services. *MMWR: Morbidity and Mortality Weekly Review CDC Surveillance Summaries Surveillance for Waterborne-Disease Outbreaks United States, 1997–1998* 49 no. SS-4 (2000). http://www.cdc.gov/mmwr/PDF/ss/ss4904.pdf.

# H. Infectious Disease Worldwide: Present Issues, Emerging Concerns

## OVERVIEW

Infectious diseases represent a continuing threat to all persons, regardless of age, sex, lifestyle, ethnic background, and socioeconomic status.[1] Today, infectious diseases account for more than 13 million deaths a year and for one in two deaths in developing countries. According to the World Health Organization, infectious diseases were responsible for 25% of all deaths in 1998.[2] These diseases can also be contributory to cancer, cardiovascular, and respiratory/digestive deaths, raising the actual percentage of deaths due to infectious diseases even more. They are the main causes of death in low-income countries. In 1998 they caused almost two-thirds (63%) of deaths among children ages 0–4 years and almost half (48%) of premature deaths of persons ages 0–44 years.

**Emerging Infectious Diseases** Within this context, new and re-emerging infections constitute particularly challenging microbial threats to health. Infections such as AIDS and haemorraghic fever have affected millions.[3] Today, it is increasingly common for individuals to know someone who has suffered from a new or re-emerging infectious disease. The incidence of these infections disproves predictions earlier last century that infectious diseases would soon be eliminated as a public health problem.[4]

New and re-emerging infections constitute particularly challenging microbial threats to global health because of certain factors that facilitate their emergence or re-emergence, their etiology, and their diversity.

The World Health Organization (WHO) recognizes five factors believed to cause the emergence or re-emergence of infectious diseases. These include "rapid and intense international travel"; "overcrowding in cities with poor sanitation"; "substantially increased international travel in food, mass distribution of food and unhygienic food preparation practices"; "increased exposure of humans to disease vectors and reservoirs in nature"; and "alteration of the environment and climatic changes which have a direct impact on the composition and size of the population of inset vectors and animal reservoirs."[5] Other factors include a deteriorating public health infrastructure that is unable to cope with the needs of the population.

**Drug-Resistant Infections** The rapidly growing number of bacteria, paraviruses, viruses, and fungi becoming resistant to an increasing range of antibiotics present another emerging public health problem. Antimicrobial resistance can develop in any type of microbe or germ. Specifically, microbes can develop resistance to specific medicines; drug resistance happens when microbes develop ways to survive the use of medicines meant to kill or weaken them. If a microbe is resistant to many drugs, treating the infections it causes can become difficult or even impossible. Additionally, someone with an infection that is resistant to a certain medicine can pass that resistant infection to another person. In this way, a hard-to-treat illness can be spread from person to person. In some cases, the illness can lead to serious disability or death. A common misconception is that a person's body becomes resistant to specific drugs; however, it is microbes, not people, that become resistant to the drugs.

As long as antimicrobial drugs are used, drug resistance will remain a challenge. By undermining the control and prevention of infectious diseases, the emergence of drug resistance is reversing advances of the previous 50 years. As we enter the twenty-first century, many important drug choices for the treatment of common infections are becoming increasingly limited, expensive, and, in some cases, nonexistent.

A WHO Fact Sheet on the subject notes, "In many regions, the low cost, first choice antibiotics have lost their power to clear infections . . . increasing the cost and length of treatment of many common diseases. . . . Further problems stem from the use of antimicrobial substances in food animal production."[6]

Infections caused by drug-resistant organisms prolong illness and, if not treated in time with expensive alternative antimicrobial agents, can cause death. Additionally, if drugs cannot be replaced as they lose their effectiveness or if the emergence and spread of drug resistance cannot be limited, some diseases might become untreatable, as they were in the pre-antibiotic era.

New, re-emerging, and drug-resistant infections place a substantial economic burden on health-care systems worldwide. It is increasingly clear that, in order to be strong and effective, our national and international public health systems must be both flexible and well prepared to respond to these challenges

## SURVEILLANCE

**General Global Surveillance** The status of infectious diseases worldwide is monitored by the World Health Organization (WHO), in addition to other organizations and associations. The lead agency in international health, WHO was created in 1948 and today includes over 190 member states. WHO's goal is to foster the attainment by all peoples—especially the poor and most vulnerable—of the highest possible standards of health. WHO has the mandate to lead and coordinate global surveillance. This includes setting international epidemic surveillance standards, providing technical assistance to member states in surveillance activities, training in field epidemiology, and strengthening laboratory capacity and laboratory networks. WHO's Outbreak Verification network is linked to the WHO global surveillance system, a worldwide network of laboratories and reporting sites that collects information on reported and rumored outbreaks nationally and worldwide. Once confirmed, information is made available immediately on the World Wide Web, and WHO forms partnerships to investigate and contain those outbreaks that could spread internationally and require concerted action.

WHO also maintains international collaborating networks such as the cholera task force that coordinates preparedness and response to cholera epidemics and the International Coordinating Group (ICG) on Vaccine Prevention for Epidemic Meningitis Control. In addition, WHO ensures international coordination of epidemic response, particularly for diseases of international public health importance or for countries that lack the capacity to respond to an epidemic themselves. Responses can range from investigating the cause of an epidemic, to verifying and disseminating information, and to providing needed equipment and laboratory supplies. General WHO information can be accessed at www.who.int.

**New and Emerging Disease Surveillance** The CDC tracks new and emerging diseases worldwide to provide an early warning system of diseases that might become a new threat to humans. Although many of these diseases are in developing countries that lack proper sanitation, industrialized countries like the United States are by no means immune from new or re-emerging infectious disease.

In the early 1990s, the National Academy of Science Institute of Medicine published a report that emphasized the ongoing threat of emerging infectious diseases, and CDC developed a strategy to respond to this threat. A central feature of this strategy was the establishment of the Emerging Infections Program (EIP) in nine sites across the United States (California, Colorado, Connecticut, Georgia, New York, Maryland, Minnesota, Oregon, and Tennessee). The goals of the EIP network are to improve national surveillance for new and emerging infectious diseases, conduct appropriate epidemiologic and laboratory research, develop prevention and control measures, and strengthen the national public health infrastructure.

Information relative to tracking trends and analyzing new and reemerging infectious disease issues around the world is disseminated by the CDC through its peer-reviewed journal *Emerging Infectious Diseases*, published since 1995 by the National Center for Infectious Diseases.[7]

In 1995, a resolution of the World Health Assembly (WHA) urged all member states to strengthen surveillance for infectious diseases in order to promptly detect re-emerging diseases and identity new infectious diseases. This resolution led to WHO's establishment of the Division of Emerging and Other Communicable Diseases Surveillance and Control (EMC), whose mission is to strengthen national and international capacity in the surveillance and control of communicable diseases, including those that represent new, emerging, and re-emerging public health problems.

In general, tracking trends and analyzing new and reemerging infectious diseases around the world are significantly more challenging tasks for researchers and scientists than monitoring more established infectious diseases. Disease information in peer-reviewed journals often takes the form of news and notes (synopses, research highlights, dispatches, letters, book reviews, etc.) and comprehensive data on specific diseases are often difficult to come by.

## PREVENTION AND CONTROL

CDC's plan to combat today's infectious diseases and prevent those of tomorrow is described in *Preventing*

*Emerging Infectious Diseases: A Strategy for the 21st Century*.[8] Released in 1998, this plan represents the second phase of the effort launched in 1994 with the publication of CDC's *Addressing Emerging Infectious Disease Threats: A Prevention Strategy for the United States*.[9]

The objectives of the plan are organized under four goals: surveillance and response, applied research, infrastructure and training, and prevention and control. Under each objective, the plan describes in detail the many public health activities that must be conducted to implement CDC's strategy. To accomplish these goals, objectives, and activities, nine categories of problems that cause human suffering and place a burden on society are targeted. These categories include antimicrobial resistance; foodborne and vectorborne diseases; vectorborne and zoonotic diseases; diseases transmitted through blood transfusions or blood products; chronic diseases caused by infectious agents; vaccine development and use; diseases of persons with impaired host defenses; diseases of pregnant women and newborns; and diseases of travelers, immigrants, and refugees. Anticipated outcomes are also provided in the plan.

CDC decided to update its strategy for addressing emerging infectious diseases because of progress in implementing the highest priorities in the 1994 plan as well as several recent developments. These developments include emerging threats, scientific findings, tools and technologies, changes in health care delivery, and public and policy issues.

## HIGHLIGHTED DISEASES

WHO has identified seven diseases as either new or prone to causing epidemics. These include African trypanosomiasis, cholera, dengue and dengue haemorrhagic fever, HIV/AIDS, meningococcal disease, plague, and yellow fever.

**African Trypanosomiasis** Human African trypanosomiasis, known as sleeping sickness, is a parasitic disease transmitted to humans by tsetse flies. It occurs only in sub-Saharan Africa, in regions where tsetse flies are endemic.

The early phase of the disease entails bouts of fever, headaches, and pains in the joints and itching. The second, known as the neurological phase, begins when the parasite crosses the blood-brain barrier and infects the central nervous system. This is when the characteristic signs and symptoms of the disease appear: confusion, sensory disturbances, and poor coordination. Disturbance of the sleep cycle, which gives the disease its name, is the most important feature. Without treatment, the disease is fatal. If the patient does not receive treatment before the onset of the second phase, neurological damage is irreversible even after treatment.

There have been three severe epidemics in Africa over the last century: one between 1896 and 1906, mostly in Uganda and the Congo Basin; one in 1920 in several African countries; and one that began in 1970 and is still in progress. Sleeping sickness threatens over 60 million people in 36 countries of sub-Saharan Africa.[10] Only 3–4 million people at risk are under surveillance, with regular examination or access to a health center that can provide screening.[11]

**Cholera** An acute diarrheal illness caused by infection of the intestine with the bacterium *Vibrio cholera*, cholera has been very rare in industrialized nations for the last 100 years; however, the disease is still common today in other parts of the world, including the Indian subcontinent and sub-Saharan Africa. The emergence of a new serotype, *Vibrio cholerae* O139, permits the organism to continue to spread and cause disease even in populations protected by traditional cholera vaccination or by antibodies generated in response to previous exposure to other serotypes of the same organism. First detected in India in 1992, *Vibrio cholerae* O139 has since been reported in at least seven countries in Asia. If not adequately monitored, food preparation and distribution can cause serious infectious diseases in industrialized countries today, as illustrated by three recent outbreaks of *Vibrio cholerae* in 1991, 1994, and 1997.[12]

**Dengue and Dengue Haemorrhagic Fevers** A mosquito-borne infection that in recent years has become a major international public health concern, dengue is caused by four virusus and transmitted to humans by mosquitoes. It is characterized by fever, rash, and muscle and joint pain. Although incapacitating, it is rarely fatal.

Dengue haemorrhagic fever is caused when when several of the dengue viruses are present simultaneously or when a person who first contracted dengue fever from one virus contracts it again from another of the four viruses. Initial symptoms are similar to dengue fever, but after a few days the patient goes into a shock-like state that is frequently fatal.

Dengue fever and dengue haemorrhagic fever (DHF) occur in over 100 countries and territories. They threaten the health of more than 2.5 billion people in tropical and subtropical areas of Africa, the Americas, the Eastern Mediterranean, Southeast Asia, and the Western Pacific. Prior to 1970 only nine countries in the world had experienced DHF epidemics; by 1995 the number had increased more than fourfold. In 1998, a total of 1.2 million cases of dengue and DHF were reported to WHO, including 15,000 deaths. Globally, the annual number of infections is much higher than is indicated by the number of reported cases. Based on statistical modeling methods, there are an estimated 51 million infections each year.[13]

**Human Immunodeficiency Virus (HIV)** Acquired immunodeficiency disease, or AIDS, is perhaps the most dramatic recent example of an important new infectious disease that has made and continues to make headlines and raise public concern. The disease is believed to be caused by a previously unidentified virus, a member of the family of retroviruses, which has been named the human immunodeficiency virus, or HIV. Note that HIV was first isolated in 1983. Shortly after the retrovirus that causes AIDS was identified in 1984, a blood test to detect the antibodies to HIV was developed in 1985. This advance helped researchers discover that persons who had developed AIDS were only the "tip of the iceberg" of a much larger epidemic of HIV infection. The "iceberg" is perhaps best represented by the following global estimates of the HIV/AIDS epidemic as of the end of 1999: as of the end of 1999, 5.4 million people newly infected with HIV; 34.3 million people living with HIV/AIDS; 2.8 million AIDS deaths; 18.8 million total number of AIDS deaths since the beginning of the epidemic; and 13.2 million total number of AIDS orphans[14] since the beginning of the epidemic.[15]

**Meningococcal Disease** Meningococcal meningitis is a severe form of meningitis. It is the only form of bacterial meningitis that causes epidemics.[16] The disease is spread by direct contact, from respiratory droplets from coughing or sneezing. Meningococcal meningitis is characterized by sudden onset of intense headache, fever, nausea, vomiting, skin rash, and stiff neck. Even with appropriate drugs, 10%–20% of people with the disease die, often within hours of the onset of symptoms.

Meningococcal meningitis occurs worldwide, but devastating, large-scale epidemics have mainly been in the dry sub-Saharan regions of Africa, designated the "African meningitis belt," a region extending from Ethiopia in the east to Senegal in the west. Since the mid-1990s, epidemics in this area have been on an unprecedented scale. While the highest disease rates are found in young children, during epidemics older children, teenagers, and young adults are also affected. The most recent meningococcal meningitis pandemic, which began in 1996, has so far resulted in approximately 300,000 cases, primarily in Nigeria, Burkina Faso, Mali, and Niger.

**Plague** Plague is an infectious disease of animals and humans caused by a bacterium named *Yersinia pestis*. People usually get plague from being bitten by a rodent flea that is carrying the plague bacterium or by direct contact with infected tissues or fluids from handling sick or dead animals. Enlarged, tender lymph nodes, fever, chills, and prostration characterize bubonic plague. Today, modern antibiotics are effective against plague; but if an infected person is not treated promptly, the disease is likely to cause illness or death.

Millions of people in Europe died from plague in the Middle Ages, when flea-infested rats inhabited human homes and places of work. Wild rodents in certain areas around the world are infected with plague, and outbreaks in people in rural communities or in cities are usually associated with infected rats and rat fleas that live in the home. In the United States, the last urban plague epidemic occurred in Los Angeles in 1924–1925. Since then human plague in the United States has occurred as mostly scattered cases in rural areas. Globally, the World Health Organization reports 1,000 to 3,000 cases of plague per year.[17]

**Yellow Fever** Yellow fever is a tropical disease caused by the yellow fever virus, which belongs to the *Flavivirus* group. Transmitted by the bite of mosquitoes, it is characterized by fever, headache, muscle ache, shivers, and nausea and/or vomiting. The "yellow" in the name is explained by the jaundice that affects some patients.

Threat of yellow fever is present in 33 countries in Africa and nine in South America. It is also endemic in several Caribbean islands. Yellow fever is an example of a disease for which an effective vaccine exists, but because it is not widely used in many areas at risk, epidemics continue to occur. Since the mid-1980s there has been a steady increase in the number of cases or countries reporting cases, yet the true number of cases occurring could be many times higher, as outbreaks generally occur in remote areas and miss the attention of health services.

## TABLE OVERVIEW

**H1.1–H1.2. Global Estimates and Surveillance** Data presented here include estimates for 1999 of deaths by cause, sex, and mortality stratum in WHO regions—Africa, the Americas, the Eastern Mediterranean, Europe, Southeast Asia, and the Western Pacific (Table H.1)—and estimates for 1999 of the burden of disease in disability-adjusted life years (DALYs) by cause, sex, and mortality stratum in WHO regions (Table H.2). These tables present concepts and measures that lay the empirical basis for assessing health system performance worldwide.

In Table H.1, causes of death for the 14 subgroups and the world have been estimated based on data from national vital registration systems that capture 16.7 million deaths annually. Data is provided for communicable diseases, maternal and perinatal conditions, and nutritional deficiencies as well as for noncommunicable conditions. Estimates of the cause of death patterns are based on information from sample registration systems, population laboratories, and epidemiological analyses of specific conditions.[18] Additionally, cause of death data have been carefully analyzed to take into account incomplete coverage of vital registration in countries and the likely differences in cause of death patterns that would be expected in the uncovered and often poorer subpopulations.[19] Special attention has been paid to problems of misattribution or miscoding of causes of death in cardiovascular diseases, cancer, injuries, and general ill-defined categories.[20]

In Table H.2, estimates of the burden of disease using disability-adjusted life years (DALYs) as a measure of the health gap in the world in 1999 are provided. DALYs, along with disability-adjusted life expectancy, are summary measures of population health.[21] DALYs are a type of health measure that states the difference between a population's health and a normative goal of living in full health. DALYs have been estimated based on cause of death information for each region and on regional assessments of the epidemiology of major disabling conditions. In this table, data are provided for communicable diseases, maternal and perinatal conditions, and nutritional deficiencies, as well as for noncommunicable conditions.

**H2.1–H2.27. Targeted Diseases** Data for nine infectious epidemic diseases that either are new or volatile or pose an important public health threat are provided next. These diseases include African trypanosomiasis, cholera, dengue and dengue haemorrhagic fever, HIV/AIDS, meningococcal disease, plague, and yellow fever.

## NOTES

1. Institute of Medicine, *Emerging Infections: Microbial Threats to Health in the United States* (Washington, DC: National Academy Press, 1992).
2. The leading causes of death in 1998 were cardiovascular diseases (31%), infectious diseases (25%), cancers (13%), injuries (11%), maternal (5%), respiratory and digestive (9%), and other (6%).
3. Pathogens recognized since 1973.
4. M. Burnet, *Natural history of infectious disease* (Cambridge, England: Cambridge University Press, 1963).
5. *Emerging and Re-Emerging Infectious Diseases*, WHO Fact Sheet No. 97, revised August 1998, http://www.who.int/inf-fs/fact097.html. The CDC recognizes similar causes. Centers for Disease Control and Prevention, "Preventing Emerging Infectious Diseases: A Strategy for the 21st Century: Overview of the Updated CDC Plan," *MMWR* 47, no. RR-15 (1998): 1.
6. *Emerging and Re-Emerging Infectious Diseases*, WHO Fact Sheet No 97.
7. The series, "Emerging Infectious Diseases," was introduced in the April 16, 1993, issue of *MMWR* (42, no. 14). The first article in this series updated an ongoing investigation of an outbreak of *E. coli* O157:H7 in the western United States. Subsequent articles address these diseases, as well as surveillance, control, and prevention efforts by health-care providers and public health officials.
8. CDC, "Preventing Emerging Infectious Diseases: A Strategy for the 21st Century."
9. CDC, *Addressing Emerging Infectious Disease Threats: A Prevention Strategy for the United States* (Atlanta, GA: U.S. Department of Health and Human Services, Public Health Service, 1994).
10. See WHO Information Fact Sheet "African Trypanosomiasis or Sleeping Sickness" at http://www.who.int/inf-fs/en/fact259.html
11. Ibid.
12. In Italy in 1997 the outbreak was traced to a seafood salad packaged in that country. An outbreak in Indiana in 1994 was associated with food transported from El Salvador, and an outbreak in Maryland in 1991 with imported frozen conconut milk.
13. See http://www.who.int/ctd/dengue/disease.htm and WHO Information Fact Sheet No. 117, revised November 1998, "*Dengue and Dengue Haemorrhagic Fever*," at http://www/who/int/inf-fs/en/fact117.html
14. Defined as children who lost their mother or both parents to AIDS when they were under the age of 15.
15. Joint United Nations Programme on HIV/AIDS. *Report on the Global HIV/AIDS Epidemic June 2000*. Joint United Nations Programme on HIV/AIDS. Geneva, Switzerland. (2001). http://www.unaids.org/epidemic_update/report/Epi_report.pdf.
16. WHO Information Fact Sheet No. 105, revised December 1998, *Epidemic Meningococcal Disease*, at http://www.who.int/inf-fs/en/fact105.html.
17. See http://www.cdc.gov/ncidod/dvbid/plague/index.htm and http://www.cdc.gov/ncidod/dvbid/plague/facts.htm.
18. See the *Explanatory Notes* that accompany the *Statistical Annex* to the *World Health Report 2000*.
19. World Health Organization, *World Health Report 2000* (Geneva: World Health Organization, 2000), 145. Internet: http://www.who.int/whr/2000/en/report.htm
20. Ibid.
21. C.J.L. Murray, J. Salomon, and C. Mathers. *A critical review of summary measures of population health*, GPE Discussion Paper No. 2 (Geneva: World Health Organization, 2000).

## Table H1.1. Deaths from Infectious and Parasitic Disease, by Cause, Sex, and Mortality Stratum in WHO Regions,[a] Estimates for 2000

| Cause[b] | SEX | | | | | | Africa | | The Americas | | |
|---|---|---|---|---|---|---|---|---|---|---|---|
| | | | | | | | Mortality stratum | | Mortality stratum | | |
| | Both sexes | | Males | | Females | | High child, high adult | High child, very high adult | Very low child, very low adult | Low child, low adult | High child, high adult |
| *Population (000s)* | *6 045 172* | | *3 045 372* | | *2 999 800* | | *294 099* | *345 533* | *325 186* | *430 951* | *71 235* |
| | (000) | *% total* | (000) | *% total* | (000) | *% total* | (000) | (000) | (000) | (000) | (000) |
| **Infectious and parasitic diseases** | **10 457** | 18.8 | **5 637** | 19.0 | **4 819** | 18.5 | **1 969** | **3 467** | **60** | **213** | **93** |
| Tuberculosis | **1 660** | 3.0 | **1 048** | 3.5 | **613** | 2.4 | **146** | **235** | **2** | **33** | **22** |
| STDs excluding HIV | **217** | 0.4 | **119** | 0.4 | **97** | 0.4 | **43** | **58** | **0** | **1** | **0** |
| Syphilis | **197** | 0.4 | **118** | 0.4 | **79** | 0.3 | **42** | **56** | **0** | **0** | **0** |
| Chlamydia | **7** | 0.0 | **0** | 0.0 | **7** | 0.0 | **1** | **1** | **0** | **0** | **0** |
| Gonorrhoea | **4** | 0.0 | **0** | 0.0 | **4** | 0.0 | **1** | **1** | **0** | **0** | **0** |
| HIV/AIDS | **2 943** | 5.3 | **1 500** | 5.0 | **1 443** | 5.6 | **517** | **1 875** | **15** | **34** | **23** |
| Diarrhoeal diseases | **2 124** | 3.8 | **1 178** | 4.0 | **946** | 3.6 | **272** | **433** | **2** | **49** | **27** |
| Childhood diseases | **1 385** | 2.5 | **693** | 2.3 | **692** | 2.7 | **432** | **308** | **0** | **2** | **6** |
| Pertussis | **296** | 0.5 | **148** | 0.5 | **148** | 0.6 | **92** | **74** | **0** | **1** | **6** |
| Poliomyelitis | **1** | 0.0 | **0** | 0.0 | **0** | 0.0 | **0** | **0** | **0** | **0** | **0** |
| Diphtheria | **3** | 0.0 | **2** | 0.0 | **2** | 0.0 | **1** | **1** | **0** | **0** | **0** |
| Measles | **777** | 1.4 | **388** | 1.3 | **388** | 1.5 | **264** | **188** | **0** | **0** | **0** |
| Tetanus | **309** | 0.6 | **154** | 0.5 | **154** | 0.6 | **75** | **45** | **0** | **1** | **1** |
| Meningitis | **156** | 0.3 | **87** | 0.3 | **69** | 0.3 | **19** | **23** | **1** | **9** | **1** |
| Hepatitis[c] | **128** | 0.2 | **70** | 0.2 | **57** | 0.2 | **15** | **18** | **5** | **3** | **1** |
| Malaria | **1 080** | 1.9 | **522** | 1.8 | **558** | 2.1 | **489** | **477** | **0** | **1** | **1** |
| Tropical diseases | **124** | 0.2 | **76** | 0.3 | **48** | 0.2 | **33** | **30** | **0** | **20** | **3** |
| Trypanosomiasis | **50** | 0.1 | **32** | 0.1 | **18** | 0.1 | **25** | **24** | **0** | **0** | **0** |
| Chagas disease | **21** | 0.0 | **12** | 0.0 | **9** | 0.0 | **0** | **0** | **0** | **18** | **3** |
| Schistosomiasis | **11** | 0.0 | **8** | 0.0 | **3** | 0.0 | **3** | **2** | **0** | **1** | **0** |
| Leishmaniasis | **41** | 0.1 | **23** | 0.1 | **18** | 0.1 | **5** | **4** | **0** | **0** | **0** |
| Lymphatic filariasis | **0** | 0.0 | **0** | 0.0 | **0** | 0.0 | **0** | **0** | **0** | **0** | **0** |
| Onchocerciasis | **0** | 0.0 | **0** | 0.0 | **0** | 0.0 | **0** | **0** | **0** | **0** | **0** |
| Leprosy | **2** | 0.0 | **2** | 0.0 | **1** | 0.0 | **0** | **0** | **0** | **0** | **0** |
| Dengue | **12** | 0.0 | **8** | 0.0 | **4** | 0.0 | **0** | **0** | **0** | **0** | **0** |
| Japanese encephalitis | **4** | 0.0 | **1** | 0.0 | **2** | 0.0 | **0** | **0** | **0** | **0** | **0** |
| Trachoma | **0** | 0.0 | **0** | 0.0 | **0** | 0.0 | **0** | **0** | **0** | **0** | **0** |
| Intestinal nematode infections | **17** | 0.0 | **9** | 0.0 | **8** | 0.0 | **1** | **2** | **0** | **2** | **1** |
| Ascariasis | **6** | 0.0 | **3** | 0.0 | **3** | 0.0 | **0** | **1** | **0** | **1** | **0** |
| Trichuriasis | **2** | 0.0 | **1** | 0.0 | **1** | 0.0 | **0** | **0** | **0** | **0** | **0** |
| Hookworm disease | **6** | 0.0 | **4** | 0.0 | **2** | 0.0 | **1** | **1** | **0** | **0** | **0** |

[a] See list of Member States by WHO Region in Appendix

[b] Estimates for specific causes may not sum to broader causes groupings due to omission of residual categories.

## Table H1.1. *(Continued)*

| Cause[b] | Eastern Mediterranean Mortality stratum | | Europe Mortality stratum | | | South-East Asia Mortality stratum | | Western Pacific Mortality Stratum | |
|---|---|---|---|---|---|---|---|---|---|
| | Low child, low adult | High child, high adult | Very low child, very low adult | Low child, low adult | Low child, high adult | Low child, low adult | High child, high adult | Very low child, very low adult | Low child, low adult |
| *Population (000s)* | *139 071* | *342 584* | *411 910* | *218 473* | *243 192* | *293 821* | *1 241 813* | *154 358* | *1 532 946* |
| | (000) | (000) | (000) | (000) | (000) | (000) | (000) | (000) | (000) |
| **Infectious and parasitic diseases** | 84 | 836 | 49 | 85 | 86 | 332 | 2 540 | 25 | 618 |
| Tuberculosis | 7 | 129 | 6 | 19 | 49 | 157 | 517 | 6 | 336 |
| STDs excluding HIV | 0 | 12 | 0 | 2 | 1 | 1 | 95 | 0 | 3 |
| Syphilis | 0 | 10 | 0 | 1 | 0 | 1 | 85 | 0 | 2 |
| Chlamydia | 0 | 0 | 0 | 0 | 0 | 0 | 4 | 0 | 0 |
| Gonorrhoea | 0 | 0 | 0 | 0 | 0 | 0 | 2 | 0 | 0 |
| HIV/AIDS | 0 | 54 | 10 | 1 | 10 | 37 | 334 | 0 | 32 |
| Diarrhoeal diseases | 24 | 262 | 2 | 27 | 4 | 30 | 921 | 1 | 71 |
| Childhood diseases | 1 | 196 | 0 | 8 | 0 | 43 | 337 | 0 | 52 |
| Pertussis | 0 | 57 | 0 | 0 | 0 | 1 | 62 | 0 | 2 |
| Poliomyelitis | 0 | 0 | 0 | 0 | 0 | 0 | 0 | 0 | 0 |
| Diphtheria | 0 | 0 | 0 | 0 | 0 | 0 | 1 | 0 | 0 |
| Measles | 0 | 81 | 0 | 7 | 0 | 34 | 168 | 0 | 34 |
| Tetanus | 0 | 57 | 0 | 0 | 0 | 8 | 105 | 0 | 17 |
| Meningitis | 2 | 22 | 2 | 7 | 5 | 12 | 42 | 1 | 11 |
| Hepatitis[c] | 3 | 7 | 4 | 5 | 2 | 5 | 32 | 5 | 22 |
| Malaria | 0 | 47 | 0 | 0 | 0 | 8 | 43 | 0 | 13 |
| Tropical diseases | 1 | 5 | 0 | 0 | 0 | 0 | 30 | 0 | 2 |
| Trypanosomiasis | 0 | 1 | 0 | 0 | 0 | 0 | 0 | 0 | 0 |
| Chagas disease | 0 | 0 | 0 | 0 | 0 | 0 | 0 | 0 | 0 |
| Schistosomiasis | 1 | 2 | 0 | 0 | 0 | 0 | 0 | 0 | 2 |
| Leishmaniasis | 0 | 2 | 0 | 0 | 0 | 0 | 30 | 0 | 0 |
| Lymphatic filariasis | 0 | 0 | 0 | 0 | 0 | 0 | 0 | 0 | 0 |
| Onchocerciasis | 0 | 0 | 0 | 0 | 0 | 0 | 0 | 0 | 0 |
| Leprosy | 0 | 0 | 0 | 0 | 0 | 0 | 1 | 0 | 0 |
| Dengue | 0 | 1 | 0 | 0 | 0 | 1 | 10 | 0 | 1 |
| Japanese encephalitis | 0 | 0 | 0 | 0 | 0 | 0 | 0 | 0 | 3 |
| Trachoma | 0 | 0 | 0 | 0 | 0 | 0 | 0 | 0 | 0 |
| Intestinal nematode infections | 0 | 2 | 0 | 0 | 0 | 1 | 5 | 0 | 3 |
| Ascariasis | 0 | 1 | 0 | 0 | 0 | 0 | 1 | 0 | 1 |
| Trichuriasis | 0 | 0 | 0 | 0 | 0 | 0 | 0 | 0 | 1 |
| Hookworm disease | 0 | 0 | 0 | 0 | 0 | 0 | 3 | 0 | 0 |

[a] See list of Member States by WHO Region and mortality stratum (pp.168-169).

[b] Estimates for specific causes may not sum to broader causes groupings due to omission of residual categories.

*Source*: World Health Organization. *World Health Report 2000* (Geneva: World Health Organization, 2000). http://www.who.int/whr/2000/en/report.htm.

## Table H1.2. Burden of Disease in Disability-Adjusted Life Years (DALYs), by Cause, Sex, and Mortality Stratum in WHO Regions.[a] Estimates for 2000

| | SEX | | | | | | AFRICA | | THE AMERICAS | | |
|---|---|---|---|---|---|---|---|---|---|---|---|
| | | | | | | | Mortality stratum | | Mortality stratum | | |
| Cause[b] | Both sexes | | Males | | Females | | High child, high adult | High child, very high adult | Very low child, very low adult | Low child, low adult | High child, high adult |
| Population (000) | 6 045 172 | | 3 045 372 | | 2 999 800 | | *294 099* | *345 533* | *325 186* | *430 951* | *71 235* |
| | (000) | % total | (000) | % total | (000) | % total | (000) | (000) | (000) | (000) | (000) |
| **Infectious and parasitic diseases** | **340 176** | **23.1** | **173 704** | **22.7** | **166 473** | **23.6** | **68 459** | **114 085** | **1 478** | **7 820** | **3 058** |
| Tuberculosis | 35 792 | 2.4 | 21 829 | 2.9 | 13 962 | 2.0 | 3 754 | 6 034 | 20 | 633 | 482 |
| STDs excluding HIV | 15 839 | 1.1 | 5 808 | 0.8 | 10 031 | 1.4 | 2 837 | 3 351 | 110 | 601 | 98 |
| Syphilis | 5 574 | 0.4 | 3 095 | 0.4 | 2 479 | 0.4 | 1 353 | 1 817 | 1 | 23 | 4 |
| Chlamydia | 6 128 | 0.4 | 902 | 0.1 | 5 226 | 0.7 | 829 | 837 | 91 | 389 | 63 |
| Gonorrhoea | 3 919 | 0.3 | 1 758 | 0.2 | 2 161 | 0.3 | 655 | 693 | 16 | 186 | 31 |
| HIV/AIDS | 90 392 | 6.1 | 44 366 | 5.8 | 46 026 | 6.5 | 15 605 | 57 046 | 504 | 1 145 | 714 |
| Diarrhoeal diseases | 62 227 | 4.2 | 32 399 | 4.2 | 29 828 | 4.2 | 8 070 | 13 424 | 108 | 1 838 | 882 |
| Childhood diseases | 50 380 | 3.4 | 25 151 | 3.3 | 25 229 | 3.6 | 15 396 | 11 043 | 50 | 202 | 256 |
| Pertussis | 12 768 | 0.9 | 6 369 | 0.8 | 6 398 | 0.9 | 3 612 | 2 922 | 50 | 178 | 236 |
| Poliomyelitis | 184 | 0.0 | 95 | 0.0 | 89 | 0.0 | 16 | 7 | 0 | 6 | 1 |
| Diphtheria | 114 | 0.0 | 61 | 0.0 | 53 | 0.0 | 24 | 23 | 0 | 2 | 0 |
| Measles | 27 549 | 1.9 | 13 755 | 1.8 | 13 793 | 2.0 | 9 344 | 6 646 | 0 | 2 | 3 |
| Tetanus | 9 766 | 0.7 | 4 870 | 0.6 | 4 895 | 0.7 | 2 400 | 1 446 | 0 | 14 | 17 |
| Meningitis | 5 751 | 0.4 | 3 011 | 0.4 | 2 740 | 0.4 | 698 | 817 | 47 | 437 | 46 |
| Hepatitis[c] | 2 739 | 0.2 | 1 400 | 0.2 | 1 339 | 0.2 | 334 | 444 | 82 | 59 | 35 |
| Malaria | 40 213 | 2.7 | 19 237 | 2.5 | 20 976 | 3.0 | 17 916 | 17 832 | 1 | 83 | 27 |
| Tropical diseases | 12 289 | 0.8 | 8 271 | 1.1 | 4 018 | 0.6 | 3 051 | 3 012 | 9 | 701 | 109 |
| Trypanosomiasis | 1 585 | 0.1 | 1 013 | 0.1 | 572 | 0.1 | 804 | 754 | 0 | 0 | 0 |
| Chagas disease | 680 | 0.0 | 360 | 0.0 | 320 | 0.0 | 0 | 0 | 7 | 582 | 91 |
| Schistosomiasis | 1 713 | 0.1 | 1 037 | 0.1 | 676 | 0.1 | 648 | 724 | 1 | 70 | 9 |
| Leishmaniasis | 1 810 | 0.1 | 1 067 | 0.1 | 744 | 0.1 | 222 | 173 | 1 | 41 | 5 |
| Lymphatic filariasis | 5 549 | 0.4 | 4 245 | 0.6 | 1 304 | 0.2 | 894 | 966 | 0 | 8 | 1 |
| Onchocerciasis | 951 | 0.1 | 549 | 0.1 | 402 | 0.1 | 484 | 395 | 0 | 1 | 2 |
| Leprosy | 141 | 0.0 | 76 | 0.0 | 65 | 0.0 | 8 | 8 | 0 | 15 | 0 |
| Dengue | 433 | 0.0 | 286 | 0.0 | 147 | 0.0 | 2 | 4 | 0 | 3 | 7 |
| Japanese encephalitis | 426 | 0.0 | 207 | 0.0 | 219 | 0.0 | 0 | 0 | 0 | 0 | 0 |
| Trachoma | 1 181 | 0.1 | 319 | 0.0 | 862 | 0.1 | 212 | 232 | 0 | 0 | 0 |
| Intestinal nematode infections | 4 811 | 0.3 | 2 461 | 0.3 | 2 350 | 0.3 | 289 | 364 | 11 | 549 | 123 |
| Ascariasis | 1 252 | 0.1 | 636 | 0.1 | 616 | 0.1 | 48 | 70 | 3 | 168 | 27 |
| Trichuriasis | 1 640 | 0.1 | 836 | 0.1 | 803 | 0.1 | 50 | 70 | 5 | 239 | 46 |
| Hookworm disease | 1 829 | 0.1 | 939 | 0.1 | 890 | 0.1 | 191 | 222 | 3 | 125 | 20 |

[a] See list of Member States by WHO Region in Appendix

[b] Estimates for specific causes may not sum to broader causes groupings due to omission of residual categories.

## Table H1.2. *(Continued)*

| | EASTERN MEDITERRANEAN Mortality stratum | | EUROPE Mortality stratum | | | SOUTH-EAST ASIA Mortality stratum | | WESTERN PACIFIC Mortality stratum | |
|---|---|---|---|---|---|---|---|---|---|
| Cause[b] | Low child, low adult | High child, high adult | Very low child, very low adult | Low child, low adult | Low child, high adult | Low child, low adult | High child, high adult | Very low child, very low adult | Low child, low adult |
| Population (000) | *139 071* | *342 584* | *411 910* | *218 473* | *243 192* | *293 821* | *1 241 813* | *154 358* | *1 532 946* |
| | (000) | (000) | (000) | (000) | (000) | (000) | (000) | (000) | (000) |
| **Infectious and parasitic diseases** | **2 965** | **28 474** | **1 097** | **3 118** | **2 608** | **9 745** | **76 637** | **397** | **20 234** |
| Tuberculosis | 176 | 2 775 | 63 | 444 | 1 096 | 3 063 | 11 929 | 53 | 5 272 |
| STDs excluding HIV | 79 | 1 150 | 122 | 201 | 194 | 541 | 5 981 | 51 | 521 |
| Syphilis | 3 | 316 | 1 | 24 | 4 | 33 | 1 932 | 1 | 62 |
| Chlamydia | 51 | 463 | 105 | 120 | 140 | 291 | 2 442 | 41 | 266 |
| Gonorrhoea | 20 | 313 | 15 | 35 | 38 | 215 | 1 505 | 8 | 189 |
| HIV/AIDS | 2 | 1 784 | 307 | 36 | 421 | 1 198 | 10 279 | 11 | 1 340 |
| Diarrhoeal diseases | 815 | 8 358 | 109 | 963 | 166 | 976 | 22 387 | 45 | 4 084 |
| Childhood diseases | 63 | 6 934 | 66 | 332 | 34 | 1 599 | 12 128 | 37 | 2 240 |
| Pertussis | 42 | 2 204 | 63 | 63 | 29 | 133 | 2 737 | 36 | 462 |
| Poliomyelitis | 5 | 16 | 1 | 5 | 1 | 11 | 62 | 0 | 52 |
| Diphtheria | 0 | 16 | 0 | 6 | 1 | 4 | 35 | 0 | 4 |
| Measles | 10 | 2 882 | 1 | 252 | 2 | 1 212 | 5 989 | 1 | 1 206 |
| Tetanus | 7 | 1 816 | 1 | 6 | 1 | 239 | 3 306 | 0 | 516 |
| Meningitis | 71 | 800 | 66 | 206 | 125 | 442 | 1 429 | 14 | 555 |
| Hepatitis[c] | 73 | 181 | 45 | 142 | 46 | 98 | 756 | 56 | 389 |
| Malaria | 47 | 1 898 | 2 | 19 | 0 | 292 | 1 582 | 2 | 514 |
| Tropical diseases | 62 | 846 | 0 | 7 | 0 | 242 | 3 772 | 4 | 472 |
| Trypanosomiasis | 0 | 26 | 0 | 0 | 0 | 0 | 0 | 0 | 0 |
| Chagas disease | 0 | 0 | 0 | 0 | 0 | 0 | 0 | 0 | 0 |
| Schistosomiasis | 43 | 154 | 0 | 0 | 0 | 3 | 1 | 0 | 60 |
| Leishmaniasis | 16 | 124 | 0 | 6 | 0 | 6 | 1 210 | 0 | 9 |
| Lymphatic filariasis | 4 | 473 | 0 | 1 | 0 | 233 | 2 562 | 4 | 403 |
| Onchocerciasis | 0 | 69 | 0 | 0 | 0 | 0 | 0 | 0 | 0 |
| Leprosy | 0 | 12 | 0 | 0 | 0 | 7 | 83 | 0 | 6 |
| Dengue | 0 | 19 | 0 | 0 | 0 | 25 | 346 | 0 | 26 |
| Japanese encephalitis | 0 | 6 | 0 | 0 | 0 | 22 | 61 | 0 | 336 |
| Trachoma | 71 | 108 | 0 | 0 | 0 | 24 | 50 | 0 | 484 |
| Intestinal nematode infections | 47 | 248 | 0 | 8 | 1 | 469 | 1 044 | 6 | 1 651 |
| Ascariasis | 20 | 83 | 0 | 7 | 0 | 114 | 123 | 1 | 588 |
| Trichuriasis | 1 | 31 | 0 | 0 | 0 | 194 | 202 | 2 | 799 |
| Hookworm disease | 26 | 134 | 0 | 0 | 0 | 160 | 703 | 2 | 242 |
| **Respiratory infections** | **1 279** | **10 120** | **676** | **2 264** | **951** | **3 456** | **29 005** | **381** | **14 387** |
| Lower respiratory infections | 1 212 | 9 929 | 612 | 2 182 | 894 | 3 350 | 28 134 | 358 | 13 316 |
| Upper respiratory infections | 28 | 77 | 28 | 48 | 31 | 38 | 528 | 10 | 741 |
| Otitis media | 40 | 115 | 37 | 34 | 27 | 69 | 343 | 13 | 330 |

[a] See list of Member States by WHO Region in Appendix

[b] Estimates for specific causes may not sum to broader causes groupings due to omission of residual categories.

*Source*: World Health Organization. *World Health Report 2000* (Geneva: World Health Organization, 2000). http://www.who.int/whr/2000/en/report.htm.

## Table H2.1. African Trypanosomiasis, Cases Reported to WHO, Number of Countries Reporting, and Population Screened, 1990–1998

| | 1990 | 1991 | 1992 | 1993 | 1994 | 1995 | 1996 | 1997 | 1998 |
|---|---|---|---|---|---|---|---|---|---|
| Angola | 1,498 | 2,094 | 2,406 | 1,796 | 1,274 | 2,478 | 6,726 | 8,291 | 6,610 |
| Benin | 0 | 0 | 2 | 1 | 0 | 0 | 0 | 0 | 0 |
| Botswana | | | | | | | | | |
| Burkina Faso | 27 | 27 | 20 | 2 | 18 | 13 | 12 | 2 | |
| Burundi | | | | | | | | | |
| Cameroon | 65 | 41 | 22 | 16 | 12 | 8 | 9 | 6 | 55 |
| Central African Republic | 118 | 535 | 365 | 264 | 362 | 673 | 434 | 708 | 1,069 |
| Chad | 20 | 212 | 133 | 65 | 213 | 401 | 178 | 131 | 134 |
| Congo | 580 | 703 | 727 | 754 | 418 | 475 | 474 | 142 | 201 |
| Cote d'Ivoire | 365 | 349 | 456 | 462 | 404 | 596 | | 18 | 21 |
| Dem. Rep. of the Congo | 7,712 | 5,824 | 7,757 | 11,384 | 19,340 | 18,158 | 19,342 | 25,200 | 27,044 |
| Equatorial Guinea | 28 | 30 | 85 | 32 | 62 | 38 | 46 | 68 | 59 |
| Gabon | 43 | 32 | 18 | 94 | 85 | 41 | | 11 | 6 |
| Gambia | | | | | | | | | |
| Ghana | 4 | 6 | 16 | | | | | | |
| Guinea | 41 | 29 | 24 | 27 | 26 | 33 | 47 | 92 | 57 |
| Guinea-Bissau | | | | | | | | | |
| Kenya | 90 | 7 | 2 | 2 | 1 | 0 | 0 | 6 | 20 |
| Mali | | | | 27 | 17 | 11 | 5 | 0 | 0 |
| Mozambique | 3 | 7 | 24 | 10 | 16 | | | | |
| Niger | | | | | | | | | |
| Nigeria | | | | | | | | | |
| Rwanda | | | | | | | | | |
| Senegal | | | | | | | | | |
| Sierra Leone | | | | | | | | | |
| Sudan | 67 | 58 | 28 | 62 | 69 | 56 | 157 | 737 | |
| United Rep. of Tanzania | 180 | 466 | 513 | 303 | 319 | 422 | 400 | 508 | 194 |
| Togo | 2 | 0 | 0 | 0 | 0 | 3 | 0 | 1 | |
| Uganda | 2,667 | 2,481 | 1,126 | 1,770 | 1,891 | 1,200 | 1,125 | 1,300 | 677 |
| Zambia | | | | | | | | | |
| Total no. of cases | 13,510 | 12,901 | 13,724 | 17,071 | 24,527 | 24,606 | 28,955 | 37,221 | 36,147 |

*Source*: World Health Organization, Department of Communicable Disease Surveillance and Response. *WHO Report on Global Surveillance of Epidemic-prone Infectious Diseases* (2000). http://www.who.int/emc-documents/surveillance/whocdscsrisr20001c.html#english.

## Table H2.2. Cholera, Cases and Total Number of Deaths Reported to WHO, Africa, 1990–1998

| | 1990 | 1991 | 1992 | 1993 | 1994 | 1995 | 1996 | 1997 | 1998 |
|---|---|---|---|---|---|---|---|---|---|
| Algeria | 1,293 | 1,991 | 69 | | 118 | | | | |
| Angola | 9,527 | 8,590 | 3,608 | | 3,443 | 3,295 | 1,306 | | |
| Benin | | 7,474 | 413 | 10 | 187 | 203 | 6,190 | 778 | 206 |
| Burkina Faso | | 537 | | | | 1,451 | 425 | | 1,036 |
| Burundi | 82 | 3 | 479 | 78 | 562 | 2,297 | 418 | 1,959 | 1,067 |
| Cameroon | 16 | 4,026 | 1,268 | 648 | 527 | 615 | 5,796 | 1,709 | 4,603 |
| Cape Verde | | | | | 128 | 12,913 | 426 | | 133 |
| Central African Republic | | | | | | | | 443 | 4,095 |
| Chad | | 13,915 | | | 1,094 | | 7,830 | 8,801 | 22 |
| Comoros | | | | | | | | | 7,300 |
| Congo | | | | | | | | 275 | 3,222 |
| Cote d'Ivoire | | 604 | 37 | 724 | 1,108 | 4,993 | 1,345 | | |
| Dem. Rep. of the Congo | 468 | 4,066 | 1,949 | 986 | 58,057 | 553 | 7,888 | 2,421 | 34,899 |
| Djibouti | | | | 10,055 | 1,122 | | | 2,424 | 164 |
| Equatorial Guinea | | | | | | | | | |
| Ethiopia | | | | | | | | | |
| Gabon | | | | | | | | | |
| Gambia | | | | | 1 | 15 | 7 | | |
| Ghana | 2,937 | 13,172 | 228 | 1,448 | 2,267 | 4,698 | 1,665 | 379 | 3,426 |
| Guinea | | | | | 31,415 | 6,506 | 287 | | 881 |
| Guinea Bissau | | | | | 15,296 | 119 | 8,397 | 20,555 | 126 |
| Kenya | | | 3,388 | | 880 | 1,543 | 482 | 17,200 | 22,432 |
| Liberia | | 132 | | | 764 | 3,420 | 8,922 | 91 | 2,123 |
| Libyan Arab Jamahiriya | | | | | | 22 | | | |
| Madagascar | | | | | | | | | |
| Malawi | 13,457 | 8,088 | 298 | 25,193 | 107 | 1 | 1 | 130 | 1,745 |
| Mali | | | | | | 2,048 | 5,723 | 6 | |
| Mauritania | | | | | | | 4,534 | 462 | |
| Morocco | | | | | 6 | | | | |
| Mozambique | 4,152 | 7,847 | 30,802 | 19,803 | 692 | | | 8,739 | 42,672 |
| Niger | | 3,238 | | | 732 | 264 | 3,957 | 259 | |
| Nigeria | | 59,478 | 7,671 | 4,160 | 2,859 | 1,059 | 12,374 | 1,322 | 3,464 |
| Rwanda | | 679 | 530 | 568 | 10 | 3 | 106 | 274 | 3,220 |
| Sao Tome and Principe | 804 | 3 | | | | | | | |
| Senegal | | | | | | 3,222 | 16,107 | 371 | |
| Sierra Leone | | | | | 9,709 | 10,285 | | | 2,096 |
| Somalia | | | | | 27,904 | 9,255 | 10,274 | 6,814 | 4,404 |
| South Africa | | 10 | 11 | 78 | 4 | | | | 20 |
| Sudan | | | | | | | | | |
| Swaziland | | | 2,281 | | | | 2 | | 7 |
| Togo | | 2,396 | 753 | 19 | 47 | 65 | 146 | 42 | 3,217 |
| Tunisia | | | | | | | | | |
| Uganda | | 279 | 5,072 | | 704 | 538 | 291 | 2,610 | 49,514 |
| United Republic of Tanzania | 2,230 | 5,676 | 18,526 | 792 | 2,240 | 1,698 | 1,464 | 40,249 | 14,488 |
| Zambia | 3,717 | 13,154 | 11,659 | 6,766 | | | 2,172 | 36 | 171 |
| Zimbabwe | | | 2,039 | 5,385 | | | | | 995 |
| Total no. of cases | 38,683 | 155,358 | 91,081 | 76,713 | 161,983 | 71,081 | 108,535 | 118,349 | 211,748 |
| Total no. of deaths | 2,288 | 13,998 | 5,291 | 2,532 | 8,128 | 3,024 | 6,216 | 5,853 | 9,856 |
| No. of countries reporting | 11 | 22 | 20 | 16 | 28 | 26 | 28 | 25 | 29 |

*Source*: World Health Organization, Department of Communicable Disease Surveillance and Response. *WHO Report on Global Surveillance of Epidemic-prone Infectious Diseases* (2000). http://www.who.int/emc-documents/surveillance/whocdscsrisr20001c.html#english.

## Table H2.3. Cholera, Cases and Total Number of Deaths Reported to WHO, the Americas, 1991–1998

| | 1991 | 1992 | 1993 | 1994 | 1995 | 1996 | 1997 | 1998 |
|---|---|---|---|---|---|---|---|---|
| Argentina | | 553 | 2,080 | 889 | 188 | 474 | 637 | 12 |
| Belize | | 159 | 135 | 6 | 19 | 26 | 2 | 28 |
| Bolivia | 206 | 22,260 | 10,134 | 2,710 | 2,293 | 2,847 | 1,632 | 466 |
| Brazil | 1,567 | 30,309 | 59,212 | 49,455 | 15,915 | 4,634 | 2,881 | 2,571 |
| Canada | 2 | 4 | 6 | 2 | 7 | 2 | | 2 |
| Chile | 41 | 73 | 32 | 1 | | 1 | 4 | 24 |
| Colombia | 11,979 | 15,129 | 230 | 996 | 1,922 | 4,428 | 1,508 | 442 |
| Costa Rica | | 12 | 14 | 38 | 24 | 19 | 1 | |
| Ecuador | 46,320 | 31,870 | 6,833 | 1,785 | 2,160 | 1,059 | 65 | 3,724 |
| El Salvador | 947 | 8,106 | 6,573 | 11,739 | 2,923 | 182 | 0 | 8 |
| French Guiana | 1 | 16 | 2 | 2 | | | | |
| Guatemala | 3,674 | 15,395 | 30,604 | 5,282 | 7,970 | 1,568 | 1,263 | 5,970 |
| Guyana | | 576 | 66 | | | | | |
| Honduras | 11 | 384 | 4,007 | 4,965 | 4,717 | 708 | 90 | 306 |
| Mexico | 2,690 | 8,162 | 10,712 | 4,059 | 16,430 | 1,088 | 2,356 | 71 |
| Nicaragua | 1 | 3,067 | 6,631 | 7,821 | 8,825 | 2,813 | 1,283 | 1,437 |
| Panama | 1,178 | 2,416 | 42 | | | | | |
| Paraguay | | | 3 | | | 4 | | |
| Peru | 322,562 | 212,642 | 71,448 | 23,887 | 22,397 | 4,518 | 3,483 | 41,717 |
| Suriname | | 12 | | | | | | |
| United States of America | 26 | 102 | 19 | 47 | 19 | 3 | 4 | 15 |
| Venezuela | 15 | 2,842 | 409 | | | 269 | 2,551 | 313 |
| Total no. of cases | 391,220 | 354,089 | 209,192 | 113,684 | 85,809 | 24,643 | 17,760 | 57,106 |
| Total no. of deaths | 4,002 | 2,401 | 2,438 | 1,107 | 845 | 351 | 225 | 558 |
| No. of countries reporting | 16 | 21 | 21 | 17 | 15 | 18 | 16 | 16 |

*Source*: World Health Organization, Department of Communicable Disease Surveillance and Response. *WHO Report on Global Surveillance of Epidemic-prone Infectious Diseases* (2000). http://www.who.int/emc-documents/surveillance/whocdscsrisr20001c.html#english.

## Table H2.4. Cholera, Cases and Total Number of Deaths Reported to WHO, Asia, 1990–1998

| | 1990 | 1991 | 1992 | 1993 | 1994 | 1995 | 1996 | 1997 | 1998 |
|---|---|---|---|---|---|---|---|---|---|
| Afghanistan | | | | 37,046 | 38,735 | 19,903 | | 4,170 | 10,000 |
| Armenia | | | | | | | | | 25 |
| Azerbaijan | | | | | 9 | | | | |
| Bahrain | | | | | | | | | |
| Bangladesh | | | | 12 | | | | | |
| Bhutan | | 422 | 494 | | | 25 | | | 19 |
| Brunei Darussalam | | | | | | | | | |
| Cambodia | | 770 | 1,229 | 2,252 | 3,085 | 4,190 | 740 | 155 | 1,197 |
| China | 639 | 205 | 580 | 11,717 | 34,821 | 10,344 | 312 | 1,163 | |
| Dem. People's Republic of Korea | | | | | | | | | |
| Georgia | | | | 8 | | | | | |
| Hong Kong SAR | 5 | 5 | 3 | 30 | 56 | 6 | 4 | 14 | 71 |
| India | 3,583 | 6,993 | 6,911 | 9,437 | 4,973 | 3,315 | 4,396 | 2,768 | 7,151 |
| Indonesia | 155 | 6,202 | 25 | 3,564 | 47 | | | 66 | |
| Iran (Islamic Republic of) | 178 | 1,880 | 97 | 1,347 | 15 | 2,177 | | 1,106 | 270 |
| Iraq | | 877 | 97 | 280 | 838 | 820 | | | 53 |
| Israel | | | | | | | | | |
| Japan | 73 | 90 | 46 | 89 | 91 | 321 | 39 | 89 | 60 |
| Jordan | 2 | | | | | | | | |
| Kazakhstan | | | | 74 | 3 | 8 | | 4 | |
| Kuwait | | | | 1 | | | | 1 | |
| Kyrgyzstan | | | | | 4 | | | | |
| Lao People's Dem. Republic | | | | 5,521 | 9,640 | 1,365 | 720 | | |
| Lebanon | | | | 344 | 3 | | | | |
| Maldives | | | | | | | | | |
| Macao SAR | 1 | | | | | | | | 8 |
| Malaysia | 2,071 | 506 | 474 | 995 | 534 | 2,209 | 1,486 | 389 | 1,304 |
| Mongolia | | | | | | | 177 | | |
| Myanmar | 24 | 924 | 826 | 1,758 | 421 | 1,296 | | | |
| Nepal | 23,888 | 30,648 | 764 | 31 | 32 | 157 | 274 | 245 | 1,745 |
| Oman | | | | | | | | | |
| Pakistan | | | | 12,092 | | | | | |
| Philippines | | | 345 | 708 | 3,340 | 847 | 1,402 | 605 | 729 |
| Republic of Korea | | 113 | 6 | 5 | 34 | 74 | 7 | 10 | |
| Saudi Arabia | | | | | | | | | |
| Singapore | 26 | 34 | 17 | 24 | 41 | 14 | 19 | 19 | 31 |
| Syrian Arab Republic | | | | | | | | | |
| Sri Lanka | | 70 | 121 | 1 | | | | 430 | 1,536 |
| Tajikistan | | | | 165 | 10 | | | | |
| Thailand | | | | | 3,487 | | | | |
| Turkey | | | | | | | | | |
| Turkmenistan | | | | | 1 | | | 55 | |
| United Arab Emirates | | | | | | | | | |
| Uzbekistan | | | | | 1 | | | | |
| Viet Nam | 358 | 52 | 4,260 | 3,361 | 5,776 | 6,088 | 566 | 4 | 13 |
| West Bank and Gaza Strip | | | | | 103 | | | | |
| Yemen | | | 4 | | | | | | |
| Total no. of cases | 31,003 | 49,791 | 16,299 | 90,862 | 106,100 | 53,159 | 10,142 | 11,293 | 24,212 |
| Total no. of deaths | 628 | 1,286 | 372 | 1,809 | 1,393 | 1,158 | 122 | 196 | 172 |
| No. of countries reporting | 13 | 16 | 18 | 25 | 26 | 18 | 13 | 18 | 16 |

*Source*: World Health Organization, Department of Communicable Disease Surveillance and Response. *WHO Report on Global Surveillance of Epidemic-prone Infectious Diseases* (2000). http://www.who.int/emc-documents/surveillance/whocdscsrisr20001c.html#english.

## Table H2.5. Cholera, Cases and Total Number of Deaths Reported to WHO, Europe, 1990–1998

| | 1990 | 1991 | 1992 | 1993 | 1994 | 1995 | 1996 | 1997 | 1998 |
|---|---|---|---|---|---|---|---|---|---|
| Albania | | | | | 626 | | | | |
| Andorra | | | | 1 | | | | | |
| Austria | 2 | | | 1 | 1 | | | | 1 |
| Belarus | | | | | 3 | 3 | | | |
| Belgium | | | 1 | 1 | 1 | | | | |
| Czechoslovakia [1] | | | | | | | | | |
| Denmark | 1 | | | 2 | 2 | 3 | | | |
| Estonia | | | | 2 | | | | | 1 |
| Finland | | | | | 2 | 1 | | | |
| France | 6 | | | 5 | 4 | 5 | 6 | 3 | 2 |
| Germany | 1 | 7 | 1 | 1 | 5 | 1 | | 2 | 5 |
| Greece | | | | 1 | | | | | |
| Hungary | | | | | | | | 1 | |
| Italy | | | | | 12 | 1 | | | 2 |
| Netherlands | 3 | | | 2 | 1 | 9 | 3 | 2 | 4 |
| Norway | | | | | | 1 | | | 2 |
| Poland | | | | | 1 | | | | |
| Portugal | | | | | 1 | 1 | | | |
| Republic of Moldova | | | | 1 | 8 | 240 | | | |
| Romania | 270 | 226 | 3 | 15 | 80 | 118 | | | |
| Russian Federation | | 3 | 6 | 23 | 1,048 | 9 | 1 | 4 | 10 |
| Spain | 11 | 1 | | 3 | 1 | 6 | 1 | | |
| Sweden | | | 1 | | 1 | 2 | 1 | | |
| Switzerland | | | 1 | 2 | | 2 | | | 2 |
| United Kingdom of G.B and N.I. | 6 | 8 | 5 | 13 | 18 | 10 | 13 | 6 | 18 |
| Ukraine | 49 | 75 | | | 813 | 525 | | | |
| Yugoslavia | | | | | 2 | | | | |
| Total no. of cases | 349 | 320 | 18 | 73 | 2,630 | 937 | 25 | 18 | 47 |
| Total no. of deaths | 2 | 9 | 0 | 0 | 0 | 0 | 0 | 1 | 0 |
| No. of countries reporting | 9 | 6 | 7 | 15 | 20 | 17 | 6 | 6 | 10 |

[1] Czechoslovakia dissolved on 31 December 1992.

*Source*: World Health Organization, Department of Communicable Disease Surveillance and Response. *WHO Report on Global Surveillance of Epidemic-prone Infectious Diseases* (2000). http://www.who.int/emc-documents/surveillance/whocdscsrisr20001c.html#english.

**Table H2.6. Cholera, Cases and Total Number of Deaths Reported to WHO, Oceania, 1990–1998**

| | 1990 | 1991 | 1992 | 1993 | 1994 | 1995 | 1996 | 1997 | 1998 |
|---|---|---|---|---|---|---|---|---|---|
| Australia | 2 | | 3 | 5 | 3 | 5 | 2 | 2 | 5 |
| Guam | 1 | | | | 1 | | 1 | | 2 |
| Kiribati | | | | | | | | | |
| Northern Mariana Islands | | | | | | | 1 | 3 | |
| Micronesia (Federated States o | 34 | | | | | | | | |
| Nauru | | | | | | | | | |
| Papua New Guinea | | | | | | | | | |
| New Zealand | 3 | | | | 2 | 2 | | | 1 |
| Samoa | | | | | | | | | |
| Trust Territories of the Pacific [1] | | | | | | | | | |
| Tuvalu | 27 | | 293 | | | | | | |
| Total no. of cases | 67 | | 296 | 5 | 6 | 7 | 4 | 5 | 8 |
| Total no. of deaths | 1 | | 8 | 0 | 0 | 0 | 0 | 0 | 0 |
| No. of countries reporting | 5 | 0 | 2 | 1 | 3 | 2 | 3 | 2 | 3 |
| [1]The Trust Territories of the Pacific consisted of the Federated States of Micronesia, Marshall Islands, Palau, and the Northern Mariana Islands. | | | | | | | | | |

*Source*: World Health Organization, Department of Communicable Disease Surveillance and Response. *WHO Report on Global Surveillance of Epidemic-prone Infectious Diseases* (2000). http://www.who.int/emc-documents/surveillance/whocdscsrisr20001c.html#english.

## Table H2.7. Dengue Fever, Cases Reported to WHO, the Americas, 1990–1998

| | 1990 | 1991 | 1992 | 1993 | 1994 | 1995 | 1996 | 1997 | 1998 |
|---|---|---|---|---|---|---|---|---|---|
| Anguilla | 12 | 0 | 0 | | | 4 | 1 | 0 | 0 |
| Antigua | 1 | 1 | 0 | | | 56 | 12 | 9 | 4 |
| Aruba | 0 | 0 | 0 | | | 37 | 10 | 0 | |
| Bahamas | 2 | 0 | 0 | | | 1 | 0 | 0 | 126 |
| Barbados | 236 | 21 | 4 | 55 | 114 | 976 | 130 | 199 | 610 |
| Belize | 2 | 0 | 0 | | | 107 | 0 | 210 | 17 |
| Bermuda | | | | | | 0 | 0 | 0 | 0 |
| Bolivia | 0 | 0 | 0 | 0 | 0 | | 52 | 223 | 49 |
| Bonaire | 0 | 0 | 0 | | | | | | |
| Brazil | 40,642 | 97,209 | 3,501 | 6,915 | 54,453 | 124,887 | 175,751 | 254,942 | 530,578 |
| British Virgin Islands | 3 | 1 | 2 | 0 | 0 | 9 | 0 | 0 | 1 |
| Cayman Islands | | | | | | 1 | 0 | 0 | 1 |
| Colombia | 17,389 | 15,103 | 20,130 | 25,585 | 27,885 | 51,059 | 33,155 | 14,958 | 43,855 |
| Costa Rica | 0 | 0 | | 4,612 | 13,929 | 5,134 | 2,307 | 14,267 | 2,290 |
| Cuba | 0 | 0 | 0 | 0 | 0 | | | 3,012 | |
| Dominica | 6 | 12 | 0 | 0 | 1 | 293 | 3 | 0 | 7 |
| Dominican Republic | 39 | 24 | 105 | 138 | 1,211 | 249 | 89 | 64 | 3,049 |
| Ecuador | 2,109 | 302 | 454 | 9,015 | 8,145 | 6,607 | 5,189 | 284 | 4,219 |
| El Salvador | 2,381 | 1,273 | 884 | 245 | 281 | 9,658 | 790 | 348 | 1,354 |
| French Guiana | 29 | 269 | 569 | 178 | 164 | 896 | 364 | 851 | 534 |
| Grenada | 3 | 1 | 1 | 1 | 5 | 74 | 6 | 22 | |
| Guadeloupe | 12 | 51 | 75 | 0 | 0 | 156 | 186 | 0 | |
| Guatemala | 5,757 | 10,968 | 1,286 | 1,907 | 2,872 | 3,980 | 3,679 | 5,379 | 1,593 |
| Guyana | 3 | 0 | 2 | 0 | 1 | 0 | 0 | 0 | 42 |
| Haiti | | 0 | 0 | | 0 | 0 | 0 | | |
| Honduras | 1,700 | 5,303 | 2,113 | 2,847 | 3,055 | 27,575 | 5,047 | 11,730 | 22,218 |
| Jamaica | 9 | 5 | 296 | 0 | 4 | 1,884 | 46 | 16 | 68 |
| Martinique | 4 | 0 | 38 | 0 | 0 | 519 | 430 | 235 | 44 |
| Mexico | 14,485 | 7,158 | 8,131 | 2,899 | 6,770 | 17,088 | 20,687 | 35,108 | 23,639 |
| Montserrat | 0 | 0 | 0 | | 15 | 75 | 3 | | 0 |
| Netherlands Antilles | | | | | | | | | |
| Nicaragua | 4,137 | 1,885 | 4,936 | 8,938 | 20,469 | 19,260 | 2,792 | 3,126 | 13,592 |
| Panama | 0 | 0 | 0 | 14 | 790 | 3,083 | 811 | 1,710 | 2,717 |
| Paraguay | 0 | 0 | 0 | 0 | 0 | | 0 | | |
| Puerto Rico | 9,450 | 10,305 | 13,000 | 6,600 | 22,000 | 6,765 | 4,655 | 6,955 | 14,828 |
| Peru | 7,858 | 714 | 1,971 | 897 | 1,478 | 2,732 | 6,395 | 1,151 | 988 |
| St. Kitts and Nevis | 0 | 8 | 0 | 1 | 8 | 27 | 6 | 0 | |
| St. Lucia | 2 | 4 | 0 | 5 | 0 | 52 | 65 | 14 | 3 |
| St. Martin | 0 | 0 | 0 | | | | | | |
| St. Vincent | 9 | 1 | 7 | 7 | 2 | 224 | 190 | 3 | 112 |
| Suriname | 16 | 40 | 24 | 171 | 75 | 344 | 677 | 90 | 1,230 |
| Trinidad and Tobago | 526 | 36 | 116 | 268 | 48 | 312 | 3,983 | 1,357 | 2,792 |
| Turks and Caicos Islands | 0 | 0 | 0 | 0 | 0 | 0 | 0 | 0 | |
| United States of America | 102 | 25 | 68 | 57 | 91 | 7 | 0 | | 0 |
| Venezuela | 10,962 | 6,559 | 2,707 | 9,059 | 15,046 | 32,280 | 9,180 | 33,654 | 37,586 |
| Virgin Islands (USA) | 339 | 62 | 48 | 0 | 0 | 0 | 0 | 0 | 0 |
| Other Caribbean islands | | | | 500 | 275 | | | | |
| Total no. of cases | 118,225 | 157,340 | 60,468 | 80,914 | 179,187 | 316,411 | 276,691 | 389,917 | 708,146 |
| No. of countries reporting | 42 | 43 | 42 | 35 | 37 | 40 | 42 | 39 | 35 |

*Source*: World Health Organization, Department of Communicable Disease Surveillance and Response. *WHO Report on Global Surveillance of Epidemic-prone Infectious Diseases* (2000). http://www.who.int/emc-documents/surveillance/whocdscsrisr20001c.html#english.

## Table H2.8. Dengue Haemorrhagic Fever, Cases Reported to WHO, the Americas, 1990–1998

| | 1990 | 1991 | 1992 | 1993 | 1994 | 1995 | 1996 | 1997 | 1998 |
|---|---|---|---|---|---|---|---|---|---|
| Argentina | | | | | | | | | |
| Aruba | | | | | | | | | |
| Barbados | | | | | | 2 | | 3 | |
| Brazil | 274 | 188 | | | 24 | 105 | 2 | 35 | 89 |
| Belize | | | | | | | | | 1 |
| Bermuda | | | | | | | | | |
| Bolivia | | | | | | | | | 0 |
| Cayman Islands | | | | | | | | | |
| Colombia | 39 | 96 | 493 | 303 | 568 | 1,028 | 1,757 | 3,330 | 5,276 |
| Costa Rica | | | | | | 1 | | | |
| Cuba | | | | | | | | 205 | |
| Curacao | | | | | | | | | |
| Dominica | | | | | | 11 | | | |
| Dominican Republic | 2 | 7 | 2 | 4 | 100 | 38 | 17 | 3 | 176 |
| El Salvador | | 1 | 0 | 3 | 0 | 129 | 1 | | 2 |
| French Guiana | | | 38 | 2 | 1 | 1 | 6 | 3 | 1 |
| Grenada | | | | | | 1 | | | |
| Guadeloupe | | | | | | 7 | | | |
| Guatemala | | | | | | 1 | 19 | 6 | 1 |
| Haiti | | | | | | | | | |
| Honduras | | 16 | 1 | 1 | 4 | 15 | 0 | | 18 |
| Jamaica | | | | | | 108 | | | |
| Martinique | | | | | | 3 | | 15 | |
| Mexico | | 2 | | | 30 | 539 | 884 | 239 | 372 |
| Montserrat | | | | | | | | | |
| Nicaragua | | | 559 | 97 | 249 | 806 | 49 | 68 | 432 |
| Panama | | | | | | 3 | | | 1 |
| Puerto Rico | 6 | 14 | 9 | 8 | 137 | 24 | 24 | 62 | 133 |
| St. Lucia | | | | | | | | 1 | 1 |
| Suriname | | | | 7 | 1 | | | | 11 |
| Trinidad and Tobago | | | | | | | | 39 | 189 |
| Venezuela | 3,325 | 1,980 | 649 | 2,884 | 3,607 | 5,380 | 1,680 | 6,300 | 5,723 |
| | | | | | | | | | |
| Total no. of cases | 3,646 | 2,304 | 1,751 | 3,309 | 4,721 | 8,202 | 4,439 | 10,309 | 12,426 |
| No. of countries reporting | 5 | 8 | 8 | 9 | 11 | 19 | 11 | 14 | 18 |

*Source*: World Health Organization, Department of Communicable Disease Surveillance and Response. *WHO Report on Global Surveillance of Epidemic-prone Infectious Diseases* (2000). http://www.who.int/emc-documents/surveillance/whocdscsrisr20001c.html#english.

## Table H2.9. Dengue Fever and Dengue Haemorrhagic Fever, Cases Reported to WHO, Asia, 1990–1998

| | 1990 | 1991 | 1992 | 1993 | 1994 | 1995 | 1996 | 1997 | 1998 |
|---|---|---|---|---|---|---|---|---|---|
| Bangladesh | | | | | | | | | |
| Cambodia | 7,247 | 1,882 | 4,695 | 3,913 | 1,498 | 10,199 | 1,433 | 4,224 | 16,216 |
| China | 376 | 902 | 46,095 | 359 | 2 | 6,114 | 13 | 647 | 15 |
| India | | 6,291 | 2,683 | 11,125 | 7,494 | 7,847 | 16,517 | 1,177 | 707 |
| Indonesia | 22,807 | 21,120 | 17,620 | 17,418 | 18,783 | 35,102 | 44,650 | 30,730 | 71,087 |
| Lao People's Dem. Rep. | 60 | | 138 | 343 | 2,585 | 7,781 | 8,197 | 1,536 | 3,755 |
| Malaysia | 4,880 | 6,628 | 5,473 | 5,589 | 3,133 | 6,543 | 14,255 | 19,544 | 27,370 |
| Maldives | 0 | 0 | 0 | 0 | 0 | 0 | 0 | 0 | 2,000 |
| Myanmar | 6,318 | 8,055 | 1,685 | 2,279 | 11,647 | 2,477 | 1,655 | 3,993 | 8,978 |
| Philippines | 588 | 1,865 | 3,980 | 5,715 | 5,603 | 7,413 | 13,614 | 12,811 | 31,829 |
| Saudi Arabia | | | | | 315 | | | | |
| Singapore | 1,733 | 2,179 | 2,878 | 837 | 1,216 | 2,008 | 3,128 | 4,300 | 5,183 |
| Sri Lanka | 1,350 | 1,048 | 656 | 750 | 582 | 440 | 1,298 | 980 | 800 |
| Thailand | 92,002 | 43,511 | 41,125 | 67,017 | 51,688 | 59,911 | 38,109 | 99,150 | 126,348 |
| Viet Nam | 37,569 | 111,817 | 51,311 | 53,674 | 44,944 | 80,447 | 89,963 | 108,000 | 150,898 |
| Total no. of cases | 174,930 | 205,298 | 178,339 | 169,019 | 149,490 | 226,282 | 232,832 | 287,092 | 445,186 |
| No. of countries reporting | 12 | 12 | 13 | 13 | 14 | 13 | 13 | 13 | 13 |

*Source*: World Health Organization, Department of Communicable Disease Surveillance and Response. *WHO Report on Global Surveillance of Epidemic-prone Infectious Diseases* (2000). http://www.who.int/emc-documents/surveillance/whocdscsrisr20001c.html#english.

## Table H2.10. Dengue Fever and Dengue Haemorrhagic Fever, Cases Reported to WHO, Oceania, 1990–1998

| | 1990 | 1991 | 1992 | 1993 | 1994 | 1995 | 1996 | 1997 | 1998 |
|---|---|---|---|---|---|---|---|---|---|
| American Samoa | | | 0 | 0 | 246 | 0 | 49 | | |
| Australia | | 46 | 366 | 690 | 17 | 34 | 43 | 205 | 500 |
| Cook Islands | 5 | 833 | 5 | 0 | 0 | 786 | 2 | 1,075 | |
| Fiji | 1,461 | | 349 | 39 | 0 | 27 | | | 24,780 |
| French Polynesia | | | 593 | 355 | 0 | 208 | | | |
| Guam | | | | | 0 | | | 1 | 2 |
| Kiribati | 0 | 0 | 0 | 0 | 0 | | | | |
| Marshall Islands | | | | | 0 | | | | |
| Micronesia (Fed. States of) | | | | 0 | 0 | 20 | | | 275 |
| Nauru | | | | | 0 | 0 | | | |
| New Caledonia | 92 | 16 | 10 | 0 | 0 | 1,820 | | 154 | 2,618 |
| New Zealand | | | | | | | 11 | | |
| Niue | | | | 0 | 0 | 0 | | | |
| Palau | | | | 0 | 0 | 636 | | | |
| Papua New Guinea | | 475 | | | | 0 | | | |
| Samoa | | | 3 | 2 | | 278 | 1,013 | 163 | 49 |
| Tokelau | | | 0 | 0 | 0 | | | | |
| Tonga | 896 | 115 | 35 | 8 | 0 | | 3 | | 460 |
| Tuvalu | | | 811 | | 0 | 0 | | | |
| Vanuatu | 52 | | 113 | 27 | 16 | | | | 131 |
| Wallis and Futuna | | | 0 | 0 | | 3 | | | 395 |
| Total no. of cases | 2,506 | 1,485 | 2,285 | 1,121 | 279 | 3,812 | 1,121 | 1,598 | 29,210 |
| No. of countries reporting | 6 | 6 | 13 | 15 | 17 | 14 | 6 | 5 | 9 |

*Source*: World Health Organization, Department of Communicable Disease Surveillance and Response. *WHO Report on Global Surveillance of Epidemic-prone Infectious Diseases* (2000). http://www.who.int/emc-documents/surveillance/whocdscsrisr20001c.html#english.

**Table H2.11. Global Summary of the HIV/AIDS Epidemic, December 2000**

| | | |
|---|---|---|
| **People newly infected with HIV in 2000** | **Total** | **5.3 million** |
| | Adults | 4.7 million |
| | *Women* | *2.2 million* |
| | Children <15 years | 600 000 |
| **Number of people living with HIV/AIDS** | **Total** | **36.1 million** |
| | Adults | 34.7 million |
| | *Women* | *16.4 million* |
| | Children <15 years | 1.4 million |
| **AIDS deaths in 2000** | **Total** | **3 million** |
| | Adults | 2.5 million |
| | *Women* | *1.3 million* |
| | Children <15 years | 500 000 |
| **Total number of AIDS deaths since the beginning of the epidemic** | **Total** | **21.8 million** |
| | Adults | 17.5 million |
| | *Women* | *9 million* |
| | Children <15 years | 4.3 million |

*Source*: Joint United Nations Programme on HIV/AIDS. World Health Organization. *AIDS Epidemic Update: December 2000.* Joint United Nations Programme on HIV/AIDS. Geneva, 2001. http://www.wnaids.org/wac/2000/wad00/files/WAD_epidemic_report.PDF.

## Table H2.12. Regional HIV/AIDS Statistics and Features, end of 1999[1]

| | *Epidemic started* | *Adults & children living with HIV/AIDS* | *Adults & children newly infected with HIV in 1999* | *Adult prevalence rate (2)* | *% HIV positive women* | *Main mode(s) of transmission for those living with HIV/AIDS* |
|---|---|---|---|---|---|---|
| Sub-Saharan Africa | late '70s – early '80s | 24.5 million | 4 million | 8.57% | 55% | Hetero |
| North Africa and Middle East | late '80s | 220 000 | 20 000 | 0.12% | 20% | IDU, Hetero |
| South and South- East Asia | Late '80s | 5.6 million | 800 000 | 0.54% | 35% | Hetero, IDU |
| East Asia and Pacific | Late '80s | 530 000 | 120 000 | 0.06% | 13% | IDU, Hetero, MSM |
| Latin America | Late '70s – early '80s | 1.3 million | 150 000 | 0.49% | 25% | MSM, IDU, Hetero |
| Caribbean | Late '70s – early '80s | 360 000 | 60 000 | 2.11% | 35% | Hetero, MSM |
| Eastern Europe and Central Asia | early '90s | 420 000 | 130 000 | 0.21% | 25% | IDU |
| Western Europe | late '70s – early '80s | 520 000 | 30 000 | 0.23% | 25% | MSM, IDU |
| North America | late '70s – early '80s | 900 000 | 45 000 | 0.58% | 20% | MSM, IDU, Hetero |
| Australia and New Zealand | late '70s – early '80s | 15 000 | 500 | 0.13% | 10% | MSM, IDU |
| **Total** | | **34.3 million** | **5.4 million** | **1.07%** | **47%** | |

(1) Source: Report on the global HIV/AIDS epidemic, UNAIDS/CO.13E.

(2) The proportion of adults (15-49 years of age) living with HIV/AIDS in 1998 using 1999 population numbers.

*Source*: World Health Organization, Department of Communicable Disease Surveillance and Response. *WHO Report on Global Surveillance of Epidemic-prone Infectious Diseases* (2000). http://www.who.int/emc-documents/surveillance/whocdscsrisr20001c.html#english.

## Table H2.13. AIDS, Cases Reported to WHO, Africa, 1979–1999[1]

| | 1979-1996 | 1997 | 1998 | 1999 | Total (2 | Last report |
|---|---|---|---|---|---|---|
| Algeria | 298 | 39 | 49 | 24 | 410 | 15/Nov/99 |
| Angola | 1,510 | 416 | 507 | | 2,433 | 26/Mar/99 |
| Benin | 1,783 | 1,030 | | | 2,813 | 06/Jun/98 |
| Botswana | 4,815 | 2,335 | 2,992 | | 10,142 | 10/Jun/99 |
| Burkina Faso | 9,136 | 2,216 | 2,166 | | 13,518 | 11/Jun/99 |
| Burundi | 8,776 | 470 | 581 | 2,187 | 12,014 | 30/Jun/99 |
| Cameroon | 9,626 | 3,950 | 5,410 | | 18,986 | 29/Oct/99 |
| Cape Verde | 187 | 39 | 43 | | 269 | 29/Jan/99 |
| Central African Republic | 7,016 | 0 | | | 7,016 | 30/May/97 |
| Chad | 5,239 | 2,753 | 2,129 | | 10,121 | 03/Jun/99 |
| Comoros | 15 | 3 | 2 | | 20 | 12/Oct/99 |
| Congo | 10,223 | 0 | | | 10,223 | 06/Sep/96 |
| Cote d'Ivoire | 37,898 | 5,949 | 5,685 | | 49,532 | 30/Aug/99 |
| Dem. Rep. of the Congo | 38,841 | 4,948 | 3,746 | 22 | 47,557 | 20/Oct/99 |
| Djibouti | 1,238 | 434 | 111 | | 1,783 | 06/Apr/99 |
| Egypt | 143 | 25 | 33 | 14 | 215 | 04/Aug/99 |
| Equatorial Guinea | 231 | 90 | | | 321 | 03/Nov/98 |
| Eritrea | 2,917 | 1,260 | 1,610 | 1,086 | 6,873 | 30/Jun/99 |
| Ethiopia | 21,579 | 7,981 | 8,314 | | 37,874 | 04/Jul/99 |
| Gabon | 1,660 | 0 | | | 1,660 | 31/Dec/97 |
| Gambia | 437 | 74 | 126 | | 637 | 15/Jun/99 |
| Ghana | 20,859 | 3,833 | 4,854 | | 29,546 | 20/May/99 |
| Guinea | 3,080 | 1,005 | 1,222 | | 5,307 | 14/Jun/99 |
| Guinea-Bissau | 823 | 0 | | | 823 | 31/Oct/96 |
| Kenya | 74,042 | 4,885 | 2,565 | | 81,492 | 28/Sep/98 |
| Lesotho | 1,872 | 2,203 | 3,242 | | 7,317 | 31/Dec/98 |
| Liberia | 128 | 104 | 40 | | 272 | 26/Oct/98 |
| Libyan Arab Jamahiriya | 20 | 7 | 5 | | 32 | 25/May/99 |
| Madagascar | 29 | 6 | 2 | | 37 | 07/Oct/99 |
| Malawi | 47,270 | 3,705 | | | 50,975 | 21/May/98 |
| Mali | 3,642 | 711 | 620 | 290 | 5,263 | 14/Oct/99 |
| Mauritania | 532 | | | | 532 | 31/May/97 |
| Mauritius | 34 | 7 | 5 | 4 | 50 | 12/Nov/99 |
| Morocco | 372 | 92 | 93 | | 557 | 24/Feb/99 |
| Mozambique | 4,826 | 1,661 | 4,376 | | 10,863 | 25/Mar/99 |
| Namibia | 5,977 | 807 | | | 6,784 | 30/Sep/99 |
| Niger | 3,002 | 217 | 425 | | 3,644 | 11/Jun/99 |
| Nigeria | 6,057 | 745 | 18,490 | 984 | 26,276 | 13/Sep/99 |
| Reunion | 166 | 0 | | | 166 | 31/Dec/95 |
| Rwanda | 14,553 | 1,350 | | | 15,903 | 31/Dec/97 |
| Sao Tome and Principe | 24 | 11 | 25 | 10 | 70 | 14/Oct/99 |
| Senegal | 1,982 | 411 | 151 | 144 | 2,688 | 30/Sep/99 |
| Seychelles | 23 | 4 | 5 | | 32 | 09/Jun/99 |
| Sierra Leone | 224 | 67 | 26 | | 317 | 21/Aug/98 |
| Somalia | 13 | - | - | - | 13 | 05/Oct/99 |
| South Africa | 12,825 | | | | 12,825 | 30/Oct/96 |
| Sudan | 1,562 | 270 | 511 | 392 | 2,735 | 05/Oct/99 |
| Swaziland | 1,329 | 1,466 | 733 | | 3,528 | 15/Jul/99 |
| Togo | 7,993 | 1,211 | 1,623 | | 10,827 | 08/Mar/99 |
| Tunisia | 393 | 62 | 44 | 20 | 519 | 21/Jul/99 |

## Table H2.13. *(Continued)*

| | | | | | | |
|---|---|---|---|---|---|---|
| Uganda | 51,344 | 1,962 | 1,406 | | 54,712 | 31/Mar/99 |
| United Rep. of Tanzania | 92,593 | 10,592 | 8,867 | | 112,052 | 11/Aug/99 |
| Zambia | 43,266 | 1,676 | | | 44,942 | 31/Jul/97 |
| Zimbabwe | 63,937 | 6,732 | 4,113 | | 74,782 | 30/Nov/98 |
| | | | | | | |
| Total no. of cases | 628,360 | 79,814 | 86,947 | 5,177 | 800,298 | |
| No. of countries reporting | 54 | 51 | 40 | 12 | 54 | |

(1) AIDS cases reported to WHO as of 15 November 1999.

(2) Total includes cases with unknown date of reporting.

-. No AIDS surveillance.

*Source*: World Health Organization, Department of Communicable Disease Surveillance and Response. *WHO Report on Global Surveillance of Epidemic-prone Infectious Diseases* (2000). http://www.who.int/emc-documents/surveillance/whocdscsrisr20001c.html#english.

## Table H2.14. AIDS, Cases Reported to WHO, the Americas, 1979–1999[1]

| | 1979-1996 | 1997 | 1998 | 1999 | Total (2) | Last report |
|---|---|---|---|---|---|---|
| Anguilla | 5 | 0 | | | 5 | 30/Dec/95 |
| Antigua and Barbuda | 87 | 7 | 2 | | 96 | 31/May/99 |
| Argentina | 11,357 | 2,058 | 1,492 | 259 | 15,166 | 01/Oct/99 |
| Aruba | 22 | 2 | | | 24 | 30/Apr/97 |
| Bahamas | 2,475 | 389 | 234 | | 3,098 | 28/Feb/99 |
| Barbados | 762 | 113 | 168 | | 1,043 | 16/Sep/99 |
| Belize | 198 | 0 | | | 198 | 30/Apr/97 |
| Bermuda | 322 | 13 | 5 | 6 | 346 | 15/Nov/99 |
| Bolivia | 149 | 21 | 9 | | 179 | 16/Apr/98 |
| Brazil | 120,576 | 17,187 | 7,564 | | 145,327 | 30/Nov/98 |
| British Virgin Islands | 12 | 3 | 1 | 0 | 16 | 31/Oct/98 |
| Canada | 15,386 | 444 | 105 | | 15,935 | 31/Aug/98 |
| Cayman Islands | 21 | 1 | 2 | | 24 | 31/May/99 |
| Chile | 1,976 | 435 | 366 | 44 | 2,821 | 31/Mar/99 |
| Colombia | 7,844 | 589 | | | 8,433 | 31/Dec/97 |
| Costa Rica | 1,166 | 233 | 162 | 19 | 1,580 | 31/May/99 |
| Cuba | 578 | 128 | 140 | | 846 | 31/Aug/99 |
| Dominica | 51 | 19 | 12 | 5 | 87 | 15/Nov/99 |
| Dominican Republic | 4,021 | 392 | 320 | | 4,733 | 10/Sep/99 |
| Ecuador | 610 | 128 | 134 | | 872 | 28/Feb/98 |
| El Salvador | 1,823 | 409 | 146 | | 2,378 | 15/Nov/99 |
| French Guiana | 606 | 35 | | | 641 | 31/Dec/97 |
| Grenada | 99 | 4 | | | 103 | 30/Nov/97 |
| Guadeloupe | 752 | 38 | | | 790 | 31/Dec/97 |
| Guatemala | 1,639 | 760 | 993 | | 3,392 | 31/Aug/99 |
| Guyana | 842 | 115 | 96 | | 1,053 | 31/Oct/98 |
| Haiti | 4,967 | 3,932 | | | 8,899 | 28/Feb/99 |
| Honduras | 7,288 | 929 | | | 8,217 | 28/Jan/98 |
| Jamaica | 2,060 | 370 | 320 | 225 | 2,975 | 31/May/99 |
| Martinique | 413 | 23 | | | 436 | 31/Dec/97 |
| Mexico | 34,406 | 3,364 | 1,905 | | 39,675 | 31/May/99 |
| Montserrat | 7 | 0 | 1 | | 8 | 31/May/99 |
| Neth. Antilles and Aruba | 233 | 0 | | | 233 | 31/Mar/96 |
| Nicaragua | 152 | 18 | 10 | 2 | 182 | 30/Apr/99 |
| Panama | 1,357 | 341 | 195 | 49 | 1,942 | 15/Nov/99 |
| Paraguay | 294 | 96 | 34 | | 424 | 15/Jul/98 |
| Peru | 6,618 | 1,058 | 954 | 310 | 8,940 | 30/Sep/99 |
| Saint Kitts and Nevis | 54 | 4 | | | 58 | 08/Sep/97 |
| Saint Lucia | 90 | 15 | 6 | | 111 | 28/Feb/99 |
| Saint Vincent & the Grenadines | 87 | 24 | 28 | | 139 | 31/Dec/98 |
| Suriname | 211 | 0 | | | 211 | 31/Dec/96 |
| Trinidad and Tobago | 2,495 | 118 | | | 2,613 | 02/Jul/97 |
| Turks and Caicos Islands | 39 | 0 | | | 39 | 03/Nov/93 |
| United States of America | 622,898 | 50,000 | 44,532 | | 717,430 | 15/Nov/99 |
| Uruguay | 840 | 173 | 180 | | 1,193 | 22/Sep/99 |
| Venezuela | 7,088 | 194 | | | 7,282 | 24/Apr/98 |
| Total no. of cases | 864,976 | 84,182 | 60,116 | 919 | 1,010,193 | |
| No. of countries reporting | 46 | 46 | 30 | 10 | 46 | |

1 AIDS cases reported to WHO as of 15 November 1999.

2 Total includes cases with unknown date of reporting.

*Source*: World Health Organization, Department of Communicable Disease Surveillance and Response. *WHO Report on Global Surveillance of Epidemic-prone Infectious Diseases* (2000). http://www.who.int/emc-documents/surveillance/whocdscsrisr20001c.html#english.

## Table H2.15. AIDS, Cases Reported to WHO, Asia, 1979–1999[1]

| | 1979-1996 | 1997 | 1998 | 1999 | Total (2) | Last report |
|---|---|---|---|---|---|---|
| Afghanistan | - | - | - | - | - | 17/Oct/99 |
| Armenia | 10 | 2 | 2 | 1 | 15 | 02/Nov/99 |
| Azerbaijan | 4 | 5 | 3 | 0 | 12 | 02/Nov/99 |
| Bahrain | 40 | 15 | 11 | 4 | 70 | 28/Jun/99 |
| Bangladesh | 7 | 3 | 0 | | 10 | 31/Mar/98 |
| Bhutan | 0 | | | | 0 | 30/Nov/96 |
| Brunei Darussalam | 10 | 2 | 0 | 0 | 12 | 31/Jul/99 |
| Cambodia | 1,312 | 572 | 1,494 | 1,456 | 4,834 | 30/Jun/99 |
| China | 155 | 126 | 136 | 2 | 419 | 15/Oct/99 |
| Cyprus | 75 | 10 | 6 | 6 | 97 | 09/Aug/99 |
| Dem. Peoples Rep. of Korea | 0 | 0 | | | 0 | 30/Nov/96 |
| Georgia | 16 | 6 | 2 | 3 | 27 | 02/Nov/99 |
| Hong Kong SAR | 245 | 64 | 63 | 37 | 409 | 30/Jun/99 |
| India | 5,182 | 2,108 | 1,148 | | 8,438 | 31/Aug/99 |
| Indonesia | 119 | 34 | 74 | 38 | 265 | 15/Nov/99 |
| Iran (Islamic Republic of) | 154 | 40 | 21 | | 215 | 25/Jan/99 |
| Iraq | 102 | 2 | 4 | 0 | 108 | 18/Apr/99 |
| Israel | 420 | 45 | 36 | 47 | 548 | 02/Nov/99 |
| Japan | 1,437 | 250 | 231 | 148 | 2,066 | 27/Jun/99 |
| Jordan | 47 | 12 | 11 | 1 | 71 | 10/Aug/99 |
| Kazakhstan | 7 | 8 | 9 | 1 | 25 | 02/Nov/99 |
| Korea, Republic of | 63 | 33 | 37 | 14 | 147 | 10/Oct/99 |
| Kuwait | 24 | 2 | 19 | 1 | 46 | 18/May/99 |
| Kyrgyzstan | 19 | 2 | 6 | | 27 | 30/Jun/98 |
| Lao People's Dem. Rep. | 30 | 48 | 27 | | 105 | 07/Oct/99 |
| Lebanon | 104 | 8 | 35 | | 147 | 02/Mar/99 |
| Macao SAR | 9 | 2 | 4 | 2 | 17 | 30/Jun/99 |
| Malaysia | 911 | 568 | 875 | 540 | 2,894 | 30/Jun/99 |
| Maldives | 4 | 1 | 0 | | 5 | 30/Apr/97 |
| Mongolia | 0 | 0 | 0 | 1 | 1 | 04/Aug/99 |
| Myanmar | 1,783 | 554 | 231 | | 2,568 | 31/Mar/98 |
| Nepal | 118 | 101 | 42 | | 261 | 30/Jun/99 |
| Oman | 288 | 36 | 33 | 10 | 367 | 11/Aug/99 |
| Pakistan | 128 | 19 | 23 | 3 | 173 | 24/May/99 |
| Philippines | 299 | 23 | 41 | 41 | 404 | 11/Oct/99 |
| Qatar | 84 | 4 | 1 | 4 | 93 | 10/Jun/99 |
| Saudi Arabia | 237 | 112 | 39 | 26 | 414 | 01/Aug/99 |
| Singapore | 271 | 88 | 125 | 61 | 545 | 15/Oct/99 |
| Sri Lanka | 69 | 9 | 15 | | 93 | 11/Feb/99 |
| Syrian Arab Republic | 45 | 8 | 8 | 4 | 65 | 28/Jul/99 |
| Tajikistan | - | - | - | - | - | 02/Nov/99 |
| Thailand | 63,158 | 26,000 | 25,847 | 13,601 | 128,606 | 31/Oct/99 |
| Turkey | 221 | 33 | 34 | 16 | 304 | 02/Nov/99 |
| Turkmenistan | 1 | 0 | | | 1 | 30/Nov/95 |
| United Arab Emirates | 8 | | | | 8 | 28/Feb/91 |
| Uzbekistan | 4 | 1 | 2 | 0 | 7 | 02/Nov/99 |
| Viet Nam | 1,082 | 400 | 935 | 319 | 2,736 | 07/Aug/99 |
| West Bank and Gaza Strip | 20 | 9 | 3 | 1 | 33 | 21/Aug/99 |
| Yemen | 82 | 40 | 34 | | 156 | 25/Feb/99 |
| Total no. of cases | 78,404 | 31,405 | 31,667 | 16,388 | 157,864 | |
| No. of countries reporting | 47 | 45 | 43 | 32 | 47 | |

1 AIDS cases reported to WHO as of 15 November 1999.
2 Total includes cases with unknown date of reporting.
-: No AIDS surveillance.

*Source*: World Health Organization, Department of Communicable Disease Surveillance and Response. *WHO Report on Global Surveillance of Epidemic-prone Infectious Diseases* (2000). http://www.who.int/emc-documents/surveillance/whocdscsrisr20001c.html#english.

## Table H2.16. AIDS, Cases Reported to WHO, Europe, 1979–1999[1]

| | 1979-1996 | 1997 | 1998 | 1999 | Total (2) | Last report |
|---|---|---|---|---|---|---|
| Albania | 8 | 2 | 1 | 0 | 11 | 02/Nov/99 |
| Austria | 1,643 | 130 | 110 | 32 | 1,915 | 02/Nov/99 |
| Belarus | 15 | 2 | 4 | 2 | 23 | 02/Nov/99 |
| Belgium | 2,213 | 136 | 166 | 84 | 2,599 | 02/Nov/99 |
| Bosnia and Herzegovina | 17 | 0 | | | 17 | 25/Jun/97 |
| Bulgaria | 45 | 8 | 3 | 4 | 60 | 02/Nov/99 |
| Croatia | 108 | 12 | 17 | 7 | 144 | 02/Nov/99 |
| Czech Republic | 90 | 21 | 8 | 6 | 125 | 02/Nov/99 |
| Denmark | 1,994 | 108 | 71 | 43 | 2,216 | 02/Nov/99 |
| Estonia | 14 | 3 | 4 | 1 | 22 | 02/Nov/99 |
| Finland | 251 | 17 | 20 | 6 | 294 | 02/Nov/99 |
| France | 44,559 | 2,836 | 2,026 | | 49,421 | 02/Nov/99 |
| Germany | 15,615 | 1,414 | 922 | 288 | 18,239 | 02/Nov/99 |
| Greece | 1,501 | 238 | 143 | 82 | 1,964 | 02/Nov/99 |
| Hungary | 245 | 32 | 35 | 16 | 328 | 02/Nov/99 |
| Iceland | 41 | 2 | 2 | 5 | 50 | 02/Nov/99 |
| Ireland | 578 | 31 | 41 | 24 | 674 | 02/Nov/99 |
| Italy | 37,139 | 3,782 | 2,484 | 1,111 | 44,516 | 02/Nov/99 |
| Latvia | 17 | 3 | 11 | 6 | 37 | 02/Nov/99 |
| Lithuania | 11 | 3 | 8 | 4 | 26 | 02/Nov/99 |
| Luxembourg | 117 | 10 | 10 | 2 | 139 | 02/Nov/99 |
| Malta | 41 | 2 | 4 | 0 | 47 | 02/Nov/99 |
| Monaco | 39 | 1 | 0 | 0 | 40 | 02/Nov/99 |
| Netherlands | 4,288 | 342 | 291 | 133 | 5,054 | 02/Nov/99 |
| Norway | 561 | 38 | 39 | 0 | 638 | 02/Nov/99 |
| Poland | 477 | 117 | 132 | 68 | 794 | 02/Nov/99 |
| Portugal | 3,781 | 919 | 888 | 432 | 6,020 | 02/Nov/99 |
| Republic of Moldova | 7 | 10 | 4 | 2 | 23 | 02/Nov/99 |
| Romania | 4,485 | 650 | 645 | 148 | 5,928 | 02/Nov/99 |
| Russian Federation | 255 | 13 | 98 | 29 | 395 | 02/Nov/99 |
| San Marino | 4 | 4 | 4 | 2 | 14 | 02/Nov/99 |
| Slovakia | 13 | 5 | 3 | 1 | 22 | 02/Nov/99 |
| Slovenia | 60 | 1 | 14 | 6 | 81 | 02/Nov/99 |
| Spain | 42,783 | 6,068 | 4,202 | 1,911 | 54,964 | 02/Nov/99 |
| Sweden | 1,481 | 77 | 63 | 42 | 1,663 | 02/Nov/99 |
| Switzerland | 5,527 | 567 | 428 | 119 | 6,641 | 02/Nov/99 |
| The F.Y.R. of Macedonia | 23 | 0 | 3 | 3 | 29 | 02/Nov/99 |
| Ukraine | 226 | 193 | 287 | 316 | 1,022 | 02/Nov/99 |
| United Kingdom of G.B. anc | 13,682 | 1,379 | 964 | 412 | 16,437 | 02/Nov/99 |
| Yugoslavia | 608 | 56 | 114 | 28 | 806 | 02/Nov/99 |
| Total no. of cases | 184,562 | 19,232 | 14,269 | 5,375 | 223,438 | |
| No. of countries reporting | 40 | 40 | 39 | 38 | 40 | |

1 AIDS cases reported to WHO as of 15 November 1999.

2 Total includes cases with unknown date of reporting.

*Source*: World Health Organization, Department of Communicable Disease Surveillance and Response. *WHO Report on Global Surveillance of Epidemic-prone Infectious Diseases* (2000). http://www.who.int/emc-documents/surveillance/whocdscsrisr20001c.html#english.

## Table H2.17. AIDS, Cases Reported to WHO, Oceania, 1979–1999[1]

| | 1979-1996 | 1997 | 1998 | 1999 | Total (2) | Last report |
|---|---|---|---|---|---|---|
| American Samoa | 0 | 0 | 0 | | 0 | 27/Sep/98 |
| Australia | 7,466 | 357 | 273 | 44 | 8,140 | 30/Jun/99 |
| Cook Islands | 0 | 0 | 0 | | 0 | 28/Sep/98 |
| Fiji | 8 | 0 | 0 | | 8 | 11/Aug/98 |
| French Polynesia | 54 | 0 | 0 | | 54 | 02-Sep-98 |
| Guam | 42 | 5 | 7 | 6 | 60 | 31/Jul/99 |
| Kiribati | 3 | 1 | 2 | | 6 | 31/Jul/99 |
| Mariana Islands | 7 | 1 | 0 | | 8 | 15/Apr/98 |
| Marshall Islands | 2 | 0 | 0 | | 2 | 27/Feb/98 |
| Micronesia (Federated States of) | 2 | 0 | 0 | | 2 | 01/Apr/98 |
| Nauru | 0 | 0 | 0 | | 0 | 20/Oct/97 |
| New Caledonia and Dependencies | 55 | 8 | 3 | 1 | 67 | 12/Jul/99 |
| New Zealand | 615 | 31 | 26 | 9 | 681 | 30/Jun/99 |
| Niue | 0 | 0 | 0 | | 0 | 08/Sep/98 |
| Palau | 1 | 0 | 0 | | 1 | 28/Feb/98 |
| Papua New Guinea | 225 | 120 | 232 | 41 | 618 | 31/Mar/99 |
| Samoa | 6 | 0 | 0 | | 6 | 28/Sep/98 |
| Solomon Islands | 0 | 0 | 0 | | 0 | 03/Aug/97 |
| Tokelau | 0 | 0 | | | 0 | 02/Sep/97 |
| Tonga | 13 | 0 | 1 | | 14 | 03/Sep/98 |
| Tuvalu | 0 | 0 | 0 | | 0 | 08/Oct/97 |
| Vanuatu | 0 | 0 | 0 | | 0 | 21/Sep/98 |
| Wallis and Futuna Islands | 1 | 0 | 0 | | 1 | 17/Aug/98 |
| Total no. of cases | 8,500 | 523 | 544 | 101 | 9,668 | |
| No. of countries reporting | 23 | 23 | 22 | 5 | 23 | |

1 AIDS cases reported to WHO as of 15 November 1999.
2 Total includes cases with unknown date of reporting.

*Source*: World Health Organization, Department of Communicable Disease Surveillance and Response. *WHO Report on Global Surveillance of Epidemic-prone Infectious Diseases* (2000). http://www.who.int/emc-documents/surveillance/whocdscsrisr20001c.html#english.

## Table H2.18. Meningococcal Disease, Cases Reported to WHO, Africa, 1990–1999

| | 1990 | 1991 | 1992 | 1993 | 1994 | 1995 | 1996 | 1997 | 1998 | 1999 |
|---|---|---|---|---|---|---|---|---|---|---|
| Algeria | 722 | 267 | 529 | 549 | 483 | ... | ... | 6 | 418 | 1,337 |
| Angola | 823 | 1,106 | 1,440 | 2,260 | 3,310 | 1,007 | | | 1,266 | 29 |
| Benin | 425 | 688 | | 2,146 | 1,377 | 1,294 | 1,775 | 442 | 1,115 | 346 |
| Botswana | 83 | 97 | | | | | | | | 35 |
| Burkina Faso | 2,499 | 2,057 | 2,034 | 2,094 | 823 | 2,595 | 42,129 | 22,305 | 5,629 | 3,215 |
| Burundi | 37 | 546 | 2,739 | | 42 | | 138 | 33 | 91 | 71 |
| Cameroon | 2,684 | 2,625 | 27,752 | 5,372 | 578 | | 178 | 572 | 2,887 | 2,272 |
| Cap Verde | 89 | 41 | 40 | 204 | 144 | | | | | |
| Central African Republic | 784 | 538 | 1,226 | 472 | | | 155 | 10 | 245 | 757 |
| Chad | 8,189 | 885 | 2,392 | 2,901 | 948 | 30 | 1,079 | 1,123 | 7,964 | 2,540 |
| Comoros | | | | | | | | | | 1 |
| Congo | 0 | | 0 | 0 | 0 | | | | | |
| Cote d'Ivoire | | | | | | | | 5 | 3 | 94 |
| Dem. Rep. of the Congo | 88 | | | 102 | | 48 | 86 | 1,327 | 1,991 | 3,200 |
| Djibouti | 22 | 31 | 5 | | | | 47 | | 0 | |
| Egypt | 2,986 | 1,646 | 1,165 | 896 | 800 | 671 | 661 | 156 | 489 | 402 |
| Equatorial Guinea | | | | | | | | | | |
| Eritrea | | | | | | | | 7 | 1 | 3 |
| Ethiopia | 2,537 | | | 78 | | 247 | 771 | | | 175 |
| Gabon | 135 | | | | | | | | | |
| Gambia | 49 | | | | | | | 1,390 | | |
| Ghana | 530 | 578 | 1,542 | 1,564 | 2,173 | 26 | 479 | 19,055 | 1,049 | 527 |
| Guinea | 799 | 829 | 403 | 1,578 | 2,130 | 238 | 89 | 51 | 58 | 507 |
| Guinea-Bissau | | | | | 30 | | | | 114 | 2,836 |
| Kenya | | | | | | | | | | 146 |
| Lesotho | | | | | | | | | | 0 |
| Liberia | | | | 135 | 640 | | | | 101 | 114 |
| Libyan Arab Jamahiriya | 28 | 15 | 25 | 68 | | | | | 0 | |
| Madagascar | | | | | | | | | | |
| Malawi | | | | | | | 269 | | | |
| Mali | 1,054 | | | | | 1,199 | 7,254 | 11,228 | 2,704 | 1,038 |
| Mauritania | 48 | 197 | 23 | 34 | | | 0 | 32 | 18 | 259 |

### Table H2.18. *(Continued)*

| | 1990 | 1991 | 1992 | 1993 | 1994 | 1995 | 1996 | 1997 | 1998 | 1999 |
|---|---|---|---|---|---|---|---|---|---|---|
| Mauritius | 2 | 4 | 1 | 0 | 2 | | | 1 | | |
| Morocco | 826 | 529 | 226 | 405 | 462 | 341 | 349 | 217 | 439 | 96 |
| Mozambique | 65 | 87 | | | | 34 | 5,291 | 1,276 | 462 | 255 |
| Namibia | | 130 | 364 | 104 | 2,773 | 76 | | | | |
| Niger | 2,262 | 4,208 | 8,171 | 11,025 | 11,838 | 43,203 | 16,145 | 4,910 | 2,328 | 5,510 |
| Nigeria | 6,842 | 6,991 | 6,418 | 4,209 | 5,298 | 7,376 | 108,568 | 3,229 | 5,948 | 1,946 |
| Reunion (France) | 2 | | | | | | | | | |
| Rwanda | 180 | | 1,100 | 1,560 | | | | 10 | 291 | 62 |
| Sao Tome and Principe | ... | | | | | | | | 0 | |
| Senegal | ... | | | 0 | 0 | 41 | 11 | 13 | 977 | 4,939 |
| Seychelles | 5 | 16 | 6 | 10 | 7 | | | | | |
| Sierra Leone | | | | | | 157 | | | | 8 |
| Somalia | | | | | | | | | 0 | |
| South Africa | 850 | 760 | 510 | 87 | | | | | | |
| Sudan | 1,326 | 737 | 716 | 1,147 | 391 | 276 | 340 | 297 | 697 | 33,313 |
| Swaziland | | | | | | | | | | |
| Togo | 158 | | | 339 | 228 | 619 | 693 | 3,262 | 335 | 249 |
| Tunisia | 459 | 430 | 451 | 422 | 325 | 278 | | | 0 | |
| Uganda | 3,498 | 1,529 | 1,079 | 1,230 | | | | | | |
| United Rep.of Tanzania | 686 | 6,923 | 4,279 | 2,289 | | | 1,286 | 194 | | 372 |
| Zambia | 1,772 | 3,272 | 3,622 | 2,092 | | | 1,897 | 130 | 122 | 100 |
| Zimbabwe | 31 | 118 | 29 | | | | | 58 | 77 | 10 |
| Total no. of cases | 43,575 | 37,880 | 68,287 | 45,372 | 34,802 | 59,756 | 189,690 | 71,339 | 37,819 | 66,764 |
| No. of countries reporting | 38 | 30 | 29 | 32 | 24 | 20 | 24 | 28 | 33 | 35 |

*Source*: World Health Organization, Department of Communicable Disease Surveillance and Response. *WHO Report on Global Surveillance of Epidemic-prone Infectious Diseases* (2000). http://www.who.int/emc-documents/surveillance/whocdscsrisr20001c.html#english.

## Table H2.19. Meningococcal Disease, Cases Reported to WHO, the Americas, 1990–1999

| | 1990 | 1991 | 1992 | 1993 | 1994 | 1995 | 1996 | 1997 | 1998 |
|---|---|---|---|---|---|---|---|---|---|
| Antigua and Barbuda | | | | | | | | | |
| Bahamas | | | | | | | | | 3,114 |
| Barbados | | | | | | | | | |
| Belize | | | | | | | | | 1 |
| Bermuda | | | | | | | | | 0 |
| Bolivia | | | | | | | | | |
| Brazil | | | 702 | 863 | 971 | 1,106 | | | 149 |
| Canada | 429 | 419 | 443 | 379 | 334 | 281 | 185 | | 126 |
| Cayman Islands | 0 | 1 | 0 | 0 | | | | | |
| Chile | 257 | 322 | 391 | 490 | | | | | 536 |
| Colombia | 143 | 248 | 197 | 53 | | | | | 148 |
| Costa Rica | | | | | | | | | |
| Cuba | | | | | | | | | 42 |
| Dominica | | | | | | | | | |
| Ecuador | | | | | | | | | |
| El Salavador | | | | | | | | | 9 |
| French Guiana | | | | | | | | | |
| Grenada | | | | | | | | | |
| Guadeloupe | | | | | | | | | |
| Guatemala | | | | | | | | | 2 |
| Haiti | | | | | | | | | |
| Honduras | 3 | 5 | 3 | | | | | | 0 |
| Jamaica | | | | | | | | | |
| Martinique | | | | | | | | | |
| Mexico | | | | | | | | | 0 |
| Nicaragua | | | | | | | | | 55 |
| Panama | 112 | 54 | 40 | 31 | | | | | 20 |
| Paraguay | 5 | 12 | 25 | 17 | | | | | 7 |
| Peru | | | | | | | | | 84 |
| Puerto Rico | | | | | | | | | |
| Saint Kitts and Nevis | | | | | | | | | |
| Suriname | | | | | | | | | |
| Trinidad and Tobago | 3 | 2 | 6 | 4 | | | | | 13 |
| Turks and Caicos Islands | | | | | | | | | |
| United States of America | 2,451 | 2,130 | 2,134 | 2,637 | 2,886 | 3,243 | 3,437 | | 2,633 |
| Uruguay | 107 | 86 | 87 | | | | | | 12 |
| Venezuela | | 36 | 55 | 43 | 73 | | | | |
| Total no. of cases | 3,510 | 3,315 | 4,083 | 4,517 | 4,264 | 4,630 | 3,622 | | 6,951 |
| No. of countries reporting | 10 | 11 | 12 | 10 | 4 | 3 | 2 | 0 | 19 |

*Source*: World Health Organization, Department of Communicable Disease Surveillance and Response. *WHO Report on Global Surveillance of Epidemic-prone Infectious Diseases* (2000). http://www.who.int/emc-documents/surveillance/whocdscsrisr20001c.html#english.

## Table H2.20. Meningococcal Disease, Cases Reported to WHO, Asia, 1990–1999

| | 1990 | 1991 | 1992 | 1993 | 1994 | 1995 | 1996 | 1997 | 1998 |
|---|---|---|---|---|---|---|---|---|---|
| Afghanistan | | | | | | | | | 27 |
| Bahrain | 4 | 0 | 10 | 1 | 2 | 0 | 8 | | 15 |
| Bhutan | | | | | | | | | |
| Brunei Darussalam | | | | | | 3 | | | |
| Cambodia | | | | | | | | | |
| China | | | | 5,000 | 5,863 | 5,771 | 5,730 | 4,751 | |
| Cyprus | 2 | 0 | 0 | 1 | 0 | 4 | 8 | | 0 |
| Hong Kong SAR | | 2 | 1 | 0 | 3 | 1 | 2 | | |
| India | 16,757 | 11,995 | 8,112 | | | | 3,460 | 4,443 | 4,297 |
| Iran (Islamic Republic of) | 500 | 546 | 281 | 322 | 306 | 156 | 102 | 45 | 304 |
| Iraq | | 5,792 | 4,534 | 3,923 | 3,427 | 211 | 131 | 188 | 40 |
| Israel | 67 | 52 | 71 | 104 | 81 | 78 | 51 | | 92 |
| Japan | | 10 | 11 | 7 | 6 | 3 | 4 | 5 | 6 |
| Jordan | 58 | 29 | 39 | 45 | 35 | 44 | 27 | | 37 |
| Kuwait | 15 | 4 | 6 | 7 | 6 | 9 | | 16 | 49 |
| Kyrgyzstan | | | | | | 298 | 478 | 336 | |
| Lao People's Dem. Republic | | | 258 | 481 | 561 | 860 | 1,103 | | |
| Lebanon | | | 3 | 5 | 20 | 54 | | | 9 |
| Macao SAR | | 0 | 0 | 0 | 0 | | | | |
| Malaysia | | | | | | | | | |
| Maldives | | | | | | 1 | 0 | 3 | 3 |
| Mongolia | 776 | 748 | 411 | 393 | 3,084 | 2,739 | 881 | 480 | 263 |
| Myanmar | | | 143 | | | 65 | | | 3 |
| Nepal | 703 | 786 | 759 | | | | | | 18 |
| Oman | | 27 | 7 | 15 | 2 | 4 | 7 | | 4 |
| Pakistan | 5,309 | 5,143 | 5,505 | | | 6,621 | 7,998 | | 0 |
| Philippines | | | | | | | | | |
| Qatar | 1 | 0 | 1 | | | 8 | 10 | | 8 |
| Republic of Korea | | | | | | | | | 13 |
| Saudi Arabia | 101 | 74 | 88 | 52 | 30 | 58 | 38 | | 40 |
| Singapore | | | | | | | | | |
| Sri Lanka | 36 | 68 | 89 | 41 | 70 | 61 | 68 | 54 | 71 |
| Syrian Arab Republic | 478 | 232 | 443 | 285 | 371 | 190 | 190 | | 0 |
| Thailand | 23 | 25 | 28 | | | 75 | 71 | 60 | 68 |
| Turkey | 2,030 | 1,878 | | | 1,195 | 1,071 | | | |
| United Arab Emirates | 73 | 62 | 47 | 166 | 56 | 14 | 10 | | 23 |
| Viet Nam | | 1,846 | 1,917 | 1,794 | 2,272 | 2,236 | 1,468 | | |
| West Bank and Gaza Strip | 11 | 2 | 4 | 2 | 7 | 0 | 2 | | 0 |
| Yemen | | | 646 | 433 | | | | | 0 |
| Total no. of cases | 26,944 | 29,321 | 23,414 | 13,077 | 17,397 | 20,635 | 21,847 | 10,381 | 5,390 |
| No. of countries reporting | 18 | 24 | 27 | 22 | 22 | 28 | 24 | 11 | 26 |

*Source*: World Health Organization, Department of Communicable Disease Surveillance and Response. *WHO Report on Global Surveillance of Epidemic-prone Infectious Diseases* (2000). http://www.who.int/emc-documents/surveillance/whocdscsrisr20001c.html#english.

## Table H2.21. Meningococcal Disease, Cases Reported to WHO, Europe, 1990–1999

| | 1990 | 1991 | 1992 | 1993 | 1994 | 1995 | 1996 | 1997 | 1998 |
|---|---|---|---|---|---|---|---|---|---|
| Albania | 86 | 97 | | | 103 | 42 | | | |
| Austria | 49 | 38 | | | 60 | 81 | 98 | | |
| Belgium | 45 | 39 | | | 121 | 193 | 210 | | 9 |
| Bulgaria | 80 | 102 | | | | | | | 82 |
| Croatia | | | | | | | | | 52 |
| Czech Republic | | | | 193 | 195 | 232 | 216 | | 73 |
| Czechoslovakia [1] | 98 | 90 | | | | | | | |
| Denmark | 201 | 183 | 226 | | 220 | 235 | 226 | | |
| Estonia | | | | | | 24 | 18 | | 7 |
| Finland | 31 | 29 | | | 42 | | 76 | | 54 |
| France | 426 | 429 | 442 | | 365 | 310 | 364 | | |
| Germany | 807 | 813 | | | 708 | 655 | 687 | 809 | 729 |
| Greece | 131 | 69 | | | | 143 | 79 | | |
| Hungary | 34 | 41 | | | | | 20 | 12 | 26 |
| Iceland | 6 | 12 | | | 26 | 22 | 17 | | |
| Ireland | | | | | 95 | 271 | 199 | | |
| Italy | 309 | 141 | | | 63 | 138 | 164 | | 113 |
| Latvia | 97 | 62 | | | 17 | 43 | 45 | | 8 |
| Lithuania | 112 | 103 | | | | | | | 16 |
| Luxembourg | | | | | | | | | |
| Malta | 2 | 1 | | | 3 | 4 | 10 | | 29 |
| Monaco | 0 | 1 | | | | | | | |
| Netherlands | 505 | 443 | 518 | 563 | 422 | 460 | 583 | | 505 |
| Norway | 171 | 163 | 197 | 126 | 102 | 158 | 138 | | |
| Poland | 3,952 | 3,713 | | | 176 | 167 | 145 | 142 | |
| Portugal | 221 | 181 | | | | 183 | 172 | | 126 |
| Romania | | | | | 13 | 11 | 15 | | |
| Russian Federation | 6,615 | 5,860 | 5,167 | | | 3,839 | | | |
| Slovakia | | | | | 12 | 29 | 98 | | 87 |
| Slovenia | | | | | 12 | 9 | 11 | | 4 |
| Spain | 1,258 | 1,308 | 1,377 | | 255 | 970 | 1481 | | |
| Sweden | 102 | 130 | 114 | 88 | 66 | 99 | 84 | | |
| Switzerland | 121 | 143 | 106 | 120 | 104 | 119 | 95 | | 121 |
| United Kingdom | 1,415 | 1,390 | 1,559 | 1,651 | 1,541 | 2,097 | 1,777 | | |
| Yugoslavia | 472 | 320 | | | | | | | |
| Total no. of cases | 17,346 | 15,901 | 9,706 | 2,741 | 4,721 | 10,534 | 7,028 | 963 | 2,041 |
| No. of countries reporting | 27 | 27 | 9 | 6 | 23 | 26 | 26 | 3 | 17 |

[1] Czechoslovakia dissolved on 31 December 1992.

*Source*: World Health Organization, Department of Communicable Disease Surveillance and Response. *WHO Report on Global Surveillance of Epidemic-prone Infectious Diseases* (2000). http://www.who.int/emc-documents/surveillance/whocdscsrisr20001c.html#english.

## Table H2.22. Meningococcal Disease, Cases Reported to WHO, Oceania, 1990–1999

| | 1990 | 1991 | 1992 | 1993 | 1994 | 1995 | 1996 | 1997 | 1998 |
|---|---|---|---|---|---|---|---|---|---|
| American Samoa | | 1 | 0 | | 0 | | | | |
| Australia | 295 | 285 | 292 | 378 | 383 | 382 | 426 | | 421 |
| Cook Islands | | 4 | 4 | 4 | 4 | | 6 | | |
| Fiji | | 75 | 57 | 195 | 89 | | | | |
| French Polynesia | | 72 | 74 | 47 | 21 | | | | |
| Guam | | 11 | 25 | 19 | 23 | 15 | 10 | | |
| Kiribati | | 6 | 38 | 48 | 32 | | | | |
| Marshall Islands | | | 3 | 8 | 7 | | | | |
| Micronesia (Fed. States of) | | 5 | | 3 | | | | | |
| Nauru | | 1 | | | 2 | | | | |
| New Caledonia | | 104 | 123 | 84 | 73 | | | | |
| New Zealand | | | | | | | 87 | | |
| Niue | | 1 | 0 | 1 | 0 | | 2 | | |
| Northern Mariana Islands | | 1 | 1 | 2 | 0 | | | | |
| Palau | | | | | 2 | | | | |
| Papua New Guinea | | 1,575 | 1,593 | 1,676 | 1,651 | 1,517 | | | |
| Samoa | | 39 | 44 | 35 | 36 | | | | |
| Solomon Islands | | 47 | 55 | 54 | 93 | 50 | 4 | | |
| Tokelau | | | 1 | 0 | 0 | | | | |
| Tonga | | 2 | 1 | 0 | 1 | | | | |
| Tuvalu | | 2 | | | | | | | |
| Vanuatu | | 15 | 35 | 21 | 15 | | | | |
| Wallis and Futuna | | 1 | 2 | 5 | 9 | | | | |
| Total no. of cases | | 2,247 | 2,348 | 2,580 | 2,441 | 1,964 | 535 | | 421 |
| No. of countries reporting | 1 | 19 | 18 | 18 | 20 | 4 | 6 | 0 | 1 |

*Source*: World Health Organization, Department of Communicable Disease Surveillance and Response. *WHO Report on Global Surveillance of Epidemic-prone Infectious Diseases* (2000). http://www.who.int/emc-documents/surveillance/whocdscsrisr20001c.html#english.

## Table H2.23. Plague, Cases and Total Number of Deaths Reported to WHO, Africa, 1990–1998

| | 1990 | 1991 | 1992 | 1993 | 1994 | 1995 | 1996 | 1997 | 1998 |
|---|---|---|---|---|---|---|---|---|---|
| Angola | | | | | | | | | |
| Botswana | 70 | | | | | | | | |
| Burkina Faso | | | | | | | | | |
| Cameroon | | | | | | | | | |
| Dem. Rep. of the Congo | | 289 | 390 | 636 | 82 | 582 | | | |
| Guinea | | | | | | | | | |
| Kenya | 44 | | | | | | | | |
| Lesotho | | | | | | | | | |
| Libyan Arab Jamahiriya | | | | | | | | | |
| Madagascar 1 | 226 | 137 | 198 | 147 | 126 | 1,147 | 1,629 | 2,863 | 677 |
| Malawi | | | | | 9 | | | 582 | |
| Mozambique | | | | | 216 | | | 825 | 430 |
| Namibia | | | | | | | | | |
| South Africa | | | | | | | | | |
| Uganda | | | | 167 | | | | | 49 |
| United Rep. of Tanzania 1 | 364 | 1,293 | 16 | 18 | 444 | 831 | 947 | 504 | |
| Zambia | | | | | | | | 319 | |
| Zimbabwe | | | | | 392 | | | 8 | 5 |
| Total no. of cases | 704 | 1,719 | 604 | 968 | 1,269 | 2,560 | 2,576 | 5,101 | 1,161 |
| Total no. of deaths | 98 | 118 | 168 | 130 | 106 | 123 | 173 | 261 | 61 |
| No. of countries reporting | 4 | 3 | 3 | 4 | 6 | 3 | 2 | 6 | 4 |

1 Includes suspected cases.

*Source*: World Health Organization, Department of Communicable Disease Surveillance and Response. *WHO Report on Global Surveillance of Epidemic-prone Infectious Diseases* (2000). http://www.who.int/emc-documents/surveillance/whocdscsrisr20001c.html#english.

## Table H2.24. Plague, Cases and Total Number of Deaths Reported to WHO, Americas, 1990–1998

| | 1990 | 1991 | 1992 | 1993 | 1994 | 1995 | 1996 | 1997 | 1998 |
|---|---|---|---|---|---|---|---|---|---|
| Argentina | | | | | | | | | |
| Bolivia | 10 | | | | | | 26 | 1 | |
| Brazil | 18 | 10 | 25 | | 4 | 9 | 1 | | |
| Ecuador | | | | | | | | | 11 |
| El Salvador | | | | | | | | | |
| Peru | 18 | | 120 | 611 | 420 | 97 | 23 | 39 | 8 |
| United States of America | 2 | 11 | 13 | 10 | 14 | 9 | 5 | 4 | 8 |
| Venezuela | | | | | | | | | |
| | | | | | | | | | |
| Total no. of cases | 48 | 21 | 158 | 621 | 438 | 115 | 55 | 44 | 27 |
| Total no. of deaths | 6 | | 6 | 32 | 21 | 3 | 6 | 1 | 11 |
| No. of countries reporting | 4 | 2 | 3 | 2 | 3 | 3 | 4 | 3 | 3 |

*Source*: World Health Organization, Department of Communicable Disease Surveillance and Response. *WHO Report on Global Surveillance of Epidemic-prone Infectious Diseases* (2000). http://www.who.int/emc-documents/surveillance/whocdscsrisr20001c.html#english.

## Table H2.25. Plague, Cases and Total Number of Deaths Reported to WHO, Asia, 1990–1998

| | 1990 | 1991 | 1992 | 1993 | 1994 | 1995 | 1996 | 1997 | 1998 |
|---|---|---|---|---|---|---|---|---|---|
| China | 75 | 29 | 35 | 13 | 7 | 8 | 98 | 43 | |
| Cambodia | | | | | | | | | |
| India | | | | | 876 | | | | |
| Indonesia | | | | | | | | 6 | |
| Iran | | | | | | | | | |
| Kazakhstan | 4 | 1 | | 3 | | | | 1 | |
| Lao People's Dem. Rep. | | | | | | 7 | 3 | | |
| Mongolia | 15 | 3 | 12 | 21 | | 1 | 6 | 4 | 8 |
| Myanmar | 6 | 100 | 528 | 87 | 6 | | | | |
| Nepal | | | | | | | | | |
| Philippines | | | | | | | | | |
| Viet Nam [1] | 405 | 94 | 437 | 481 | 339 | 170 | 279 | 220 | |
| | | | | | | | | | |
| Total no. of cases | 505 | 227 | 1,012 | 605 | 1,228 | 186 | 386 | 274 | 8 |
| Total no. of deaths | 29 | 15 | 30 | 28 | 85 | 11 | 26 | 12 | 5 |
| No. of countries reporting | 5 | 5 | 4 | 5 | 4 | 4 | 4 | 5 | 1 |

[1] Includes suspected cases.

*Source*: World Health Organization, Department of Communicable Disease Surveillance and Response. *WHO Report on Global Surveillance of Epidemic-prone Infectious Diseases* (2000). http://www.who.int/emc-documents/surveillance/whocdscsrisr20001c.html#english.

## Table H2.26. Yellow Fever, Number of Cases and Total Number of Deaths Reported to WHO, Africa, 1990–1998

| | 1990 | 1991 | 1992 | 1993 | 1994 | 1995 | 1996 | 1997 | 1998 |
|---|---|---|---|---|---|---|---|---|---|
| Angola | | | | | | | | | |
| Benin | | | | | | | 120 | 18 | 6 |
| Burkina Faso | | | | | | | | | 2 |
| Cameroon | 173 | | | | 10 | | | | |
| Central African Republic | | | | | | | | | |
| Congo | | | | | | | | | |
| Cote d'Ivoire | | | | | | | | 11 | |
| Dem. Rep. of the Congo | | | | | | | | | |
| Equatorial Guinea | | | | | | | | | |
| Ethiopia | | | | | | | | | |
| Gabon | | | | | 28 | 16 | | | |
| Gambia | | | | | | | | | |
| Ghana | | | | 39 | 79 | | 27 | 6 | |
| Guinea | | | | | | | | | |
| Guinea Bissau | | | | | | | | | |
| Kenya | | | 27 | 27 | 7 | 3 | | | |
| Liberia | | | | | | 360 | | 3 | 25 |
| Mali | | | | | | | | | |
| Mauritania | | | | | | | | | |
| Niger | | | | | | | | | |
| Nigeria | 4,075 | 2,561 | 149 | 152 | 1,227 | | | 7 | |
| Senegal | | | | | | 79 | 128 | | |
| Sierra Leone | | | | | | 1 | 4 | | |
| Sudan | | | | | | | | | |
| Togo | | | | | | | | | |
| Uganda | | | | | | | | | |
| Total no. of cases | 4,248 | 2,561 | 176 | 218 | 1,351 | 459 | 279 | 45 | 33 |
| Total no. of deaths | 341 | 661 | 21 | 38 | 452 | 34 | 141 | 9 | 10 |
| No. of countries reporting | 2 | 1 | 2 | 3 | 5 | 5 | 4 | 5 | 3 |

*Source*: World Health Organization, Department of Communicable Disease Surveillance and Response. *WHO Report on Global Surveillance of Epidemic-prone Infectious Diseases* (2000). http://www.who.int/emc-documents/surveillance/whocdscsrisr20001c.html#english.

**Table H2.27. Yellow Fever, Number of Cases and Total Number of Deaths reported to WHO, the Americas, 1990–1998**

| | 1990 | 1991 | 1992 | 1993 | 1994 | 1995 | 1996 | 1997 | 1998 |
|---|---|---|---|---|---|---|---|---|---|
| Argentina | | | | | | | | | |
| Bolivia | 50 | 91 | 22 | 18 | 7 | 15 | 30 | 63 | 57 |
| Brazil | 2 | 15 | 12 | 83 | 19 | 4 | 15 | 3 | 34 |
| Colombia | 7 | 4 | 2 | 1 | 2 | 3 | 8 | 6 | 0 |
| Costa Rica | | | | | | | | | |
| Ecuador | 12 | 14 | 16 | 1 | | 1 | 8 | 31 | 3 |
| French Guiana | | | | | | | | | 1 |
| Guatemala | | | | | | | | | |
| Guyana | | | | | | | | | |
| Honduras | | | | | | | | | |
| Nicaragua | | | | | | | | | |
| Panama | | | | | | | | | |
| Paraguay | | | | | | | | | |
| Peru | 17 | 27 | 67 | 89 | 61 | 499 | 86 | 44 | 160 |
| Suriname | | | | | | | | | |
| Trinidad and Tobago | | | | | | | | | |
| Venezuela | | | | | | | | | 14 |
| United States of America | | | | | | | 1 | | |
| Total no. of cases | 88 | 151 | 119 | 192 | 89 | 522 | 148 | 147 | 269 |
| Total no. of deaths | 69 | 90 | 81 | 81 | 40 | 213 | 81 | 80 | 109 |
| No. of countries reporting | 5 | 5 | 5 | 5 | 4 | 5 | 6 | 5 | 7 |

*Source*: World Health Organization, Department of Communicable Disease Surveillance and Response. *WHO Report on Global Surveillance of Epidemic-prone Infectious Diseases* (2000). http://www.who.int/emc-documents/surveillance/whocdscsrisr20001c.html#english.

# I. Vaccine-Preventable Diseases

## OVERVIEW

The statistics are staggering: More than 11 million children under age five die each year in developing countries; nearly three-quarters of these deaths result from infectious diseases.[1] The World Health Organization estimates that the deaths of at least 4 million of these children are linked to their lack of access to vaccines. The U.S. General Accounting Office (GAO) found that although global immunization coverage for six diseases originally targeted by the World Health Organization (diphtheria, measles, pertussis, polio, tetanus, and tuberculosis) has improved significantly since the mid-1970s, coverage rates are low for children living in the poorest countries, particularly in urban slums and remote rural areas. Several interrelated factors are credited with having limited the availability of vaccines for children in the developing world, including (1) an inadequate health infrastructure; (2) the relatively higher cost of vaccines recently recommended by the World Health Organization; (3) insufficient information on disease burden and vaccine efficiency; and (4) changing priorities of international donors.

What would happen if we stopped vaccinations? Vaccines are responsible for the control of many infectious diseases that were once common. They have reduced, and in some cases eliminated, many diseases that routinely killed or harmed many infants, children, and adults. However, the viruses and bacteria that cause vaccine-preventable disease and death still exist and can be passed on to people who are not protected by vaccines. Vaccine-preventable diseases have a costly impact, resulting in doctor's visits, hospitalizations, and premature deaths. Sick children can also cause parents to lose time from work. What would happen if we stopped vaccines? We would experience a massive resurgence of infectious diseases that are now considered vaccine preventable.

## VACCINES

A suspension of infectious agents, or some part of them, given for the purpose of establishing resistance to an infectious disease, vaccines function to stimulate an immune response in the body by creating antibodies or activated T-lymphocytes capable of controlling the organism. The result is more or less permanent protection against a disease. An attack of smallpox or diphtheria, for example, usually leaves the recovered patient permanently immune to those diseases. As a result of infection, the body succeeds in building up its own defenses, so that a new infection causes no illness. A successful vaccine does the same thing without risk of illness.

Vaccines are of four general classes: those containing living attenuated[2] infectious organisms; those containing infectious agents killed by physical or chemical means; those containing soluble toxins of microorganisms, sometimes used as such, but generally forming toxoids; and those containing substances extracted from infectious agents. An understanding of individual vaccines involves knowledge of their preparation, dosing schedule, lower age limit, and booster interval.

## SELECTED VACCINE ROSTER

In this millennium, the roster of vaccines continues to grow, underscoring the role of vaccines in the prevention of infectious diseases. This subsection focuses on selected vaccines for diseases on which the United States and the world community provide data: cholera, diphtheria, *heamophilus influenza* type b (Hib), hepatitis B, meningitis, pertussis, plague, rabies, tetanus, tuberculosis, typhoid, and yellow fever. Missing from this roster is the smallpox vaccine. Made from lymph of cowpox vesicles obtained from healthy bovine animals, the smallpox vaccine is no longer used because smallpox has been eradicated. However, new fears of possible terrorist attacks utilizing the smallpox virus have renewed interest in the smallpox vaccine.

**Cholera** An acute diarrheal illness caused by infection of the intestine with the bacterium *Vibrio cholera*, cholera has been very rare in industrialized nations for the last 100 years; however, the disease is still common today in other parts of the world. Prepared from killed *Vibrio cholerae*, the cholera vaccine is administered every 3–6 months for those who remain in epidemic areas. Only those traveling to countries where cholera is present need to be vaccinated. Whole-cell vaccines provide partial protection for 3–6 months. The vaccine does not protect against *Vibrio cholerae* O 139.[3]

**Diphtheria** A respiratory disease caused by bacteria, diphtheria is spread by coughing and sneezing or by direct contact with secretions from the respiratory tract of infectious individuals. Symptoms include the gradual onset of a sore throat and low-grade fever. Complications include airway constriction, coma, and death if not treated. Note that it frequently causes heart and nerve problems.

The diphtheria toxoid (contained in DTP, DTaP, DT, or Td vaccines) can prevent this disease. In the 1920s, diphtheria was a major cause of illness and death for children in the United States. With vaccine development in 1923, new cases of diphtheria began to fall in the United States, until in 1998 only one case had been reported. If immunization were stopped in the United States, the country might experience a situation similar to the newly independent states of the former Soviet Union. With the breakdown of public health services in this area, diphtheria epidemics began in 1990, fueled by persons who were not properly vaccinated. From 1990 to 1998, more than 150,000 cases and 5,000 deaths were reported.[4]

***Haemophilus Influenza* Type b (Hib)** A severe bacterial infection, occurring primarily in infants, *Haemophilus influenza* type b (Hib) is spread by coughing and sneezing. Symptoms include skin and throat infections, meningitis, pneumonia, sepsis, and arthritis. The vaccine is prepared from the bacterial polysaccharide or polysaccharide converted to protein and is given to children between 18 months and 2 years.

**Hepatitis A** A disease of the liver caused by hepatitis A virus, hepatitis A is spread most often by the fecal-oral route. There are potentially no symptoms with this disease; the likelihood of symptoms increases with the person's age. If present, symptoms include yellow skin or eyes, tiredness, stomachache, loss of appetite, or nausea. The hepatitis A vaccine is prepared from inactivated hepatitis A viral antigen. The CDC recommends that children in states with at least 20 cases out of 100,000 population receive the vaccination.

**Hepatitis B** A disease of the liver caused by hepatitis B virus, hepatitis B is spread through contact with the blood of an infected person or by having sex with an infected person. There are potentially no symptoms when first infected. If present, symptoms include yellow skin or eyes, tiredness, stomachache, loss of appetite, nausea, or joint pain. Prepared from inactivated hepatitis B viral antigen, the hepatitis B vaccine is recommended for all persons at risk of contracting the virus, such as health professionals. The vaccine is expensive and is given to those at high risk of developing the disease who do not show evidence of immunity to the virus.

**Measles** An acute viral infectious disease,[5] measles is transmitted by coughing and sneezing. Considered highly contagious, measles is a systemic infection. The measles virus was first isolated in 1954; the first measles vaccines were licensed in 1963. The only measles virus vaccine now available in the United States is a live virus available as a single antigen preparation or combined with rubella vaccine or combined with mumps and rubella vaccines. Vaccination is a key component of the world health community's campaign to eradicate the disease.

**Meningitis** An inflammation of the membranes of the spinal cord or brain, meningitis is caused by various infectious agents, including viruses and protozoa, but bacteria produce the most serious forms of the disease. Prepared from bacterial polysaccharides from certain types of meningococci, the meningococcal vaccine is highly effective in preventing the disease. It is indicated for people travelling in epidemic areas.

**Mumps** A disease of the lymph nodes caused by a virus, mumps is transmitted by coughing and sneezing. Symptoms include fever, headache, muscle ache, and swelling of the lymph nodes close to the jaw. Complications include meningitis, inflammation of the pancreas, and deafness (usually permanent). Mumps is usually a mild viral disease. However, rare conditions such as swelling of the brain, nerves, and spinal cord can lead to serious side effects such as paralysis, seizures, and fluid in the brain. Mumps virus was isolated in 1945, and an inactivated vaccine was developed in 1948. The currently used live virus was licensed in 1967. Mumps vaccine is available as a single antigen preparation or combined with rubella vaccine or combined with measles and rubella vaccines. Mumps vaccine is recommended for all infants 12 months old and older and for susceptible adolescents and adults without documented evidence of mumps immunity.

**Pertussis** Pertussis, or whooping cough, is a highly contagious respiratory disease transmitted through coughing or sneezing. Caused by the bacterium *Bordetella pertussis*, it is characterized by spasms of severe coughing (paroxysms). In infants, pertussis can cause pneumonia and lead to brain damage, seizures, and mental retardation. Since the introduction of a vaccine in 1926, the disease had become rare in the United States; however, cases continue to occur throughout the world. A recent study found that, in eight countries where immunization coverage was reduced, incidence rates of pertussis surged to 10 to 100 times the rates in countries where vaccination rates were sustained.[6] Immunization generally takes place in infancy with the DPT vaccine (see Diphtheria).

**Plague** A word once used to describe any widespread contagious disease associated with a high death rate, "plague" is now applied specifically to the highly fatal disease caused by *Yersinia pestis* infection. Made from a crude fraction of killed plague bacilli for immunization against plague, the plague vaccine is recommended for those traveling to Southeast Asia, persons who work closely with wild rodents in plague areas, and laboratory personnel working with *Yersinia pestis* organisms.

**Poliomyelitis** A disease of the lymphatic and nervous systems, polio is transmitted by contact with an infected person. Two types of poliovirus vaccine are highly effective in producing immunity to poliovirus. Trivalent oral poliovirus vaccine (OPV) is prepared from three types of live poliovirus. Injectable killed vaccine (IPV) is made from three types of inactivated polioviruses. OPV has been the vaccine of choice in the United States and most other countries of the world since it was licensed in 1963. The world health community is currently conducting a campaign to vaccine all infants and children in an effort to eradicate the disease.

Until January 1, 2000, OPV was recommended for most children in the United States. OPV helped us rid the country of polio, and is still used in many parts of the world. Both vaccines give immunity to polio, but OPV has two benefits—intestinal immunity and secondary spread, that is, it is better at keeping the disease from spreading to other people. However, for a few people (about one in 2.4 million), OPV actually causes polio. (Polio associated with use of the live oral poliovirus vaccine is called vaccine-associated paralytic polio, or VAPP.) The polio shot (IPV) does not cause polio. In 1997, to decrease the risk for VAPP while maintaining the benefits of OPV, the Advisory Committee on Immunization Practices (ACIP) recommended a sequential schedule of inactivated polio vaccine followed by OPV.[7] Since 1997, the global eradication initiative has progressed rapidly, and the likelihood of poliovirus importation into the United States has decreased substantially. In addition, since 1997, the sequential schedule has been well accepted. No declines in childhood vaccination coverage were observed, despite the need for additional injections.[8] On the basis of these data, on June 17, 1999, to eliminate the risk for VAPP, the ACIP recommended an all-IPV schedule for routine childhood polio vaccination in the United States. A new all inactivated polio vaccine schedule and new vaccine information statements (VISs) were published by the Centers for Disease Control and Prevention on January 1, 2000; these documents reflect the new recommendations. The ACIP recommends that OPV should be used only for the following special circumstances: mass vaccination campaigns to control outbreaks of paralytic polio; unvaccinated children who will be traveling in less than four weeks to areas where polio is endemic; children of parents who do not accept the recommended number of vaccine injections.

**Rabies** A preventable viral disease of mammals most often transmitted through the bite of a rabid animal, rabies virus infects the central nervous system, causing encephalopathy and ultimately death. The inactivated virus vaccine is prepared from fixed rabies virus grown in human diploid cell tissue culture. It is used for individuals in high-risk occupations and those in endemic areas.

**Tetanus** Tetanus is an acute, often fatal, disease caused by an exotoxin produced by *Clostridium tetani.* The bacteria that cause tetanus are widely distributed in soil and street dust, are found in the waste of many animals, and are very resistant to heat and germ-killing cleaners. *C. tetani* usually enters the body through a break in the skin such as a wound. Symptoms include lockjaw, fever, elevated blood pressure, and severe muscle spasms that can cause fractures (breaks) of the spine and long bones. Death is a complication in one-third of cases, especially in people over age 50. Immunization from tetanus is generally given to all children as part of a diphtheria, tetanus, and pertussis vaccine (DTP or DtaP).

**Tuberculosis** TB, or tuberculosis, is a disease caused by bacteria called *Mycobacterium tuberculosis.* The bacteria can attach to any part of the body, but they usually attack the lungs. BCG or Bacille Calmette-Guerin, a preparation of a dried, living culture of *Mycobacterium tuberculosis*, is a vaccine for TB. Named after the French scientists Calmette and Guerin, this vaccine is not widely used in the United States, but it is often administered in areas with a high incidence of tuberculosis. It is used in prophylactic vaccination of infants against tuberculosis. It is also used in adults who are at high and unavoidable risk of becoming infected with tuberculosis.

**Typhoid** An acute infectious disease caused by the bacterium *Salmonella typhi*, typhoid is characterized by fever, headache, abdominal pain, and diarrhea. Made of killed *Salmonella typhii* organisms for immunizing against typhoid, the typhoid vaccine may not be effective if the person receives unusually large doses of the live organism at time of exposure. Immunization with the typhoid vaccine is indicated when a person has come into contact with a known typhoid carrier, if there is an outbreak of typhoid fever, or prior to traveling to an area where typhoid is endemic.

**Yellow Fever** Yellow fever is an acute infectious disease characterized by jaundice, fever, headache, muscle ache, shivers, and nausea and/or vomiting. Made from a live attenuated strain of yellow fever virus, the yellow fever vaccine is required for all persons traveling in or living in areas where yellow fever is present.

## TABLE OVERVIEW

**I1.1–I1.2. Vaccines and Vaccine Development** The first table in this set presents a chronology of vaccine development and use. I1.2 focuses on vaccine development or licensure in the United States from 1798 to 1998.

**I2.1–I2.7. Incidence of Disease** Incidence is the focus of the next suite of tables. Table I2.1 shows baseline twentieth-century annual morbidity and 1998 provisional morbidity from nine diseases with vaccines recommended before 1990 for universal use in children in the United States. Companion tables show global annual reported incidence, 1980–1999, for diphtheria, pertussis, human rabies, neonatal tetanus, total tetanus, and yellow fever. Incidences of vaccine-preventable diseases that the World Health Organization classifies as volatile or an important heath threat—cholera, meningococcal disease, plague, and yellow fever—are found in Section H. Incidences of those that the world health community has targeted for elimination—measles and polio—are found in Section J.

**I3.1–I3.9. Immunization Coverage** The complementary data in the next series provide global summaries of immunization coverage for the following vaccines: BCG (Bacille Calmette-Guerin) [TB] vaccine); DTP3 (third dose of diphtheria toxoid, tetanus toxoid, and pertussis vaccine); HepB3 (third dose of hepatitis B vaccine); MCV (measles-containing vaccine); POL3 (third dose of polio vaccine); TT2plus (second and subsequent dose of tetanus toxoid); and YFV (yellow fever vaccine). Coverage estimates are based on reported coverage from WHO member states. Table I3.8 presents global and regional summaries of percentage vaccination coverage, by antigen and with associated range, from 1990 to 1999.

**I4.1–I4.2. U.S. Childhood Immunization** Childhood immunization in the United States is the focus of the next two tables. Table I4.1 shows the percentage of U.S. children aged 19–35 months vaccinated for selected diseases by poverty status, race, and Hispanic origin. Table I4.2 depicts vaccination coverage levels among children aged 19–35 months, by selected vaccines, from 1995 to 1999.

**I5.1–I5.3. Vaccination in Developing Countries** The first table in this suite shows overall immunization rates for countries, grouped by region for 1991–1997. The next table presents immunization coverage rates in the poorest countries, with and without conflict, during the same period. Table I5.3, showing immunization coverage for measles and tuberculosis in sub-Saharan Africa for the same period, concludes this cluster.

**I6. Spending** The final table in this chapter shows UNICEF expenditures on vaccine procurement as a proportion of total immunization expenditures from 1990 to 1998.

## NOTES

1. General Accounting Office. *Global Health Factors Contributing to Low Vaccination Rates in Developing Countries*. General Accounting Office. Washington, DC. 1999.
2. Attenuated generally means diluted; however, for the purposes of this discussion, attenuated is defined as the reduced virulence of pathogenic microorganisms, and attenuation is defined not merely as dilution, but also as a lessening of virulence. This may be accomplished with bacteria and viruses by heating, drying, treating with chemicals, passing through another organism, or culturing under unfavorable conditions.
3. Note that at the present time, the manufacture and sale of the only licensed cholera vaccine in the United States (Wyeth-Ayerst) has been discontinued. It has not been recommended for travelers because of the brief and incomplete immunity it offers. No cholera vaccination requirements exist for entry or exit in any country. Two recently developed vaccines for cholera are licensed and available in other countries (Dukoral, Biotec AB, and Mutacol, Berna). Both vaccines appear to provide a somewhat better immunity and fewer side effects than the previously available vaccine. However, neither of these two vaccines is recommended for travelers or available in the United States.
4. From the National Immunization Program's "What Would Happen if we Stopped Vaccinations?" http://www.cdc.gov/nip/publications/fs/gen/WhatIfStop.htm
5. The measles virus is a paramyxovirus, genus *Morbillivirus*.
6. E.J. Gangarosa et al., "Impact of Anti-Vaccine Movements on Pertussis Control: The Untold Story," *Lancet* 351 (1998): 356–61.
7. Centers for Disease Control and Prevention. Poliomyelitis prevention in the United States: introduction of a sequential schedule of inactivated poliovirus vaccine followed by oral poliovirus vaccine. *MMWR: Morbidity and Mortality Weekly Report* 1997 46, no. RR-3.
8. Centers for Disease Control and Prevention. Impact of the sequential IPV. OPV schedule on vaccination coverage levels. *MMWR: Morbidity and Mortality Weekly Report* 1998 47:1017–19.

## Table I1.1. Vaccine Usage

**1. The date of introduction of the first generation of vaccines for use in humans*.**

1798 Smallpox
1885 Rabies
1897 Plague
1923 Diphtheria
1926 Pertussis
1927 Tuberculosis (BCG)
1928 Tetanus
1935 Yellow Fever
1955 Injectable Polio Vaccine (IPV)
1962 Oral Polio Vaccine (OPV)
1963 Measles
1967 Mumps
1970 Rubella
1981 Hepatitis B

**2. Vaccines used in national immunization programmes up to 1974.**

**Smallpox**
BCG
Diphtheria toxoid
Tetanus toxoid
Pertussis
IPV then OPV
Measles

**3. Vaccines used by the Expanded Programme on Immunization from 1974 onwards.**

- BCG
- Polio
- DTP
- Measles*

*Added Later*

- Yellow Fever (in endemic countries)
- Hepatitis B
- Many industrialized countries now use measles, mumps and rubella combines vaccine (MMR)

*This list is not exhaustive.

*Source*: World Health Organization. Diseases and Vaccines. *The History of Vaccination*. http://www.who.int/vaccines-diseases/history/history.htm.

## Table I1.2. Vaccine-Preventable Diseases, by Year of Vaccine Development or Licensure—United States, 1798–1998

| Disease | Year | Disease | Year |
|---|---|---|---|
| Smallpox* | 1798† | Rubella* | 1969§ |
| Rabies | 1885† | Anthrax | 1970§ |
| Typhoid | 1896† | Meningitis | 1975§ |
| Cholera | 1896† | Pneumonia | 1977§ |
| Plague | 1897† | Adenovirus | 1980§ |
| Diphtheria* | 1923† | Hepatitis B* | 1981§ |
| Pertussis* | 1926† | *Haemophilus influenzae* type b* | 1985§ |
| Tetanus* | 1927† | Japanese encephalitis | 1992§ |
| Tuberculosis | 1927† | Hepatitis A | 1995§ |
| Influenza | 1945§ | Varicella* | 1995§ |
| Yellow fever | 1953§ | Lyme disease | 1998§ |
| Poliomyelitis* | 1955§ | Rotavirus* | 1998§ |
| Measles* | 1963§ | | |
| Mumps* | 1967§ | | |

*Vaccine recommended for universal use in U.S. children. For smallpox, routine vaccination was ended in 1971.
†Vaccine developed (i.e., first published results of vaccine usage).
§Vaccine licensed for use in United States.
*Source*: Center for Disease Control and Prevention. U.S. Department of Health and Human Services. "Ten Great Public Health Achievements—United States, 1900–1999." *MMWR: Morbidity and Mortality Weekly Review* 48 no. 12 (April 2, 1999). ftp://ftp.cdc.gov/pub/Publications/mmwr/wk/mm4812.pdf.

## Table I2.1. Baseline 20th-Century Annual Morbidity and 1998 Provisional Morbidity from Nine Diseases with Vaccines Recommended before 1990 for Universal Use in Children—United States

| Disease | Baseline 20th century annual morbidity | 1998 Provisional morbidity | % Decrease |
|---|---|---|---|
| Smallpox | 48,164* | 0 | 100% |
| Diphtheria | 175,885† | 1 | 100%§ |
| Pertussis | 147,271¶ | 6,279 | 95.7% |
| Tetanus | 1,314** | 34 | 97.4% |
| Poliomyelitis (paralytic) | 16,316†† | 0§§ | 100% |
| Measles | 503,282¶¶ | 89 | 100%§ |
| Mumps | 152,209*** | 606 | 99.6% |
| Rubella | 47,745††† | 345 | 99.3% |
| *Congenital rubella syndrome* | *823§§§* | 5 | *99.4%* |
| *Haemophilus influenzae* type b | 20,000¶¶¶ | 54**** | 99.7% |

*Average annual number of cases during 1900–1904 (1).
†Average annual number of reported cases during 1920–1922, 3 years before vaccine development.
§Rounded to nearest tenth.
¶Average annual number of reported cases during 1922–1925, 4 years before vaccine development.
** Estimated number of cases based on reported number of deaths during 1922–1926 assuming a case-fatality rate of 90%.
††Average annual number of reported cases during 1951–1954, 4 years before vaccine licensure.
§§Excludes one case of vaccine-associated polio reported inn 1998.
¶¶Average annual number of reported cases during 1956–1962, 5 years before vaccine licensure.
*** Number of reported cases in 1968, the first year reporting began and the first year after vaccine licensure.
†††Average number of reported cases during 1966–1968, 3 years before vaccine licensure.
§§§Estimated number of cases based on seroprevalence data in the population and on the risk that women infected during a childbearing year would have a fetus with congenital rubella syndrome (*7*).
¶¶¶Estimated number of cases from population-based surveillance studies before vaccine licensure in 1985 (*8*).
****Excludes 71 cases of *Haemophilus influenzae* disease of unknown serotype.
*Source*: Center for Disease Control and Prevention. U.S. Department of Health and Human Services. "Ten Great Public Health Achievements—United States, 1900–1999." *MMWR: Morbidity and Mortality Weekly Review* 48 no. 12 (April 2, 1999). ftp://ftp.cdc.gov/pub/Publications/mmwr/wk/mm4812.pdf.

## Table I2.2. Diphtheria Global Annual Reported Incidence, 1980–1999

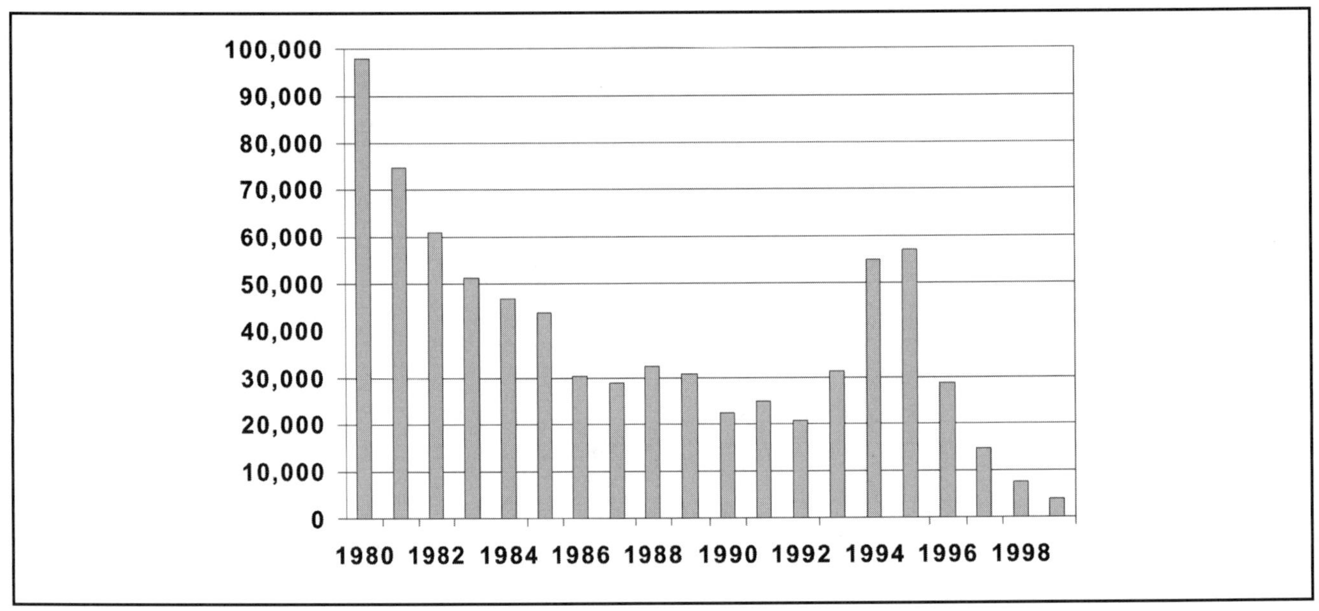


*Source*: Department of Vaccines and Biologicals. *WHO vaccine preventable diseases 2000 global summaries* (Geneva: World Health Organization, 2000). http://www.who.int/vaccines-documents/DocsPDF00/www542.pdf.

## Table I2.3. Pertussis Global Annual Reported Incidence, 1980–1999

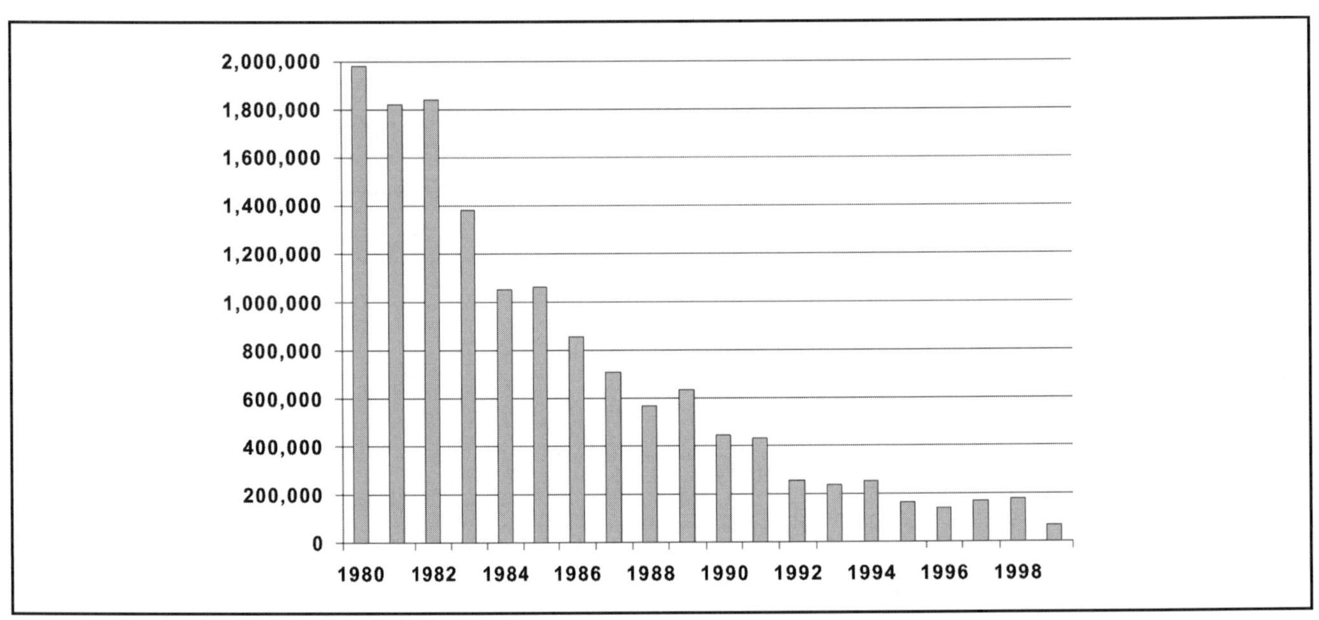


*Source*: Department of Vaccines and Biologicals. *WHO vaccine preventable diseases 2000 global summaries* (Geneva: World Health Organization, 2000). http://www.who.int/vaccines-documents/DocsPDF00/www542.pdf.

## Table I2.4. Human Rabies Cases, Latin America, 1980–1997

| Countries by Subregion | 1980 | 1981 | 1982 | 1983 | 1984 | 1985 | 1986 | 1987 | 1988 | 1989 | 1990 | 1991 | 1992 | 1993 | 1994 | 1995 | 1996 | 1997 | Total |
|---|---|---|---|---|---|---|---|---|---|---|---|---|---|---|---|---|---|---|---|
| **LATIN AMERICA** | 283 | 351 | 332 | 258 | 267 | 243 | 205 | 192 | 224 | 268 | 251 | 212 | 224 | 213 | 144 | 150 | 179 | 114 | 4110 |
| ***Andean Area*** | ***50*** | ***111*** | ***119*** | ***75*** | ***67*** | ***62*** | ***38*** | ***51*** | ***65*** | ***130*** | ***95*** | ***75*** | ***92*** | ***88*** | ***60*** | ***63*** | ***94*** | ***42*** | ***1377*** |
| Bolivia | 11 | 6 | 13 | 17 | 3 | 7 | 8 | 16 | 17 | 11 | 8 | 11 | 25 | 16 | 6 | 8 | 3 | 11 | 197 |
| Colombia | 9 | 27 | 18 | --- | 11 | 13 | 10 | 10 | 14 | 15 | 12 | 5 | 8 | 5 | 2 | 9 | 3 | 5 | 176 |
| Ecuador | 18 | 33 | 44 | 34 | 15 | 16 | 10 | 8 | 13 | 24 | 12 | 20 | 36 | 31 | 11 | 20 | 65 | 9 | 419 |
| Peru | 6 | 29 | 34 | 21 | 32 | 22 | 7 | 14 | 20 | 79 | 62 | 37 | 22 | 34 | 41 | 21 | 19 | 12 | 512 |
| Venezuela | 6 | 16 | 10 | 3 | 6 | 4 | 3 | 3 | 1 | 1 | 1 | 2 | 1 | 2 | 0 | 5 | 4 | 5 | 73 |
| ***Southern Cone*** | *6* | *8* | *3* | *2* | *5* | *3* | *9* | *5* | *3* | *0* | *2* | *5* | *3* | *3* | *2* | *4* | *7* | *6* | *76* |
| Argentina | 0 | 3 | 1 | 1 | 3 | 0 | 0 | 0 | 0 | 0 | 0 | 0 | 0 | 0 | 1 | 0 | 0 | 1 | 10 |
| Chile | 0 | 0 | 0 | 0 | 0 | 0 | 0 | 0 | 0 | 0 | 0 | 0 | 0 | 0 | 0 | 0 | 1 | 0 | 1 |
| Paraguay | 6 | 5 | 2 | 1 | 2 | 3 | 9 | 5 | 3 | 0 | 2 | 5 | 3 | 3 | 1 | 4 | 6 | 5 | 65 |
| Uruguay | 0 | 0 | 0 | 0 | 0 | 0 | 0 | 0 | 0 | 0 | 0 | 0 | 0 | 0 | 0 | 0 | 0 | 0 | 0 |
| **Brazil** | 155 | 138 | 125 | 99 | 78 | 52 | 33 | 37 | 37 | 50 | 73 | 70 | 60 | 50 | 22 | 31 | 25 | 25 | 1160 |
| **Countries by Subregion** | **1980** | **1981** | **1982** | **1983** | **1984** | **1985** | **1986** | **1987** | **1988** | **1989** | **1990** | **1991** | **1992** | **1993** | **1994** | **1995** | **1996** | **1997** | **Total** |
| ***Central America*** | ***26*** | ***25*** | ***38*** | ***30*** | ***43*** | ***36*** | ***28*** | ***35*** | ***41*** | ***22*** | ***9*** | ***8*** | ***30*** | ***37*** | ***30*** | ***17*** | ***21*** | ***17*** | ***493*** |
| Belize | 0 | 0 | 0 | 0 | 0 | 0 | 0 | 0 | 2 | 3 | 0 | 0 | 0 | 0 | 0 | 0 | 0 | 0 | 5 |
| Costa Rica | 0 | 0 | 0 | 0 | 0 | 0 | 0 | 0 | 0 | 0 | 0 | 0 | 0 | 0 | 0 | 0 | 0 | 0 | 0 |
| El Salvador | 11 | 10 | 12 | 21 | 33 | 24 | 11 | 15 | 26 | 1 | 3 | 7 | 19 | 15 | 13 | 7 | 12 | 10 | 250 |
| Guatemala | 5 | 3 | 10 | 5 | 4 | 7 | 10 | 12 | 11 | 13 | 3 | 1 | 6 | 20 | 13 | 8 | 8 | 6 | 145 |
| Honduras | 5 | 10 | 11 | 3 | 6 | 5 | 5 | 4 | 1 | 4 | 2 | 0 | 2 | 0 | 1 | 2 | 0 | 1 | 62 |
| Nicaragua | 5 | 2 | 5 | 1 | 0 | 0 | 2 | 4 | 1 | 1 | 1 | 0 | 3 | 2 | 1 | 0 | 1 | 0 | 29 |
| Panama | 0 | 0 | 0 | 0 | 0 | 0 | 0 | 0 | 0 | 0 | 0 | 0 | 0 | 0 | 2 | 0 | 0 | 0 | 2 |
| **Mexico** | 40 | 59 | 45 | 47 | 63 | 84 | 85 | 60 | 72 | 65 | 69 | 48 | 35 | 29 | 25 | 31 | 22 | 23 | 902 |
| ***Latin Caribbean*** | ***6*** | ***10*** | ***2*** | ***5*** | ***11*** | ***6*** | ***12*** | ***4*** | ***6*** | ***1*** | ***3*** | ***6*** | ***4*** | ***6*** | ***5*** | ***4*** | ***10*** | ***1*** | ***102*** |
| Cuba | 0 | 0 | 0 | 0 | 0 | 0 | 0 | 0 | 0 | 0 | 1 | 1 | 0 | 1 | 0 | 1 | 0 | 0 | 4 |
| Haiti | 2 | 8 | 1 | 0 | 1 | 2 | 4 | 1 | 3 | 1 | 1 | 3 | 3 | 4 | 3 | 2 | 7 | 0 | 46 |
| Puerto Rico | 0 | 0 | 0 | 0 | 0 | 0 | 0 | 0 | 0 | 0 | 0 | 0 | 0 | 0 | 0 | 0 | 0 | 0 | 0 |
| Dominican Rep. | 4 | 2 | 1 | 5 | 10 | 4 | 8 | 3 | 3 | 0 | 1 | 2 | 1 | 1 | 2 | 1 | 3 | 1 | 52 |

—-Not available.

*Source*: Regional Information System for Epidemiological Surveillance of Rabies INPPAZ-PAHO/WHO, Talcahuano, 1660 Martinez, Buenos Aires, Argentina PANAFTOSA-PAHO/WHO, Caixa Postal 598, Rio de Janeiro, 200001-970, Brazil. http://www.who.int/emc/diseases/zoo/PAHO_data/humanlatinamerica.html.

## Table I2.5. Human Rabies Cases, Caribbean and North America, 1980–1997

| Countries by Subregion | 1980 | 1981 | 1982 | 1983 | 1984 | 1985 | 1986 | 1987 | 1988 | 1989 | 1990 | 1991 | 1992 | 1993 | 1994 | 1995 | 1996 | 1997 | Total |
|---|---|---|---|---|---|---|---|---|---|---|---|---|---|---|---|---|---|---|---|
| **CARIBBEAN** | 0 | 0 | 0 | 0 | 0 | 0 | 0 | 0 | 0 | 0 | 0 | 0 | 0 | 0 | 0 | 0 | 0 | 0 | 0 |
| Anguilla | 0 | 0 | 0 | 0 | 0 | 0 | 0 | 0 | 0 | 0 | 0 | 0 | 0 | 0 | 0 | 0 | 0 | 0 | 0 |
| Antigua and Barbuda | 0 | 0 | 0 | 0 | 0 | 0 | 0 | 0 | 0 | 0 | 0 | 0 | 0 | 0 | 0 | 0 | 0 | 0 | 0 |
| Aruba | 0 | 0 | 0 | 0 | 0 | 0 | 0 | 0 | 0 | 0 | 0 | 0 | 0 | 0 | 0 | 0 | 0 | 0 | 0 |
| Bahamas | 0 | 0 | 0 | 0 | 0 | 0 | 0 | 0 | 0 | 0 | 0 | 0 | 0 | 0 | 0 | 0 | 0 | 0 | 0 |
| Barbados | 0 | 0 | 0 | 0 | 0 | 0 | 0 | 0 | 0 | 0 | 0 | 0 | 0 | 0 | 0 | 0 | 0 | 0 | 0 |
| Bonaire | 0 | 0 | 0 | 0 | 0 | 0 | 0 | 0 | 0 | 0 | 0 | 0 | 0 | 0 | 0 | 0 | 0 | 0 | 0 |
| Curazao | 0 | 0 | 0 | 0 | 0 | 0 | 0 | 0 | 0 | 0 | 0 | 0 | 0 | 0 | 0 | 0 | 0 | 0 | 0 |
| Dominica | 0 | 0 | 0 | 0 | 0 | 0 | 0 | 0 | 0 | 0 | 0 | 0 | 0 | 0 | 0 | 0 | 0 | 0 | 0 |
| Grenada | 0 | 0 | 0 | 0 | 0 | 0 | 0 | 0 | 0 | 0 | 0 | 0 | 0 | 0 | 0 | 0 | 0 | 0 | 0 |
| Guadalupe | 0 | 0 | 0 | 0 | 0 | 0 | 0 | 0 | 0 | 0 | 0 | 0 | 0 | 0 | 0 | 0 | 0 | 0 | 0 |
| French Guiana | 0 | 0 | 0 | 0 | 0 | 0 | 0 | 0 | 0 | 0 | 0 | 0 | 0 | 0 | 0 | 0 | 0 | 0 | 0 |
| Guyana | 0 | 0 | 0 | 0 | 0 | 0 | 0 | 0 | 0 | 0 | 0 | 0 | 0 | 0 | 0 | 0 | 0 | 0 | 0 |
| Caiman islands | 0 | 0 | 0 | 0 | 0 | 0 | 0 | 0 | 0 | 0 | 0 | 0 | 0 | 0 | 0 | 0 | 0 | 0 | 0 |
| Turks and Caicos | 0 | 0 | 0 | 0 | 0 | 0 | 0 | 0 | 0 | 0 | 0 | 0 | 0 | 0 | 0 | 0 | 0 | 0 | 0 |
| British Virgin Islands | 0 | 0 | 0 | 0 | 0 | 0 | 0 | 0 | 0 | 0 | 0 | 0 | 0 | 0 | 0 | 0 | 0 | 0 | 0 |
| Jamaica | 0 | 0 | 0 | 0 | 0 | 0 | 0 | 0 | 0 | 0 | 0 | 0 | 0 | 0 | 0 | 0 | 0 | 0 | 0 |
| Martinica | 0 | 0 | 0 | 0 | 0 | 0 | 0 | 0 | 0 | 0 | 0 | 0 | 0 | 0 | 0 | 0 | 0 | 0 | 0 |
| Montserrat | 0 | 0 | 0 | 0 | 0 | 0 | 0 | 0 | 0 | 0 | 0 | 0 | 0 | 0 | 0 | 0 | 0 | 0 | 0 |
| Saint Kitts - Nevis | 0 | 0 | 0 | 0 | 0 | 0 | 0 | 0 | 0 | 0 | 0 | 0 | 0 | 0 | 0 | 0 | 0 | 0 | 0 |
| St. Eustaquio | 0 | 0 | 0 | 0 | 0 | 0 | 0 | 0 | 0 | 0 | 0 | 0 | 0 | 0 | 0 | 0 | 0 | 0 | 0 |
| St. Martín | 0 | 0 | 0 | 0 | 0 | 0 | 0 | 0 | 0 | 0 | 0 | 0 | 0 | 0 | 0 | 0 | 0 | 0 | 0 |
| St. Vincent and Grenadines | 0 | 0 | 0 | 0 | 0 | 0 | 0 | 0 | 0 | 0 | 0 | 0 | 0 | 0 | 0 | 0 | 0 | 0 | 0 |
| St. Lucia | 0 | 0 | 0 | 0 | 0 | 0 | 0 | 0 | 0 | 0 | 0 | 0 | 0 | 0 | 0 | 0 | 0 | 0 | 0 |
| Suriname | 0 | 0 | 0 | 0 | 0 | 0 | 0 | 0 | 0 | 0 | 0 | 0 | 0 | 0 | 0 | 0 | 0 | 0 | 0 |
| Trinidad and Tobago | 0 | 0 | 0 | 0 | 0 | 0 | 0 | 0 | 0 | 0 | 0 | 0 | 0 | 0 | 0 | 0 | 0 | 0 | 0 |

| Countries by Subregion | 1980 | 1981 | 1982 | 1983 | 1984 | 1985 | 1986 | 1987 | 1988 | 1989 | 1990 | 1991 | 1992 | 1993 | 1994 | 1995 | 1996 | 1997 | Total |
|---|---|---|---|---|---|---|---|---|---|---|---|---|---|---|---|---|---|---|---|
| **NORTH AMERICA** | 0 | 1 | 0 | 0 | 1 | 1 | 0 | 1 | 0 | 1 | 1 | 3 | 1 | 3 | 6 | 4 | 4 | 4 | 31 |
| Bermuda | 0 | 0 | 0 | 0 | 0 | 0 | 0 | 0 | 0 | 0 | 0 | 0 | 0 | 0 | 0 | 0 | 0 | 0 | 0 |
| Canada | 0 | 0 | 0 | 0 | 1 | 1 | 0 | 0 | 0 | 0 | 0 | 0 | 0 | 0 | 0 | 0 | 0 | 0 | 2 |
| United States | 0 | 1 | 0 | 0 | 0 | 0 | 0 | 1 | 0 | 1 | 1 | 3 | 1 | 3 | 6 | 4 | 4 | 4 | 29 |
| **TOTAL** | 283 | 352 | 332 | 258 | 268 | 244 | 205 | 193 | 224 | 269 | 252 | 215 | 225 | 216 | 150 | 154 | 183 | 118 | 4141 |

—-Not available.

*Source*: Regional Information System for Epidemiological Surveillance of Rabies INPPAZ-PAHO/WHO, Talcahuano, 1660 Martinez, Buenos Aires, Argentina PANAFTOSA-PAHO/WHO, Caixa Postal 598, Rio de Janeiro, 200001-970, Brazil. http://www.who.int/emc/diseases/zoo/PAHO_data/humanrabiescaribbean.html.

## Table I2.6. Neonatal Tetanus Global Annual Reported Incidence, 1980–1999

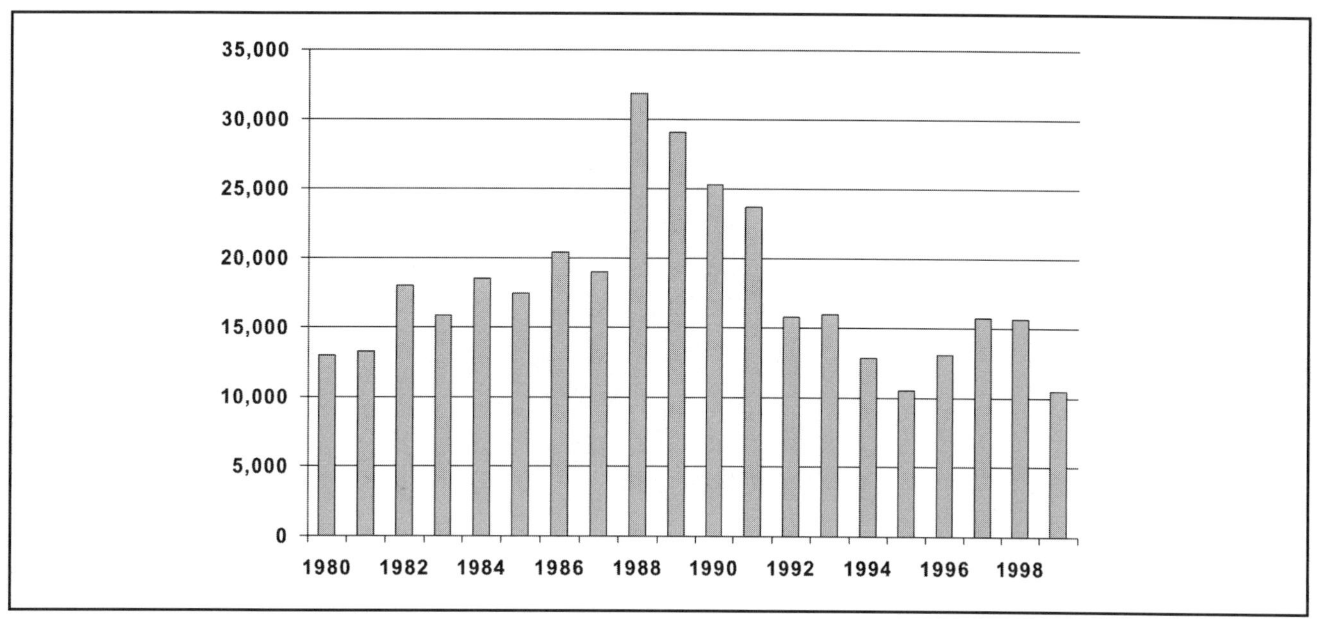


*Source*: Department of Vaccines and Biologicals. *WHO vaccine preventable diseases 2000 global summaries* (Geneva: World Health Organization, 2000). http://www.who.int/vaccines-documents/DocsPDF00/www542.pdf.

## Table I2.7. Total Tetanus Global Annual Reported Incidence, 1980–1999

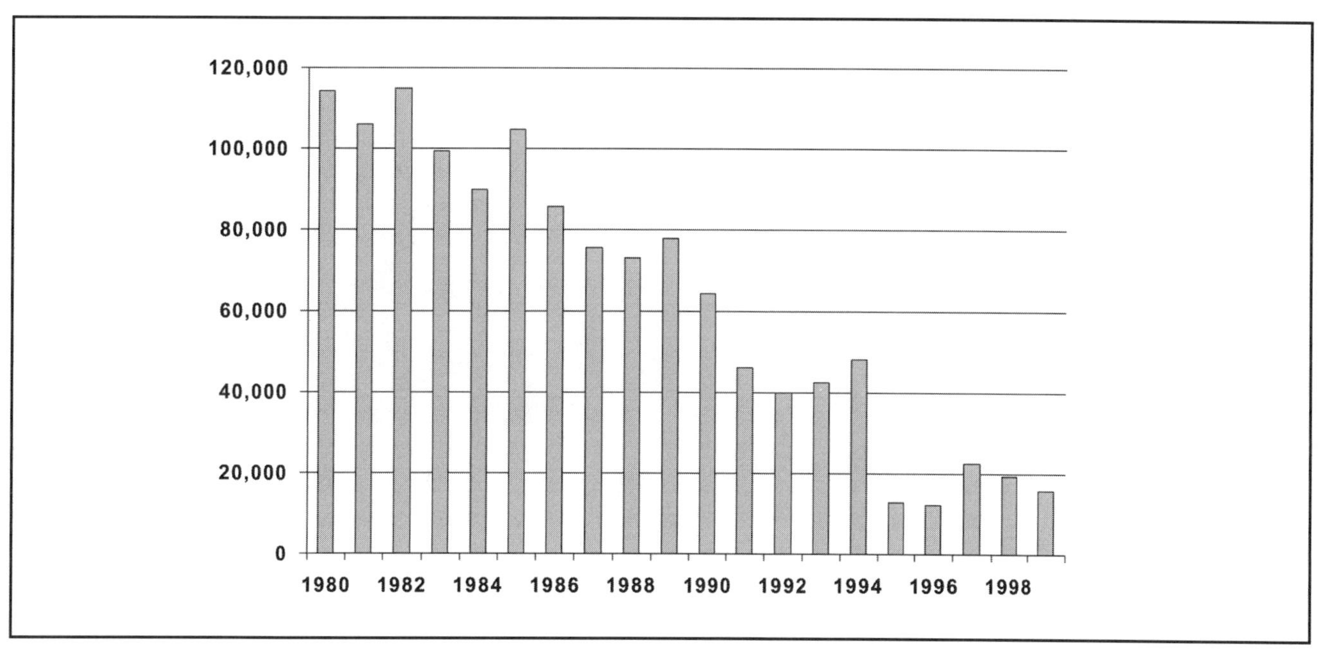


*Source*: Department of Vaccines and Biologicals. *WHO vaccine preventable diseases 2000 global summaries* (Geneva: World Health Organization, 2000). http://www.who.int/vaccines-documents/DocsPDF00/www542.pdf.

**Table I3.1. BCG (Tuberculosis) Global Annual Coverage, 1980–1999**

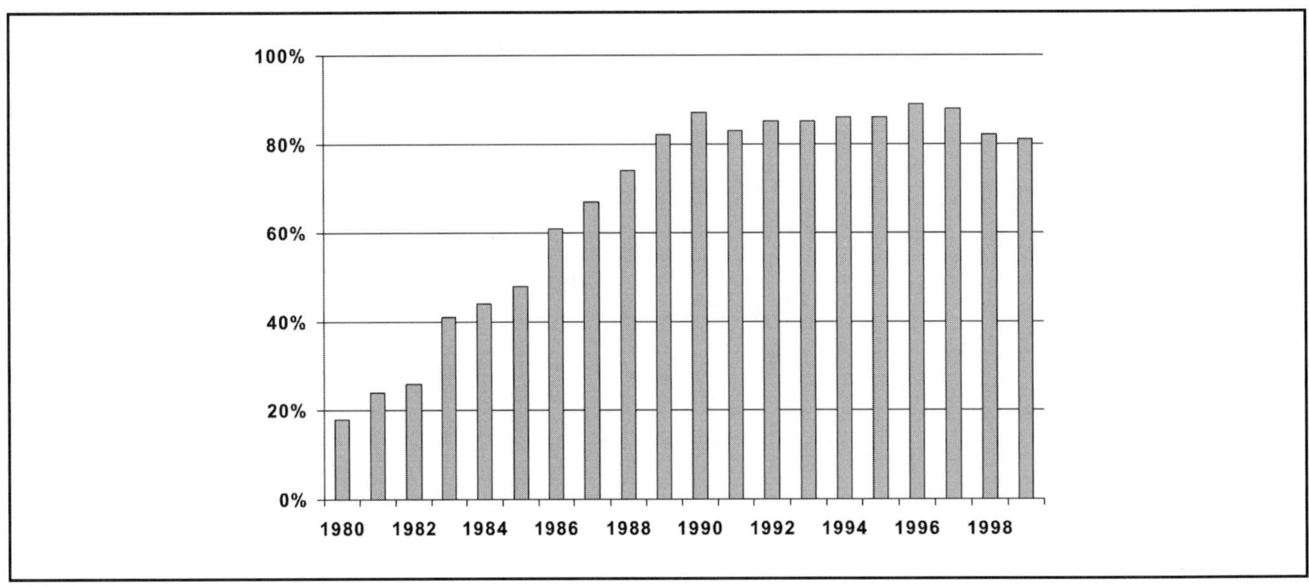


*Source*: Department of Vaccines and Biologicals. *WHO vaccine preventable diseases 2000 global summaries* (Geneva: World Health Organization, 2000). http://www.who.int/vaccines-documents/DocsPDF00/www542.pdf.

**Table I3.2. DTP3 (Diphtheria, Tetanus, Pertussis) Global Annual Coverage, 1980–1999**

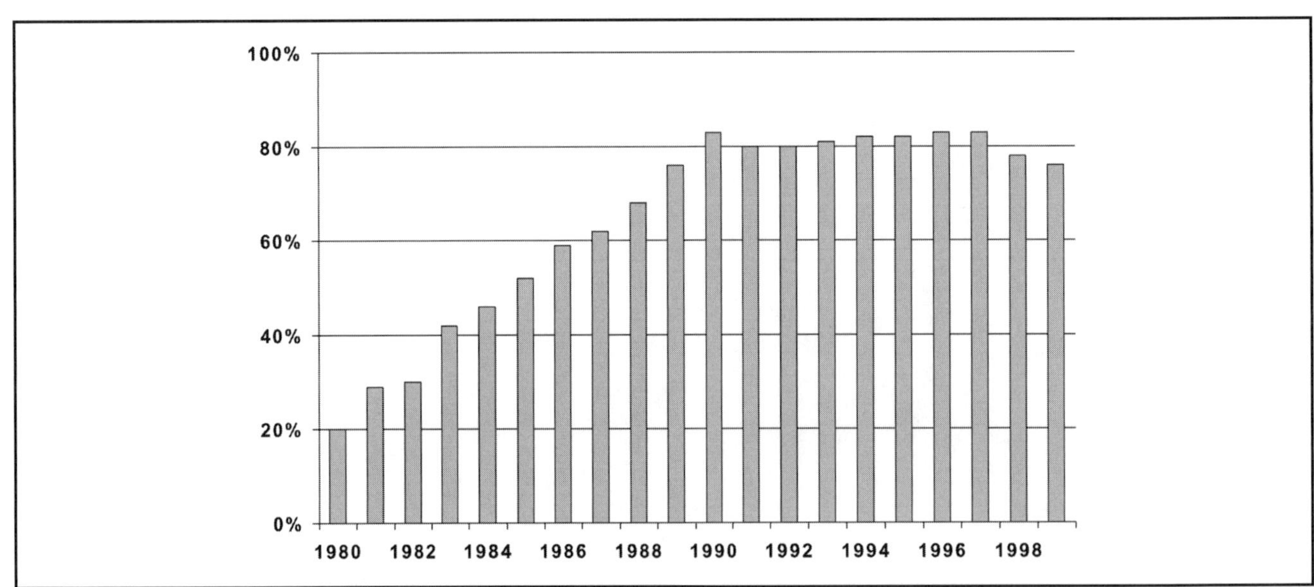


*Source*: Department of Vaccines and Biologicals. *WHO vaccine preventable diseases 2000 global summaries* (Geneva: World Health Organization, 2000). http://www.who.int/vaccines-documents/DocsPDF00/www542.pdf.

**Table I3.3. HepB3 (Hepatitis B) Global Annual Coverage, 1980–1999**

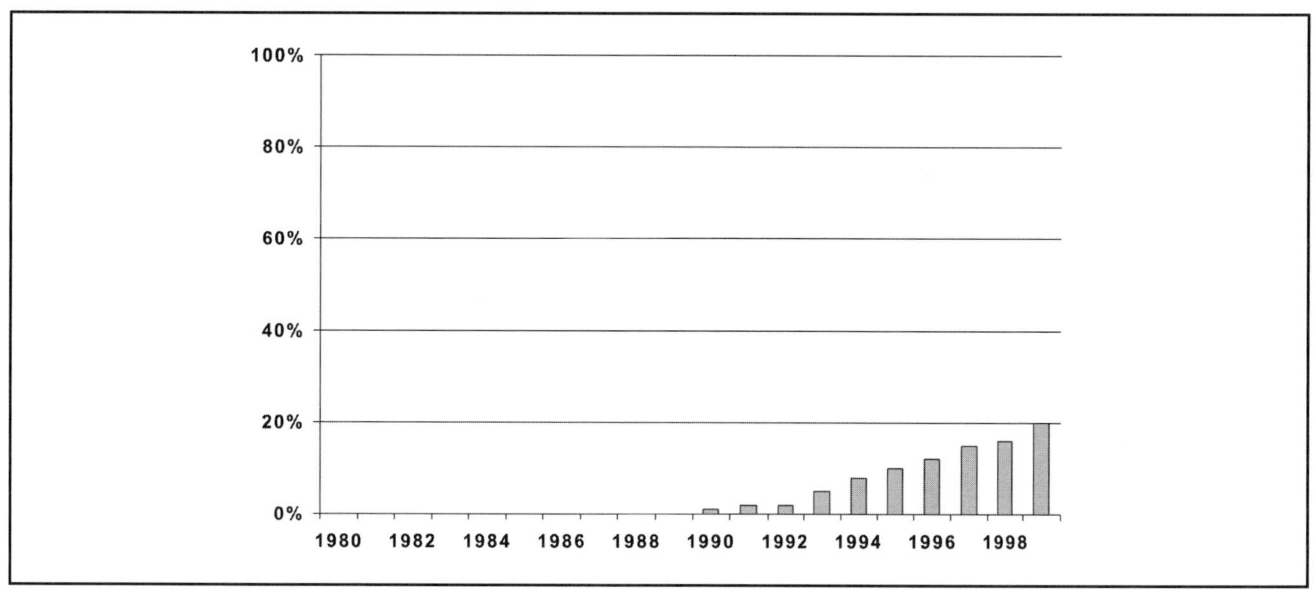


*Source*: Department of Vaccines and Biologicals. *WHO vaccine preventable diseases 2000 global summaries* (Geneva: World Health Organization, 2000). http://www.who.int/vaccines-documents/DocsPDF00/www542.pdf.

**Table I3.4. MCV (Measles-Containing Vaccine) Global Annual Coverage, 1980–1999**

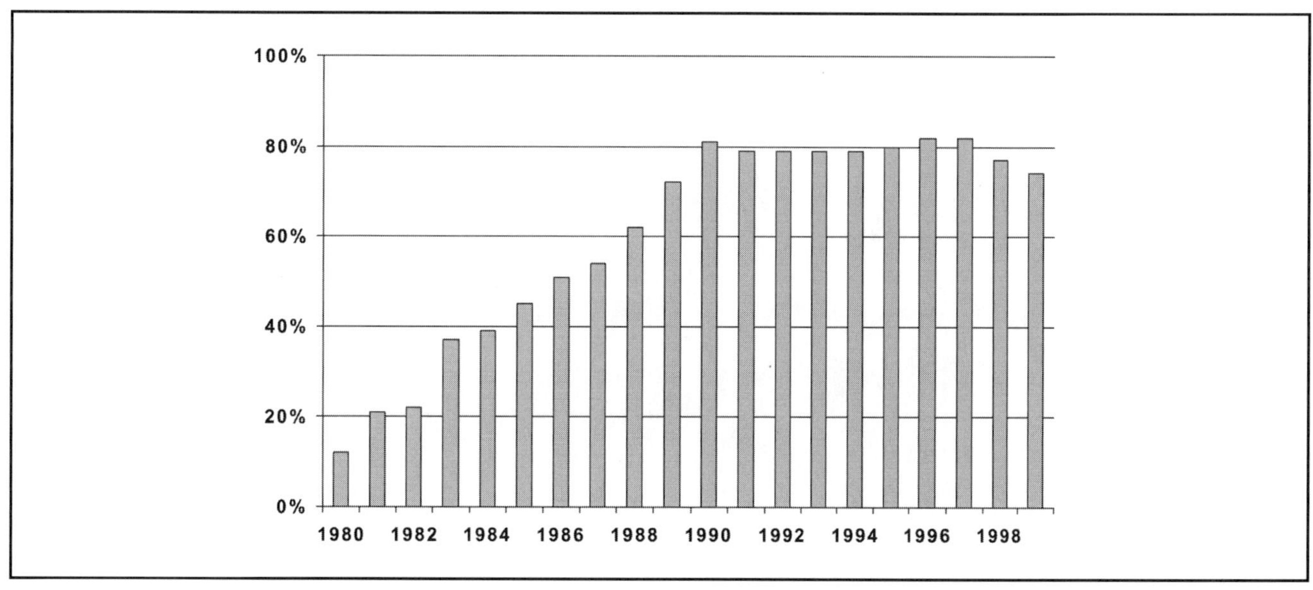


*Source*: Department of Vaccines and Biologicals. *WHO vaccine preventable diseases 2000 global summaries* (Geneva: World Health Organization, 2000). http://www.who.int/vaccines-documents/DocsPDF00/www542.pdf.

## Table I3.5. Global Measles Vaccine Coverage and Reported Measles Cases, 1980–1999

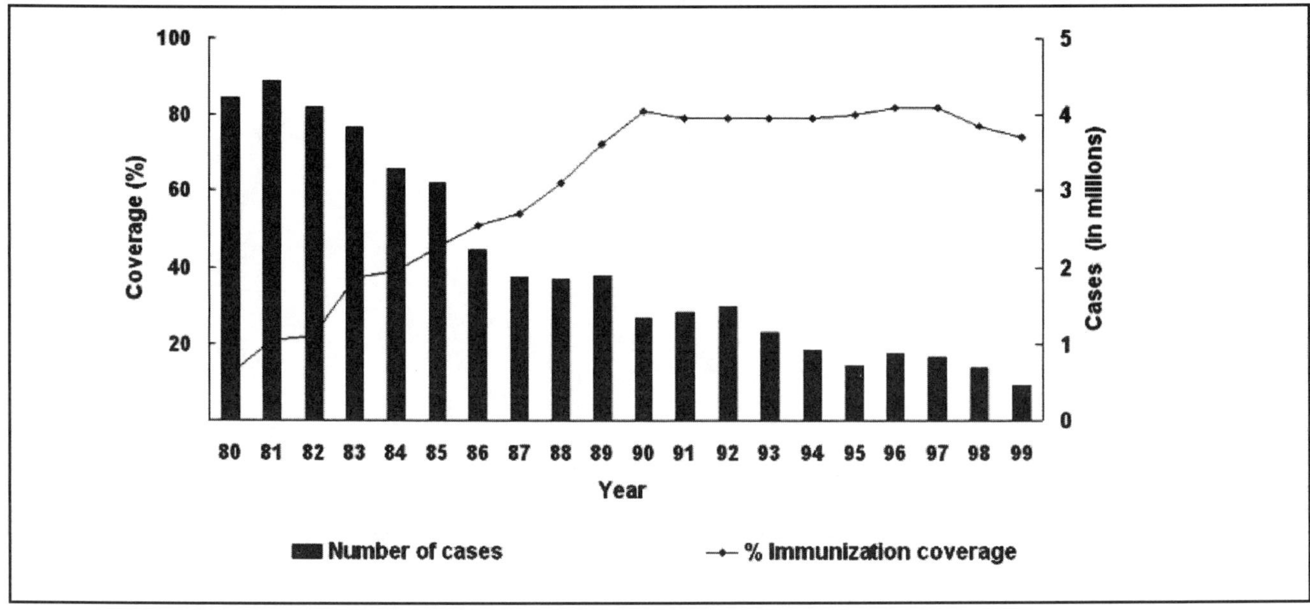


*Source*: Department of Vaccines and Biologicals Vaccine Assessment and Monitoring Team. *Vaccines, Immunization and Biologicals*. Geneva: World Health Organization, 2001. http://www.who.int/vaccines-surveillance/graphics/htmls/measlescascov.htm.

## Table I3.6. POL3 (Polio Vaccine) Global Annual Coverage, 1980–1999

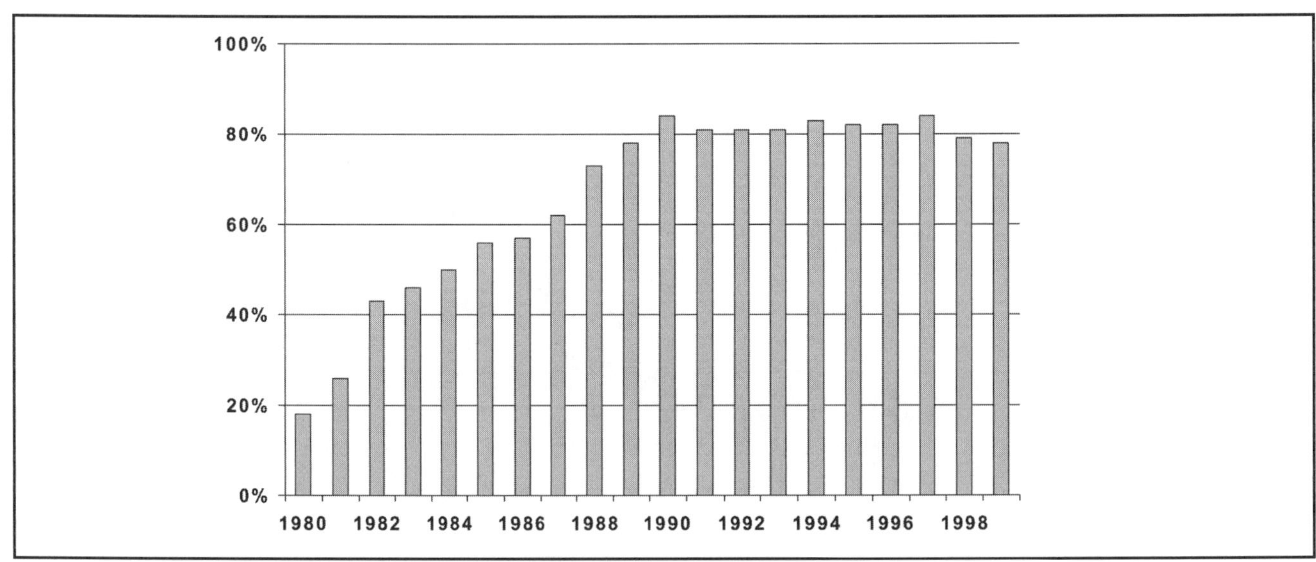


*Source*: Department of Vaccines and Biologicals. *WHO vaccine preventable diseases 2000 global summaries* (Geneva: World Health Organization, 2000). http://www.who.int/vaccines-documents/DocsPDF00/www542.pdf.

## Table I3.7. TT2plus (Second and Subsequent Dose of Tetanus Toxoid) Global Annual Coverage, 1980–1999

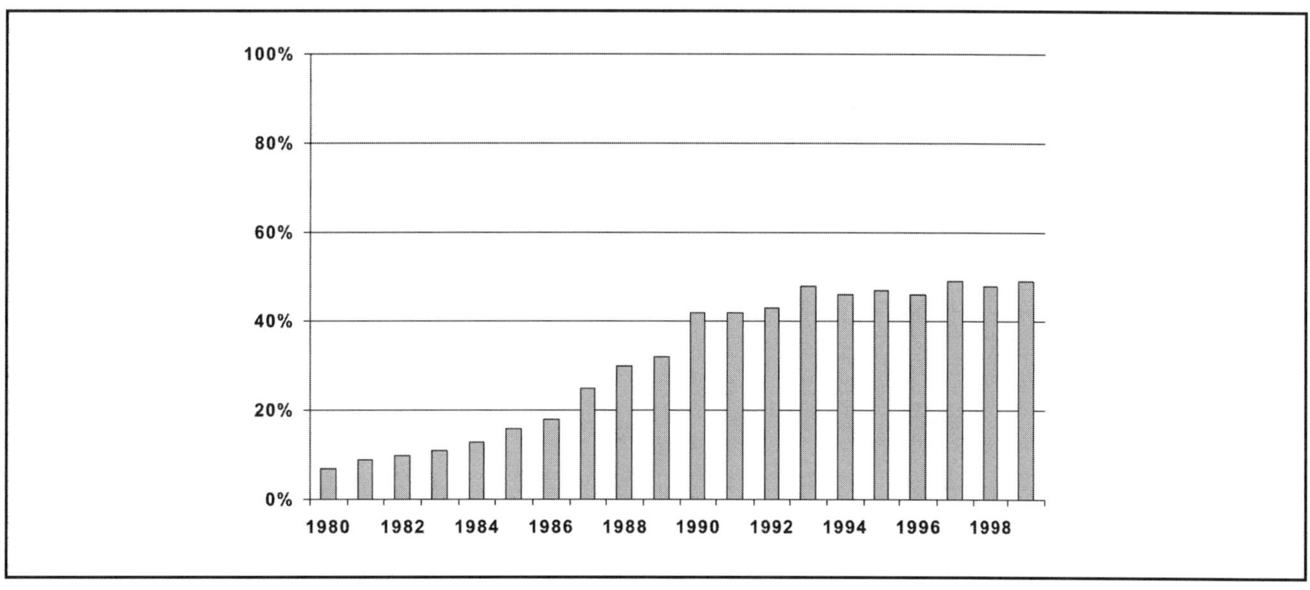


*Source*: Department of Vaccines and Biologicals. *WHO vaccine preventable diseases 2000 global summaries* (Geneva: World Health Organization, 2000). http://www.who.int/vaccines-documents/DocsPDF00/www542.pdf.

## Table I3.8. YFV (Yellow Fever Vaccine) Global Annual Coverage, 1980–1999

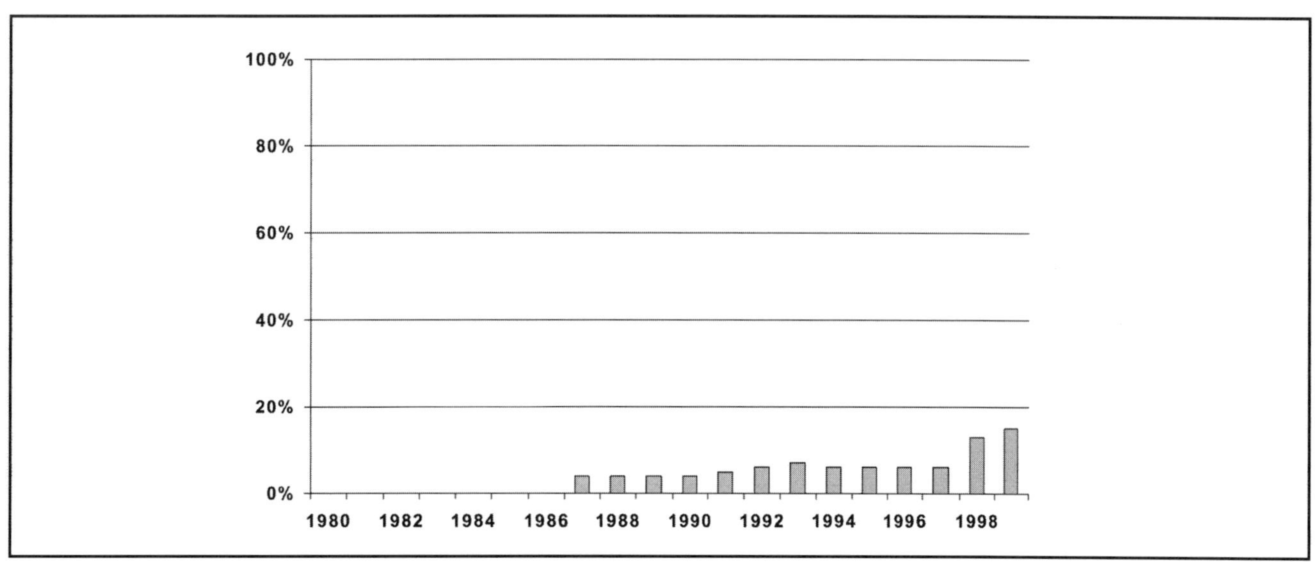


*Source*: Department of Vaccines and Biologicals. *WHO vaccine preventable diseases 2000 global summaries* (Geneva: World Health Organization, 2000). http://www.who.int/vaccines-documents/DocsPDF00/www542.pdf.

## Table I3.9. Immunization Coverage, Global and Regional Summaries of Percent Vaccination Coverage, by Antigen and with Associated Range, from 1990 to 1999

**BCG**

| | 1990 | 1991 | 1992 | 1993 | 1994 | 1995 | 1996 | 1997 | 1998 | 1999 |
|---|---|---|---|---|---|---|---|---|---|---|
| AFRO | 71 | 61 | 61 | 59 | 64 | 68 | 69 | 68 | 64 | 65 |
| | (70-72) | (60-62) | (60-63) | (59-60) | (63-66) | (68-69) | (69-70) | (66-69) | (62-65) | (59-70) |
| AMRO | 80 | 81 | 88 | 93 | 91 | 95 | 96 | 95 | 94 | 93 |
| | (79-80) | (81-82) | (87-88) | (92-93) | (91-92) | (95-96) | (95-96) | (94-95) | (93-94) | (93-94) |
| EMRO | 86 | 81 | 82 | 82 | 78 | 77 | 86 | 85 | 85 | 88 |
| | (85-88) | (80-84) | (80-85) | (81-85) | (77-81) | (75-81) | (85-88) | (84-88) | (85-87) | (88-90) |
| EURO | 70 | 72 | 72 | 73 | 78 | 79 | 80 | 80 | 81 | 81 |
| | (65-75) | (71-73) | (69-76) | (69-77) | (77-80) | (74-81) | (75-83) | (74-83) | (72-88) | (67-94) |
| SEARO | 97 | 91 | 96 | 95 | 98 | 96 | 97 | 97 | 82 | 83 |
| | (97-97) | (91-92) | (96-97) | (95-96) | (97-98) | (96-97) | (96-97) | (96-97) | (81-82) | (83-84) |
| WPRO | 96 | 94 | 92 | 92 | 93 | 92 | 95 | 94 | 93 | 85 |
| | (95-96) | (93-95) | (92-93) | (91-92) | (92-94) | (91-93) | (94-96) | (93-95) | (92-94) | (82-88) |
| Global | 87 | 83 | 85 | 85 | 86 | 86 | 89 | 88 | 82 | 81 |
| | (86-88) | (82-84) | (84-86) | (84-86) | (85-87) | (85-87) | (87-89) | (86-89) | (81-84) | (78-84) |

**DTP3**

| | 1990 | 1991 | 1992 | 1993 | 1994 | 1995 | 1996 | 1997 | 1998 | 1999 |
|---|---|---|---|---|---|---|---|---|---|---|
| AFRO | 55 | 48 | 47 | 48 | 52 | 55 | 53 | 54 | 50 | 50 |
| | (54-55) | (47-49) | (46-49) | (47-48) | (52-53) | (54-55) | (53-54) | (53-55) | (50-51) | (46-55) |
| AMRO | 76 | 79 | 79 | 81 | 83 | 87 | 86 | 86 | 88 | 89 |
| | (73-78) | (76-81) | (78-79) | (81-82) | (83-84) | (87-88) | (86-87) | (86-87) | (87-88) | (88-90) |
| EMRO | 80 | 77 | 77 | 76 | 73 | 72 | 79 | 79 | 80 | 80 |
| | (79-81) | (76-77) | (76-78) | (75-77) | (72-73) | (71-73) | (79-80) | (79-80) | (80-81) | (79-81) |
| EURO | 79 | 86 | 86 | 84 | 89 | 89 | 93 | 92 | 91 | 91 |
| | (79-80) | (85-86) | (85-86) | (84-85) | (88-89) | (88-90) | (92-93) | (92-93) | (87-95) | (80-98) |
| SEARO | 94 | 89 | 90 | 91 | 92 | 90 | 89 | 90 | 73 | 76 |
| | (93-94) | (89-90) | (90-91) | (91-92) | (92-93) | (89-90) | (89-90) | (89-91) | (73-74) | (75-76) |
| WPRO | 93 | 92 | 92 | 92 | 91 | 90 | 94 | 93 | 94 | 84 |
| | (93-94) | (92-93) | (91-92) | (91-93) | (90-92) | (90-91) | (93-94) | (92-93) | (93-95) | (81-87) |
| Global | 83 | 80 | 80 | 81 | 82 | 82 | 83 | 83 | 78 | 76 |
| | (82-83) | (80-81) | (80-81) | (80-81) | (81-82) | (81-82) | (82-83) | (82-84) | (77-79) | (74-79) |

**HepB3**

| | 1990 | 1991 | 1992 | 1993 | 1994 | 1995 | 1996 | 1997 | 1998 | 1999 |
|---|---|---|---|---|---|---|---|---|---|---|
| AFRO | 0 | 0 | 0 | 0 | 0 | 0 | 0 | 1 | 1 | 1 |
| | (0-0) | (0-0) | (0-0) | (0-0) | (0-0) | (0-0) | (0-1) | (0-1) | (1-1) | (1-1) |
| AMRO | 0 | 0 | 0 | 4 | 11 | 17 | 21 | 32 | 36 | 53 |
| | (0-0) | (0-0) | (0-0) | (4-4) | (11-11) | (17-17) | (21-21) | (32-33) | (36-37) | (52-54) |
| EMRO | 3 | 4 | 5 | 15 | 27 | 28 | 30 | 34 | 31 | 35 |
| | (3-3) | (4-4) | (5-5) | (15-15) | (27-28) | (28-28) | (30-30) | (34-34) | (31-32) | (35-35) |
| EURO | 4 | 8 | 9 | 10 | 11 | 11 | 16 | 22 | 24 | 27 |
| | (4-4) | (8-8) | (9-9) | (10-10) | (11-11) | (10-11) | (16-17) | (21-23) | (23-25) | (26-29) |
| SEARO | 0 | 0 | 0 | 3 | 6 | 9 | 11 | 12 | 12 | 13 |
| | (0-0) | (0-0) | (0-0) | (3-4) | (4-8) | (9-9) | (11-11) | (11-12) | (11-13) | (13-13) |
| WPRO | 0 | 2 | 2 | 3 | 3 | 5 | 5 | 8 | 12 | 13 |
| | (0-0) | (2-2) | (2-3) | (3-3) | (3-3) | (5-5) | (5-6) | (7-8) | (12-12) | (12-14) |
| Global | 1 | 2 | 2 | 5 | 8 | 10 | 12 | 15 | 16 | 20 |
| | (1-1) | (2-2) | (2-2) | (5-5) | (7-8) | (10-10) | (12-12) | (15-15) | (16-17) | (19-20) |

**Table I3.9. *(Continued)***

MCV

| | 1990 | 1991 | 1992 | 1993 | 1994 | 1995 | 1996 | 1997 | 1998 | 1999 |
|---|---|---|---|---|---|---|---|---|---|---|
| AFRO | 52 (51-53) | 50 (50-51) | 47 (46-48) | 48 (47-48) | 53 (52-54) | 57 (56-57) | 55 (54-55) | 58 (57-58) | 51 (51-52) | 51 (46-56) |
| AMRO | 80 (78-83) | 82 (79-84) | 83 (82-83) | 83 (83-84) | 84 (83-84) | 88 (87-88) | 86 (86-87) | 89 (88-89) | 91 (91-92) | 90 (89-91) |
| EMRO | 75 (75-76) | 74 (74-75) | 76 (75-77) | 74 (73-75) | 75 (74-76) | 72 (71-73) | 80 (79-81) | 81 (80-81) | 79 (79-80) | 82 (81-83) |
| EURO | 80 (76-84) | 82 (77-86) | 81 (81-82) | 83 (82-84) | 83 (82-84) | 84 (83-85) | 87 (87-88) | 89 (88-89) | 88 (80-95) | 88 (74-98) |
| SEARO | 88 (87-88) | 84 (83-84) | 86 (86-87) | 88 (87-88) | 87 (87-88) | 84 (83-84) | 85 (84-85) | 84 (84-85) | 69 (69-70) | 64 (64-65) |
| WPRO | 93 (92-93) | 92 (92-93) | 91 (90-91) | 91 (90-91) | 88 (87-89) | 92 (91-92) | 95 (94-96) | 94 (93-94) | 94 (93-95) | 86 (81-88) |
| Global | 81 (79-82) | 79 (78-80) | 79 (78-80) | 79 (79-80) | 79 (79-80) | 80 (80-81) | 82 (81-82) | 82 (82-83) | 77 (76-78) | 74 (70-76) |

POL3

| | 1990 | 1991 | 1992 | 1993 | 1994 | 1995 | 1996 | 1997 | 1998 | 1999 |
|---|---|---|---|---|---|---|---|---|---|---|
| AFRO | 55 (55-56) | 48 (47-49) | 47 (47-48) | 48 (47-48) | 52 (52-53) | 55 (54-55) | 47 (46-47) | 54 (53-55) | 51 (49-52) | 49 (45-54) |
| AMRO | 86 (82-90) | 84 (80-88) | 83 (82-83) | 83 (83-84) | 86 (85-86) | 86 (86-87) | 87 (86-87) | 88 (87-89) | 88 (87-89) | 87 (86-88) |
| EMRO | 80 (79-80) | 77 (76-77) | 77 (76-78) | 76 (75-77) | 73 (72-74) | 72 (70-73) | 79 (79-80) | 80 (79-80) | 82 (82-83) | 80 (79-81) |
| EURO | 81 (81-82) | 84 (84-85) | 86 (85-86) | 84 (83-85) | 89 (89-90) | 88 (87-89) | 93 (93-94) | 93 (92-94) | 93 (90-94) | 93 (85-97) |
| SEARO | 94 (94-95) | 89 (89-90) | 91 (91-92) | 92 (92-93) | 93 (92-93) | 91 (91-92) | 91 (90-91) | 91 (91-92) | 76 (75-76) | 78 (77-78) |
| WPRO | 94 (93-94) | 93 (92-94) | 92 (91-93) | 92 (91-93) | 92 (92-93) | 93 (92-93) | 95 (94-95) | 95 (94-95) | 95 (94-96) | 89 (86-91) |
| Global | 84 (83-85) | 81 (80-82) | 81 (81-82) | 81 (81-82) | 83 (82-83) | 82 (82-83) | 82 (82-83) | 84 (83-84) | 79 (78-80) | 78 (75-79) |

TT2plus

| | 1990 | 1991 | 1992 | 1993 | 1994 | 1995 | 1996 | 1997 | 1998 | 1999 |
|---|---|---|---|---|---|---|---|---|---|---|
| AFRO | 36 (35-37) | 26 (26-27) | 30 (28-31) | 35 (34-36) | 32 (31-33) | 35 (34-35) | 32 (31-32) | 42 (40-45) | 36 (32-40) | 41 (34-48) |
| AMRO | 39 (34-43) | 40 (37-43) | 36 (29-43) | 38 (26-49) | 36 (23-51) | 35 (20-51) | 34 (17-53) | 32 (15-54) | 31 (12-58) | 30 (9-62) |
| EMRO | 45 (44-46) | 47 (46-48) | 45 (44-46) | 53 (52-54) | 47 (45-48) | 47 (45-49) | 48 (47-50) | 51 (49-52) | 52 (51-53) | 51 (50-53) |
| EURO | 14 (14-14) | 81 (81-82) | 78 (77-78) | 78 (77-78) | 43 (42-43) | 42 (41-42) | 45 (44-45) | 48 (48-49) | 48 (21-75) | 48 (18-80) |
| SEARO | 74 (73-74) | 75 (74-75) | 75 (74-75) | 76 (76-77) | 78 (78-79) | 76 (76-77) | 75 (75-76) | 79 (78-80) | 79 (79-80) | 79 (79-80) |
| WPRO | 7 (7-7) | 7 (7-7) | 11 (11-12) | 20 (20-21) | 19 (19-20) | 21 (16-25) | 21 (15-27) | 21 (14-28) | 20 (10-29) | 20 (10-31) |
| Global | 42 (41-43) | 42 (41-43) | 43 (42-44) | 48 (46-50) | 46 (44-49) | 47 (43-50) | 46 (42-50) | 49 (45-54) | 48 (42-54) | 49 (42-57) |

**Table I3.9. *(Continued)***

YFV

| | 1990 | 1991 | 1992 | 1993 | 1994 | 1995 | 1996 | 1997 | 1998 | 1999 |
|---|---|---|---|---|---|---|---|---|---|---|
| AFRO | 6 (5-7) | 7 (7-7) | 8 (8-9) | 10 (8-11) | 8 (7-11) | 9 (7-12) | 9 (6-14) | 9 (6-15) | 9 (7-15) | 11 (8-19) |
| AMRO | 0 (0-0) | 0 (0-0) | 0 (0-0) | 0 (0-0) | 0 (0-0) | 0 (0-0) | 0 (0-0) | 0 (0-0) | 28 (28-29) | 28 |
| EMRO | 0 (0-0) | 0 (0-0) | 0 (0-0) | 0 (0-0) | 0 (0-0) | 0 (0-0) | 0 (0-0) | 0 (0-0) | 0 (0-0) | 0 (0-0) |
| Global | 4 (3-4) | 5 (5-5) | 6 (6-6) | 7 (6-7) | 6 (5-8) | 6 (5-9) | 6 (4-10) | 6 (4-10) | 13 (12-18) | 15 (12-21) |

BCG (Bacille Calmete-Guerin vaccine) = TB vaccine
DTP3 = third dose of diphtheria toxoid, tetanus toxoid, and pertussis vaccine
HepB3 = third dose of hepatitis B vaccine
MCV = measles-containing vaccine
POL3 = third dose of polio vaccine
TT2plus = second and subsequent dose of tetanus toxoid
YFV = Yellow fever vaccine
*Source*: Department of Vaccines and Biologicals. *WHO vaccine preventable diseases 2000 global summaries* (Geneva: World Health Organization, 2000). http://www.who.int/vaccines-documents/DocsPDF00/www542.pdf

**Table I4.1. Childhood Immunization: Percentage of Children Aged 19–35 Months Vaccinated for Selected Diseases, by Poverty Status, Race, and Hispanic Origin, 1994–1998**

| | Total | | | | | Below poverty | | | | | At or above poverty | | | | |
|---|---|---|---|---|---|---|---|---|---|---|---|---|---|---|---|
| Characteristic | 1994 | 1995 | 1996 | 1997 | 1998 | 1994 | 1995 | 1996 | 1997 | 1998 | 1994 | 1995 | 1996 | 1997 | 1998 |
| **Total** | | | | | | | | | | | | | | | |
| Combined series (4:3:1:3)[a] | 69 | 74 | 77 | 76 | 79 | 61 | 67 | 69 | 71 | 74 | 72 | 77 | 80 | 79 | 82 |
| Combined series (4:3:1)[b] | 75 | 76 | 78 | 78 | 81 | 66 | 67 | 71 | 73 | 76 | 77 | 79 | 81 | 80 | 83 |
| DTP (4 doses or more)[c] | 76 | 79 | 81 | 81 | 84 | 69 | 71 | 73 | 76 | 80 | 79 | 81 | 84 | 84 | 86 |
| Polio (3 doses or more) | 83 | 88 | 91 | 91 | 91 | 78 | 84 | 88 | 90 | 90 | 85 | 89 | 92 | 92 | 92 |
| Measles-containing[d] | 89 | 90 | 91 | 91 | 92 | 87 | 85 | 87 | 86 | 90 | 90 | 91 | 92 | 92 | 93 |
| Hib (3 doses or more)[e] | 86 | 92 | 92 | 93 | 93 | 81 | 88 | 88 | 90 | 91 | 88 | 93 | 93 | 94 | 95 |
| Hepatitis B (3 doses or more)[f] | 37 | 68 | 82 | 84 | 87 | 25 | 64 | 78 | 80 | 85 | 41 | 69 | 83 | 85 | 88 |
| Varicella[g] | - | - | 12 | 26 | 43 | - | - | 5 | 17 | 41 | - | - | 15 | 29 | 44 |
| **White, non-Hispanic** | | | | | | | | | | | | | | | |
| Combined series (4:3:1:3)[a] | 72 | 77 | 79 | 79 | 82 | - | 68 | 68 | 70 | 77 | - | 79 | 81 | 76 | 83 |
| Combined series (4:3:1)[b] | 78 | 79 | 80 | 80 | 83 | - | - | 70 | 73 | 79 | - | - | 82 | 82 | 84 |
| DTP (4 doses or more)[c] | 80 | 81 | 83 | 84 | 87 | - | - | 72 | 76 | 82 | - | - | 85 | 85 | 88 |
| Polio (3 doses or more) | 85 | 89 | 92 | 92 | 92 | - | - | 88 | 90 | 91 | - | - | 93 | 92 | 93 |
| Measles-containing[d] | 90 | 91 | 92 | 92 | 93 | - | - | 86 | 85 | 91 | - | - | 93 | 93 | 94 |
| Hib (3 doses or more)[e] | 87 | 93 | 93 | 94 | 95 | - | - | 87 | 90 | 92 | - | - | 94 | 95 | 96 |
| Hepatitis B (3 doses or more)[f] | 40 | 68 | 82 | 85 | 88 | - | - | 75 | 80 | 87 | - | - | 83 | 85 | 88 |
| Varicella[g] | - | - | 15 | 28 | 42 | - | - | 6 | 17 | 37 | - | - | 16 | 29 | 43 |
| **Black, non-Hispanic** | | | | | | | | | | | | | | | |
| Combined series (4:3:1:3)[a] | 67 | 70 | 74 | 73 | 73 | - | 66 | 70 | 72 | 72 | - | 75 | 78 | 80 | 74 |
| Combined series (4:3:1)[b] | 70 | 72 | 76 | 74 | 74 | - | - | 73 | 72 | 74 | - | - | 80 | 78 | 76 |
| DTP (4 doses or more)[c] | 72 | 74 | 79 | 78 | 77 | - | - | 75 | 76 | 77 | - | - | 82 | 80 | 79 |
| Polio (3 doses or more) | 79 | 84 | 90 | 90 | 88 | - | - | 88 | 90 | 88 | - | - | 92 | 91 | 87 |
| Measles-containing[d] | 86 | 86 | 89 | 90 | 89 | - | - | 88 | 88 | 89 | - | - | 91 | 92 | 90 |
| Hib (3 doses or more)[e] | 85 | 89 | 90 | 92 | 90 | - | - | 87 | 92 | 90 | - | - | 92 | 94 | 90 |
| Hepatitis B (3 doses or more)[f] | 29 | 65 | 82 | 83 | 84 | - | - | 79 | 82 | 86 | - | - | 86 | 84 | 83 |
| Varicella[g] | - | - | 9 | 21 | 42 | - | - | 3 | 16 | 40 | - | - | 13 | 27 | 44 |
| **Hispanic[h]** | | | | | | | | | | | | | | | |
| Combined series (4:3:1:3)[a] | 62 | 69 | 71 | 72 | 75 | - | 65 | 68 | 71 | 73 | - | 72 | 74 | 77 | 79 |
| Combined series (4:3:1)[b] | 68 | 72 | 73 | 74 | 77 | - | - | 70 | 72 | 76 | - | - | 75 | 77 | 80 |
| DTP (4 doses or more)[c] | 70 | 75 | 77 | 77 | 81 | - | - | 73 | 75 | 79 | - | - | 79 | 80 | 83 |
| Polio (3 doses or more) | 81 | 87 | 89 | 90 | 89 | - | - | 88 | 89 | 90 | - | - | 90 | 90 | 90 |
| Measles-containing[d] | 88 | 88 | 88 | 88 | 91 | - | - | 88 | 86 | 91 | - | - | 89 | 89 | 93 |
| Hib (3 doses or more)[e] | 84 | 90 | 89 | 90 | 92 | - | - | 88 | 89 | 92 | - | - | 90 | 92 | 94 |
| Hepatitis B (3 doses or more)[f] | 33 | 69 | 80 | 81 | 86 | - | - | 79 | 79 | 83 | - | - | 82 | 84 | 88 |
| Varicella[g] | - | - | 8 | 22 | 47 | - | - | 6 | 18 | 44 | - | - | 11 | 25 | 48 |

- = not available

[a]The 4:3:1:3 combined series consists of 4 doses of diphtheria and tetanus toxoids and pertussis vaccine (DTP), 3 doses of polio vaccine, 1 dose of a measles-containing vaccine (MCV), and 3 doses of *Haemophilus influenzae* type b (Hib) vaccine.

[b]The 4:3:1 combined series consists of 4 doses of diphtheria and tetanus toxoids and pertussis vaccine (DTP), 3 doses of polio vaccine, and 1 dose of a measles-containing vaccine (MCV).

[c]Diphtheria and tetanus toxoids and pertussis vaccine.

[d]Respondents were asked about measles-containing vaccine, including MMR (measles-mumps-rubella) vaccine.

[e]*Haemophilus influenzae* type b (Hib) vaccine.

[f]The percentage of children 19 to 35 months of age who received 3 doses of hepatitis B vaccine was low in 1994, because universal infant vaccination with a 3-dose series was not recommended until November 1991.

[g]Recommended in July 1996. Administered on or after the first birthday.

[h]Persons of Hispanic origin may be of any race.

*Source*: Federal Interagency Forum on Child and Family Statistics. *America's Children: Key National Indicators of Well-Being, 2000.* Federal Interagency Forum on Child and Family Statistics (Washington, DC: U.S. Government Printing Office, 2000). http://www.childstats.gov/ac2000/ac00.asp.

## Table I4.2. Vaccination Coverage Levels among Children Aged 19–35 Months, by Selected Vaccines—National Immunization Survey, United States, 1995–1999

| Vaccine/Dose | 1995* % | 1995* (95% CI††) | 1996† % | 1996† (95% CI) | 1997§ % | 1997§ (95% CI) | 1998¶ % | 1998¶ (95% CI) | 1999** % | 1999** (95% CI) |
|---|---|---|---|---|---|---|---|---|---|---|
| DTP§§ | | | | | | | | | | |
| 3 Doses | 94.7 | (±0.6) | 95.0 | (±0.4) | 95.5 | (±0.4) | 95.6 | (±0.5) | 95.9 | (±0.4) |
| 4 Doses | 78.5 | (±1.0) | 81.1 | (±0.7) | 81.5 | (±0.7) | 83.9 | (±0.8) | 83.3 | (±0.8) |
| Poliovirus | | | | | | | | | | |
| 3 Doses | 87.9 | (±0.8) | 91.1 | (±0.5) | 90.8 | (±0.5) | 90.8 | (±0.7) | 89.6 | (±0.6) |
| Hib¶¶ | | | | | | | | | | |
| 3 Doses | 91.7 | (±0.6) | 91.7 | (±0.5) | 92.7 | (±0.5) | 93.4 | (±0.6) | 93.5 | (±0.5) |
| MMR*** | | | | | | | | | | |
| 1 Dose | 87.8 | (±0.7) | 90.7 | (±0.5) | 90.5 | (±0.7) | 92.0 | (±0.6) | 91.5 | (±0.6) |
| Hepatitis B | | | | | | | | | | |
| 3 Doses | 68.0 | (±1.0) | 81.8 | (±0.7) | 83.7 | (±0.6) | 87.0 | (±0.7) | 88.1 | (±0.7) |
| Varicella | | | | | | | | | | |
| 1 Dose | NA††† | | NA | | 25.9 | (±0.7) | 43.2 | (±1.0) | 59.4 | (±1.0) |
| Combined series | | | | | | | | | | |
| 4 DTP/3 Polio/1 MCV§§§ | 76.2 | (±1.0) | 78.4 | (±0.8) | 77.9 | (±0.7) | 80.6 | (±0.9) | 79.9 | (±0.8) |
| 4 DTP/3 Polio/1 MCV/3 Hib¶¶¶ | 74.2 | (±1.0) | 76.5 | (±0.8) | 76.2 | (±0.8) | 79.2 | (±0.9) | 78.4 | (±0.9) |

* Children in this survey period were born during February 1992–May 1994.
†Children in this survey period were born during February 1993–May 1995.
§Children in this survey period were born during February 1994–May 1996.
¶Children in this survey period were born during February 1995–May 1997.
** Children in this survey period were born during February 1996–May 1998.
††Confidence interval.
§§Includes diphtheria and tetanus toxoids and pertussis vaccine (DTP), diphtheria and tetanus toxoids (DT), and diphtheria and tetanus toxoids and a cellular pertussis vaccine.
¶¶*Haemophilus influenzae* type b vaccine (Hib).
*** Previous reports of vaccination coverage were for measles-containing vaccine (MCV); the above reflects coverage with measles-mumps-rubella vaccine (MMR).
†††Data not available in this reporting period. Data collection for varicella vaccine began July 1996.
§§§Four doses of DTP/DT, three doses of poliovirus vaccine, and one dose of MCV.
¶¶¶Four doses of DTP/DT, three doses of poliovirus vaccine, one dose of MCV, and three doses of Hib.
*Source*: Center for Disease Control and Prevention. U.S. Department of Health and Human Services. "National, State and Urban Area Vaccination Coverage Levels Among Children Aged 19–35 Months—United States, 1999." *MMWR: Morbidity and Mortality Weekly Review* 49 no. 26 (April 2, 1999). http://www.cdc.gov/mmwr/PDF/wk/mm4926.pdf.

## Table I5.1. Overall Immunization Coverage Rates for Countries, Grouped by Region, 1991–1997

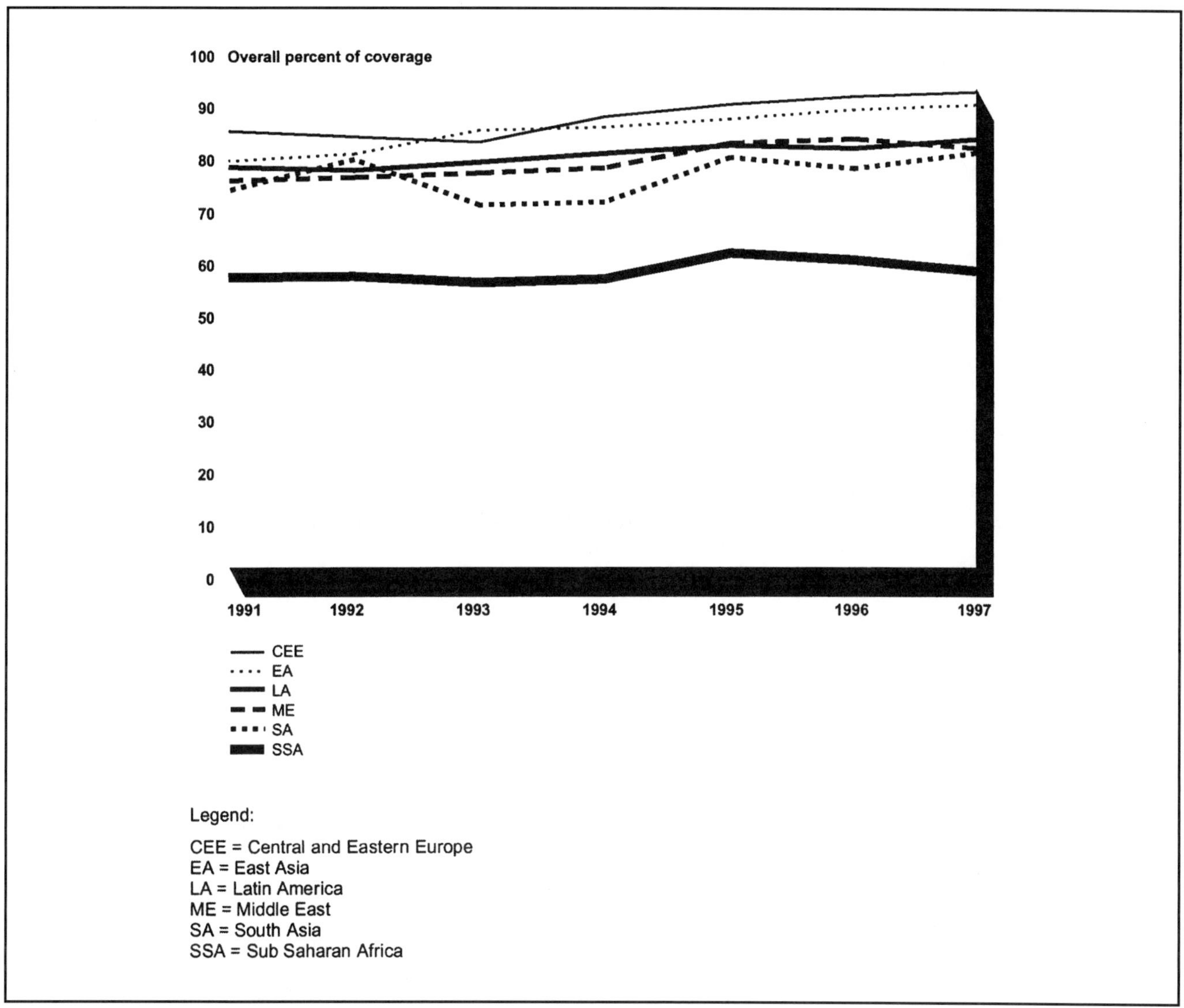


Note: Immunization coverage for diphtheria, measles, pertussis, tetanus, tuberculosis, and polio.

*Source*: General Accounting Office. *Global Health: Factors Contributing to Low Vaccination Rates in Developing Countries* (Washington, DC: U.S. General Accounting Office, 1999). http://www.gao.gov/archive/2000/ns00004.pdf.

## Table I5.2. Immunization Coverage Rates in the Poorest Countries, with and without Conflict, 1991–1997

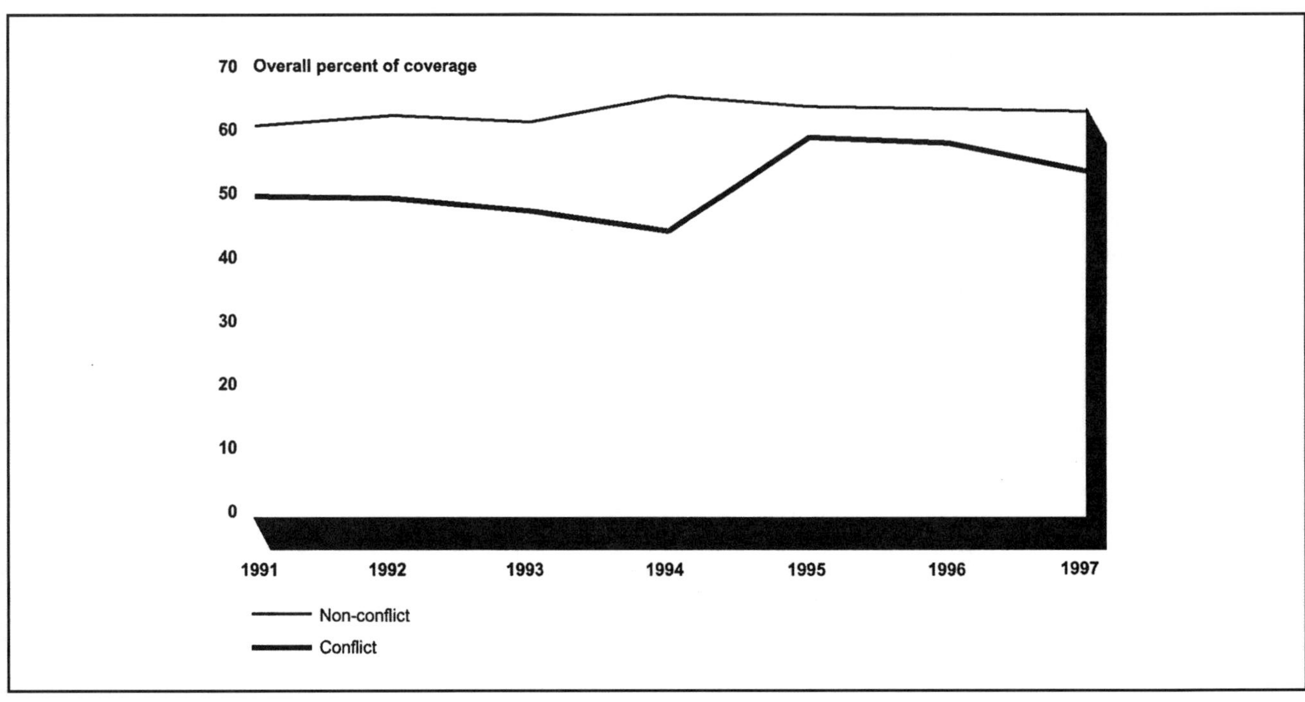


Note: Immunization coverage for diphtheria, measles, pertussis, tetanus, tuberculosis, and polio.
*Source*: General Accounting Office. *Global Health: Factors Contributing to Low Vaccination Rates in Developing Countries* (Washington, DC: U.S. General Accounting Office, 1999). http://www.gao.gov/archive/2000/ns00004.pdf.

## Table I5.3. Immunization Coverage Rates for Measles and Tuberculosis in sub-Saharan Africa, 1991–1997

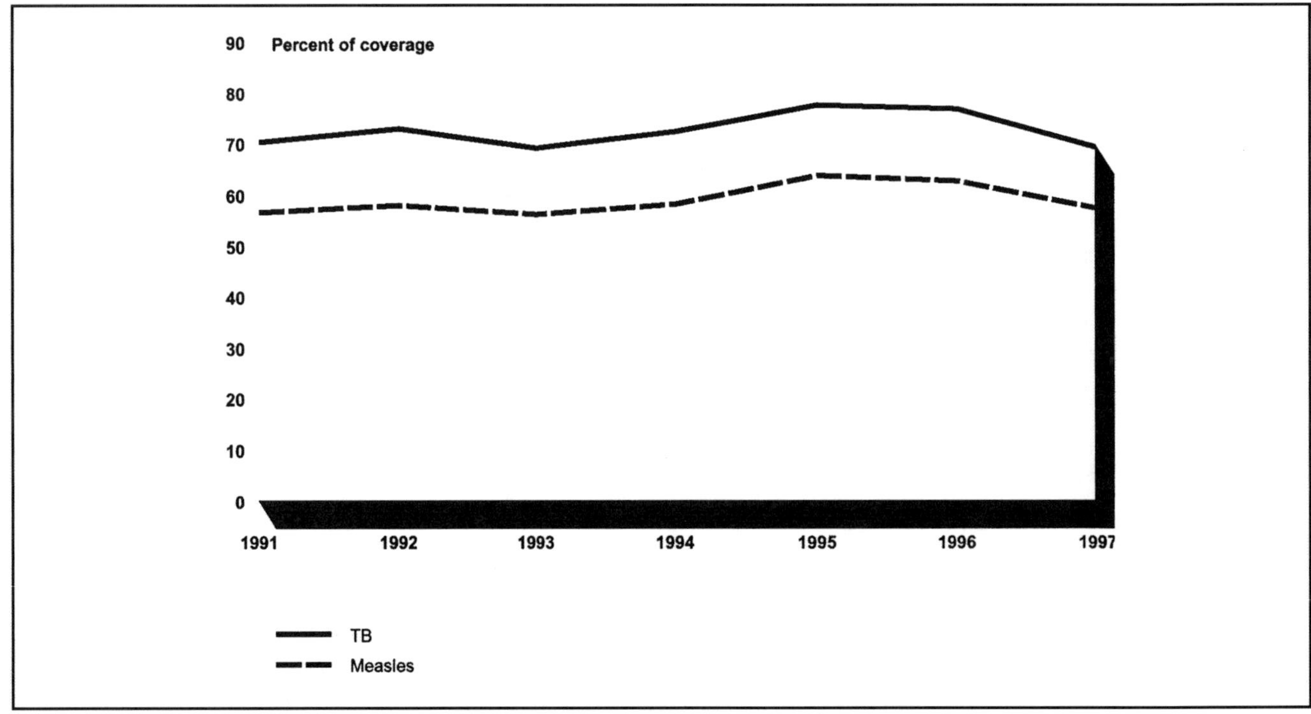


*Source*: General Accounting Office. *Global Health: Factors Contributing to Low Vaccination Rates in Developing Countries* (Washington, DC: U.S. General Accounting Office, 1999). http://www.gao.gov/archive/2000/ns00004.pdf.

**Table I6. UNICEF Expenditures on Immunization, 1990–1998**

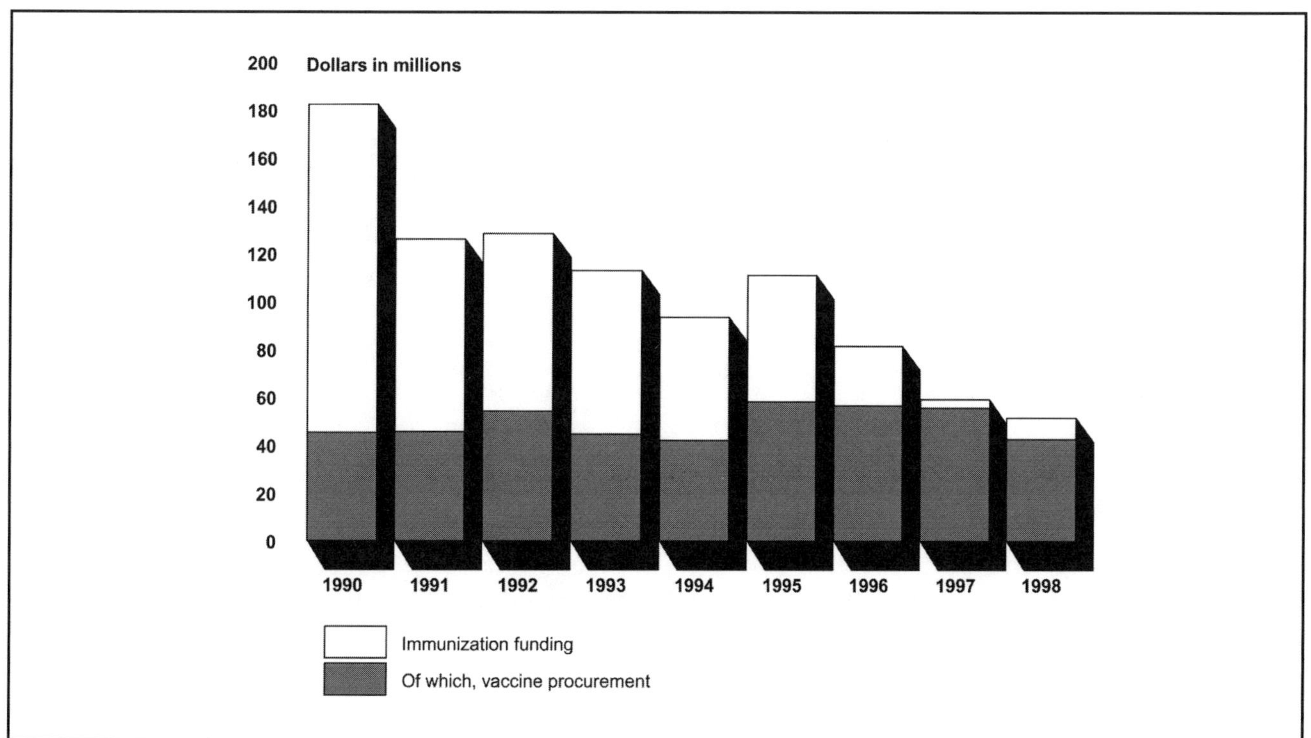


Note: Expenditures are in constant 1997 dollars (in millions). UNICEF officials note that recent data coding changes may slightly increase the spending totals for 1997 and 1998.

*Source*: General Accounting Office. *Global Health: Factors Contributing to Low Vaccination Rates in Developing Countries* (Washington, DC: U.S. General Accounting Office, 1999). http://www.gao.gov/archive/2000/ns00004.pdf.

# J. Infectious Disease Elimination and Eradication

## OVERVIEW

The declaration in 1980 by the Thirty-third World Health Assembly that smallpox had been eradicated globally reawakened interest in disease elimination and eradication as a public health strategy. Ten years later, the World Health Organization (WHO) inaugurated the Polio Eradication Initiative; and by the end of the century, the world was on the brink of eradicating this disease forever. In early 2000 Dr. Gro Harlem Brundtland, Director General of WHO, noted that three major areas of the world were polio-free: Europe, the Americas, and the Western Pacific Region, which includes China. Had the initiative not been launched, he maintained, 3 million children who today can walk and play might otherwise have been crippled with polio.[1] WHO launched the Final Push for Polio Eradication, billed as "Every Child Counts," in January 2000. At that time only 30 polio-infected countries remained, five of which were in Asia. Currently, WHO has officially targeted seven infectious diseases endemic in the developing world for global eradication: Chagas disease, dracunculiasis (Guinea worm disease), leprosy, lymphatic filariasis, measles, onchocerciasis, and polio.

An understanding of disease control helps set the stage for understanding of disease eradication and elimination. Disease control refers to the reduction of disease incidence, prevalence, morbidity, or mortality to a locally acceptable level as a result of deliberate efforts; continued intervention measures are required to maintain the reduction. Control measures usually depend on routine services being instituted and maintained in a long-term perspective.

Evolving naturally from disease control, the ultimate goals of public health are elimination, eradication, and extinction. The elimination of disease refers to the reduction to zero of the incidence of a specified disease in a defined geographical area as a result of deliberate efforts; continued intervention measures are required. Disease elimination is contrasted to the elimination of infections—the reduction to zero of the incidence of infection caused by a specific agent in a defined geographical area as a result of deliberate efforts; continued measures to prevent re-establishment of transmission are required.

In contrast to elimination, eradication has been defined as extinction of the disease pathogen[2]; as elimination of the occurrence of a given disease, even in the absence of all preventive measures[3]; as control of an infection to the point at which transmission ceases within a specified area[4]; and as reduction of the worldwide incidence of a disease to zero as a result of deliberate efforts, obviating the necessity for further control measures[5]. Eradication activities are characterized as time-limited, often intensive, targeted, and organized in circumscribed programs with campaign elements as prominent features. In general, strategies for disease control, elimination, and eradication are derived primarily from the epidemiological characteristics of the disease, the intervention available, the logistical requirements, and the resource needs.

Finally, disease extinction occurs when the specific infectious agent no longer exists in nature or in the laboratory; to date, there are no examples of extinction.

## DISEASE CONTROL AND ELIMINATION

Progress toward disease elimination or eradication is attributable to several factors. First among these are efforts by U.S. and international public health authorities to enhance surveillance for individual diseases, to investigate disease outbreaks, and to design and implement preventive measures. Today information on diagnosis, treatment, and prevention of individual diseases is more widely available to public health authorities worldwide than it was in the past. The fact that the public is better educated about preventive measures also contributes to progress toward disease elimination or eradication. Ongoing campaigns designed to eliminate or eradicate the individual disease have also helped progress. Partners, peace, and a mobilized and confident workforce are critical to the success of these campaigns. Funding is also key to these efforts; toward this end, and as important as the contributions of advocates, health workers, and volunteers, are individual donors and donor companies, foundations, and state, local, national, and international governments.

## THE DISEASES

**Chagas Disease** Also called American trypanosomiasis, Chagas disease is an infection caused by the parasite *Trypanosoma cruzi*. Reduviid bugs, or "kissing bugs," live in cracks and holes of substandard housing found in South and Central America. Insects become infected after biting an animal or person who already has Chagas disease. Infection is spread to humans when an infected bug deposits feces on a person's skin, usually while the person is sleeping at night. The person accidentally rubs the feces into the bite wound, an open cut, the eyes, or the mouth. Chagas disease primarily affects low-income people living in rural areas. Many people get infection during childhood. The early stage of infection usually is not severe, but sometimes it can cause death, particularly in infants. However, in about one-third of those who get the infection, chronic symptoms develop after 10–20 years. For these persons who develop chronic symptoms, life expectancy decreases by an average of 9 years.

**Dracunculiasis** More commonly known as Guinea worm disease, dracunculiasis is caused by the parasite *Dracunculus medinensis*. Infection affects poor communities in remote parts of Africa that do not have safe water to drink. People get infected with Guinea worm disease by drinking water contaminated with Dracunculus larvae. In the water, the larvae are swallowed by small copepods, "water fleas." The worms mature inside the water flea and become infective in about 10 days. Once the worms have matured inside the water flea, any person who swallows contaminated water becomes infected. Once inside the body, the stomach acid digests the water flea, but not the Guinea worm. For the next year, the Guinea worm then grows to a full-size adult. Adult worms can grow up to 3 feet long and are as wide as a spaghetti noodle. After a year, the worm will migrate to the surface of the body. As the worm migrates, a blister develops on the skin where the worm will emerge. This blister will eventually rupture, causing a very painful burning sensation. For relief, persons will immerse the affected skin into water. The temperature change causes the blister to erupt, exposing the worm. When someone with a Guinea worm ulcer enters the water, the adult female emerges from the wound and releases a milky white liquid containing millions of immature worms into the water, thus contaminating the water supply.

Infected persons usually do not have symptoms until about 1 year after they drink contaminated water. A few days to hours before the worm emerges, the person may develop a fever, swelling, and pain in the area. More than 90% of the worms appear on the legs and feet, but may occur anywhere on the body. Without medical care, ulcers may take many weeks to heal, often becoming infected. This causes disabling complications, such as locked joints or permanent crippling. Each time a worm emerges, the victim is often unable to work and resume daily activities for an average of 3 months.

**Leprosy** Leprosy, caused by a bacillus, *Mycobacterium leprae*, is transmitted via droplets from the nose and mouth during close and frequent contacts with untreated, infected persons. It is not highly infectious. *M. leprae* multiples very slowly, and the incubation period of the disease is about five years. Symptoms can take as long as 20 years to appear. Leprosy mainly affects the skin and nerves. If untreated, there can be progressive and permanent damage to the skin, nerves, limbs, and eyes. Treatment provided in the early stages averts disability.

**Lymphatic Filariasis** Lymphatic filariasis is a parasitic disease caused by microscopic, thread-like worms. The adult worms live only in the human lymph system. The disease spreads from person to person by mosquito bites. When a mosquito bites a person who has lymphatic filariasis, microscopic worms circulating in the person's blood enter and infect the mosquito, which, in turn, infects other people it bites. Many mosquito bites over several months are needed to get lymphatic filariasis. People living or staying for a long time in tropical or subtropical areas where the disease is common are at the greatest risk for infection.

The disease is usually not life threatening, but it can permanently damage the lymph system and kidneys. Because the lymph system does not work properly, fluid collects and causes swelling in the arms, breasts, legs, and for men, the genital area. The swelling and the decreased function of the lymph system make it difficult for the body to fight germs and infections, resulting in increased bacterial infections in the skin and lymph system. This causes hardening and thickening of the skin, which is called elephantiasis. Lymphatic filariasis is a leading cause of permanent and long-term disability worldwide. People with the disease can suffer pain, disfigurement, and sexual disability.

**Measles** A highly contagious viral illness that occurs throughout the world, measles is caused by a paramyxovirus, genus *Morbillivirus*. Measles transmission is primarily person to person via large respiratory droplets. Measles is highly communicable, with >90% secondary attack rates among susceptible persons. Measles may be transmitted from 4 days prior to 4 days after rash onset. The incubation period of measles, from exposure to prodrome, averages 10–12 days. From exposure to rash onset averages 14 days. The prodrome lasts 2–4 days. It is characterized by fever, which increases in stepwise fashion, often peaking as high as 103° to 105°; cough, or coryza (runny nose), or conjunctivitis; and Koplik spots. The measles rash is a maculopapular eruption that usually lasts 5–6 days. Other symptoms of measles include anorexia, diarrhea, especially in infants, and generalized lymphadenopathy.

**Onchocerciasis** Onchocerciasis is caused by *Onchocerca volvulus*, a parasitic worm that lives for up to 14 years in the human body. Each adult female worm, thin but more than ½ meter in length, produces millions of microfilariae (microscopic larvae) that migrate throughout the body and give rise to a variety of symptoms: serious visual impairment, including blindness; rashes, lesions, intense itching, and depigmentation of the skin; lymphadenitis, which results in hanging groins and elephantiasis of the genitals; and general debilitation. Onchocerciasis manifestations begin to occur in infected persons 1 to 3 years after the injection of infective larvae. Microfilariae produced in one person are carried to another by the blackfly.

The world's second leading infectious cause of blindness, onchocerciasis is present in 36 countries of Africa, the Arabian peninsula and the Americas. As a public health problem the disease is most closely associated with Africa, where it constitutes a serious obstacle to socioeconomic development. Onchocerciasis is often called "river blindness" because of its most extreme manifestation and because the blackfly vector abounds in fertile riverside areas, which frequently remain uninhabited for fear of infection.

**Poliomyelitis** Poliovirus is a member of the enterovirus subgroup, family *Picornaviridae*. Person-to-person spread of poliovirus via the fecal-oral route is the most important route of transmission, although the oral-oral route may account for some cases. The incubation period for poliomyelitis is commonly 6–20 days, with a range of from 3 to 35 days. The response to poliovirus infection is highly variable and has been categorized based on the severity of clinical presentation. Up to 95% of all polio infections are inapparent or subclinical without symptoms. Approximately 4%–8% of polio infections consist of a minor, nonspecific illness without clinical or laboratory evidence of central nervous system invasion. This syndrome, known as abortive poliomyelitis, is characterized by complete recovery in less than a week. Nonparalytic aseptic meningitis (symptoms of stiffness of the neck, back, and/or legs), usually following several days after a prodrome similar to that of minor illness, occurs in 1%–2% of polio infections. Increased or abnormal sensations can also occur. Typically these symptoms will last from 2 to 10 days, followed by complete recovery. Less than 2% of all polio infections result in flaccid paralysis. Paralytic symptoms generally begin 1–10 days after prodromal (early) symptoms and progress for 2–3 days. Generally, no further paralysis occurs after the temperature returns to normal. Many persons with paralytic poliomyelitis recover completely, and muscle function returns to some degree in most. Patients with weakness or paralysis 12 months after onset will usually be left with permanent residua.

**Smallpox** Variola virus is the etiological agent of smallpox. During the smallpox era, the only known reservoir for the virus was humans; no known animal or insect reservoirs or vectors existed. The most frequent mode of transmission was person to person, spread through direct deposit of infective droplets onto the nasal, oral, or pharyngeal mucosal membranes or the alveoli of the lungs from close, face-to-face contact with an infectious person. Indirect spread (i.e., not requiring face-to-face contact with an infectious person) through fine-particle aerosols or a fomite (any substance that adheres to and transmits infectious material) containing the virus was less common. Symptoms of smallpox begin 12–14 days after exposure. Two to three days before the eruption of the characteristic rash, the victim experiences high fever, malaise, and severe headache and backache. This preeruptive stage is followed by the appearance of a maculopapular rash that progresses to papules 1–2 days after the rash appears; the appearance of vesicles, pustules, and scab lesions follow. As the skin lesions heal, the scabs separate and pitted scarring gradually develops. Smallpox patients are most infectious during the first week of the rash, when the oral mucosa lesions ulcerate and release substantial amounts of virus into the saliva. A patient is no longer infectious after all scabs have separated.

## TABLE OVERVIEW

**J1.1–J1.2. Target Dates and Cost of Eradication** The first table in this cluster summarizes the goals and estimated cost of eradication or elimination of the seven diseases targeted by the World Health Organization. The second table summarizes U.S. spending for the eradication of these diseases for fiscal 1997, the latest year for which figures are available.

**J2.1–J2.7. Diseases Targeted for Elimination or Eradication** The tables in this cluster summarize epidemiological data for those diseases targeted for elimination or eradication: Chagas' disease (*Trypanosoma cruzi*), dracunculiasis, leprosy, measles, and poliomyelitis. International data is not available for lymphatic filariasis and onchoceriasis. The cluster also includes historical data on smallpox.

## NOTES

1. "Final Push for Polio Eradication in Year 2000—Every Child Counts." Dr. Gro Harlem Brundtland, New Delhi, India, 6 January 2000.
2. T.A. Cockburn, "Eradication of Infectious Diseases." *Science* 133 no. 3458 (Apr. 7, 1961): 1050–1058.
3. F.L. Soper, "Problems to Be Solved if the Eradication of Tuberculosis Is to Be Realized," *American Journal of Public Health* 52 (1962): 734–745.
4. J.M. Andrews and A.D. Langmuir, "The Philosophy of Disease Eradication," *American Journal of Public Health* 53 (1963): 1–6.
5. CDC, "Recommendations of the International Task Force for Disease Eradication," *Morbidity and Mortality Weekly Report* 42, no. RR-16 (1993): 1–38.

## Table J1.1. WHO Estimated Target Dates and Costs for Eradicating or Eliminating Selected Diseases as of December 1997

| Disease | Goal | Target date | Estimate cost* ($ million) |
|---|---|---|---|
| Dracunculiasis | Eradication | 2011** | $40 |
| Polio | Eradication | 2000*** | $1,600 |
| Leprosy | Elimination | 2000 | $225 |
| Measles | Eradication | 2010 | $4,900 |
| Onchocarciasis | Elimination | 2010 | $143 |
| Changas' disease | Elimination | 2010 | $391 |
| Lymphatic filariasis | Elimination | 2030 | $228 |
| | | | |
| *These costs represent projected public expenditures by national governments and donor countries for eradication or elimination campaigns. Costs are in 1997 dollars. | | | |
| **WHO expects that all but two countries will be free of dracunculiasis by 2005 | | | |
| ***Certification is expected by 2005 | | | |

*Source*: United States General Accounting Office, *Infectious Diseases: Soundness of World Health Organization Estimates for Eradication or Elimination* (Washington, DC: General Accounting Office, 1998).

## Table J1.2. U.S. Spending on Diseases to Be Eradicated or Eliminated, Fiscal Year 1997

| Disease | Domestic programs ($ millions) | )verseas programs ($ millions) | Total ($ millions) |
|---|---|---|---|
| Dracunculiasis | 0 | 0.7 | 0.7 |
| Polio | 230 | 74.2 | $304 |
| Leprosy | 20 | 0 | $20 |
| Measles | 50 | 11.7 | $62 |
| Onchocarciasis | 0 | 3.5 | $4 |
| Changas' disease | 0 | 0.4 | $0 |
| Lymphatic filariasis | 0 | 0.6 | $1 |
| **Total** | **300** | **91.1** | **391.1** |

*Source*: United States General Accounting Office, *Infectious Diseases: Soundness of World Health Organization Estimates for Eradication or Elimination*. (Washington, DC: General Accounting Office, 1998).

**Table J2.1. Human Infection by *Trypanosoma cruzi* and Reduction of Incidence, Southern Cone Initiative, 1983–1999**

| Country | Age group (Years) | Infection in 1983 (Rates x 100) | Infection in 1999 (Rates x 100) | Reduction of Incidence (%) |
|---|---|---|---|---|
| Argentina | 18 | 4.5 | 1.2 | 85.0 |
| Brazil | 7-14 | 18.5 | 0.17 | 96.0 |
| Bolivia | 1-4 | 33.9 | ND | ND |
| Chile | 0-10 | 5.4 | 0.14 | 99.0 |
| Paraguay | 18 | 9.3 | 3.9 | 60.0 |
| Uruguay | 6-12 | 2.5 | 0.06 | 99.0 |

*Source*: World Health Organization, *Chagas* (Web site). ttp://www.who.int/ctd/chagas/epidemio.htm.

**Table J2.2. Dracunculiasis, Recent Epidemiological Data**

| Year | 1992 | 1993 | 1994 | 1995 | 1996 | 1997 | 1998 | 1999** |
|---|---|---|---|---|---|---|---|---|
| Country | | | | | | | | |
| Benin | 4315 | 16334 | 4302 | 2273 | 1427 | 855 | 695* | 492 |
| Burkina Faso | 11784 | 8281 | 6861 | 6281 | 3241 | 1898 | 2227 | 2160 |
| Cameroon | 127 | 72 | 30 | 15 | 17 | 19* | 23* | 8* |
| CAR | 0 | 0 | 1 | 18 | 9 | 5 | 34 | 10* |
| Chad | 156 | 1231 | 640 | 149 | 127 | 25 | 3 | 1* |
| Côte d'Ivoire | 0 | 8034 | 5061 | 3801 | 2794 | 1254 | 1414* | 485 |
| India | 1081 | 755 | 371 | 60 | 9 | 0 | 0 | 0 |
| Kenya | 0 | 35 | 53 | 23 | 0 | 6* | 7* | 1* |
| Mali | 16024 | 12011 | 5581 | 4218 | 2402 | 1099 | 650* | 405 |
| Mauritania | 1557 | 5882 | 5029 | 1762 | 562 | 388 | 379* | 214 |
| Niger | 32829 | 25346 | 18562 | 13821 | 2956 | 3030 | 2700* | 1920 |
| Nigeria | 183169 | 75752 | 39774 | 16374 | 12282 | 12590 | 13420* | 13237 |
| Togo | 8179 | 10349 | 5044 | 2073 | 1626 | 1762 | 2128* | 1589 |
| Uganda | 126369 | 42852 | 10425 | 4810 | 1455 | 1374 | 1061* | 321 |
| Yemen | 0 | 0 | 106 | 82 | 62 | 7 | 0 | 0 |
| Ethiopia | 303 | 1120 | 1252 | 514 | 371 | 451 | 365* | 247 |
| Ghana | 33464 | 17918 | 8432 | 8894 | 4877 | 8921 | 5473* | 9027 |
| Senegal | 728 | 815 | 195 | 76 | 19 | 4 | 0 | 0 |
| Sudan | 2447 | 2984 | 53271 | 64608 | 118578 | 43596 | 47997* | 59860 |
| Pakistan | 23 | 2 | 0 | 0 | 0 | 0 | 0 | 0 |
| TOTAL | 422555 | 229773 | 164990 | 129852 | 152814 | 77863 | 78557* | 89966* |

* Including imported cases.

** Provisional data, based on reports received through December, 1999.

*Source*: World Health, Organization, *Dracunculiasis* (Web site). http://www.wHO.int/ctd/dracun/epidemio.htm.

## Table J2.3. Registered Prevalence of Leprosy and Detection Rate in the Top 11 Endemic Countries, Start of 2000[a]

| Country | Registered Cases at start of 2000 | Prevalence per 10 000 | New cases detected during 1999 | Detection rate per 100 000 population |
|---|---|---|---|---|
| India | 495 073 | 5.0 | 537 956 | 54.3 |
| Brazil (b) | 78 068 | 4.3 | 42 055 | 25.9 |
| Myanmar | 28 404 | 5.9 | 30 479 | 62.9 |
| Indonesia | 23 156 | 1.1 | 17 477 | 8.3 |
| Nepal | 13 572 | 5.7 | 18 693 | 78.7 |
| Madagascar | 7 865 | 4.7 | 8 704 | 51.6 |
| Ethiopia(b) | 7 764 | 1.3 | 4 457 | 7.4 |
| Mozambique | 7 403 | 3.9 | 5 488 | 28.7 |
| Congo DR(b) | 5 031 | 1.0 | 4 221 | 8.6 |
| Tanzania | 4 701 | 1.4 | 5 081 | 15.4 |
| Guinea | 1 559 | 2.0 | 2 475 | 32.0 |
| **Total** | **672 596** | **4.1** | **677 086** | **41.7** |

a)The top 11 endemic countries included in the above table have the following characteristics: (i) they have a prevalence of 1 or more than 1 in 10 000 population, and (ii) the number of prevalent leprosy cases is more than 5 000, or the number of newly detected cases is more than 2 000.

b)1999 information

Last Update: 14 December 2000

*Source*: World Health Organization., *The most endemic countries in 2000* (Web site). http://www.who.int/lep/l3.htm.

## Table J2.4. Measles Global Annual Reported Incidence, 1980–1999

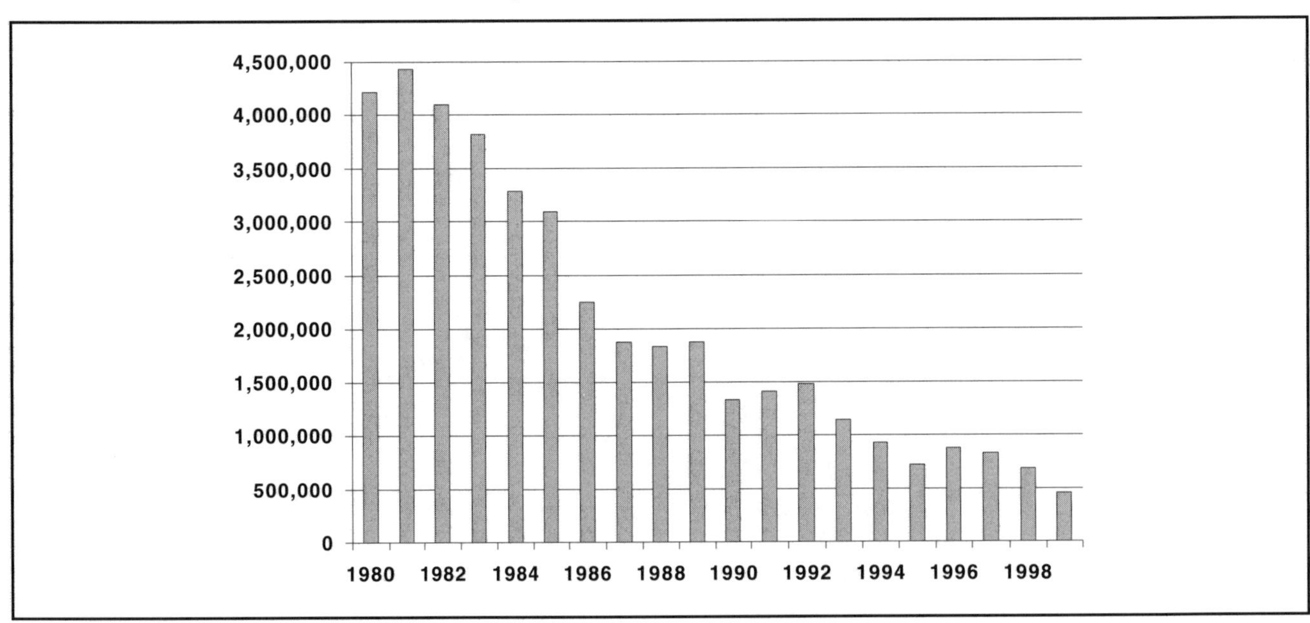


*Source*: World Health Organization, Department of Vaccines and Biologicals, *WHO Vaccine Preventable Diseases: Monitoring System 2000 Global Summary* (Geneva: World Health Organization, 2000). Available on the Internet at http://www.who.int/vaccines-documents/GlobalSummary/GlobalSummary.pdf.

## Table J2.5. Polio Global Annual Reported Incidence, 1980–1999

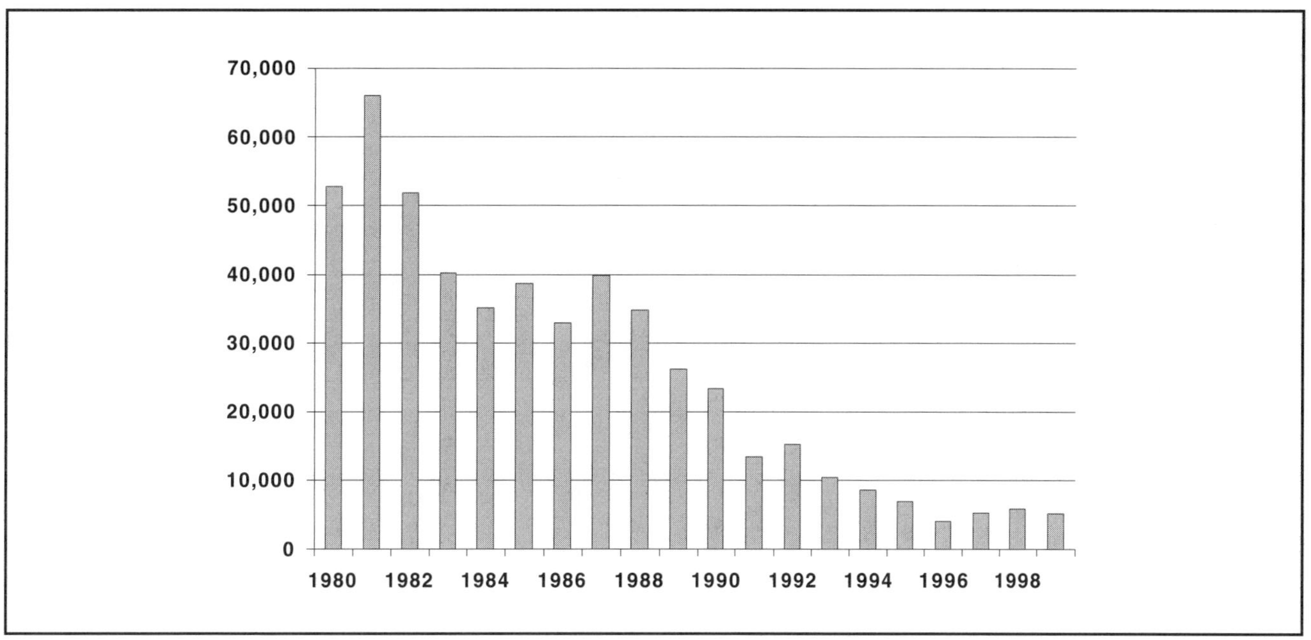


*Source*: World Health Organization, Department of Vaccines and Biologicals, *WHO Vaccine Preventable Diseases: Monitoring System 2000 Global Summary* (Geneva: World Health Organization, 2000). Available on the Internet at http://www.who.int/vaccines-documents/GlobalSummary/GlobalSummary.pdf.

## Table J2.6. Smallpox Cases in the United States, 1920–1950

| Year | Number of Cases | Number of Deaths |
|---|---|---|
| 1920 | 102 128 | 498 |
| 1921 | 102 787 | 620 |
| 1922 | 33 378 | 607 |
| 1923 | 30 907 | 126 |
| 1924 | 56 591 | 871 |
| 1925 | 39 572 | 707 |
| 1926 | 33 732 | 376 |
| 1927 | 37 600 | 138 |
| 1928 | 39 396 | 129 |
| 1929 | 42 282 | 137 |
| 1930 | 48 907 | 165 |
| 1931 | 30 233 | 93 |
| 1932 | 11 224 | 38 |
| 1933 | 6 491 | 39 |
| 1934 | 5 371 | 24 |
| 1935 | 7 957 | 25 |
| 1936 | 7 834 | 35 |
| 1937 | 11 673 | 34 |
| 1938 | 14 939 | 48 |
| 1939 | 9 877 | 41 |
| 1940 | 2 795 | 14 |
| 1941 | 1 396 | 12 |
| 1942 | 865 | 2 |
| 1943 | 765 | 8 |
| 1944 | 397 | 9 |
| 1945 | 346 | 12 |
| 1946 | 337 | 25 |
| 1947 | 176 | 5 |
| 1948 | 57 | 5 |
| 1949 | 49 | 2 |
| 1950 | 39 | 0 |

*Source*: Jack W. Hopkins, *The Eradication of Smallpox: Organizational Learning and Innovation in Health* (Boulder: Westview Press, 1989).

## Table J2.7. Smallpox Cases Reported in World, by Year, 1920–1979

| | Cases |
|---|---|
| 1920 | 401,318 |
| 1921 | 303,850 |
| 1922 | 190,159 |
| 1923 | 174,799 |
| 1924 | 186,354 |
| 1925 | 284,845 |
| 1926 | 324,125 |
| 1927 | 327,289 |
| 1928 | 272,529 |
| 1929 | 267,322 |
| 1930 | 360,575 |
| 1931 | 182,829 |
| 1932 | 211,274 |
| 1933 | 328,212 |
| 1934 | 327,373 |
| 1935 | 331,151 |
| 1936 | 263,579 |
| 1937 | 149,184 |
| 1938 | 144,042 |
| 1939 | 186,393 |
| 1940 | 235,820 |
| 1941 | 195,863 |
| 1942 | 124,504 |
| 1943 | 210,358 |
| 1944 | 407,525 |
| 1945 | 405,833 |
| 1946 | 302,694 |
| 1947 | 163,375 |
| 1948 | 161,893 |
| 1949 | 632,858 |
| 1950 | 426,006 |
| 1951 | 554,756 |
| 1952 | 167,085 |
| 1953 | 94,135 |
| 1954 | 99,232 |
| 1955 | 91,823 |
| 1956 | 96,089 |
| 1957 | 156,652 |
| 1958 | 280,475 |
| 1959 | 96,270 |
| 1960 | 67,148 |
| 1961 | 90,555 |
| 1962 | 98,757 |
| 1963 | 133,504 |
| 1964 | 76,198 |
| 1965 | 122,280 |
| 1966 | 92,799 |
| 1967 | 131,697 |
| 1968 | 80,024 |
| 1969 | 54,202 |

*Source*: World Health Organization, *The Global Eradication of Smallpox: Final Report of the Global Commission for the Certification of Smallpox Eradication* (Geneva): World Health Organization, December 1979.

# K. Bioterrorism and Biological Warfare

## OVERVIEW

An intentional attack with a biological agent, bioterrorism is one of the most formidable of the growing roster of emerging infectious diseases. Prior to September 11, 2001, the clandestine release of infectious agents and the specter of biological weapons use were considered little more than theoretical possibilities. On September 11, 2001, however, the United States was attacked with, as President George W. Bush noted, "deliberate and massive cruelty."[1] Images of fire, ashes, and bent steel were seen worldwide. The attacks were followed by anthrax mailings over the course of the fall.

Today the clandestine release of infectious agents and the specter of biological weapons use constitute a public health threat of enormous magnitude. Today bioterrorism and bioweapons constitute new and increasingly critical policy priorities for public health and medical communities worldwide. Note that as recently as 1998 the U. S. Federal Bureau of Investigation (FBI) issued some statistics that appear to indicate a trend towards greater use of nuclear, biological, and chemical weapons.[2] For these reasons, and although surveillance of bioterrorism has only recently begun at the federal level, and that data on this phenomenon are few, this *Handbook* would be incomplete without discussion of bioterrorism. Discussion includes a review of recent events, definitions of key terms, overview of diagnostic challenges, facts about two critical agents[3] that remain in the media spotlight, and concludes with a review of the status of surveillance and prevention.

**Recent Events** Recent events in the United States, Iraq, Japan, and Russia, cast an ominous shadow and are proof that large scale bioterrorism could happen.

In the fall of 2001, anthrax mailings in the United States raised the public's awareness of health threats arising from exposure to biological agents. As of November 14, 2001, a total of 22 cases of anthrax has met the Centers for Disease Control and Prevention case definition;[4] 10 were confirmed inhalational anthrax, and 12 (seven confirmed and five suspected) were cutaneous anthrax.[5] Confirmed anthrax cases[6] include workers at American Media, Inc., Boca Raton, FL; NBC, ABC and CBS in Manhattan; West Trenton, New Jersey post office; Hamilton Township mail center, also in New Jersey; Brentwood mail center in Washington, DC; the Department of State Annex mail center, in Sterling, VA; and the Manhattan Eye, Ear & Throat Hospital. (Further information about anthrax is presented below.) Note too that anthrax contamination had forced the closure of the largest of the United States' Senate's office buildings, the Hart Office Building, for more than three months in the fall and early winter, 2001–2002.

After the Gulf War, Iraq was discovered to have a large biological weapons program. In 1995, Iraq confirmed that it had produced, filled, and deployed bombs, rockets, and aircraft spray tanks containing *Bacillus anthracis* and botulinum toxin.

In the same year, the Japanese cult, Aum Shinrikyo, released the nerve gas Sarin in the Tokyo subway. The cult also had plans for biological terrorism, and in its arsenal were large quantities of nutrient media, botulinum toxin, anthrax cultures, and drone aircraft equipped with spray tanks. Members of this group had traveled to Zaire in 1992 to obtain samples of Ebola virus for weapons development. Aum Shinrikyo demonstrated that terrorist groups now exist with resources comparable to those of some governments.

Also of recent concern is the status of one of Russia's largest and most sophisticated former bioweapons facilities, called Vector, in Koltsovo, Novosibirsk. Writing in the journal *Emerging Infectious Diseases*, D. A. Henderson states

> Through the early 1990s, this was a 4,000-person, 30-building facility with ample biosafety level 4 laboratory facilities, used for the isolation of both specimens and human cases. Situated on an open plain surrounded by electric fences and protected by an elite guard, the facility housed the smallpox virus as well as Ebola, Marburg, and the hemorrhagic

fever viruses (e.g., Machupo and Crimean-Congo). A visit in the autumn of 1997 found a half empty facility protected by a handful of guards who had not been paid for months. (P. Jahrling, pers. comm., 1998).[7]

**Key Terms** Unlike chemical terrorism, which is immediately obvious, bioterrorism "may appear insidiously, with primary care providers witnessing the first cases."[8] An understanding of biological agents is key to understanding the epidemiology of bioterrorism. Specifically, "A biological agent is commonly portrayed as a genetically engineered organism resistant to all known vaccines and drugs, highly contagious, and able to harm thousands of people."[9] The Centers for Disease Control and Prevention categorizes biological agents by priority into Category A, B and C.[10] High-priority agents include organisms that pose a risk to national security because they can be easily disseminated or transmitted person-to-person; cause high mortality, with potential for major public health impact; might cause public panic and social disruption; and require special action for public health preparedness. Category A agents include variola major (smallpox); *Bacillus anthracis* (anthrax); *Yersinia pestis* (plague); *Clostribium botulinum* toxin (botulism); *Francisella tularensis* (tularaemia); filoviruses (Ebola hemorrhagic fever and Marburg hemorrhagic fever); and arenaviruses (Lass and Junin [Argenine hemorrhagive fever]).

Category B, or second priority agents, include those that are moderately easy to disseminate; cause moderate morbidity and low mortality; and require specific enhancements of CDC's diagnostic capacity and enhanced disease surveillance. Category B agents include *Coxiella burnetti* (Q fever); *Brucella* species (brucellosis); *Burkholderia mallei* (glanders); alphaviruses (Venezuelan encephalomyelitis, eastern and western equine encephalomyelitis); ricin toxin from *Ricinus communis* (castor beans); *Staphylococcus* enterotoxin B. A subset of List B agents includes pathogens that are food- or waterborne: *Salmonella* species; *Shigella dysenteriae; Escherichia coli* O 157:H7; *Vibrio cholerae*; and *Cryptosporidium parvum*.

Third highest priority agents include emerging pathogens that could be engineered for mass dissemination in the future because of availability; ease of production and dissemination; and potential for high morbidity and mortality and major health impact. Category C agents include Nipah virus; hantaviruses, tickborne hemorrhagic fever viruses; tickborne encephalitis viruses; yellow fever; and multidrug-resistant tuberculosis.

Epidemiologists and others report that biological attacks may not follow an expected pattern. They caution that "a small outbreak of an illness could be an early warning of a more serious attack. . . . "[11] They advise that "any small or large outbreak of disease should be evaluated as a potential bioterrorist attack."[12]

Biological warfare—that in which disease-producing microorganisms, toxins, or organic biocides (a substance capable of destroying living organisms) are deliberately used to destroy, injure, or immobilize livestock, vegetation, or human life, is contrasted with chemical warfare—the tactics and technique of conducting warfare by use of toxic chemical agents. Chemical agents that might be used by terrorists range from warfare agents to toxic chemicals commonly used in industry. Categories of chemical agents include nerve agents (tabun, sarin, soman, GF, VX); blood agents (hydrogen cyanide, cyanogen chloride); blister agents (lewisite, ntirogen and sulfur mustards, phosgene oxime); heavy metals (arsenic, lead, mercury); volatile toxins (benzene, chloroform, trihalomethanes); pulmonary agents (phosgene, chlorine, vinyl chloride); incapacitating agents (BZ); pesticides; dioxins, furans, and polychlorinated biphenyls (PCBs); explosive nitro compounds and oxidizers (ammonium nitrate combined with fuel oil); flammable industrial gases and liquids (gasoline and propane); poison industrial gases, liquids, and solids (cyanides, nitriles); and corrosive industrial acids and bases (nitric acid, sulfuric acids).

Note too the phenomena of biocrimes, the illicit use of biological agents by criminals and terrorists. Of concern here are instances in which a perpetrator or perpetrators used, acquired, or threatened to use a biological agent with the intent of inflicting mass casualties to achieve ideological, revenge, or "religious" goals, often hard to understand by laypersons and terrorism experts alike.

Of relevance here too is the concept of weapons of mass destruction. The U.S. Department of Defense defines a weapon of mass destruction to include nuclear, biological, and chemical weapons, but the legal definition is different. "The Violent Crime Control and Law Enforcement Act of 1994" defines a weapon of mass destruction to include "any destructive device as defined in section 921" of Title 18 of the U.S. Code. According to section 921, a destructive device is any type of weapon which will, or which may be readily converted to, expel a projectile by the action of an explosive or other propellant, and which has any barrel with a bore of more than one-half inch in diameter; any bomb, grenade, any rocket having a propellant charge of more than four ounces; missile having an explosive or incendiary charge of more than one-quarter ounce; mine; or similar device. To the Federal Bureau of Investigation, then, a weapon of mass destruction is basically any destructive device, including a great many that clearly cannot cause mass destruction and that have nothing to do with nuclear, biological, and chemical weapons cases.

## DIAGNOSIS

Differential diagnosis of an outbreak is advised as a first course of action. Many epidemiologic clues or indicators may point to the intentional use of a biological agent, including

> 1) the presence of a large epidemic, with greater case loads than expected, especially in a discrete population.
> 2) More severe disease than expected for a given pathogen, as well as unusual routes of exposure. . . .
> 3) A disease that is unusual for a given geographic area, is found outside the normal transmission season, or is impossible to transmit naturally in the absence of the normal vector for transmission.
> 4) Multiple simultaneous epidemics of different disease.
> 5) A disease outbreak with zoonotic as well as human consequences, as many of the potential threat agents are pathogenic to animals.
> 6) Unusual strains or variants of organisms or antimicrobial resistance patterns disparate from those circulating.
> 7) Higher attack rates in those exposed in certain areas. . . .
> 8) intelligence that an adversary has access to a particular agent or agents.
> 9) Claims by a terrorist of the release of a biological agent.
> 10) Direct evidence of the release of an agent, with findings of equipment, munitions, or tampering.[13]

Of the long list of potential pathogens, D. A. Henderson comments

> only a handful are reasonably easy to prepare and disperse and can inflict sufficiently severe disease to paralyze a city and perhaps a nation. In April 1994, Anatoliy Vorobyov, A Russian bioweapons expert, presented to a working group of the National Academy of Sciences the conclusions of Russian experts as to the agents most likely to be used. Smallpox headed the list followed closely by anthrax and plague.[14]

None of these agents has so far effectively been deployed as a biological weapon. However, the magnitude of the problems that would be associated with the release of smallpox and anthrax were vividly demonstrated by two epidemics of smallpox in Europe during the 1970s and by an accidental release of aerosolized anthrax from a Russian bioweapons facility in 1979.

**In the Media Spotlight: *Bacillus anthracis* (anthrax)** The Centers for Disease Control and Prevention defines a confirmed case of anthrax as (1) a clinically compatible case of cutaneous, inhalational, or gastrointestinal illness that is laboratory confirmed by isolation of B. antracis from an affected tissue or site or (2) other laboratory evidence of B. antracis infection bases on at least two supportive laboratory tests.

Cutaneous anthrax is the most common naturally occurring type of infection (>95%) and usually occurs after skin contact with contaminated meat, wool, hides, or leather from infected animals. The incubation period ranges from 1–12 days. The skin infection begins as a small papule, progresses to a vesicle in 1–2 days followed by a necrotic ulcer. The lesion is usually painless, but patients also may have fever, malaise, headache, and regional lymphadenopathy. Most (about 95%) anthrax infections occur when the bacterium enters a cut or abrasion on the skin. Skin infection begins as a raised bump that resembles a spider bite, but (within 1–2 days) it develops into a vesicle and then a painless ulcer, usually 1–3 cm in diameter, with a characteristic black necrotic (dying) area in the center. Lymph glands in the adjacent area may swell. About 20% of untreated cases of cutaneous anthrax will result in death. Deaths are rare if patients are given appropriate antimicrobial therapy. Early treatment of cutaneous anthrax is usually curative. Patients with cutaneous anthrax have reported case fatality rates of 20% without antibiotic treatment and less than 1% with it.[15]

Inhalational anthrax is the most lethal form of anthrax. Anthrax spores must be aerosolized in order to cause inhalational anthrax. The number of spores that cause human infection is unknown. The incubation period of inhalational anthrax among humans is unclear, but it is reported to range from 1 to 7 days, possibly ranging up to 60 days. It resembles a viral respiratory illness and initial symptoms include sore throat, mild fever, muscle aches and malaise. These symptoms may progress to respiratory failure and shock with meningitis frequently developing. Early treatment is important for recovery. Although case fatality estimates for inhalational anthrax are based on incomplete information, the rate is extremely high, approximately 75%, even with all possible supportive care including appropriate antibiotics. Estimates of the impact of the delay in post-exposure prophylaxis are not known.[16]

Gastrointestinal anthrax usually follows the consumption of raw or undercooked contaminated meat and has an incubation period of 1 to 7 days. It is associated with severe abdominal distress followed by fever and signs of septicemia. The disease can take an oropharyngeal or abdominal form. Involvement of the pharynx is usually characterized by lesions at the base of the tongue, sore throat, dysphagia, fever, and regional lymphadenopathy. Lower bowel inflammation usually causes nausea, loss of appetite, vomiting and fever, followed by abdominal pain, vomiting blood, and bloody diarrhea. As with cutaneous and inhalational anthrax, early treatment is important for recovery. For gastrointestinal anthrax, the case-fatality rate is estimated to be 25%–60% and the effect of early antibiotic treatment on that case-fatality rate is not defined.[17]

People should watch for the following symptoms: fever (temperature greater than 100 degrees F) and flu-like symptoms, and a sore, especially on the face, arms or hands, that starts as a raised bump and develops into a painless ulcer with a black area in the center. The fever may be accompanied by chills or night sweats. Flu-like symptoms include a cough (usually non-productive cough), chest discomfort, shortness of breath, fatigue, muscle aches, sore throat, followed by difficulty swallowing, enlarged lymph nodes, headache, nausea, loss of appetite, abdominal distress, vomiting, or diarrhea.

Before 2001, the last case of cutaneous anthrax in the United States occurred in North Dakota in 2000. It was the only case since 1992.[18]

Note that there is no screening test for anthrax; the only way exposure can be determined is through a public health investigation. Nasal swabs and environmental tests are used to determine the extent of exposure in a given building or workplace; they are not tests to determine whether an individual should be treated. Note too that anthrax is not contagious; the illness cannot be transmitted from person to person. Therefore, there is no need to quarantine individuals suspected of being exposed to anthrax or to immunize or treat contacts of persons ill with anthrax, such as household contacts, friends, or coworkers, unless they also were also exposed to the same source of infection.

With regards to prevention, note that a vaccine has been developed for anthrax that is protective against invasive disease; it is currently only recommended for high-risk populations. CDC and academic partners are continuing to support the development of the next generation of anthrax vaccines. The Advisory Committee on Immunization Practices (ACIP) has recommended anthrax vaccination for the following groups: persons who work directly with the organism in the laboratory; persons who work with imported animal hides or furs in areas where standards are insufficient to prevent exposure to anthrax spores; persons who handle potentially infected animal products in high-incidence areas; and military personnel deployed to areas with high risk for exposure to the organism.

The anthrax crisis in the United States in the fall of 2001 precipitated an overwhelming demand from the American public and professionals for up-to-date and accurate information on health threats arising from exposure to biological, chemical, or radiological agents. In response to this demand the Centers for Disease Control and Prevention redesigned its Web site on bioterrorism resources (www.bt.cdc.gov). The redesigned site is the official federal site for medical, laboratory, and public health professionals to reference when providing information to the public and for updates on protocols related to health threats such as anthrax.

In response to the mailings, Congress in December 2001 set aside $500 million to help the United States Postal Service, walloped by steep drops in revenue and mail volume, safeguard its customers, employees and the mail itself against bioterrorist attacks. In March of 2002, the Postal Service announced plans to use a highly sophisticated technology—polymerase chain reaction,[19] to detect anthrax and other biohazards in the mail virtually as it is being sorted. By the end of September 2002, the Service plans to install the PCR systems at 292 facilities across the country. The Service also plans to spend $245 million to retrofit its high speed sorters, adding a system that will vacuum up air near the mail and feed it through a filter to capture any harmful bacteria. Today, fear of anthrax contamination remains high, fueled in part by the fact that scientists and bioinformatics experts still cannot pinpoint the source of the microbes used in the anthrax mailings.

**In the Media Spotlight: Variola major (smallpox)** Caused by the variola virus, smallpox is spread from one person to another by infected saliva droplets that expose a susceptible person having face-to-face contact with the ill person. Persons with smallpox are most infectious during the first week of illness when the largest amount of virus is present in saliva. However, some risk of transmission lasts until all scabs have fallen off.

The incubation period is about 12 days (range: 7 to 17 days) following exposure. Initial symptoms include high fever, fatigue, and head and backaches. A characteristic rash, most prominent on the face, arms, and legs, follows in 2–3 days. The rash starts with flat red lesions that evolve at the same rate. Lesions become pus-filled and begin to crust early in the second week. Scabs develop and then separate and fall off after about 3–4 weeks. The majority of patients with smallpox recover, but death occurs in up to 30% of cases.

There is no proven treatment for smallpox but research to evaluate new antiviral agents is ongoing. Patients with smallpox can benefit from supportive therapy (intravenous fluids, medicine to control fever or pain, etc.) and antibiotics for secondary bacterial infections that occur.

Smallpox infection was eliminated from the world in 1977. Routine vaccination against smallpox ended in 1972. The level of immunity, if any, among persons who were vaccinated before 1972 is uncertain; therefore, these persons are assumed to be susceptive. Vaccination against smallpox is not recommended to prevent the disease in the general public and is therefore not available. In people exposed to smallpox, the vaccine can lessen the severity of or even prevent illness if given within 4 days after exposure. Vaccine against smallpox contains another live virus called vaccinia. The vaccine does not contain smallpox virus. The United States currently has an emergency supply of smallpox vaccine.

As of this writing, a debate is underway as to the pros and cons of the resumption of smallpox vaccination. Scientists agree that smallpox vaccine knowledge is lacking among physicians and the public: misinformation about the vaccine is widespread. The first vaccine to be developed (in 1796), the smallpox vaccine is considered to be the most dangerous. Unlike most other immunizations, smallpox vaccine can harm recipients and their contacts. Current guidelines, published in June 2001, do not recommend smallpox vaccine for the public. Vaccination is limited chiefly to laboratory workers directly involved with smallpox virus or its close virological cousins. The limits were based largely on the lack of enough vaccine. At the time, the government had only 15 million doses. But in the wake of the anthrax attacks in the fall 2001, the government expanded its stockpile of smallpox vaccine. Despite the fact that there is no information to suggest that a smallpox attack is likely, there is a tremendous demand for smallpox vaccine, including parents and health-care and other workers who would be the first to respond in an attack.

## SURVEILLANCE

Formal surveillance for potential bioterrorism agents began in January 1999, when CDC established the Bioterrorism Preparedness and Response Program to improve the public health ability to detect and respond to biological and chemical terrorism. Members of this program are working with the FBI and other federal agencies to develop an organized response to suspect and confirm biological events. The program focuses on state-level preparedness for early clinical and laboratory detection, which is essential to ensure a prompt response to a bioterrorist attack (e.g., by providing prophylactic medicines or vaccines). Its initial activities are aimed at what are seen as critical agents, as defined in an earlier note. These critical agents and their associated diseases include variola major (smallpox), *Bacillus anthracis* (anthrax), *Yersinia pestis* (plague), *Francisella tularensis* (tularemia), *Clostridium botulinum* (botulism), and the viral hemorrhagic fevers (e.g., arenaviruses and filoviruses).

Several other agents, including ones that cause food and waterborne disease, have been identified but require less broad-based preparedness efforts. An important part of preparedness is defining the natural epidemiology of diseases that can be caused by critical agents, including anthrax and plague, which are nationally notifiable diseases.

**Prevention** The prospect of domestic bioterrorism is of increasing concern to a wide spectrum of individuals nationwide. Today it is generally understood that the United States is vulnerable to both biological and chemical terrorism. Today, too, it is generally understood that biological terrorism is more likely than ever before and far more threatening than either explosives or chemicals. Today we know that preventing or controlling bioterrorism will be extremely difficult. The fact that the detection or interdiction of those intending to use biological weapons is next to impossible poses additional challenges. In the United States today it is widely understood that substantial resources at the federal, state, and local levels are required to mount a credible and meaningful response. Educating the public and policy makers about bioterrorism is required for longer-term solutions, as is the building of a global consensus condemning the use of biological weapons.

Today it is probably safe to say that the public health infrastructure is better prepared than it was prior to the fall of 2001 to prevent illness and injury that would result from biological and chemical terrorism, especially a covert terrorist attack. In the United States, preparedness activities and prevention efforts are multifaceted. Federal Emergency Management Agency and the Centers for Disease Control and Prevention occupy center stage in the preparation for a possible bioterrorism threat.

In a bioterrorist event, the Department of Health and Human Services has special responsibilities, including detecting the disease, investigating the outbreak, and providing stockpiled pharmaceuticals and emergency supplies in the large amounts needed. President Bush has named the Federal Emergency Management Agency to coordinate federal response efforts in the event of chemical, biological or nuclear terrorism.

The Centers for Disease Control and Prevention has developed a strategic plan to address the deliberate dissemination of biological or chemical agents. The plan contains recommendations to reduce United States' vulnerability to biological and chemical terrorism—preparedness planning, detection and surveillance, laboratory analysis, emergency response, and communication systems.[20] Training and research are integral components for achieving these recommendations. The success of the plan hinges on strengthening the relationships between medical and public health professionals and on building new partnerships with emergency management, the military, and law enforcement professionals.

Reliable information is undisputedly the key to preparedness: for information on the public health aspects of bioterrorism see the Centers for Disease Control and Prevention's *Bioterrorism Preparedness and Response* Web site. The site provides information about chemical and biological agents, press releases, training, contacts, and other important information dealing with the public health aspects of bioterrorism, preparedness, and response. As concerns biological agents/diseases, the information provided for selected infectious diseases includes case definition, basic laboratory protocols for the presumptive identification of causative agents, prevention guidelines, and fact sheets or FAQs (frequently asked questions).

Additionally, and as regards bioterrorism reports, CDC acknowledges that the ability to recognize a bioterrorism hoax is an important part of preparedness, and has taken steps to educate the public. CDC advises persons that if they are not sure whether a bioterrorism report is true or not, to check with credible sources, such as CDC's Health-Related Hoaxes and Rumors Web Site at http://www.cdc.gov/hoax_rumors.htm. A number of Internet sites are available regarding urban legends and hoaxes, such as the Urban Legend Reference Page at http://www.snopes2.com and the Computer Incident Advisory Committee and Department of Energy's HoaxBusters site at http://hoaxbusters.ciac.org. The HoaxBuster's site also offers a guide for recognizing Internet hoax at http://hoaxbusters.ciac.org/HBHoaxInfo.html#identify.

Efforts in the United States to deal with possible incidents involving bioweapons in the civilian sector have begun only recently and have made only limited progress.

The prospect of global bioterrorism, like that of domestic bioterrorism, is also of increasing concern to a wide spectrum of individuals worldwide. Today the CDC is cooperating with international health organizations like the World Health Organization (WHO) to help authorities in other countries investigate cases of what appear to be bioterrorism-related diseases. Requests for information regarding bioterrorism-related issues outside the United States should be directed to the International Team of CDC's Emergency Operations Center (email, eocinternational@cdc.gov). In the event of a suspected or confirmed bioterrorist attack outside the United States, CDC would respond to a request for assistance from the World Health Organization or a International Ministry of Health. CDC's role in an international team responding to a bioterrorist attack would be determined by the specific needs identified by the World Health Organization and the host country or countries.

## TABLE OVERVIEW

Trends in bioagent cases since 1900 are presented in Table K1. State supporters of terrorism and nuclear, biological, and chemical programs are presented in Table K2. The U.S. Department of State suspects that all of the countries listed possess biological weapons programs; six possess chemical weapons programs; and four have nuclear weapons programs.

Today, anthrax and plague are nationally notifiable diseases. The last case of naturally occurring anthrax in the United States was reported in 1992. Cases of anthrax and plague are shown in Tables K3 and K4. Finally, two tables depict incidences of smallpox, both in the United States and globally, Tables K5 and K6.

## NOTES

1. Taken from President George W. Bush's address at a prayer service on Friday, September 14, 2001 at the Washington National Cathedral.
2. "Reno, FBI Head Warn of Terrorism," *Associated Press*, April 23, 1998, 4:44 A.M. feed; Tim Weiner, "U.S. May Stockpile Medicine for Terrorist Attack," *New York Times*, April 23, 1998.
3. Critical agents are defined as those that are associated with high case fatality, can be disseminated to a large population, can cause social disruption because of public perception, and require preparedness efforts.
4. Centers for Disease Control and Prevention. "Update: Investigation of Anthrax Associated with Intentional Exposure and Interim Public Health Guidelines." October 2001. *MMWR: Morbidity and Mortality Weekly Report* 2001, 50:889–93.

5. Centers for Disease Control and Prevention. "Update: Investigation of Bioterrorism-related anthrax, 2001." November 2001. *MMWR: Mobidity and Mortality Weekly Report* 2001, 50:1008–1010.
6. Cases were confirmed by the Centers for Disease Control and Prevention. The status of the victims varies; several have died. Other suspected cases remain unconfirmed as of this writing by the CDC. They include workers at the *New York Post* and a second NBC worker.
7. D. A. Henderson. Bioterrorism as a Public Health Threat. Emerging Infectious Diseases. Vol. 4, no. 3, July–September 1998.
8. J. A. Pavlin. Epidemiology of Bioterrorism. Emerging Infectious Diseases.
9. Ibid.
10. Ibid.
11. Ibid.
12. Ibid.
13. Ibid.
14. D. A. Henderson, Bioterrorism as a Public Health Threat. Emerging Infectious Diseases. Vol. 4, no. 3 (July—September 1998) p. 488–92.
15. Centers for Disease Control and Prevention. Facts about Anthrax. http://www.bt.cdc.gov/DocumentsApp/faqanthrax.asp. Accessed March 13, 2002.
16. Ibid.
17. Centers for Disease Control and Prevention. Facts about Anthrax. http://www.bt.cdc.gov/DocumentsApp/faqanthrax.asp. Accessed March 13, 2002.
18. To find out more about this case, see "Human Anthrax Associated with an Epizootic Among Livestock—North Dakota, 2000" (MMWR 2000; 5[32]:677).
19. Polymerase chain reaction is a laboratory method used to detect and amplify genetic material from organisms. It can be used to diagnose disease by identifying genetic material (DNA) commonly found in all *Bacillus anthracis* strains or it can be used to subtype the organism by amplifying specific genetic material and comparing it with known strains of B. anthracis to se if it matches of if it is different. When PCR is used for subtyping (a laboratory process to identify different subtypes of organisms), the amplified genetic material is usually further analyzed by other molecular methods, such as DNA sequencing.
20. Full details may be found in Centers for Disease Control and Prevention. Biological and Chemical Terrorism: Strategic Plan for Preparedness and Response. Recommendations of the CDC Strategic Planning Workgroup. MMWR 2000;49 (No. RR-4).

**Table K1. Trends in Bioagent Cases, 1900–1999**

| | Terrorist | Criminal | Other/ Uncertain | Total |
|---|---|---|---|---|
| 1990-1999 | 19 | 40 | 94 | 153 |
| 1980-1989 | 3 | 6 | 0 | 9 |
| 1970-1979 | 3 | 2 | 3 | 8 |
| 1960-1969 | 0 | 1 | 0 | 1 |
| 1950-1959 | 1 | 0 | 0 | 1 |
| 1940-1949 | 1 | 0 | 0 | 1 |
| 1930-1939 | 0 | 3 | 0 | 3 |
| 1920-1929 | 0 | 0 | 0 | 0 |
| 1910-1919 | 0 | 3 | 0 | 3 |
| 1900-1909 | 0 | 1 | 0 | 1 |
| Totals | 27 | 56 | 97 | 180 |

*Source*: W. Seth Carus, *Bioterrorism and Biocrimes: The Illicit Use of Biological Agents Since 1900.* Working Paper. Center for Counterprofileration Research, National Defense University, Washington, DC. (February 2001 revision). http://www.ndu.edu/ndu/centercounter/Full_Doc.pdf.

**Table K2. State Supporters of Terrorism and NBC Programs**

| *State Supporters of Terrorism* | *Nuclear Program* | *CW Program* | *BW Program* |
|---|---|---|---|
| Cuba | None | None | Confirmed |
| Iraq | Confirmed | Confirmed | Confirmed |
| Iran | Confirmed | Confirmed | Confirmed |
| Libya | Confirmed | Confirmed | Confirmed |
| North Korea | Confirmed | Confirmed | Confirmed |
| Sudan | None | Confirmed | Confirmed |
| Syria | None | Confirmed | Confirmed |

*Source*: Robert G. Joseph, and John F. Reichart, *Deterrence and Defense in a Nuclear, Biological, and Chemical Environment*. Center for Counterproliferation Research, National Defense University, Washington, DC (1999). http://www.ndu.edu/inss/books/017.pdf.

## Table K3. Anthrax Cases in the United States, 1990–1999

| Year | Number |
|---|---|
| 1990 | 0 |
| 1991 | 0 |
| 1992 | 1 |
| 1993 | 0 |
| 1994 | 0 |
| 1995 | 0 |
| 1996 | 0 |
| 1997 | 0 |
| 1998 | 0 |
| 1999 | 0 |

*Source*: Center for Disease Control and Prevention. U.S. Department of Health and Human Services. *MMWR: Morbidity and Mortality Weekly Review Summary of Notifiable Disease. United States, 1999*. 48 no. 53 (2001). http://www.cdc.gov/mmwr/PDF/wk/mm4853.pdf.

## Table K4. Reported Cases of Plague, United States, 1980–1999

| Year | Number of Cases |
|---|---|
| 1999 | 9 |
| 1998 | 9 |
| 1997 | 4 |
| 1996 | 5 |
| 1995 | 9 |
| 1994 | 17 |
| 1993 | 10 |
| 1992 | 13 |
| 1991 | 11 |
| 1990 | 2 |
| 1989 | 4 |
| 1988 | 15 |
| 1987 | 12 |
| 1986 | 10 |
| 1985 | 17 |
| 1984 | 31 |
| 1983 | 40 |
| 1982 | 19 |
| 1981 | 13 |
| 1980 | 18 |

*Source*: Center for Disease Control and Prevention. U.S. Department of Health and Human Services. *MMWR: Morbidity and Mortality Weekly Review Summary of Notifiable Disease. United States, 1999* 48 no. 53 (2001). http://www.cdc.gov/mmwr/PDF/wk/mm4853.pdf.

**Table K5. Smallpox Cases in the United States, 1920–1950**

| Year | Number of Cases | Number of Deaths |
|---|---|---|
| 1920 | 102 128 | 498 |
| 1921 | 102 787 | 620 |
| 1922 | 33 378 | 607 |
| 1923 | 30 907 | 126 |
| 1924 | 56 591 | 871 |
| 1925 | 39 572 | 707 |
| 1926 | 33 732 | 376 |
| 1927 | 37 600 | 138 |
| 1928 | 39 396 | 129 |
| 1929 | 42 282 | 137 |
| 1930 | 48 907 | 165 |
| 1931 | 30 233 | 93 |
| 1932 | 11 224 | 38 |
| 1933 | 6 491 | 39 |
| 1934 | 5 371 | 24 |
| 1935 | 7 957 | 25 |
| 1936 | 7 834 | 35 |
| 1937 | 11 673 | 34 |
| 1938 | 14 939 | 48 |
| 1939 | 9 877 | 41 |
| 1940 | 2 795 | 14 |
| 1941 | 1 396 | 12 |
| 1942 | 865 | 2 |
| 1943 | 765 | 8 |
| 1944 | 397 | 9 |
| 1945 | 346 | 12 |
| 1946 | 337 | 25 |
| 1947 | 176 | 5 |
| 1948 | 57 | 5 |
| 1949 | 49 | 2 |
| 1950 | 39 | 0 |

*Source*: Jack W. Hopkins. *The Eradication of Smallpox: Organizational Learning and Innovation in Health*. Boulder: Westview Press, 1989.

**Table K6. World: Number of Smallpox Cases Reported, by Year, 1920–1979**

| Year | Number |
|---|---|
| 1920 | 401 318 |
| 1921 | 303 850 |
| 1922 | 190 159 |
| 1923 | 174 799 |
| 1924 | 186 354 |
| 1925 | 284 845 |
| 1926 | 324 125 |
| 1927 | 327 289 |
| 1928 | 272 529 |
| 1929 | 267 322 |
| 1930 | 360 575 |
| 1931 | 182 829 |
| 1932 | 211 274 |
| 1933 | 328 212 |
| 1934 | 327 373 |
| 1935 | 331 151 |
| 1936 | 263 579 |
| 1937 | 149 184 |
| 1938 | 144 042 |
| 1939 | 186 393 |
| 1940 | 235 820 |
| 1941 | 195 863 |
| 1942 | 124 504 |
| 1943 | 210 358 |
| 1944 | 407 525 |
| 1945 | 405 833 |
| 1946 | 302 694 |
| 1947 | 163 375 |
| 1948 | 161 893 |
| 1949 | 632 858 |
| 1950 | 426 006 |
| 1951 | 554 756 |
| 1952 | 167 085 |
| 1953 | 94 135 |
| 1954 | 99 232 |
| 1955 | 91 823 |
| 1956 | 96 089 |
| 1957 | 156 652 |
| 1958 | 280 475 |
| 1959 | 96 270 |
| 1960 | 67 148 |
| 1961 | 90 555 |

**Table K6.** ***(Continued)***

| Year | Number |
|---|---|
| 1962 | 98 757 |
| 1963 | 133 504 |
| 1964 | 76 198 |
| 1965 | 122 280 |
| 1966 | 92 799 |
| 1967 | 131 697 |
| 1968 | 80 024 |
| 1969 | 54 202 |
| 1970 | 33 706 |
| 1971 | 52 806 |
| 1972 | 65 153 |
| 1973 | 135 859 |
| 1974 | 218 367 |
| 1975 | 19 278 |
| 1976 | 954 |
| 1977 | 3 234 |
| 1978 | 2 |
| 1979 | 0 |

*Source*: World Health Organization. *The Global Eradication of Smallpox: Final Report of the Global Commission for the Certification of Smallpox Eradication*. Geneva, December 1979.

# Appendix: World Health Organization (WHO) Regions

## AFRICAN REGION (AFR)

Algeria
Angola
Benin
Botswana
Burkina Faso
Burundi
Cameroon
Cape Verde
Central African Republic
Chad
Comoros
Congo
Congo, Democratic Republic of the
Côte d'Ivoire
Equatorial Guinea
Eritrea
Ethiopia
Gabon
Gambia
Ghana
Guinea
Guinea-Bissau
Kenya
Lesotho
Liberia
Madagascar
Malawi
Mali
Mauritania
Mauritius
Mozambique
Namibia
Niger
Nigeria
Rwanda
Sao Tome
Senegal
Seychelles
Sierra Leone
South Africa
Swaziland
Tanzania
Togo
Uganda
Zambia
Zimbabwe

## REGION OF THE AMERICAS (AMR)

Antigua and Barbuda
Argentina
Bahamas
Barbados
Belize
Bolivia
Brazil
Canada
Chile
Colombia
Costa Rica
Cuba
Dominica
Dominican Republic
Ecuador
El Salvador
Grenada
Guatemala
Guyana
Haiti
Honduras
Jamaica

Mexico
Nicaragua
Panama
Paraguay
Peru
Saint Kitts
Saint Lucia
Saint Vincent and the Grenadines
Suriname
Trinidad and Tobago
United States of America
Uruguay
Venezuela

## EASTERN MEDITERRANEAN REGION (EMR)

Afghanistan
Bahrain
Cyprus
Djibouti
Egypt
Iran
Iraq
Jordan
Kuwait
Lebanon
Libya
Morocco
Oman
Pakistan
Qatar
Saudi Arabia
Somalia
Sudan
Syria
Tunisia
United Arab Emirates
Yemen

## EUROPEAN REGION (EUR)

Albania
Andorra
Armenia
Austria
Azerbaijan
Belarus
Belgium
Bosnia and Herzegovina
Bulgaria
Croatia
Czech Republic
Denmark
Estonia
Finland
France
Georgia
Germany
Greece
Hungary
Iceland
Ireland
Israel
Italy
Kazakhstan
Kyrgyzstan
Latvia
Lithuania
Luxembourg
Macedonia, The Former Yugoslav Republic of
Malta
Monaco
Netherlands
Norway
Poland
Portugal
Republic
Romania
Russian Federation
San Marino
Slovakia
Slovenia
Spain
Sweden
Switzerland
Tajikistan
Turkey
Turkmenistan
Ukraine
United Kingdom
Uzbekistan
Yugoslavia

## SOUTH-EAST ASIA REGION (SEAR)

Bangladesh
Bhutan
India
Indonesia
Maldives
Myanmar

Nepal
Sri Lanka
Thailand

## WESTERN PACIFIC REGION (WPR)

Australia
Brunei
Cambodia
China
Cook Islands
Fiji
Japan
Kiribati
Korea, Republic of
Laos
Malaysia
Marshall Islands
Micronesia, Federated States of
Mongolia
Nauru
New Zealand
Niue
Palau
Papua New Guinea
Philippines
Samoa
Singapore
Solomon Islands
Tonga
Tuvalu
Vanuatu
Viet Nam

# Glossary

**Active reporting**. See Passive reporting.

**Behavioral epidemic**. Charles Mackay, in his classic work *Extraordinary Popular Delusions and the Madness of Crowds*, described what is known as a behavioral epidemic. This phenomenon can be seen in the reactions of impressionable teenagers at a rock concert, and in a different form in movements such as Nazism, when an entire nation is gripped by destructive fanaticism. The huge increase in traffic-related deaths and injury rates during the twentieth century, which has continued into the twenty-first century, is a behavioral epidemic associated with addiction to high-speed automobiles.

**Biocrimes**. The illicit use of biological agents by criminals and terrorists. Of concern are instances in which a perpetrator or perpetrators used, acquired, or threatened to use a biological agent with the intent of inflicting mass casualties to achieve ideological, revenge, or "religious" goals, often hard to understand by laypersons and terrorism experts alike. *See* biological agent; biological warfare; bioterrorism; chemical warfare; weapons of mass destruction.

**Biological agent**. "A biological agent is commonly portrayed as a genetically engineered organism resistant to all known vaccines and drugs, highly contagious, and able to harm thousands of people."[1] *See also* biocrimes; biological warfare; bioterrorism; chemical warfare; weapons of mass destruction.

**Biological warfare**. Warfare in which disease-producing microorganisms, toxins, or organic biocides (a substance capable of destroying living organisms) are deliberately used to destroy, injure, or immobilize livestock, vegetation, or human life. *See* biocrimes; biological agent; bioterrorism; chemical warfare; weapons of mass destruction.

**Bioterrorism**. Unlike chemical terrorism, which is immediately obvious, bioterrorism "may appear insidiously, with primary care providers witnessing the first cases."[2] An understanding of biological agents is key to understanding the epidemiology of bioterrorism. Specifically, "A biological agent is commonly portrayed as a genetically engineered organism resistant to all known vaccines and drugs, highly contagious, and able to harm thousands of people."[3] However, epidemiologists and others report that biological attacks may not follow an expected pattern. They caution that "a small outbreak of an illness could be an early warning of a more serious attack."[4] They advise that "any small or large outbreak of disease should be evaluated as a potential bioterrorist attack."[5] *See* biocrimes; biological agent; biological warfare; chemical warfare; weapons of mass destruction.

**Border crosser**. Defined, in part, by the Immigration and Naturalization Service as a "nonresident alien entering the United States across the Mexican border for stays of no more than 72 hours." Border crossers may go back and forth across the border many times in a short period.

**Burden of disease**. *See* disease burden.

**Case**. Within the context of infectious diseases, an episode of a disease in a person meeting the laboratory or clinical criteria for that disease generally as defined in the document "Case Definitions for Infectious Conditions under Public Health Surveillance." For example, a case of tuberculosis is an episode of TB disease in a person meeting the laboratory or clinical criteria for TB as defined in that document. *MMWR: Morbidity and Mortality Weekly Report* 1997, 46, no. RR-10.

**Case definition**. Provide uniform criteria for public health professionals to use when reporting cases of nationally notifiable infectious diseases. Components of case definitions may include clinical description, laboratory criteria for diagnosis, and case classification. Case definitions are intended to be used for identifying and classifying cases, both of which are often done retrospectively, for national reporting purposes. Case definitions serve to increase the specificity of reporting and improve the comparability of diseases reported from different geographic areas. Case definitions are revised as necessary; new case definitions are generated as needed. Case definitions are not intended to be used as the sole criteria for establishing clinical diagnoses, determining the standard of care necessary for a particular patient, setting guidelines for quality assurance, or providing standards for reimbursement, nor are they intended to be used for public health action.

In October 1990, in collaboration with the Council of State and Territorial Epidemiologists (CSTE), CDC published "Case Definitions for Public Health Surveillance" (*MMWR* 1990, 39, no. RR-13). The definitions were approved by a full vote of the CSTE membership and also were endorsed for use by the Association of State and Territorial Public Health Laboratory Directors (ASTPHLD). This document was updated in 1997 (*MMWR* 1997, 46, no. RR-10).

**Chemical warfare**. The tactics and technique of conducting warfare by use of toxic chemical agents. Chemical agents include blistering agents (e.g., distilled mustard, lewistie, mustard gas, nitrogen mustard, phosgene oxime, ethyldichloroarsine, methyldichloroarsine), agents that damage the blood (e.g., arsine, cyanogen chloride, hydrogen chloride, hydrogen cyanide), choking/lung/pulmonary damaging agents (e.g., chlorine, diphosgene, nitrogen oxide, perflurorisobutylene, phosgene, sulfur trioxide-chlororsulfonic acid), agents that cause vomiting (e.g., adamsite, diphenylchloroarsine, diphenylcyanoarsine), nerve agents (e.g., cyclohexyl sarin, GE, sarin, soman, tabun), riot control/tear agents, defoliants, and herbicides. *See* biocrimes; biological agent; biological warfare; bioterrorism; weapons of mass destruction.

**Clinically compatible case**. In the context of case classification, a clinical syndrome generally compatible with the disease.

**Common-vehicle epidemic**. An epidemic that is due to an agent that is spread on an ongoing basis in a "vehicle" such as food, water, or air. Food-borne common-vehicle epidemics usually cause gastrointestinal disease, and are sometimes perpetuated by a carrier who is a foodhandler. Waterborne epidemics include typhoid, giardia, viral hepatitis A, and many others. The best known airborne common vehicle epidemic is Legionnaire's disease. Notorious blood-borne common vehicle epidemics have occurred since the 1980s in many countries after the blood supply became infected with HIV or Hepatitis C virus.

**Communicable disease**. A disease, the causative organism of which is transmissible from one person to another either directly or indirectly through a carrier or vector.

**Communicable disease surveillance**. *See* surveillance.

**Confirmed case**. In the context of case classification, a case that is classified as confirmed for reporting purposes.

**Counting of a case**. The process whereby a reporting area with count authority evaluates verified cases of a specific disease (e.g., assesses for case duplication). These cases are then counted for morbidity in that locality (e.g., state or county) and reported to the Centers for Disease Control and Prevention for national morbidity counting. *See* verification of a case.

**DALE**. *See* disability-adjusted life expectancy.

**DALYs**. *See* disability-adjusted life years.

**Disability-adjusted life expectancy (DALE)**. A summary measure of the burden of disability from all causes in a population, DALE is best understood as the expectation of life lived in equivalent full health.

**Disability-adjusted life years (DALYs)**. DALYs, along with disability-adjusted life expectancy (DALE), are summary measures of population health. DALYs are a measure of health gaps that state the difference between a population's health and a normative goal of living in full health.

**Disease.** A pathological condition of the body that presents a group of clinical signs and symptoms and laboratory findings peculiar to it and that sets the condition apart as an abnormal entity differing from other normal or pathological body states. The concept of disease may include a condition of illness or suffering not necessarily arising from pathological changes in the body. There is a major distinction between disease and illness in that the former is usually tangible and may even be measured, whereas illness is highly individual and personal, as with pain, suffering, and distress. A person may have a serious disease such as hypertension but have no feeling of pain or suffering and thus no illness. Conversely, a person may be extremely ill, as with hysteria or mental illness, but have no evidence of disease as measured by pathological changes in the body.

**Disease burden**. The impact of a disease or disease condition(s) on a given population or populations. Discussions of disease burden have traditionally focused on mortality data and, within this context, on premature death or disability. More recently, the focus has shifted both to the impact of non-fatal outcomes of disease on the overall health status and/or productivity of a given population or populations and to the unseen burden of disease, such as the impact of years lived with disability on the overall health status and/or productivity of a population or populations. Discussions of disease burden often focus on the global burden of disease and generally include both comparisons of the burden of disease across many different disease conditions and projections for the future.

**Disease control**. The reduction of disease incidence, prevalence, morbidity, or mortality to a locally acceptable level as a result of deliberate efforts; continued intervention measures are required to maintain the reduction. Control measures usually depend on routine services being instituted and maintained in a long-term perspective.

**Disease elimination**. The reduction to zero of the incidence of a specified disease in a defined geographical area as a result of deliberate efforts; continued intervention measures are required.

**Disease eradication**. Reduction of the worldwide incidence of a disease to zero as a result of deliberate efforts, obviating the necessity for further control measures. The extinction of the disease pathogen.

**Disease projection**. Calculation of the future of disease (incidence, prevalence, etc.).

**Disease surveillance**. The monitoring of disease. Within the context of communicable disease or diseases, the procedure of closely monitoring the contacts of individuals exposed to an infectious disease during the incubation period to prevent the spread of the disease. Surveillance is used in place of quarantine. The surveillance of a communicable disease is fundamental for disease prevention and control. Disease surveillance is used for a variety of purposes, for example, to monitor disease trends; monitor progress toward control objectives; estimate the size of a health problem; detect outbreaks of an infectious disease; evaluate interventions and preventative programs; and identify research needs. *See also* multi-disease surveillance.

**Disease trend**. The general course or tendency of a disease.

**Endemic**. The constant presence of a disease or infectious agent within a given geographic area.

**Endemic zone**. Areas where there is a potential risk of infection. For example, yellow fever endemic zones in the Americas are areas in which a potential risk of infection exists because of the presence of vectors and animal reservoirs. Some countries consider these zones "infected" areas and require an international certificate of vaccination against yellow fever from travellers arriving from these areas.

**Epidemic**. The occurrence in an area of a disease or illness to an extent greater than expected on the basis of past experience for a given population. In the case of a new disease, such as AIDS, any occurrence may be considered "epidemic." Also, a temporary prevalence of a disease.

**Epidemic intelligence**. Information on ongoing outbreaks or rumors of outbreaks worldwide. To improve international preparedness for epidemic response, it is essential to actively collect and rapidly verify this information and then to share it with the public health community.

**Epidemiologically linked case**. In the context of case classification, a case in which (a) the patient has had contact with one or more persons who have or had the disease or have been exposed to a point source of infection and (b) transmission of the agent by the usual modes of transmission is plausible. A case may be considered epidemiologically linked to a laboratory-confirmed case if at least one case in the chain of transmission is laboratory confirmed.

**Health**. A condition in which all functions of the body and mind are normally active. The World Health Organization defines health as a state of complete physical, mental, or social well-being and not merely the absence of disease or infirmity.

**Infection**. The state or condition in which the body or part of it is invaded by a pathogenic agent (microorganism or virus) that, under favorable conditions, multiples and produces injurious effects. Localized infection is usually accompanied by inflammation, but inflammation may occur without infection. The symptoms of infection are those of inflammation. The five classical symptoms listed by early medical writers are dolor (pain), calor (heat), rubor (redness), tumor (swelling), and functio laesa (disordered function).

**Infectious agent**. Something that produces infection. Also, something that is capable of being transmitted with or without contact.

**Infectious disease**. Disease resulting from the presence of a pathogenic organism in the body. Specifically, any of the many diseases or illnesses (caused by bacteria or viruses) that can be transmitted from person to person, from animal to animal, or from organism to organism, by direct or indirect contact. The *International Statistical Classification of Diseases & Related Health Problems* (ICD) defines infectious diseases to include those diseases generally recognized as communicable or transmissible as well as a few diseases of unknown but possibly infectious origin.

**Laboratory-confirmed case**. In the context of case classification, a case that is confirmed by one or more of the laboratory methods listed in the case definition under "Laboratory Criteria for Diagnosis." Although other laboratory methods can be used in clinical diagnosis, only those listed are accepted as laboratory confirmation for national reporting purposes.

**Multi-disease surveillance**. A multi-disease approach to communicable disease surveillance that involves looking at all surveillance activities in a country as a common public service. These activities involve similar functions and very often use the same structure, processes, and personnel as disease surveillance. Surveillance is based on collecting only the information that is required to achieve control objectives of diseases. Data requested may differ from disease to disease, and some diseases may have specific information needs. Features of this approach include the following: looks at surveillance as a "common" service; seeks to maintain surveillance and control functions close to one another; recognizes that different diseases may have specialized surveillance needs; uses a functional approach to communicable disease surveillance; exploits opportunities for synergy in carrying out core as well as surveillance support functions; does not require a single system solution; and is best approached by developing and strengthening surveillance networks.

**Noninfectious conditions**. As contrasted with infectious conditions, noninfectious conditions include environmental or occupational conditions, chronic diseases, adverse reproductive health events, and injuries.

**Notifiable disease**. In the United States, a notifiable disease is one for which regular, frequent, and timely information regarding individual cases is considered necessary for the prevention and control of the disease. As of 1999, 55 infectious diseases were designated as notifiable at the national level.

**Pandemic**. A worldwide epidemic affecting an exceptionally high proportion of the global population. Pandemics are contrasted to epidemics, which spread from person to person in a locality where the disease is not permanently prevalent.

**Parasitic disease**. Disease resulting from the growth and development of parasitic organisms (plants and animals) in or upon the body.

**Passive reporting**. The reporting and confirmation of cases seen in health facilities, as contrasted to active case-finding methods, where by cases are actively sought.

**Point-source epidemic**. An epidemic in which a group of people fall ill as a result of a single exposure, typically to an agent in food they have all consumed, e.g., an outbreak of acute food poisoning due to staphylococcal enterotoxin.

**Prevalence**. The number of existing cases of a disease among a total or specified population in a given period of time; usually expressed as a percentage or as the number of cases per thousand, per 10,000, and so on.

**Probable case**. In the context of case classification, a case that is classified as probable for reporting purposes.

**Prophylactic**. Something that guards against or prevents disease.

**Prophylaxis**. Measures designed to prevent the spread of disease and to preserve health; protective or preventive treatment.

**Public health**. State of health of the population of a particular community as opposed to an individual or personal health. Health services to improve and protect community health, especially preventative medicine, immunization, and sanitation.

**Quarantine**. Any isolation or restriction of movement imposed on apparently well individuals after they have been exposed to an infectious disease in an effort to control its spread. Also, the period of detention at entering a country (originally 40 days). The period of isolation following the onset of contagious disease. The place where individuals are detained for observation.

**Region of acquisition**. The region or country of infection. To track epidemiologic patterns of disease acquisition more effectively, new regional categories are periodically devised.

**Region of diagnosis**. The region or country of diagnosis.

**Reporting area**. Areas responsible for counting and reporting verified cases of a disease to the Centers for Disease Control and Prevention. Currently there are 59 reporting areas: the 50 states, District of Columbia, New York City, American Samoa, Federated States of Micronesia, Guam, Northern Mariana Islands, Puerto Rico, Republic of Palau, and the U.S. Virgin Islands.

**Subepidemic**. The morbidity that occurs within a proportion of the population infected by an epidemic.

**Supportive or presumptive laboratory results**. In the context of case classification, specified laboratory results that are consistent with the diagnosis, yet do not meet the criteria for laboratory confirmation.

**Surveillance**. The ongoing systematic collection, collation, analysis, and interpretation of data and the dissemination of information to those who need to know in order that action may be taken. Within the context of epidemiology, surveillance has been defined as the continuing scrutiny of all aspects of the occurrence and spread of a disease that are pertinent to effective control.[6] For this, systematic collection, analysis, interpretation, and dissemination of health data are essential. This includes collecting information about clinical diagnoses, laboratory diagnoses, and mortality, as well as other relevant information needed to detect and track diseases in terms of person, place, and time. Surveillance systems must detect new communicable diseases as well as recognize and track diseases that are, or have the potential to become, of major public health importance. Disease surveillance systems may be national, regional, or global and may focus on an individual disease or on multiple diseases.

**Suspect**. A person for whom there is a high index of suspicion (likely to have the disease) for active disease who is currently under evaluation for that disease. For example, in the context of tuberculosis, a person for whom there is a high index of suspicion for active TB (e.g., a known contact to an active TB case or a person with signs/symptoms consistent with TB) who is currently under evaluation for TB disease.

**Suspected case**. In the context of case classification, a case that is classified as suspected for reporting purposes.

**Universal infection control precautions**. Guidelines and procedures to protect health care workers from exposure to infection from blood and other body fluids.

**Vector-borne epidemics**. Epidemics that are spread by insect vectors; vector-borne epidemics include viruses such as dengue and viral encephalitis, which are transmitted by mosquitoes.

**Verification of a case**. The process whereby a case of a disease, after the diagnostic evaluation is complete, is reviewed at the local level (e.g., state or county) by a control official who is familiar with surveillance definitions for that particular disease; if all the criteria for a case are met, the case is then verified and eligible for counting. *See* counting of a case.

**Weapon of mass destruction**. The U.S. Department of Defense defines a weapon of mass destruction to include nuclear, biological, and chemical weapons, but the legal definition is different. "The Violent Crime Control and Law Enforcement Act of 1994" defines a weapon of mass destruction to include "any destructive device as defined in section 921" of Title 18 of the U.S. Code. According to section 921, a destructive device is "any gun with a barrel larger than half an inch, any bomb, grenade, any rocket have a propellant charge of more than four ounces." To the FBI, then, a weapon of mass destruction is basically any destructive device, including a great many that clearly cannot cause mass destruction and that have nothing to do with nuclear, biological, and chemical weapons cases. *See* biocrimes; biological warfare; bioterrorism; chemical warfare.

## NOTES

1. J.A. Pavlin. "Epidemiology of Bioterrorism." *Emerging Infectious Diseases Journal* 5, no. 4 (1999): 528–30.
2. Ibid.
3. Ibid.
4. Ibid.
5. Ibid.
6. J.M. Last, *A Dictionary of Epidemiology* (New York: Oxford University Press, 1995).

# Bibliography

## A. NATIONALLY NOTIFIABLE DISEASES


Armstrong, G.L., L.A. Conn, and R.W. Pinner, "Trends in Infectious Disease Mortality in the United States in the 20th Century." *Journal of the American Medical Association* 281, no. 1 (1999): 61–66.

Centers for Disease Control and Prevention (CDC), U.S. Department of Health and Human Services. "Case Definitions for Infectious Conditions under Public Health Surveillance." *MMWR* 46, no. RR-10 (1997). Available on the Internet at http://www.cdc.gov/mmwr/PDF/rr/rr4610.pdf. Accessed Sept. 5, 2001.

Centers for Disease Control and Prevention (CDC), U.S. Department of Health and Human Services. *CDC Surveillance Summaries*. Various reports published since January 1, 1990.

Centers for Disease Control and Prevention (CDC), U.S. Department of Health and Human Services. "Changes in National Notifiable Diseases Data Presentation." *MMWR* 45, no. 2 (1996): 41–42.

Centers for Disease Control and Prevention (CDC), U.S. Department of Health and Human Services. "National Morbidity Reporting, 1952." *CDC Bulletin* 12 (1951): 50–53.

Centers for Disease Control and Prevention (CDC), U.S. Department of Health and Human Services. "Notifiable Disease Surveillance and Notifiable Disease Statistics—United States, June 1946 and June 1996." *MMWR* 45, no. 25 (1996): 530–36. Available on the Internet at http://www.cdc.gov/mmwr/PDF/wk/mm4525.pdf. Accessed Sept. 5, 2001.

Center for Disease Control and Prevention. U.S. Department of Health and Human Services. *MMWR: Morbidity and Mortality Weekly Review Summary of Notifiable Disease, United States, 1999* 48 no. 53 (2001). http//www.cdc.gov/mmwr/PDF/wk/mm4853.pdf. Accessed Sept. 5, 2001.

Centers for Disease Control and Prevention (CDC), U.S. Department of Health and Human Services. "Ten Great Public Health Achievements—United States, 1900–1999." *MMWR* 48, no. 12 (1999): 241–43.

Etheridge, E.W. *Sentinel for Health: A History of the Centers for Disease Control*. Berkeley, CA: University of California Press, 1992.

Ewald, P.W., and G. Cochran. "Catching on to What's Catching." *Natural History* 108, no. 1 (1999): 34–37.

Hinman, A.R. "1889 to 1989: A Century of Health and Disease." *Public Health Reports* 105, no. 4 (1990): 374–80.

Koo, D., and S.F. Wetterhall. "History and Current Status of the National Notifiable Diseases Surveillance System." *Journal of Public Health Management Practice* 2 (1996): 4–10.

Sacks, J.J. "Utilization of Case Definitions and Laboratory Reporting in the Surveillance of Notifiable Communicable Diseases in the United States." *American Journal of Public Health* 75 (1985): 1420–22.

Shannon, G.W., and G.F. Pyle, *Disease and Medical Care in the United States: A Medical Atlas of the Twentieth Century*. New York: Macmillan, 1993.

Stoto, M.A., R. Behrens, and C. Rosemont, eds. *Healthy People 2000: Citizens Chart the Course*. Washington, DC: National Academy Press, 1990.

Teutsch, S.M. and R.E. Churchill, eds. *Principles and Practice of Public Health Surveillance*. New York: Oxford University Press, 1994.

Ullmann, E. "Infectious Disease Facts, Concerns, and Strategies Discussed at Fourth Annual Conference on Infectious Diseases." *AORN Journal* 68, no. 4 (1998): 667(3).

U.S. Department of Health and Human Services. *Healthy People 2000: Midcourse Review and 1995 Revisions*. Washington, DC: U.S. Government Printing Office, 1995. Available on the Internet at http://odphp.osophs.dhhs.gov/pubs/hp2000/midcours.htm. Accessed Sept. 5, 2001.

U.S. Department of Health and Human Services. *Healthy People 2000: National Health Promotion and Disease Prevention Objectives*. Washington, DC: U.S. Government Printing Office, 1990.

U.S. Department of Health and Human Services. *Healthy People 2010. 2nd ed. With Understanding and Improving Health and Objectives for Improving Health*. 2 vols. Washington, DC: U.S. Government Printing Office, 2000. Available on the Internet at http://www.health.gov/healthypeople/document/. Accessed Sept. 5, 2001.

U.S. Department of Health and Human Services. *Promoting Health/Preventing Disease: Objectives for the Nation*. Washington, DC: U.S. Department of Health and Human Services, 1980.


## B. HUMAN IMMUNODEFICIENCY VIRUS (HIV) AND ACQUIRED IMMUNODEFICIENCY SYNDROME (AIDS)


Centers for Disease Control and Prevention (CDC), U.S. Department of Health and Human Services. "1993 Revised Classification System for HIV Infection and Expanded Surveillance Case Definition for AIDS Among Adolescents and Adults." *MMWR* 41, no. RR-17 (1992).

Centers for Disease Control and Prevention (CDC), U.S. Department of Health and Human Services. "1994 Revised Classification System for Human Immunodeficiency Virus Infection in Children Less than 13 Years of Age." *MMWR* 43, no. RR-12 (1994): 1–10.

Centers for Disease Control and Prevention (CDC), U.S. Department of Health and Human Services. "Characteristics of Persons Living with AIDS at the End of 1999." *HIV/AIDS Surveillance Supplemental Report* 7, no. 1 (2001). Available on the Internet at http://www.cdc.gov/hiv/stats/hasrsupp.htm. Accessed Sept. 5, 2001.

Centers for Disease Control and Prevention (CDC), U.S. Department of Health and Human Services. "Guidelines for National Human Immunodeficiency Virus Case Surveillance, Including Monitoring for Human Immunodeficiency Virus Infection and Acquired Immunodeficiency Syndrome." *MMWR* 48, no. RR-13 (1999). Available on the Internet at http://www.cdc.gov/mmwr/PDF/rr/rr4813.pdf. Accessed Sept. 5, 2001.

Centers for Disease Control and Prevention (CDC), U.S Department of Health and Human Services. "HIV/AIDS Surveillance Report, 1999" 11(No.2). Available on the Internet at http://www.cdc.gov/hiv/stats/hasr1102.htm. Accessed Sept. 5, 2001.

Centers for Disease Control and Prevention (CDC), U.S. Department of Health and Human Services. HIV/AIDS Surveillance Report Mid-year 2000 Edition; 12(No.1). Available on the Internet at http://www.cdc.gov/hiv/stats/hasr1201.htm. Accessed Sept. 5, 2001.

Centers for Disease Control and Prevention. U.S. Department of Health and Human Services. *National HIV Prevalence Surveys, 1997*. Centers for Disease Control and Prevention. Atlanta, GA. 1998. http://www.cdc.gov/hiv/pubs/hivser97.htm. Accessed Sept. 5, 2001.

Centers for Disease Control and Prevention (CDC), U.S. Department of Health and Human Services. "Revision of the CDC Surveillance Case Definition for Acquired Immunodeficiency Syndrome." *MMWR* 36 supplement no. 15 (1987).

Centers for Disease Control and Prevention (CDC), U.S. Department of Health and Human Services. "Surveillance for AIDS-Defining Opportunistic Illnesses, 1992–1997." CDC Surveillance Summaries. *MMWR* 48, no. SS-2 (1999).

Gottlieb, M.S., et al. "Pneumocystis Pneumonia—Los Angeles." *MMWR* 30, no. 21 (1981): 250–52. June 5, 1981.

Joint United Nations Programme on HIV/AIDS (UNAIDS). *Report on the Global HIV/AIDS Epidemic—December 2000.* Geneva: UNAIDS, 2000. Available on the Internet at http://www.who.int/emc-hiv/index.html. Accessed Sept. 5, 2001.

## C. MALARIA

MacArthur, J.R., et al. "Malaria Surveillance—United States, 1997." CDC Surveillance Summaries. *MMWR* 50, no. SS-1 (2001): 25–44.

Mungai, M., et al. "Malaria Surveillance—United States, 1996." CDC Surveillance Summaries. *MMWR* 50, no. SS-1 (2001): 1–22.

World Health Organization. *Terminology of Malaria and of Malaria Eradication.* Geneva: World Health Organization, 1963.

World Health Organization. "World Malaria Situation in 1994." *Weekly Epidemiological Record* 72 (1997): 269–76.

Zucker, J.R., and C.C. Campbell. "Malaria: Principles of Prevention and Treatment." *Infectious Disease Clinics of North America* 7 (1993): 547–67.

## D. SEXUALLY TRANSMITTED DISEASES

Centers for Disease Control and Prevention (CDC), U.S. Department of Health and Human Services. "Chancroid—United States, 1981–1990: Evidence for Underreporting of Cases." CDC Surveillance Summaries. *MMWR* 41, no. SS-3 (1992): 57–61.

Centers for Disease Control and Prevention (CDC), U.S. Department of Health and Human Services. "Chlamydia Trachomatis Genital Infections—United States, 1995." *MMWR* 46, no. 9 (1997): 193–98. Available on the Internet at http://www.cdc.gov/mmwr/PDF/wk/mm4609.pdf. Accessed Sept. 5, 2001.

Centers for Disease Control and Prevention (CDC), U.S. Department of Health and Human Services. "Congenital Syphilis—United States, 1998." *MMWR* 48, no. 34 (1999): 757–61. Available on the Internet at http://www.cdc.gov/mmwr/PDF/wk/mm4834.pdf. Accessed Sept. 5, 2001.

Centers for Disease Control and Prevention (CDC), U.S. Department of Health and Human Services. "Gonorrhea—United States, 1998." *MMWR* 49, no. 24 (2000): 538–42. Available on the Internet at http://www.cdc.gov/mmwr/PDF/wk/mm4924.pdf. Accessed Sept. 5, 2001.

Centers for Disease Control and Prevention (CDC), U.S. Department of Health and Human Services. "Primary and Secondary Syphilis—United States, 1998." *MMWR* 48, no. 39 (1999): 873–78. Available on the Internet at http://www.cdc.gov/mmwr/PDF/wk/mm4839.pdf. Accessed Sept. 5, 2001.

Division of STD Prevention, Centers for Disease Control and Prevention (CDC), U.S. Department of Health and Human Services. *Sexually Transmitted Disease Surveillance 1999.* Atlanta, GA: Centers for Disease Control and Prevention (CDC), 2000.

Division of STD Prevention, Centers for Disease Control and Prevention (CDC), U.S. Department of Health and Human Services. *Sexually Transmitted Disease Surveillance 1999 Supplement: Chlamydia Prevalence Monitoring Project.* Atlanta, GA: Centers for Disease Control and Prevention (CDC), November 2000. Available on the Internet at http://www.cdc.gov/nchstp/dstd/Stats_Trends/99Chlamydia.htm. Accessed Sept. 5, 2001.

Division of STD Prevention, Centers for Disease Control and Prevention (CDC), U.S. Department of Health and Human Services. *Sexually Transmitted Diseases Surveillance 1999 Supplement: Gonococcal Isolate Surveillance Project (GISP) Annual Report, 1999.* Available on the Internet at http://www.cdc.gov/nchstp/dstd/Stats_Trends/99GISP.htm. Accessed Sept. 5, 2001.

Division of STD Prevention, Centers for Disease Control and Prevention (CDC), U.S. Department of Health and Human Services. *The National Plan to Eliminate Syphilis from the United States.* Atlanta, GA: Centers for Disease Control and Prevention (CDC), 1999.

Division of STD Prevention, Centers for Disease Control and Prevention (CDC), U.S. Department of Health and Human Services. *Sexually Transmitted Disease Surveillance Supplement 1999: Syphilis Surveillance Report.* Atlanta, GA: Centers for Disease Control and Prevention (CDC), 2000.

Institute of Medicine, Committee on Prevention and Control of Sexually Transmitted Diseases. *The Hidden Epidemic: Confronting Sexually Transmitted Diseases.* Washington, DC: National Academy Press, 1997.

## E. TUBERCULOSIS

Burwen, D.R., A.B. Bloch, L.D. Griffin, C.A. Ciesielski, H.A. Stern, and I.M. Onorato. "National Trends in the Occurrence of Tuberculosis and Acquired Immunodeficiency Syndrome." *Archives of Internal Medicine* 155, no.12 (1995): 1281–86.

Cantwell, M.F., D.E. Snider, G.M. Cauthen, and I.M. Onorato. "Epidemiology of Tuberculosis in the United States, 1985 through 1992." *Journal of the American Medical Association* 272, no. 7 (1994): 535–39.

Centers for Disease Control and Prevention (CDC), U.S. Department of Health and Human Services. "Progress toward the Elimination of Tuberculosis—United States, 1998. *MMWR* 48, no. 33 (1999): 732–36. Available on the Internet at http://www.cdc.gov/mmwr/PDF/wk/mm4833.pdf. Accessed Sept. 5, 2001.

Centers for Disease Control and Prevention (CDC), U.S. Department of Health and Human Services. *Reported Tuberculosis in the United States, 1999.* Atlanta, GA: Centers for Disease Control and Prevention (CDC), 2000. Available on the Internet at http://www.cdc.gov/nchstp/tb/surv/surv99/surv99.htm. Accessed Sept. 5, 2001.

Centers for Disease Control and Prevention (CDC), U.S. Department of Health and Human Services. "Tuberculosis Elimination Revisited: Obstacles, Opportunities, and a Renewed Commitment. Advisory Council for the Elimination of Tuberculosis (ACET). *MMWR* 48, no. RR-9 (1999).

McKenna, M.T., E. McCray, J.L. Jones, I.M. Onorato, and K.G. Castor. "The Fall after the Rise: Tuberculosis in the United States, 1991–1994." *American Journal of Public Health* 88 (1998): 1059–63.

Moore, M., I.M. Onorato, E. McCray, and K.G. Castro. Trends in Drug-Resistant Tuberculosis in the United States, 1993–1996. *Journal of the American Medical Association* 278, no. 8 (1997): 833–37.

## F. FOODBORNE DISEASES

Olsen, S.J., et al. "Surveillance for Foodborne-Disease Outbreaks—United States, 1993–1997." CDC Surveillance Summaries. *MMWR* 49, no. SS-1 (2000): 1–7.

Tauxe, R.V. "Emerging Foodborne Disease: An Evolving Public Health Challenge." *Emerging Infectious Disease* 3 (1997): 425–34.

## G. WATERBORNE DISEASES

Barwick, R.S., et al. "Surveillance for Waterborne-Disease Outbreaks—United States, 1997–1998." CDC Surveillance Summaries. *MMWR* 49, no. SS-4 (1996). Available on the Internet at http://www.cdc.gov/mmwr/PDF/ss/ss4501.pdf. Accessed Sept. 5, 2001.

Craun, G.F., ed. *Waterborne Diseases in the United States*. Boca Raton, FL: CRC Press, 1986.

## H. INFECTIOUS DISEASE WORLDWIDE: PRESENT ISSUES, EMERGING CONCERNS

Burnet, M. *Natural History of Infectious Disease*. Cambridge, England: Cambridge University Press, 1963.

Centers for Disease Control and Prevention (CDC), U.S. Department of Health and Human Services. "Emerging Infectious Diseases." *MMWR* 42, no. 14 (1993): 257.

"Control of Infectious Diseases, 1900–1999." *Journal of the American Medical Association* 282, no. 11 (1999): 1029.

Eckert, E. "Diseased Societies." *World and I* 13, no. 10 (1998): 166(8).

Garrett, L. *The Coming Plague: Newly Emerging Diseases in a World out of Balance*. New York: Farrar, Straus and Giroux, 1994.

Garvey, G. "New or Emerging Infections." In *The Columbia University College of Physicians & Surgeons Complete Home Medical Guide*, 463. 3rd ed. New York: Crown, 1995.

*The Global Infectious Disease Threat and Its Implications for the United States*. Available on the Internet at http://www.odci.gov/cia/publications/nie/report/nie99-17d.html. Accessed Sept. 5, 2001.

Kunin, C.M. "Resistance to Antimicrobial Drugs—A Worldwide Calamity." *Annals of Internal Medicine* 118, no. 7 (1993): 557–61.

Lederberg, J., R.E. Shope, and S.C. Oaks, Jr., eds. *Emerging Infections: Microbial Threats to Health in the United States*. Washington, DC: National Academy Press, 1992.

Morse, S.S., ed. *Emerging Viruses*. New York: Oxford University Press, 1993.

Murray, C.J.L., and A.D. Lopez, eds. *The Global Burden of Disease: A Comprehensive Assessment of Mortality and Disability from Diseases, Injuries and Risk Factors in 1990 and Projected to 2020*. Global Burden of Disease and Injury Series, Vol. 1. Cambridge, MA: Harvard School of Public Health on behalf of the World Health Organization and the World Bank, 1996.

Murray, C.J.L., and A.D. Lopez. *Global Health Statistics: A Compendium of Incidence, Prevalence, and Mortality Estimates for over 200 Conditions*. Cambridge, MA: Harvard School of Public Health on behalf of the World Health Organization and the World Bank, 1996.

Murray, C.J.L., and A.D. Lopez. "Progress and Direction in Refining the Global Burden of Disease Approach: Response to Williams." *Health Economics* 9 (2000): 69–82.

Murray, C.J.L., et al. *Overall Health System Achievement for 191 Countries*. GPE Discussion Paper No. 28. Geneva: WHO, 2000.

Orloski, K.A., E.B. Hayes, G.L. Campbell, and D.T. Dennis. *Surveillance for Lyme Disease—United States, 1992–1998*. CDC Surveillance Summaries. *MMWR* 49, no. SS-3 (2000): 1–11. Available on the Internet at http://www.cdc.gov/mmwr/PDF/ss/ss4903.pdf. Accessed Sept. 5, 2001.

Tandon, A., et al. *Measuring Overall Health System Performance for 191 Countries*. GPE Discussion Paper No. 30. Geneva: World Health Organization, 2000.

World Health Organization (WHO). *International Statistical Classification of Diseases & Related Health Problems (ICD)*. Available on the Internet at http://www.who.int/whosis/icd10/. Accessed Sept. 5, 2001.

World Health Organization (WHO). *Report on Infectious Diseases: Overcoming Antimicrobial Resistance*. Geneva, Switzerland: World Health Organization, 2000. Available on the Internet at http://www.who.int/infectious-disease-report/2000/index.html. Accessed on Sept. 5, 2001.

World Health Organization (WHO). *Report on Infectious Diseases: Removing Obstacles to Healthy Development*. Geneva, Switzerland: World Health Organization, 1999. Available on the Internet at http://www.who.int/infectious-disease-report/index-rpt99.html. Accessed on Sept. 5, 2001.

World Health Organization (WHO). *The WHO Report on Global Surveillance of Epidemic-Prone Infectious Diseases*. Geneva, Switzerland: World Health Organization, 2000. Available on the Internet at http://www.who.int/emc-documents/surveillance/whocdscsrisr20001c.html. Accessed Sept. 5, 2001.

World Health Organization (WHO). *The World Health Report 2000. Health Systems: Improving Performance*. Geneva, Switzerland: World Health Organization, 2000. Available on the Internet at http://www.who.int/whr/2000/en/report.htm. Accessed Sept. 5, 2001.

World Health Organization, Department of Communicable Disease Surveillance and Response. *WHO Recommended Surveillance Standards*. 2d ed. Geneva: WHO, 1999. http://www.who.int/emc-documents/surveillance/whocdscsrisr992c.html. Accessed Sept. 5, 2001.

## I. VACCINE-PREVENTABLE DISEASES

*Epidemiology and Prevention of Vaccine-Preventable Diseases*. 6th ed. Waldorf, MD: Public Health Foundation, 2nd printing, January 2001. Available on the Internet at http://www.cdc.gov/nip/publications/pink/. Accessed Sept. 5, 2001.

Fenner, F., et al. *Smallpox and Its Eradication*. Geneva, Switzerland: World Health Organization, 1988.

Plotkin, S.A., and W.A. Orenstein. *Vaccines*. 3rd ed. Philadelphia, PA: W.B. Saunders Co., 1999.

## J. INFECTIOUS DISEASE ELIMINATION AND ERADICATION

Centers for Disease Control and Prevention (CDC), U.S. Department of Health and Human Services. "Eradication: Lessons from the Past: Global Disease Elimination and Eradication as Public Health Strategies. *MMWR* 48, supplement (1999): 16–22. http://www.cdc.gov/mmwr/PDF/other/suppl48.pdf. Accessed Sept. 5, 2001.

Centers for Disease Control and Prevention (CDC), U.S. Department of Health and Human Services. "Recommendations of the International Task Force for Disease Eradication." *MMWR* 42, no. RR-16 (1993). http://www.cdc.gov/mmwr/PDF/rr/rr4216.pdf. Accessed Sept. 5, 2001.

Centers for Disease Control and Prevention (CDC), U.S. Department of Health and Human Services. "Reduced Incidence of Menstrual Toxic-Shock Syndrome—United States, 1980–1990." *MMWR* 39, no. 25 (1990): 421–23. Available on the Internet at http://www.cdc.gov/mmwr/preview/mmwrhtml/00001651.htm. Accessed Sept. 5, 2001.

Dowdle, W.R., and R.D. Hopkins, eds. *The Eradication of Infectious Diseases: Report of the Dahlem Workshop on the Eradication of Infectious Diseases*. Chichester, England: John Wiley & Sons, 1998.

*The Global Eradication of Smallpox: Final Report of the Global Commission for the Certification of Smallpox Eradication, Geneva, December 1979*. Geneva: World Health Organization, 1980.

Hinman, A.R., et al. "The Case for Global Eradication of Poliomyelitis." *Bulletin of the World Health Organization* 65, no. 6 (1987): 835–40.

Hopkins, Jack W. *The Eradication of Smallpox: Organizational Learning and Innovation in International Health*. Boulder: Westview Press, 1989.

Mahon, B.E., E.D. Mintz, K.D. Greene, J.G. Wells, and R.V. Tauxe. "Reported Cholera in the United States, 1992–1994: a Reflection of Global Changes in Cholera Epidemiology." *Journal of the American Medical Association* 276, no. 4 (1996): 307–12.

Mintz, E.D., R.V. Tauxe, and M.M. Levine. "The Global Resurgence of Cholera." In N.D. Noah and M. O'Mahony, eds. *Communicable Disease Epidemiology and Control* 63–104. Chichester, England: John Wiley & Sons, 1998.

World Health Organization. "Global Eradication of Poliomyelitis by the Year 2000." *Weekly Epidemiological Record* 63 (1988): 161–62.

## K. BIOTERRORISM AND BIOLOGICAL WARFARE

Centers for Disease Control and Prevention (CDC), U.S. Department of Health and Human Services. "Biological and Chemical Terrorism: Strategic Plan for Preparedness and Response. Recommendations of the CDC Strategic Planning Workgroup." *MMWR* 49, no. RR-10 (2000).

Centers for Disease Control and Prevention (CDC), U.S. Department of Health and Human Services. "Bioterrorism Alleging Use of Anthrax and Interim Guidelines for Management—United States, 1998." *MMWR* 48, no. 4 (1999): 69–74. Available on the Internet at http://www.cdc.gov/mmwr/PDF/wk/mm4804.pdf. Accessed Sept. 5, 2001.

Centers for Disease Control and Prevention (CDC), U.S. Department of Health and Human Services. "Surveillance for Adverse Events Associated with Anthrax Vaccination—U.S. Department of Defense, 1998–2000." *MMWR* 49, no. 16 (2000): 341–45. Available on the Internet at http://www.cdc.gov/mmwr/PDF/wk/mm4916.pdf. Accessed Sept. 5, 2001.

Davis, C.J. "Nuclear Blindness: An Overview of the Biological Weapons Programs of the Former Soviet Union and Iraq." *Emerging Infectious Disease* 5 (1999): 509–12.

Franz, D.R., P.B. Jahrling, A.M. Friedlander, et al. "Clinical Recognition and Management of Patients Exposed to Biological Warfare Agents." *Journal of the American Medical Association* 278, no. 5 (1997): 399–411.

Inglesby, T.V., D.T. Dennis, D.A. Henderson, et al. "Plague as a Biological Weapon: Medical and Public Health Management. Working Group on Civilian Biodefense" [Review]. *Journal of the American Medical Association* 283, no. 17 (2000): 2281–90.

Okumura, T., K. Suzuki, A. Fukuda, et al. "Tokyo Subway Sarin Attack: Disaster Management, Part 1: Community Emergency Response." *Academic Emergency Medicine* 5 (1998): 613–17.

Pile, J.C., et al. "Anthrax as a Potential Biological Warfare Agent." *Archives of Internal Medicine* 158, no. 5 (1998): 429–34.

Tucker, J.B. "Chemical/Biological Terrorism: Coping with a New Threat." *Politics and the Life Sciences* 15 (1996): 167–84.

## GLOSSARY

Last, J.M. *A Dictionary of Epidemiology.* New York: Oxford University Press, 1995.

Pavlin, J.A. "Epidemiology of Bioterrorism." *Emerging Infectious Diseases Journal* 5, no. 4 (1999): 528–30.

# Index

# About the Authors

SARAH B. WATSTEIN is Director for Academic User Services and Head of the James Branch Cabell Library at Virginia Commonwealth University. She is the author of *The AIDS Dictionary* (1998) and *AIDS and Women: A Sourcebook* (Oryx, 1990).

JOHN JOVANOVIC works for the government documents division of the James Branch Cabell Library, specializing in the identification and use of statistical sources.